D1558484

NEURODEGENERATIVE DISEASES

NEURODEGENERATIVE DISEASES

Unifying Principles

EDITED BY

JEFFREY L. CUMMINGS, MD, ScD
Director
Cleveland Clinic
Lou Ruvo Center for Brain Health
Las Vegas, NV

JAGAN A. PILLAI, MBBS, PhD
Cleveland Clinic
Lou Ruvo Center for Brain Health
Cleveland, OH

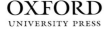

OXFORD
UNIVERSITY PRESS

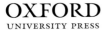

OXFORD
UNIVERSITY PRESS

Oxford University Press is a department of the University of Oxford. It furthers
the University's objective of excellence in research, scholarship, and education
by publishing worldwide. Oxford is a registered trade mark of Oxford University
Press in the UK and certain other countries.

Published in the United States of America by Oxford University Press
198 Madison Avenue, New York, NY 10016, United States of America.

Library of Congress Cataloging-in-Publication Data
Names: Cummings, Jeffrey L., 1948– , editor. | Pillai, Jagan, editor.
Title: Neurodegenerative diseases : unifying principles / edited by
Jeffrey L. Cummings, Jagan Pillai.
Other titles: Neurodegenerative diseases (Cummings)
Description: Oxford ; New York : Oxford University Press, [2017] | Includes
bibliographical references.
Identifiers: LCCN 2015038313 | ISBN 9780190233563 (alk. paper)
Subjects: | MESH: Neurodegenerative Diseases.
Classification: LCC RC522 | NLM WL 358.5 | DDC 616.8/3—dc23
LC record available at https://lccn.loc.gov/2015038313

This material is not intended to be, and should not be considered, a substitute for medical or other professional advice.
Treatment for the conditions described in this material is highly dependent on the individual circumstances. And, while
this material is designed to offer accurate information with respect to the subject matter covered and to be current as of the
time it was written, research and knowledge about medical and health issues are constantly evolving and dose schedules
for medications are being revised continually, with new side effects recognized and accounted for regularly. Readers must
therefore always check the product information and clinical procedures with the most up-to-date published product
information and data sheets provided by the manufacturers and the most recent codes of conduct and safety regulation.
The publisher and the authors make no representations or warranties to readers, express or implied, as to the accuracy
or completeness of this material. Without limiting the foregoing, the publisher and the authors make no representations
or warranties as to the accuracy or efficacy of the drug dosages mentioned in the material. The authors and the publisher
do not accept, and expressly disclaim, any responsibility for any liability, loss or risk that may be claimed or incurred as a
consequence of the use and/or application of any of the contents of this material.

9 8 7 6 5 4 3 2 1

Printed by Sheridan Books, Inc., United States of America

To my parents who woke me up

JLC – J Lee and Ellen Cummings

JP – Veera and Ayyappan Pillai

To my mentors who showed me the way

JLC – Frank Benson and Larry Ruvo

JP – Jon Siegel, Christoph Schreiner, Joe Verghese, Doug Galasko and Jeff Cummings

To my family who continue to make this journey meaningful

JC – Wife Kate and Daughter Juliana

JP – Wife Marianne and Daughter Veera

The Editors acknowledge Rhonda Heimer for her editorial assistance in assembling the book and Karthik Sreenivasan for his draft of the book cover.

CONTENTS

CONTRIBUTORS

Rahasson R. Ager, PhD
Institute for Memory Impairments
    and Neurological Disorders
University of California
Irvine, CA

Scott Ayton, PhD
Oxidation Biology Unit
Florey Institute of Neuroscience and
    Mental Health
The University of Melbourne
Parkville, Australia

David Baglietto-Vargas, PhD
Department of Neurobiology
    and Behavior
Institute for Memory Impairments
    and Neurological Disorders
University of California
Irvine, CA

Roger A. Barker, PhD
John van Geest Centre for Brain Repair
Department of Clinical Neuroscience
University of Cambridge
Cambridge, UK

Lynn M. Bekris, PhD
Cleveland Clinic
Lerner Research Institute
Genomic Medicine Institute
Cleveland, OH

Shane M. Bemiller, PhD
Stark Neurosciences Research Institute
Indiana University School
    of Medicine
Indianapolis, IN

Ilya Bezprozvanny, PhD, DSci
Department of Physiology
UT Southwestern Medical Center
Dallas, TX
Laboratory of Molecular Neurodegeneration
St. Petersburg State Polytechnical University
St. Petersburg, Russia

Ella Bossy-Wetzel, PhD
Burnett School of Biomedical Sciences
College of Medicine
University of Central Florida
Orlando, FL

Ashley I. Bush, MD, PhD
Oxidation Biology Unit
Florey Institute of Neuroscience and Mental Health
The University of Melbourne
Parkville, Australia

Paul J. Cheng-Hathaway, BA
Department of Neurosciences
Case Western Reserve University
Cleveland, OH

Jeffrey L. Cummings, MD, ScD
Director
Lou Ruvo Center for Brain Health
Neurological Institute
Cleveland Clinic
Las Vegas, NV

Janelle Drouin-Ouellet, PhD
Wallenberg Neuroscience Center and
    Lund Stem Cell Center
Department of Experimental Medical Science
Lund University
Lund, Sweden

Andreas Eigentler, MD, PhD
Institute for Neuroscience
Medical University of Innsbruck
Innsbruck, Austria

Taylor R. Jay, BS
Department of Neurosciences
Case Western Reserve University
Cleveland, OH

Andrew B. Knott, MPhil
Burnett School of Biomedical Sciences
College of Medicine
University of Central Florida
Orlando, FL

Bruce T. Lamb, PhD
Stark Neurosciences Research Institute
Indiana University School of Medicine
Indianapolis, IN

Frank M. LaFerla, PhD
Department of Neurobiology and Behavior
Institute for Memory Impairments and
    Neurological Disorders
University of California
Irvine, CA

Peng Lei, PhD
Department of Neurology, State Key Laboratory
    of Biotherapy, West China Hospital
Sichuan University, and Collaborative
    Innovation Center for Biotherapy
Sichuan, China
Florey Institute of Neuroscience
    and Mental Health
The University of Melbourne
Parkville, Victoria, Australia

James B. Leverenz, MD
Lou Ruvo Center for Brain Health
Neurological Institute
Cleveland Clinic
Cleveland, OH

Stuart A. Lipton, MD, PhD
Department of Neurosciences
Scintillon Institute
The Scripps Research Institute
University of California San Diego School
    of Medicine
La Jolla, CA

Diego F. Mastroeni, PhD
ASU-Banner Neurodegenerative Disease
    Research Center
Biodesign Institute and School of Life
    Sciences Arizona State University
Tempe, AZ

Rodrigo Medeiros, PhD
Department of Neurobiology
    and Behavior
Institute for Memory Impairments
    and Neurological Disorders
University of California
Irvine, CA

Mario F. Mendez, MD, PhD
Veterans' Affairs Neurobehavior Unit
VA Greater Los Angeles Healthcare System
Los Angeles, CA

David Morgan, PhD
Byrd Alzheimer's Institute
Department of Molecular Pharmacology
    and Physiology
Morsani College of Medicine
University of South Florida
Tampa, FL

Tomohiro Nakamura, PhD
Neurodegenerative Disease Center
Scintillon Institute
San Diego, CA
AbbVie GK
Tokyo, Japan

Roxana Nat, MD, PhD
Institute for Neuroscience
Medicine University of Innsbruck
Innsbruck, Austria

Lee E. Neilson, MD
Department of Neurology
University Hospitals
Cleveland, OH

Claudia R. Padilla, MD
Baylor AT&T Memory Center
Department of Neurology
Baylor University Medical Center
Dallas, TX

Jagan A. Pillai, MBBS, PhD
Lou Ruvo Center for Brain Health
Neurological Institute
Cleveland Clinic
Cleveland, OH

Elena Popugaeva, PhD
Laboratory of Molecular Neurodegeneration
St. Petersburg State Polytechnical University
St. Petersburg, Russia

Daniel A. Ryskamp, PhD
Department of Physiology
UT Southwestern Medical Center
Dallas, TX

Jiri G. Safar, MD
Department of Pathology
Department of Neurology
National Prion Disease Pathology
    Surveillance Center
School of Medicine, Case Western Reserve
    University
Cleveland, OH

Jonathan M. Schott
Dementia Research Centre
UCL Institute of Neurology
Queen Square
London, UK

William W. Seeley, MD
Memory and Aging Center
Departments of Neurology and Pathology
University of California
San Francisco, CA

Henrik Zetterberg, MD, PhD
Clinical Neurochemistry Laboratory
Institute of Neuroscience and Physiology
Sahlgrenska Academy at the University of
    Gothenburg
Mölndal, Sweden
Department of Molecular Neuroscience
UCL Institute of Neurology, Queen Square
London, UK

Kate Zhong, MD
Lou Ruvo Center for Brain Health
Neurological Institute
Cleveland Clinic
Las Vegas, NV

Juan Zhou, MD
Center for Cognitive Neuroscience
Neuroscience and Behavior
    Disorders Program
Duke-National University of Singapore
    Graduate Medical School
Singapore

NEURODEGENERATIVE DISEASES

1

Neurodegenerative Diseases

Evolving Unifying Principles

JEFFREY L. CUMMINGS AND JAGAN A. PILLAI

INTRODUCTION

Neurodegenerative diseases (NDDs) are among the defining public health concerns of the twenty-first century. The rise of NDDs in public health consciousness is ironically tied to public health successes of the last century, which have resulted in increasing longevity of the world's population. Between 2000 and 2050, the proportion of the world's population over the age of 60 years will double from about 11% to 22% (1). With increasing age, the likelihood of developing NDDs also increases. All NDDs are gradually progressive, disabling, and are a major threat to survival, quality of life, family integrity, and economic resources. The global burden of NDD in terms of deaths, lost productivity, and personal and family stress is enormous. Most NDD are age-related and will increase in the coming years as the global population ages (1, 2). The increase in the human, social, and economic costs of these diseases will demand huge portions of government resources if means of preventing, delaying, significantly slowing the progress, or improving the symptoms of these diseases are not found. They rob the individual of his or her memory, personality, function, and autonomy and increase dependence on others. They number among the greatest threats to the future of mankind.

NDDs are characterized by a distinct clinical syndrome of neurological deficits, behavioral changes, progressive functional decline, and motoric disturbances, underpinned by inexorable neuronal loss that is pathological for the age of the subject (Figure 1.1). NDDs include a number of brain (with or without spinal cord involvement) diseases characterized by progressive impairment of brain function and loss of activities of daily living. NDDs comprise Alzheimer's disease (AD), frontotemporal dementia (FTD), dementia with Lewy bodies (DLB), chronic traumatic encephalopathy (CTE), multiple system atrophy (MSA), progressive supranuclear palsy (PSP), corticobasal degeneration (CBD), Huntington's disease (HD), amyotrophic lateral sclerosis (ALS), progressive ataxias, and a variety of rare degenerative conditions. Phenotypes differ, but there are similarities in the general staging approach to disorders as preclinical, mild, and fully developed clinical manifestations (Figure 1.1).

Progress in the scientific understanding of NDDs has led to the recognition that there are many shared features across NDDs; the current view is that the key malefactors are proteins with altered physiochemical and neurotoxic properties. These abnormal proteins have a conformational rearrangement that endows them with a tendency to aggregate and become deposited within tissues or cellular compartments, leading to early neuronal death. This has led to the term *conformational diseases* for NDDs and a few other systemic conditions (3). The common proteins involved in conformational changes and aggregation underlying NDDs include amyloid β protein, microtubule associated protein tau (MAPT), α-synuclein, transactive response DNA-binding protein 43 (TDP-43), fused in sarcoma protein (FUS), prion protein (PrP), huntingtin, and ataxin. The aggregates and/or oligomers of these proteins appear to be toxic to neurons. This paradigm reflects knowledge accrued over a century of clinical and pathological investigations. The key advance underpinning this approach has been the use of novel stains on neuropathology specimens that have demonstrated intra- and extracellular-structural changes associated with a distinct NDD diagnosis. Neuropathology techniques have informed our understanding of NDDs and have demonstrated both variable presentations of a single pathological process and similar presentations of

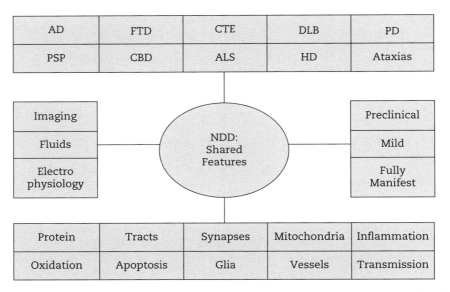

| AD | FTD | CTE | DLB | PD |
| PSP | CBD | ALS | HD | Ataxias |

Imaging		Preclinical
Fluids	NDD: Shared Features	Mild
Electro physiology		Fully Manifest

| Protein | Tracts | Synapses | Mitochondria | Inflammation |
| Oxidation | Apoptosis | Glia | Vessels | Transmission |

FIGURE 1.1. Shared features of neurodegenerative disorders (NDD). Disease (above), processes (below), biomarkers (left), and clinical phases (right).

AD: Alzheimer's disease; ALS: amyotrophic lateral sclerosis; CTE: chronic traumatic encephalopathy; CBD: corticobasal degeneration; DLB: dementia with Lewy bodies; FTD: frontotemporal dementia; HD: Huntington's disease; MSA: multiple system atrophy; PSP: progressive supranuclear palsy.

disorders with differing underlying pathological changes.

Diagnostically, similar types of biomarkers such as brain imaging are being used across NDDs. Drug development programs are searching for both transmitter-based agents that improve symptoms and disease-modifying agents that prevent, delay, or slow disease progression (4). Similar clinical trial designs are used to demonstrate drug effects in different NDDs. These convergences allow us to grasp the general concepts of neurodegeneration as manifested across a variety of disease states.

There is a recognition of the pressing problem represented by NDDs (5, 6), and significant efforts have being directed toward addressing their increasing prevalence, leading to tangible progress over the last decades (7). The diversity of approaches researching NDDs during this time has provided insights and perspectives that have made us aware of common themes shared across individual NDDs (8). These research efforts have noted recurring refrains of genetic and molecular dysfunction leading to neuronal death among NDDs. Increasingly, understanding a specific NDD impacts and illuminates our understanding across the spectrum of NDDs. It is useful to grasp this shared landscape among NDDs, as it could help enhance basic scientific understanding and

open novel therapeutic avenues. With this purpose in mind, we have developed this resource to articulate shared insights across NDDs for a new generation of students and researchers.

The principles may allow cross-disease learning and eventual cross-disease therapeutic development. This chapter establishes the premise developed throughout the book of shared principles across NDDs.

BIOLOGICAL FEATURES SHARED ACROSS NDDS

Cognitive and Brain Reserve

Symptomatic decline and progressive functional impairment can be seen as a dynamic between brain reserve and brain disease. The greater the reserve, the longer the individual will persist without symptoms. Brain reserve is produced by education, enriched life activities, and Mediterranean-type diet (9). Controlling medical illnesses that secondarily affect brain function— for example, hypertension or diabetes—will also contribute to brain health and brain reserve. This principle of cognitive or brain reserve has been demonstrated across multiple neurological diseases, including AD (10) and Parkinson's disease (PD) (11). The etiology of this phenomenon has been widely researched but is yet to be fully elucidated in mechanistic terms (12). Future efforts in better characterizing it could help develop therapeutic interventions to improve cognitive reserve across NDDs.

Brain reserve accounts for the some of the variability of phenotype/pathology findings observed. Individuals with high brain reserve will have few symptoms despite substantial pathology (e.g., amyloid burden on brain imaging), while others with more modest reserve will have greater symptom expression with lower levels of pathological changes (13).

Shared Cellular Mechanisms

Unique protein conformational changes are interconnected with multiple domains of cell dysfunction, including the following: genetic underpinnings; epigenetic modifications of the genes; post-translational RNA changes; endoplasmic reticulum-related protein modifications, including phosphorylation and ubiquitination; protein cofactors, including metal ions and chaperones; and endosomal and lysosomal clearance. Altered proteins have been further noted to disturb the ionic homeostasis and mitochondrial energetics of the cell. They trigger downstream microglial responses and neuroinflammation, contributing to the cascade of neuronal death. From a site of initial pathological seeding, proteins may spread like infectious prion diseases, leading to the spread of neurodegeneration across brain regions.

Each NDD involves a culprit protein: in AD, amyloid, tau, and TDP-43 proteins aggregate; PD has aggregated neuronal α-synuclein; MSA has glial cell α-synuclein aggregates; most FTD patients harbor either tau or TDP-43 proteins; PSP and CBD involve tau deposits; ALS involves TDP-43 and SOD-1 proteins; and DLB involves amyloid and α-synuclein proteins (Table 1.1) (4). In each case, monomers are the first molecular form generated, followed by aggregation into oligomers and eventual evolution to insoluble fibrillar proteinaceous forms. The aggregated oligomeric form of the protein appears to be associated with greater toxicity than either the monomeric or insoluble fibrillar form of the protein. Autophagy and protein processing are abnormal in these disorders, leading to mishandling of protein disposal and proteostasis.

Neurodegeneration can occur without protein misfolding. Multiple sclerosis, for example, is manifest by a combination of white matter inflammatory lesions and neurodegeneration without protein accumulation (Table 1.1).

Proteins also appear to be transmitted from cell-to-cell in a prion-like fashion across these disease states (14). Disease progression is a reflection of the progressive involvement of greater cerebral geography, and cell-to-cell transfer of the abnormal protein accounts for this progressive course (Figure 1.2). Abnormal proteins serve as templates for further production of more abnormal proteins,

TABLE 1.1. PROTEINS OF COMMON NEURODEGENERATIVE DISORDERS

Disease	Amyloid	Tau	TDP-43	α-Synuclein	Huntingtin	Prion
AD	X	X	X	X		
PD				X		
PDD				X		
DLB	X			X		
MSA				X		
FTD		X	X			
PSP		X				
CBD		X				
CTE		X				
HD					X	
CJD						X
ALS			X			

AD: Alzheimer's disease ; ALS: amyotrophic lateral sclerosis ; CBD: corticobasal degeneration; CJD: Creutzfeldt-Jakob disease; CTE: chronic traumatic encephalopathy; DLB: dementia with Lewy bodies; FTD: frontotemporal dementia; HD: Huntington's disease; MSA: multiple system atrophy; PD: Parkinson's disease; PDD: Parkinson's disease dementia; PSP: progressive supranuclear palsy.

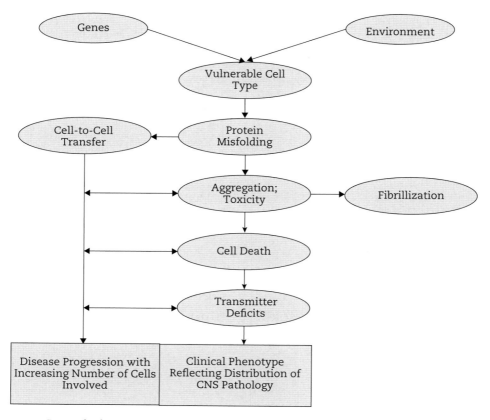

FIGURE 1.2. Process leading to neurodegeneration and clinical phenotype applicable to most NDDs.

and these eventually overwhelm normal cellular processes, leading to cell death. The proteins spread using disorder-specific networks that can be defined using functional magnetic resonance imaging (fMRI) (15). These networks provide "highways" that direct the traffic of the abnormal proteins and create the typical sequential symptomatology characteristic of each NDD (Figure 1.2).

Mitochondrial dysfunction with abnormal cellular energetics is also common across NDD (Figure 1.3) (16, 17). Mitochondrial abnormalities result in disturbed oxidative metabolism, reduced energy production, and increased free radical generation with oxidative injury. Heavy metals, such as iron, interact with these mitochondrial failures to increase oxidative injury in multiple NDDs (18). Some hypothesize that abnormalities of mitochondria may precede abnormal protein misfolding and may be responsible for the cell's inability to conduct normal protein metabolism, leading to protein accumulation. This hypothesis would place oxidative injury and mitochondrial dysfunction prior to the protein aggregation disturbances. It is consistent with the observation that in AD, preliminary amyloid beta protein

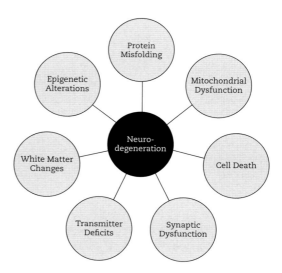

FIGURE 1.3. Pathophysiological features contributing to NDD.

disturbances are seen in high activity hubs where oxidative metabolism is greatest.

Errors in RNA processing and epigenetic abnormalities of DNA are characteristic of NDDs.

NDDs have overlapping disease-gene networks suggesting common genetic expression patterns across NDDs (19, 20). Trophic factor abnormalities with failure to maintain cell populations are seen in many NDDs. Involvement of glial cells as a primary (in MSA) abnormality or secondary mechanism is common in NDDs. Intracellular transport abnormalities with failure to maintain synaptic integrity are common across NDDs (21). These abnormalities lead to local changes, such as hippocampal abnormalities in AD, loss of cells in the substantia nigra in PD, neuronal loss in the motor system in ALS, and disruption of functional brain circuits unique to each disease state (15).

Accumulation of one type of protein in the brain may predispose to accumulation of other types of protein (22). For example, AD patients have amyloid, tau, α-synuclein, and TDP-43 aggregations. DLB and Parkinson's disease dementia (PDD) patients have aggregates of amyloid and α-synuclein.

Pathological changes in source nuclei of transmitter systems result in chemical deficiencies characteristic of NDDs. The nucleus basalis of Meynert, source nucleus of the cholinergic system, is affected in AD, PD, and DLB (23, 24). Other disorders may have deficits in non-cholinergic transmitter systems (e.g., serotonin system involvement in FTD) (Table 1.2).

Common cellular abnormalities combine with unique regional vulnerabilities to produce the characteristic phenotype of each NDD (Figure 1.2). Local degeneration produces clinically distinct abnormalities that become more

TABLE 1.2. SHARED BIOLOGICAL FEATURES OF NEURODEGENERATIVE DISORDERS (NDDs)

Class	Specific Features
Brain reserve	• Synaptic integrity • Ability to withstand concomitant pathology with fewer symptoms
Shared cellular mechanisms	• Protein misfolding • Protein aggregation • Monomer-oligomer-fibrillar types of protein • Toxic neuro-environment associated with aggregated proteins and their consequences • Cell-to-cell prion-like spread • High energy demands and cellular metabolic failure • Growth factor signaling abnormalities • Intracellular transport deficits • RNA-processing abnormalities • DNA-methylation abnormalities • Overlapping disease-gene networks • Glial cell abnormalities • Neuronal loss
Multiple type of protein accumulation	• AD has amyloid, tau, α-synuclein, and TDP-43 protein accumulation. • DLB has amyloid and α-synuclein accumulations. • Aggregation of one type of protein may represent a risk factor of aggregation of other types of protein.
Transmitter abnormalities	• Cholinergic deficits when nucleus basalis affected as in AD, PD, DLB • Other transmitter deficits reflect pathology of relevant source nuclei.
Laboratory models	• Transgenic animals with human mutations commonly used to create model systems for NDDs • Human iPS cells used for drug screening • Primates used for most human-like pharmacokinetic studies
Genetic and non-genetic forms	• Autosomal dominant disease-causing genes, usually with early onset • Risk genes with contributions to disease risk and later age of onset • Late onset forms of the disease with fewer genetic risk factors

AD: Alzheimer's disease; DLB: dementia with Lewy bodies; DMT: disease-modifying therapy; FTD: frontotemporal dementia; iPS cells: induced pluripotent stem cells; NDD: neurodegenerative disorder; PD: Parkinson's disease.

similar as the disease process spreads. The site of origin determines the first and characteristic clinical features: onset in substantia nigra leads to parkinsonism in PD; early hippocampal changes produce the episodic memory loss of AD; and striatal involvement causes the chorea of HD. Symptoms become more diverse and more severe as the diseases evolve, and patients have less distinctive features in the very advanced phase of the disease. Terminally, most patients with NDDs who do not succumb to competitive age-related mortality die of complications of pneumonia, urinary tract infections, or infections of decubitus ulcerations.

Laboratory Models of NDD

Animal models are needed to study NDDs in laboratory settings. Animal model systems provide insight into disease mechanisms, biomarkers, behavior-pathology correlations, and potential therapies. Transgenic approaches to the creation of animal models are commonly used across different NDDs. A wide variety of transgenic model organisms have been utilized including bacteria, nematodes, arthropods (*Drosophila melanogaster*), zebra fish, and rodents (mouse and rat) (25). Transgenic models tend to reliably reproduce one aspect of the NDD—such as the amyloid abnormalities of AD—but do not recapitulate the complex spectrum of disease-related abnormalities (26). In most cases, they are accelerated models that have more similarities to the autosomal dominant forms of NDD than to age-related late-onset forms of the diseases. Animal models have so far not predicted successful therapies or side effects of treatment in humans.

Human cells may be better model systems for study, and induced pluripotent stem (iPS) cells are increasingly used to study NDDs. This approach may enhance drug screening and the development of disease treatments (27–29).

Genetic and Non-Genetic Forms of NDD

NDDs have genetic and non-genetic forms. In most cases, the inherited form of the disease begins earlier in life, is more aggressive, and is associated with shortened survival. In AD, autosomal dominant forms of the disease occur with presenilin 1 (PS1), presenilin 2 (PS2), and amyloid precursor protein (APP) mutations (30). These account for a small number of cases (approximately 3%); risk factor genes (apolipoprotein e4) and non-genetic risk actors account for the majority of cases. Similarly, hereditary and environmental factors conspire in most other NDDs. HD is an exception, with only the autosomal dominant form of the disease known. The genetics of familial forms of FTD involves seven genes: the microtubule-associated protein tau (*MAPT*), progranulin (*GRN*), valosin-containing protein (*VCP*), chromatin-modifying gene 2B (*CHMP2B*), TDP-43 encoding gene (*TARBDP*), fused in sarcoma (*FUS*), and open reading frame of chromosome 9 (*C9orf72*) (31). Approximately 50% of FTD patients have no recognized genetic contribution to their illness.

Identifying the underlying protein conformational changes among NDDs has also helped clarify the relationship of genetic and clinical presentations of these diseases. *MAPT* gene is shared by PD, PSP, and frontotemporal lobar degeneration (FTLD). The gene for *C9orf72* is the most common cause of familial ALS and is also present in some FTLD and AD, suggesting a possible shared underlying cellular dysfunction.

Understanding the molecular biology and genetics of NDDs has made the field sensitive to the timeline of protein accumulation and subsequent neuronal dysfunction. A disease trajectory has been characterized for NDDs. In patients with known autosomal dominant genetic mutations, such as HD and autosomal dominant AD, the future age of onset of symptoms can be estimated even among currently asymptomatic individuals. Abnormal protein accumulation and neuronal changes related to HD and AD have been seen to predate the onset of symptoms by more than a decade among these subjects carrying the genetic mutation (32, 33). This makes it likely that an extended predementia stage is also present among individuals who develop sporadic forms of NDDs. This insight has prompted a search for clinical and biomarker changes in preclinical disease before significant neuronal damage has occurred (34, 35). Novel biochemical and imaging markers characterizing functional brain changes, neuronal network dysfunction, and molecular imaging are emerging.

CLINICAL FEATURES SHARED ACROSS NDDS

Cognitive Impairment

NDDs have clinical phenotypes comprising cognitive, neuropsychiatric, and motor manifestations (Table 1.3). The constituents of each syndrome are determined by the regional distribution of pathological changes (36).

Cognitive impairment of at least subtle severity is present in most NDDs as symptoms

TABLE 1.3. SHARED CLINICAL FEATURES OF NEURODEGENERATIVE DISORDERS (NDDs)

Class	Specific Features
Cognitive impairment	• Loss of cognitive abilities • Type of loss reflects the regional distribution of the pathological changes: FTD patients have greater executive dysfunction, AD patients have disproportionate episodic memory decline, etc.
Progressive phases	• Asymptomatic with positive state biomarkers • Prodromal, minimally symptomatic phase • Complete symptom complex
Neuropsychiatric manifestations	• Depression common among NDDs • Apathy common among NDDs • Agitation common in later stages of NDDs • Disease-specific regionally determined behavioral changes in NDDs (e.g., disinhibition in FTD, visual hallucinations in DLB)
Functional effects	• Increasing physical disability with disease progression
Age effects	• Age is a significant risk factor for most NDDs • Younger-onset forms of disease tend to have more rapid progression with shorter survival.
Terminal stages	• Patients typically succumb to complications of pneumonia, urinary tract infections, or decubitus ulcerations with infection characteristic of later stages of all NDDs.
Caregiver/family stress	• All NDDs impact family members and caregivers, compromising the quality of life of patients and their families.
Clinical trials	• Staggered start and randomized withdrawal trial designs to demonstrate disease modification • Parallel group design with biomarkers to demonstrate disease-modification • Parallel group design without biomarkers to demonstrate symptomatic, cognitive, and functional effects of drugs • Parallel group or cross-over designs to demonstrate symptomatic and behavioral effects of drugs
Biomarkers	• Genetic biomarkers to identify at-risk individuals • State biomarkers in pre-symptomatic individuals to identify persons at risk for decline • State biomarkers to support diagnostic accuracy of disease diagnosis • Target engagement biomarkers reflecting near-term mechanism of action of the test agent • Disease modifying biomarkers reflecting alterations in processes leading to cell death • Biomarkers to detect adverse safety events
Brain imaging	• Structural MRI shows atrophy appropriate for each NDD (medial temporal atrophy in AD; frontotemporal atrophy in FTD; caudate nucleus atrophy in HD; etc.). • fMRI reveals effects on brain networks characteristic of each NDD. • FDG PET shows regional hypometabolism characteristic of each disease (parietal hypometabolism in AD; frontotemporal hypometabolism in FTD; caudate nuclear hypometabolism in HD; etc.). • Molecular imaging shows molecular features characteristic of each disease (e.g., positive amyloid imaging in AD; positive tau imaging in tauopathies).
Regulatory aspects	• No approved DMT agents for NDDs: regulatory aspects evolving • Similar regulatory requirements for DMT across NDD anticipated

DLB: dementia with Lewy bodies; DMT: disease-modifying therapy; FTD: frontotemporal dementia; iPS cells: induced pluripotent stem cells.

become evident. The type and severity of cognitive impairment reflects the type and distribution of pathological changes characteristic of the disease. Cognitive decline is the hallmark of AD; the condition begins in medial temporal regions, and the principal initial phenotype features episodic memory impairment. As the disease spreads, visuospatial, language, and executive functions are compromised. FTD, as the name implies, involves frontal and temporal structures, producing a predominant executive disorder in the frontal behavioral variant and primary progressive aphasia with temporal changes. ALS patients may have an executive function disorder of variable severity. Disorders affecting basal ganglia structures—PD, PDD, PSP, CBD, MSA—disrupt frontosubcortical circuits and feature primarily mild to moderate executive dysfunction. Two disorders—FTD and CBD—are often asymmetric in brain involvement, producing unilateral or asymmetric phenomena. While clinical symptoms are recognized to reflect a brain's regional burden of pathology, they do not always indicate the molecular pathology (e.g., the frontal variant AD and the behavioral variant of FTD share the same clinical and neuropsychological presentation but have distinct molecular pathologies). Conversely, different clinical phenotypes may share a common molecular abnormality (e.g., PSP, CBD, and primary non-fluent aphasia variant of FTD have differing clinical features and regional neuropathologies but share the same underlying tau protein abnormality).

Assessment tools that could be used across all disorders would aid understanding of similarities and differences among NDDs. The National Institute of Health (NIH) Toolbox Cognitive Health Battery (NIHTB-CHB) is designed to measure neurological functions that span different disciplines, apply to diverse research questions, and measure a broad range of functions across the human life span from age three to 85. The measures can be applied across all NDDs and to normal comparison groups. The NIHTB-CHB is composed of four modules: cognition, emotion, motor, and sensory (37). Cognitive assessments of the NIHTB-CHB include measures of executive function, episodic memory, language, processing speed, working memory, and attention (38). Likewise, the National Institute of Neurological Disease and Stroke (NINDS) supported the development of a tool for the assessment of frontal-subcortical systems: Executive Abilities: Measures and Instruments for Neurobehavioral Evaluation and Research (EXAMINER) (39). This tool

includes measures of working memory, inhibition, set shifting, fluency, insight, planning, social cognition, and behavior relevant to executive and frontal lobe function. It is anticipated that this tool would be particularly useful in characterizing executive deficits in disorders such as FTD, PSP, and CBD. Use of the same tools across clinical trials would facilitate understanding of the common features and treatment responsiveness of cognitive domains across disease states.

Neuropsychiatric Manifestations

Neuropsychiatric and behavioral alterations are common across NDD (40). Apathy, depression, and agitation are especially frequent. Apathy is prominent in AD, FTD, and PSP. Depression is a common manifestation of AD, PD, DLB, HD, and CBD (41). Disinhibition is common in the behavioral variant of FTD but also occurs in AD and PSP. Psychotic phenomena such as delusions and hallucinations are characteristic of DLB and may occur in AD. Irritability and disinhibition are common in HD, and some patients exhibit compulsions. Agitation is common in most NDDs in later phases of the disease. Sleep disturbances are common in NDDs, and rapid eye movement (REM) sleep behavior disorder is characteristic of α-synucleinopathies, including PD and DLB (42). Appetite is commonly decreased in AD and increased in FTD.

Motor Manifestations

Motor abnormalities are present in most NDDs at some stage of the disease. AD is characterized by normal motor function in early and moderate stages of the disease, with paratonia and paralysis evolving late in the course. Parkinsonian syndromes are characteristic of PD, DLB, PSP, and MSA. CBD features unilateral or asymmetric dystonia and myoclonus. ALS and some forms of FTD have motor neuron disease with fasciculations and weakness. Chorea is characteristic of HD and may occur as a complication of treatment in PD.

Age Effects

A common phenomenon exhibited by many NDDs is an age-related rate of degeneration. Patients with earlier onset disease tend to progress more rapidly than those with later onset disease (43). This is evident in AD and PD and may be characteristic of other NDDs. Early onset disease often has a greater genetic contribution; it is unclear if the genetically induced changes or the age of the host or both are responsible for the more rapid decline and abbreviated disease course.

Progressive Phases

NDDs are characterized by three general phases: a period with asymptomatic disease changes in the brain; then mild symptoms not meeting the criteria for diagnosis of the full syndrome; and a final stage with characteristic manifestations meeting traditional diagnostic criteria. AD is the prototype of this progression (44). There is an initial asymptomatic period when amyloid protein changes are demonstrable on amyloid imaging or with cerebrospinal fluid (CSF) analysis. This is followed by prodromal AD, usually with episodic memory impairment and progression in biomarkers to include atrophy on magnetic resonance imaging (MRI). There is no major impairment of activities of daily living in this period, and patients do not meet criteria for dementia. Finally, cognition worsens, functional impairment occurs, and the patient meets criteria for AD dementia (45). Most NDDs are thought to follow similar disease progression trajectories.

Terminal Stages

The terminal phases of most NDDs appear to be similar. Patients are bereft of all function, paralyzed, and incontinent. They are no longer aware of their surroundings or aspects of their own biography. They succumb to pneumonia, urinary tract infections, complication of decubitus ulcerations, or age-related conditions such as stroke, cancer, or heart disease (46).

Caregiver/Family Stress

All NDDs strike families, not solely the affected individual (47). Family members are stressed by the progressive cognitive and motoric decline. Neuropsychiatric features are especially burdensome and may precipitate institutionalization. Families are concerned about the hereditary implications of the disease and whether their children and grandchildren are at increased risk for a similar disorder. Care for patients with NDDs must be delivered in the context of care for family members and caregivers. Genetic counseling, brain health/lifestyle recommendations, and psychological counseling may all have a role in the care of caregivers. These care challenges are characteristic of all NDDs.

Clinical Trials

Developing new therapies for NDD is critically important; there is not one NDD whose symptoms are adequately controlled, and none has approved disease-modifying therapy (DMT) (48). Drug development can be directed at symptoms that are produced by the disease or at the underlying disease process in an attempt to prevent, delay the onset, or slow the progression of the disorder (see Chapter 18, "Clinical Trials and Drug Development in Neurodegenerative Diseases: Unifying Principles," in this volume) (49–52).

Symptomatic therapies may address cognitive or behavioral features. An example of an agent approved by the US Food and Drug Administration (FDA) for cognition in more than one NDD is rivastigmine (53). This cholinesterase inhibitor is approved for treatment of mild-moderate cognitive impairment in PDD and for mild, moderate, and severe dementia in AD. It has been used successfully in DLB. The unifying biology that underlies this approach is the cholinergic deficit present in many NDDs; cholinergic nuclei are particularly susceptible to amyloid-related toxicity; and diseases in which amyloid is a key pathologic protein also have corresponding cholinergic deficits.

Dextromethorphan/quinidine (DM/Q; Nuedexta™) is approved for pseudobulbar affect (PBA) across neurological diseases, including NDDs. Its efficacy was shown in multiple sclerosis and ALS (54), and the FDA approved the agent for PBA in all clinical circumstances. The agent is currently in trials for agitation, disinhibition, pain, and depression and may achieve approval for other indications in NDDs.

Pimavanserin is another example of an agent that may be approved for treatment of behavioral disturbances across NDDs (55). It is poised for FDA approval for psychosis in PD and is in clinical trials for psychosis of AD. It may have applicability in psychosis, agitation, or sleep disorders in multiple NDDs.

Antidepressants, sedatives, anxiolytics, and stimulants are used across NDDs for symptoms exhibited by patients but are not approved by the FDA for these indications, are used off-label, and, in many cases, do not have efficacy studies to guide their use (56, 57).

Development of DMT is a key issue for all NDDs, and the approach to showing efficacy is similar across the NDDs. The FDA has indicated a willingness to consider evidence from two types of trial design in support of labeling that identifies the drug as disease-modifying (58). The staggered start and the randomized withdrawal designs are means of showing that treatment has altered the trajectory of the disease and has effects beyond those of symptomatic therapies (see Chapter 18, "Clinical Trials and Drug Development in Neurodegenerative

Diseases: Unifying Principles," in this volume). These designs can be applied across all NDDs; in each case, the primary outcome would differ according to disease, but the general structure of the trial would be similar. The delayed start and staggered withdrawal designs have proven difficult to implement, and most trials of DMT have chosen to rely on biomarkers instead of design-derived data. In this approach, the trial is designed to show a drug-placebo difference on a clinical outcome and a corresponding drug-placebo difference on a biomarker that supports disease-modification (e.g., less MRI atrophy in the treatment group). The trial would require disease-specific entry criteria and related clinical outcomes and a disease-specific biomarker, but the general structure of the trials would be similar across NDDs. This allows learning to be extrapolated across NDDs in terms of sample size, trial duration, biomarker performance, and regulatory approach. Anti-amyloid agents or tau-related therapeutics would be applicable in AD or tauopathies (FTD, PSP, CBD, CTE), respectively, while neuroprotective agents might be more broadly applicable across NDD.

Cross-NDD approaches become relevant when different NDDs are shown to share types of underlying cellular dysfunction, for example lysosomal dysfunction in some animal models of HD and AD (59–61), suggesting that some agents might be applied in multiple NDDs. Targeting preclinical stages of the disease is anticipated to be the focus of future clinical intervention efforts across many NDDs (59, 62). This is based on the model (described earlier) of asymptomatic, prodromal, and manifest phases of NDDs.

Biomarkers

A biomarker is defined as a characteristic that is objectively measured and evaluated as an indicator of normal biological processes, pathogenic processes, or pharmacological responses to a therapeutic intervention (63). Brain imaging (discussed later in this chapter) or patient-derived fluids (CSF, blood, urine, saliva) may provide biomarker information. In AD, CSF measures of amyloid protein, total tau protein, and hyperphosphorylated tau (p-tau) protein provide insight into disease pathophysiology and progression. Biomarkers for other NDD are less well developed, but discovery of useful biomarkers across NDD is anticipated.

Fluid biomarkers include both trait (e.g., genetic) and state (e.g., CSF markers) measures. In trials involving NDDs, genetic biomarkers can be used to identify populations (mutation carriers, risk polymorphisms), stratify recruitment,

or pre-specify data analysis. State biomarkers can support diagnosis, demonstrate target engagement (e.g., reduced CSF amyloid synthesis in AD with a secretase inhibitor) (32, 64), demonstrate disease modification in a trial, or monitor for drug toxicity (e.g., liver function tests).

Brain Imaging

Brain imaging can be used to study diverse aspects of NDDs, track changes over time, compare regional changes, and monitor side effects. Brain imaging findings differ across NDDs, but the approaches used to characterize brain structure, function, and molecular constituents are the same (Table 1.4). MRI is a versatile tool that provides information on brain structure and atrophy, cortical thickness, white matter tract integrity, biochemical characteristics (MR spectroscopy), and activity (resting state or activated with specific tasks) (65). In AD, MRI provides measures of hippocampal atrophy, whole brain atrophy, and ventricular volume useful in disease tracking and clinical trials (66) (Figure 1.4). Atrophy patterns differ in AD and FTD. MRI can also be used to monitor drug-related side effects such as amyloid-related imaging abnormalities (ARIA)

TABLE 1.4. BRAIN IMAGING TECHNIQUE APPLICABLE ACROSS NDDs

Technique	Application in NDD
MRI structural imaging	Atrophy measures
MRI diffusion tensor imaging	White matter assessment
MRI cortical thickness measures	Assess regional cortical thinning
MR spectroscopy	Assess defined chemical constituents of the brain
Resting state MR	Assess resting state activity
Functional MR	Response to cognitive challenges during imaging with regional brain activation
Fluorodeoxyglucose PET	Regional hypometabolism
Amyloid PET	Amyloid burden in brain
Tau PET	Tau protein accumulation in brian

MR: magnetic resonance; MRI: magnetic resonance imaging; PET: positron emission tomography.

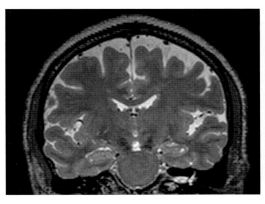
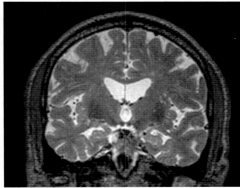

FIGURE 1.4. Magnetic resonance imaging, coronal section. Normal (left) and abnormal (right) with reduced hippocampal volume.

seen with some monoclonal antibodies used to treat AD (48).

Fluorodeoxyglucose (FDG) positron emission tomography (PET) provides a measure of regional glucose utilization (67). AD is associated with posterior cingulate and bilateral parietal hypometabolism, and FTD manifests frontotemporal hypometabolism (Figure 1.5). FDG PET can be used to assess responses to symptomatic therapies or DMT and can be used to track disease-related changes over time.

Amyloid PET shows the cortical amyloid burden characteristic of AD (32, 36) (Figure 1.6), and tau PET shows tau-related abnormalities and is being studied in AD, FTD, PSP, CBD, and CTE (68).

COMMENT

There is a wide range of NDDs, and each disorder is distinguishable on the basis of its specific biology and clinical phenotype. However, as this chapter and the ones that follow make clear, there are many similarities, overlaps, and common approaches across NDDs. Common features, such as mitochondrial and energy abnormalities, transmitter changes, apoptosis, and synaptic dysfunction, support opportunities for cross-disease learning, extrapolation across pathologies, and implementation of common lessons to interventional studies, biomarkers, and clinical care. Vigilance for possible cross-disease applications may hasten the development of new therapies for NDDs. Patients and families also share similar challenges and burdens across NDDs, and lessons derived from one may allow us to improve the quality of life in others.

Even as we recognize common threads across NDDs, intriguing questions remain. Why, for instance, are some brain regions more vulnerable

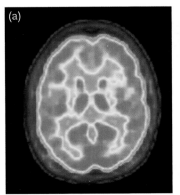
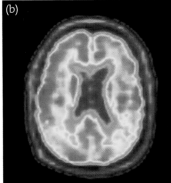
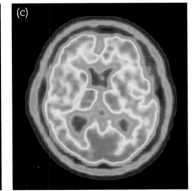

FIGURE 1.5. Fluorodeoxyglucose (FDG) positron emission tomography. Normal (a), Alzheimer's disease with reduced parietal metabolism (b), and frontotemporal dementia with reduced frontal and temporal metabolism (c).

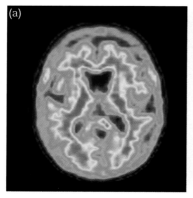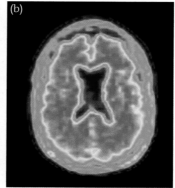

FIGURE 1.6. Amyloid positron emission tomography (PET). Normal (a), abnormal and consistent with Alzheimer's disease (b).

to specific protein misfolding disorders than others? What triggers the onset of an NDD (69–71)? To answer these questions, a better understanding of the interplay between abnormal protein processing and the molecular and genetic basis of regional brain development is crucial. With the future understanding of factors that drive disease trajectory and disease heterogeneity, distinct personalized therapeutic options may be developed for patients with NDDs.

DISCLOSURES

Dr. Pillai has no disclosures.

Dr. Cummings has provided consultation to Abbott, Acadia, Adamas, Alzheon, Anavex, Astellas, Avanir, Avid, Eisai, Forum, GE Healthcare, Genentech, Lilly, Lundbeck, Medavante Merck, Neuronetrix, Novartis, Otsuka, Pfizer, QR, Roivant, Sanofi-Aventis, Signum, Takeda, and Toyama companies. Dr. Cummings owns the copyright of the Neuropsychiatric Inventory. Dr. Cummings has stock options in Prana, Neurokos, ADAMAS, MedAvante, and QR pharma. This chapter presents drugs in development and not approved by the FDA.

REFERENCES

1. World Health Organization. *Ageing and Life Course*. Geneva: WHO; 2015.
2. Reitz C, Brayne C, Mayeux R. Epidemiology of Alzheimer disease. *Nat Rev Neurol* 2011 Mar;7: 137–152.
3. Kopito RR, Ron D. Conformational disease. *Nat Cell Biol* 2000 Nov;2:E207–E209.
4. Skovronsky DM, Lee VM, Trojanowski JQ. Neurodegenerative diseases: new concepts of pathogenesis and their therapeutic implications. *Annu Rev Pathol* 2006;1:151–170.
5. World Health Organization. First WHO ministerial conference on global action against dementia. 2015, March 16–17, 2015, Geneva, Switzerland; pp.1–68.
6. Alzheimer's Association 2014 Alzheimer's disease facts and figures. *Alzheimer's & Dementia: The Journal of the Alzheimer's* Association 10: e47–e92.
7. Young AB. Four decades of neurodegenerative disease research: how far we have come! *J Neurosci* 2009 Oct 14;29:12722–12728.
8. Institute of Medicine. *Neurodegeneration: Exploring Commonalities Across Diseases*. Workshop summary, 1st ed. Washington, DC: The National Academies Press, 2013.
9. Meng X, D'Arcy C. Education and dementia in the context of the cognitive reserve hypothesis: a systematic review with meta-analyses and qualitative analyses. *PLoS One* 2012;7:e38268.
10. Barulli D, Stern Y. Efficiency, capacity, compensation, maintenance, plasticity: emerging concepts in cognitive reserve. *Trends Cogn Sci* 2013 Oct;17:502–509.
11. Hindle JV, Martyr A, Clare L. Cognitive reserve in Parkinson's disease: a systematic review and meta-analysis. *Parkinsonism Relat Disord* 2014 Jan;20:1–7.
12. Steffener J, Stern Y. Exploring the neural basis of cognitive reserve in aging. *Biochim Biophys Acta* 2012 Mar;1822:467–473.
13. Fratiglioni L, Wang HX. Brain reserve hypothesis in dementia. *J Alzheimers Dis* 2007 Aug;12: 11–22.
14. Prusiner SB. Biology and genetics of prions causing neurodegeneration. *Annu Rev Genet* 2013;47: 601–623.
15. Greicius MD, Kimmel DL. Neuroimaging insights into network-based neurodegeneration. *Curr Opin Neurol* 2012 Dec;25:727–734.

16. Guo C, Sun L, Chen X, Zhang D. Oxidative stress, mitochondrial damage and neurodegenerative diseases. *Neural Regen Res* 2013 Jul 25;8: 2003–2014.

17. Gonzalez-Lima F, Barksdale BR, Rojas JC. Mitochondrial respiration as a target for neuroprotection and cognitive enhancement. *Biochem Pharmacol* 2014 Apr 15;88:584–593.

18. Ward RJ, Zucca FA, Duyn JH, Crichton RR, Zecca L. The role of iron in brain ageing and neurodegenerative disorders. *Lancet Neurol* 2014 Oct;13:1045–1060.

19. Forabosco P, Ramasamy A, Trabzuni D, et al. Insights into TREM2 biology by network analysis of human brain gene expression data. *Neurobiol Aging* 2013 Dec;34:2699–2714.

20. Novarino G, Fenstermaker AG, Zaki MS, et al. Exome sequencing links corticospinal motor neuron disease to common neurodegenerative disorders. *Science* 2014 Jan 31;343:506–511.

21. Gouras GK. Convergence of synapses, endosomes, and prions in the biology of neurodegenerative diseases. *Int J Cell Biol* 2013;2013:141083.

22. Rauramaa T, Pikkarainen M, Englund E, et al. TAR-DNA binding protein-43 and alterations in the hippocampus. *J Neural Transm* 2011 May;118: 683–689.

23. Bohnen NI, Kaufer DI, Ivanco LS, et al. Cortical cholinergic function is more severely affected in parkinsonian dementia than in Alzheimer disease: an in vivo positron emission tomographic study. *Arch Neurol* 2003 Dec;60:1745–1748.

24. Tiraboschi P, Hansen LA, Alford M, et al. Early and widespread cholinergic losses differentiate dementia with Lewy bodies from Alzheimer disease. *Arch Gen Psychiatry* 2002 Oct;59:946–951.

25. Gama Sosa MA, De GR, Elder GA. Modeling human neurodegenerative diseases in transgenic systems. *Hum Genet* 2012 Apr;131:535–563.

26. Sabbagh JJ, Kinney JW, Cummings JL. Alzheimer's disease biomarkers: correspondence between human studies and animal models. *Neurobiol Dis* 2013 Aug;56:116–130.

27. Choi SH, Kim YH, Hebisch M, et al. A three-dimensional human neural cell culture model of Alzheimer's disease. *Nature* 2014 Nov 13;515:274–278.

28. Cundiff PE, Anderson SA. Impact of induced pluripotent stem cells on the study of central nervous system disease. *Curr Opin Genet Dev* 2011 Jun;21:354–361.

29. Kim SU, Lee HJ, Kim YB. Neural stem cell-based treatment for neurodegenerative diseases. *Neuropathology* 2013 Oct;33:491–504.

30. Bertram L, Tanzi RE. The genetics of Alzheimer's disease. *Prog Mol Biol Transl Sci* 2012;107:79–100.

31. Nacmias B, Piaceri I, Bagnoli S, Tedde A, Piacentini S, Sorbi S. Genetics of Alzheimer's disease and frontotemporal dementia. *Curr Mol Med* 2014;14(8):985–992.

32. Bateman RJ, Xiong C, Benzinger TL, et al. Clinical and biomarker changes in dominantly inherited Alzheimer's disease. *N Engl J Med* 2012 Aug 30;367: 795–804.

33. Aylward EH, Harrington DL, Mills JA, et al. Regional atrophy associated with cognitive and motor function in prodromal Huntington disease. *J Huntingtons Dis* 2013;2:477–489.

34. Dean DC, III, Jerskey BA, Chen K, et al. Brain differences in infants at differential genetic risk for late-onset Alzheimer disease: a cross-sectional imaging study. *JAMA Neurol* 2014 Jan;71:11–22.

35. Langbaum JB, Chen K, Caselli RJ, et al. Hypometabolism in Alzheimer-affected brain regions in cognitively healthy Latino individuals carrying the apolipoprotein E epsilon4 allele. *Arch Neurol* 2010 Apr;67:462–468.

36. Fleisher AS, Chen K, Quiroz YT, et al. Florbetapir PET analysis of amyloid-beta deposition in the presenilin 1 E280A autosomal dominant Alzheimer's disease kindred: a cross-sectional study. *Lancet Neurol* 2012 Dec;11:1057–1065.

37. Weintraub S, Dikmen SS, Heaton RK, et al. The cognition battery of the NIH toolbox for assessment of neurological and behavioral function: validation in an adult sample. *J Int Neuropsychol Soc* 2014 Jul;20:567–578.

38. Weintraub S, Dikmen SS, Heaton RK, et al. Cognition assessment using the NIH Toolbox. *Neurology* 2013 Mar 12;80:S54–S64.

39. Kramer JH, Mungas D, Possin KL, et al. NIH EXAMINER: conceptualization and development of an executive function battery. *J Int Neuropsychol Soc* 2014 Jan;20:11–19.

40. Cummings JL, Mega M, Gray K, Rosenberg-Thompson S, Carusi DA, Gornbein J. The Neuropsychiatric Inventory: comprehensive assessment of psychopathology in dementia. *Neurology* 1994 Dec;44:2308–2314.

41. Cummings J, Friedman JH, Garibaldi G, et al. Apathy in neurodegenerative diseases: recommendations on the design of clinical trials. *J Geriatr Psychiatry Neurol* 2015 Mar; 28:159–173.

42. Postuma RB, Gagnon JF, Montplaisir J. Rapid eye movement sleep behavior disorder as a biomarker for neurodegeneration: the past 10 years. *Sleep Med* 2013 Aug;14:763–767.

43. Bernick C, Cummings J, Raman R, Sun X, Aisen P. Age and rate of cognitive decline in Alzheimer disease: implications for clinical trials. *Arch Neurol* 2012 Jul;69:901–905.

44. Dubois B, Feldman HH, Jacova C, et al. Advancing research diagnostic criteria for Alzheimer's disease: the IWG-2 criteria. *Lancet Neurol* 2014 Jun;13: 614–629.

45. Galasko D, Bennett D, Sano M, et al. An inventory to assess activities of daily living for clinical trials in Alzheimer's disease. The Alzheimer's Disease Cooperative Study. *Alzheimer Dis Assoc Disord* 1997;11 Suppl 2:S33-S39.

46. Mitchell SL, Teno JM, Kiely DK, et al. The clinical course of advanced dementia. *N Engl J Med* 2009 Oct 15;361:1529–1538.

47. Zarit SH. Diagnosis and management of caregiver burden in dementia. *Handb Clin Neurol* 2008;89:101–106.

48. Sperling RA, Jack CR, Jr., Black SE, et al. Amyloid-related imaging abnormalities in amyloid-modifying therapeutic trials: recommendations from the Alzheimer's Association Research Roundtable Workgroup. *Alzheimers Dement* 2011 Jul;7:367–385.

49. Morris JC. The Clinical Dementia Rating (CDR): current version and scoring rules. *Neurology* 1993 Nov;43:2412–2414.

50. Dragalin V. An introduction to adaptive designs and adaptation in CNS trials. *Eur Neuropsychopharmacol* 2011 Feb;21:153–158.

51. Elm JJ, Goetz CG, Ravina B, et al. A responsive outcome for Parkinson's disease neuroprotection futility studies. *Ann Neurol* 2005 Feb;57:197–203.

52. Tilley BC, Palesch YY, Kieburtz K, et al. Optimizing the ongoing search for new treatments for Parkinson disease: using futility designs. *Neurology* 2006 Mar 14;66:628–633.

53. Emre M, Aarsland D, Albanese A, et al. Rivastigmine for dementia associated with Parkinson's disease. *N Engl J Med* 2004 Dec 9;351: 2509–2518.

54. Pioro EP, Brooks BR, Cummings J, et al. Dextromethorphan plus ultra low-dose quinidine reduces pseudobulbar affect. *Ann Neurol* 2010 Nov; 68:693–702.

55. Cummings J, Isaacson S, Mills R, et al. Pimavanserin for patients with Parkinson's disease psychosis: a randomised, placebo-controlled phase 3 trial. *Lancet* 2014 Feb 8;383:533–540.

56. Richard IH, McDermott MP, Kurlan R, et al. A randomized, double-blind, placebo-controlled trial of antidepressants in Parkinson disease. *Neurology* 2012 Apr 17;78:1229–1236.

57. Troeung L, Egan SJ, Gasson N. A meta-analysis of randomised placebo-controlled treatment trials for depression and anxiety in Parkinson's disease. *PLoS One* 2013;8:e79510.

58. Cummings J, Gould H, Zhong K. Advances in designs for Alzheimer's disease clinical trials. *Am J Neurodegener Dis* 2012;1:205–216.

59. Postuma RB, Aarsland D, Barone P, et al. Identifying prodromal Parkinson's disease: premotor disorders in Parkinson's disease. *Mov Disord* 2012 Apr 15;27:617–626.

60. Lee JH, Yu WH, Kumar A, et al. Lysosomal proteolysis and autophagy require presenilin 1 and are disrupted by Alzheimer-related PS1 mutations. *Cell* 2010 Jun 25;141:1146–1158.

61. Martinez-Vicente M, Talloczy Z, Wong E, et al. Cargo recognition failure is responsible for inefficient autophagy in Huntington's disease. *Nat Neurosci* 2010 May;13:567–576.

62. Pillai JA, Cummings JL. Clinical trials in predementia stages of Alzheimer disease. *Med Clin North Am* 2013 May;97:439–457.

63. Cummings JL. Biomarkers in Alzheimer's disease drug development. *Alzheimers Dement* 2011 May;7:e13–e44.

64. Bateman RJ, Munsell LY, Morris JC, Swarm R, Yarasheski KE, Holtzman DM. Human amyloid-beta synthesis and clearance rates as measured in cerebrospinal fluid in vivo. *Nat Med* 2006 Jul;12: 856–861.

65. Hampel H, Prvulovic D, Teipel SJ, Bokde AL. Recent developments of functional magnetic resonance imaging research for drug development in Alzheimer's disease. *Prog Neurobiol* 2011 Dec;95:570–578.

66. Fleisher AS, Donohue M, Chen K, Brewer JB, Aisen PS. Applications of neuroimaging to disease-modification trials in Alzheimer's disease. *Behav Neurol* 2009;21:129–136.

67. Barthel H, Schroeter ML, Hoffmann KT, Sabri O. PET/MR in dementia and other neurodegenerative diseases. *Semin Nucl Med* 2015 May;45:224–233.

68. James OG, Doraiswamy PM, Borges-Neto S. PET Imaging of tau pathology in Alzheimer's disease and tauopathies. *Front Neurol* 2015;6:38.

69. Dean DC, III, Jerskey BA, Chen K, et al. Brain differences in infants at differential genetic risk for late-onset Alzheimer disease: a cross-sectional imaging study. *JAMA Neurol* 2014 Jan;71:11–22.

70. Geschwind DH, Robidoux J, Alarcon M, et al. Dementia and neurodevelopmental predisposition: cognitive dysfunction in presymptomatic subjects precedes dementia by decades in frontotemporal dementia. *Annals of Neurology* 2001;50: 741–746.

71. Geschwind DH, Miller BL. Molecular approaches to cerebral laterality: development and neurodegeneration. *Am J Med Genet* 2001 Jul 15;101:370–381.

2

Neurodegenerative Diseases as Protein Misfolding Disorders

TOMOHIRO NAKAMURA AND STUART A. LIPTON

INTRODUCTION

Many neurodegenerative diseases (NDD) manifest intra- and extracellular accumulation of misfolded proteins. For instance, in Parkinson's disease (PD), α-synuclein (α-syn) and synphilin-1 can be present in intraneuronal inclusions known as Lewy bodies and Lewy neurites. In Alzheimer's disease (AD), amyloid-β (Aβ) peptide and hyper-phosphorylated tau form extracellular amyloid plaques and intracellular neurofibrillary tangles, respectively. Protein aggregation is also a signature of polyQ disorders (e.g., Huntington's disease [HD]), amyotrophic lateral sclerosis (ALS), and prion disease, among others (1). Previously, deposits of large aggregates were thought to disrupt normal neuronal function, leading to neuronal dysfunction and death. However, more recent evidence suggests that soluble oligomers of the proteins are the most toxic species. Moreover, in the case of AD, there appears to be a lack of correlation between the amount of large, aggregated Aβ deposits or tau tangles and signs of the disease, including cognitive decline. Thus, emerging evidence points to small, soluble oligomers of misfolded proteins as the cause of synaptic dysfunction, the major pathological correlate to disease progression. In fact, the formation of larger, insoluble aggregates may in fact represent a neuroprotective response, perhaps an attempt to wall off these toxic proteins from the rest of the cell (2, 3). Structurally, toxic oligomers often expose flexible hydrophobic residues on their surfaces that facilitate aberrant and toxic interaction with other critical macromolecules (e.g., proteins and cell membranes), leading to neuronal dysfunction (4).

Protein quality control machineries, including molecular chaperones, the ubiquitin-proteasome system (UPS), and autophagy, can counterbalance the accumulation of misfolded proteins. Their ability to eliminate the neurotoxic effects of misfolded proteins, however, declines with age, contributing to the appearance of misfolded proteins in the degenerating brain. A plausible explanation for the age-dependent deterioration of the quality control machineries involves compromise of these systems by excessive generation of reactive oxygen species (ROS), such as superoxide anion ($O_2^{.-}$), and reactive nitrogen species (RNS), such as nitric oxide (NO$^.$). Such damage leads to the accumulation of misfolded proteins. Here, we focus on aberrantly increased generation of NO-related groups since this process appears to accelerate the manifestation of key neuropathological features, including protein misfolding. A well-established molecular mechanism by which NO groups affect neuronal function involves the chemical reaction of an NO moiety with the sulfhydryl (–SH) groups (or perhaps more properly thiolate anion, –S$^-$) of target proteins to form S-nitrosothiols (SNOs), a process termed S-nitrosylation (5, 6). Lipton and Stamler first discovered and characterized this redox reaction in biological systems, initially on the N-methyl-D-aspartate-type glutamate receptor (NMDAR) (7, 8). Subsequently, analogous to protein phosphorylation, a number of studies have found that the activity of potentially hundreds or even thousands of other proteins is modulated by this redox-mediated post-translational modification. In general, nitrosylating (or nitrosating) and denitrosylating (or denitrosating) enzymes catalyze the chemical reaction of putting an NO group "onto" and "off" a protein thiol.

In recent work, our group and others have shown that S-nitrosylation and further oxidation of critical cysteine residues can contribute to protein misfolding. In this chapter, we discuss recent evidence for NO-induced protein misfolding, and specifically focus on the critical roles of S-nitrosylated protein-disulfide isomerase (PDI, an endoplasmic reticulum [ER] chaperone) and parkin (a ubiquitin E3 ligase) in the accumulation of misfolded proteins in NDD (9–11). Additionally, we present the hypothesis that in sporadic forms of NDD, which constitute the vast majority of cases, pathologic protein misfolding may result from these redox post-translational changes engendered by nitrosative and/or oxidative stress. Thus, this type or post-translational modification can mimic or enhance rarer genetic variants of the disease (12).

CELL-BASED PROTEIN MISFOLDING AND QUALITY CONTROL MACHINERIES

The gradual generation and accumulation of toxic misfolded proteins cause proteotoxicity, contributing to synaptic loss and neuronal cell death. Under normal conditions, neurons utilize their quality control machinery to facilitate the clearance of misfolded proteins (Figure 2.1). For instance, molecular chaperones, such as heat-shock proteins (HSPs), glucose-regulated proteins (GRPs), and PDI, recognize mature or nascent misfolded proteins in the cytosol or ER, and assist in their refolding process to re-establish their proper structure. Additionally, if proteins are severely misfolded and damaged, they are degraded by the UPS or autophagy/lysosome pathways. Molecular chaperones also participate in the clearance of misfolded proteins by dissociating them from large aggregates for degradation by the UPS or autophagic/lysosomal system. The UPS mainly participates in the degradation of

smaller misfolded proteins. In the UPS, formation of polyubiquitin chains on a substrate protein constitutes the fundamental signal for proteasomal degradation. A cascade of enzymes catalyzes activation (E1), conjugation (E2), and ligation (E3 ligase) of ubiquitin chains to the protein, marking it for degradation via the proteasome. Individual E3 ubiquitin ligases play a key role in the recognition of specific peptide substrates (13). Finally, the 26S proteasome, comprised of the catalytic 20S core particle and two 19S regulatory subunits, recognizes polyubiquitin chains and degrades the target proteins into short peptides.

In contrast, autophagy/lysosome pathways are typically responsible for the clearance of larger protein aggregates. There are three known pathways to autophagy: macroautophagy, microautophagy, and chaperone-mediated autophagy. Among these pathways, macroautophagy represents the major pathway that eliminates aggregated inclusions or damaged cellular organelles. This process requires the sequestration of cytosolic substrates into autophagosomes that subsequently fuse with a lysosome, which contains acidic hydrolases for the degradation of proteins. In recent years, extensive studies have identified and characterized many autophagy-related proteins, including Beclin-1, p62, and LC3, all of which are involved in the regulation of autophagic processes (14).

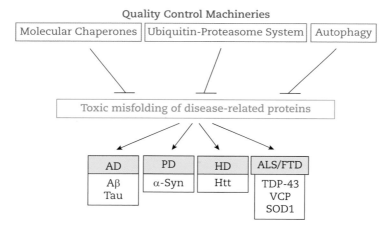

FIGURE 2.1. Cell-based quality control machinery prevents accumulation of misfolded proteins. Toxic accumulation of misfolded proteins represents a key common feature in various NDDs, including Alzheimer's disease (AD), Parkinson's disease (PD), polyglutamine (polyQ) diseases such as Huntington's disease (HD), and amyotrophic lateral sclerosis (ALS)/frontotemporal dementia (FTD). Examples of these misfolding-prone proteins include Aβ and tau in AD, α-synuclein (α-syn) in PD, mutant huntingtin (Htt) in HD (a polyQ disease), and TDP-43, VCP, and SOD1 in ALS/FTD. The quality control machinery, including molecular chaperones, the ubiquitin-proteasome system (UPS), and autophagy, decrease misfolded proteins via introduction of correct folding or degradation of the aberrantly folded proteins.

Under neuropathological conditions, decreased protein quality control leads to the disruption of normal protein homeostasis (i.e., proteostasis), resulting in the accumulation of aberrant proteins either within or outside cells. Moreover, several mutations in molecular chaperones or UPS-associated enzymes are known to contribute to neurodegeneration (15, 16). A reduction in proteasomal activity has been reported in the substantia nigra of human PD patients (17), and overexpression of the molecular chaperone HSP70 prevented neurodegeneration in vivo in models of PD (18). Additionally, recent evidence suggests that NO-related species may play a significant role in the process of protein misfolding. Consistent with this notion, increased nitrosative and oxidative stress are associated with chaperone and proteasomal dysfunction that can lead to the accumulation of misfolded aggregates (12, 19). However, until recently little was known regarding the molecular and pathogenic mechanisms underlying the contributions of NO to the accumulation of misfolded proteins. We and others recently presented (patho-)physiological and chemical evidence that S-nitrosylation and subsequent further oxidation of specific proteins can modulate the activity of the quality control systems, contributing to protein misfolding and neurotoxicity in models of neurodegenerative disorders (9–11, 20).

GENERATION OF RNS AND PROTEIN S-NITROSYLATION

Under normal, physiological conditions, brain cells produce low but sufficient levels of NO to regulate many cellular signaling pathways that support synaptic plasticity, normal development, and neuronal cell survival (21). These effects are mediated in part through the activation of guanylate cyclase to form cyclic guanosine-3',5'-monophosphate (cGMP) (22). In addition, emerging evidence suggests that a more prominent reaction of NO may be S-nitros(yl)ation of regulatory protein thiol groups (8, 19, 23). Protein S-nitrosylation results from the covalent addition of an NO group to a cysteine thiol/thiolate (RSH or RS⁻ [where R denotes an organic group]) to form an S-nitrosothiol derivative (R-SNO). A nucleophilic critical cysteine may be surrounded by acidic-basic residues, forming an SNO motif that increases the susceptibility of the sulfhydryl to S-nitrosylation (5, 24). For example, NO can exert a neuroprotective effect via S-nitrosylation of NMDARs and caspases (8, 25).

In contrast, under pathophysiological conditions, increased nitrosative/oxidative stress can result in defects in many aspects of neuronal function, thus contributing to the pathogenesis of NDD (Figure 2.2). Elevated levels of NO are neurodestructive through aberrant S-nitrosylation of matrix metalloproteinase-9 (MMP-9), glyceraldehyde 3-phosphate dehydrogenase (GAPDH), and other targets, as discussed later in this chapter (9–11, 25–32). As negative regulators of S-nitrosylation pathways, thioredoxin/thioredoxin reductase, class III alcohol dehydrogenase, PDI, and intracellular glutathione (GSH) catalyze denitrosylation of SNOs to diminish the effects of NO groups (33). Thus, these denitrosylating enzymes can possibly provide neuroprotective effects under certain conditions. Additionally, S-nitrosylation is known to be a reversible "priming" oxidation step, reacting with a vicinal (adjacent or nearby thiol if present) to form a disulfide bond between two cysteine residues (11, 30, 34). Alternatively, NO is often chemically a "good leaving group"; departure of NO from an SNO may facilitate the reaction of the free thiol with the remaining free thiol with ROS to yield a sulfenic (R-SOH) or more stable sulfinic (R-SO$_2$H) or sulfonic (R-SO$_3$H) acid derivative of the protein (10, 11, 26). While R-SO$_2$H can possibly be reduced after induction of the enzyme sulfiredoxin, R-SO$_3$H is a permanent modification without known enzymatic reversal. These stable oxidative modifications of critical cysteine thiols also may be implicated in protein misfolding. Furthermore, NO· reacts rapidly with superoxide anion (O$_2^{·-}$) to form the very toxic product peroxynitrite (ONOO⁻), which can result in disulfide formation or nitration of tyrosine residues to form another type of NO-dependent posttranslational modification, 3-nitrotyrosine (8), as discussed later in the chapter.

Concerning the production of NO in the brain, a family of NO synthases (NOSs) catalyzes the conversion of L-arginine to L-citrulline and NO. Three known NOS members produce NO in either a calcium-dependent (for neuronal NOS [nNOS, NOS-1] and endothelial NOS [eNOS, NOS-3]) or calcium-independent manner (for inducible NOS [iNOS, NOS-2]). An important signaling pathway that can stimulate nNOS activity involves the activation of NMDARs and subsequent influx of Ca^{2+} ions (23). In general, physiological synaptic NMDAR activation is essential, in part via generation of low levels of NO, for synaptic plasticity, learning, and memory. In contrast, excessive excitation of NMDARs, particularly extrasynaptic NMDARs, plays a key role in a variety of neurological disorders ranging from acute hypoxic-ischemic brain injury

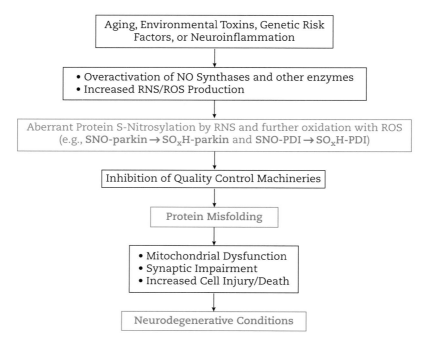

FIGURE 2.2. Possible mechanisms by which aberrantly formed S-nitrosylated proteins contribute to the accumulation of misfolded proteins and NDD. Physiological levels of NO mediate normal cell signaling and neuroprotective effects, at least in part, by S-nitrosylating NMDA-type glutamate receptors (NMDARs) and caspases, thus inhibiting their activity. In contrast, aging, environmental toxins (e.g., pesticides), genetic risk factors, or neuroinflammatory stimuli can overactivate NO synthases, such as nNOS and iNOS, as well as other enzymes such as NADPH oxidase (NOX), resulting in overproduction of RNS and ROS. Excessive levels of NO then react with thiol groups (or thiolate anion) to form abnormal SNO-proteins. Subsequent oxidation with ROS can lead to further oxidation, resulting in a series of sulfenic ($-SOH$), sulfinic ($-SO_2H$), and sulfonic acid ($-SO_3H$) derivatives. We present evidence that aberrant S-nitrosylation and further oxidation of parkin and PDI, among other specific protein targets, induce dysfunction in the protein quality control machinery, triggering accumulation of misfolded proteins. Protein misfolding can contribute to further generation of ROS/RNS, abnormal mitochondrial bioenergetics, synaptic injury, and neuronal cell death, as found in multiple NDD.

to chronic NDD. Moreover, synaptic NMDAR activity generally stimulates molecular pathways that promote neuronal survival, for example, by enhancing the expression of antioxidant enzymes (35). Conversely, excessive activation of extrasynaptic NMDARs leads to pathological production of RNS/ROS and affects additional molecular signaling pathways that contribute to neurotoxicity associated with accumulation of misfolded proteins (36–38). Additionally, a positive-feedback mechanism triggered by misfolded proteins (e.g., oligomeric Aβ peptide) can augment RNS/ROS production, in part through the hyperactivation of NMDARs, to increase nitrosative/oxidative stress (37, 38).

Numerous animal studies have suggested that NO can contribute to protein misfolding and neuronal cell injury/damage. In models of PD, pesticides, such as rotenone, paraquat, and maneb, or other environmental toxins, such as 1-methyl-4-phenyl-1,2,3,6-tetrahydropyridine (MPTP) and 6-hydroxydopamine, have been shown to specifically inhibit the mitochondrial respiratory chain. These toxins thus generate excessive ROS/RNS and recapitulate many features of sporadic PD, including degeneration of dopaminergic neurons and accumulation of aberrantly folded proteins (9–11, 39, 40). Exposure to environmental risk factors enhances vulnerability to NMDAR-mediated toxicity (i.e., excitotoxicity), thus hyperactivating NOS to produce massive amounts of NO (41). Further, inhibition of nNOS or iNOS activity via genetic ablation or pharmacological antagonism decreases protein misfolding in models of PD, consistent with the notion that NO overproduction triggers proteotoxicity (42–44). Additionally, in models of AD, deletion of the iNOS gene decreases aggregation of Aβ, suggesting that NO plays a deleterious role, although some studies have shown that iNOS activity may also be neuroprotective (45–48). These inconsistent results in AD models underscore the bifunctional aspects of NO that can serve as a neuroprotective or neurodestructive agent depending on the circumstances of its production and the proteins with which it reacts in various cell compartments. In the remaining sections of this chapter, we focus on the pathological role of NO and discuss aberrant SNO signaling pathways that contribute to protein misfolding in neurodegenerative conditions.

S-NITROSYLATION AND MOLECULAR CHAPERONES

Members of the PDI family that reside mainly within the ER represent one of the best characterized protein chaperones identified to date. In addition to its chaperone property, PDI members (especially PDIA1) can introduce structural disulfide bonds into proteins (oxidation), break disulfide bonds (reduction), and catalyze rearrangement of incorrect disulfide bonds (isomerization), thus increasing the structural stability of substrate proteins (49). A number of studies have suggested that PDIs can offer neuroprotection via decreasing protein misfolding. For example, accumulation of misfolded proteins in the ER stimulates stress response pathways, known as the unfolded protein response (UPR), that decrease protein translation and induce expression of molecular chaperones, including PDI family members (such as PDIA1 and PDIA2) and GRP78/BiP, to relieve ER stress. Severe and prolonged ER stress, however, as occurs under neurodegenerative conditions, eventually causes apoptotic cell death in neurons (50–60).

To date, at least 21 PDI family members have been identified in humans (61). Among these PDI members, PDIA1 is perhaps the most abundantly expressed form in most mammalian tissues (62). PDIA1 has four domains that are homologous to thioredoxin (TRX) (termed a, b, b', and a'). Only two of the four TRX-like domains (a and a') contain a characteristic redox-active CXXC motif, and these two-thiol/disulfide centers function as independent active sites (63–66). In contrast, the chaperone activity of PDIA1 does not require the catalytic cysteine residues of either domain (66), but all four domains (especially a') and the C-terminus of the protein contribute to this chaperone function (67, 68).

Published evidence suggests that excessive generation of NO can result in prolonged activation of the ER stress pathway (69, 70). Although the complete molecular mechanism whereby NO induces protein misfolding in the ER remains enigmatic, we initially reported finding S-nitrosylation of PDIA1 and possibly other PDIs at the active-site thiol groups in animal models of AD and PD (9). We found that exposure of neurons to neurotoxic concentrations of NMDA or rotenone results in S-nitrosylation of PDIA1 (forming SNO-PDIA1). S-Nitrosylation of PDI inhibits both its isomerase and chaperone activities (11). Moreover, we found that S-nitrosylation of PDIA1 is significantly elevated in the brains of virtually all cases examined of human sporadic AD and PD. In several models of NDD, S-nitrosylation abrogates PDIA1 activity, leading to the accumulation of polyubiquitinated/misfolded proteins (e.g., synphilin-1 and α-syn) and activation of severe ER stress (11, 71–74). Consequently, SNO-PDIA1 formation prevents its attenuation of neuronal cell death triggered by ER stress or misfolded proteins. Recent studies further demonstrated that SNO-PDIA1 exacerbates other neuropathological conditions such as ALS, stroke, prion disease, and sleep disorders (73, 75–78), suggesting that SNO-PDI formation may serve as a unifying mechanism in neurological disorders. In fact, this would make sense since PDI is important in normal protein function, and thus inhibition of PDI chaperone activity via S-nitrosylation would be expected to result in misfolding of a number of proteins.

In non-neuronal systems, S-nitrosylation has been shown to regulate the activity of other chaperone enzymes such as HSP90 and VCP (vasolin-containing protein). The HSP90 chaperone is a member of an ATPase family that assists in the stabilization of at least 200 substrate proteins, including the tumor suppressor p53 (79). NO can S-nitrosylate human HSP90 at Cys597, located at the C-terminal of the chaperone protein (80). Although Cys597 is located outside the ATPase domain, a recent study confirmed that S-nitrosylation of HSP90α at its C-terminus perturbs the conformation of the protein, influencing the ATPase domain of HSP90 (81). As a consequence of S-nitrosylation, therefore, SNO-HSP90 manifests decreased ATPase/chaperone activity. In addition, SNO-HSP90 serves as a transnitrosylase toward the androgen receptor (AR), and thus SNO-HSP90 may also regulate AR-dependent transcription (82). Moreover, S-nitrosylation of the HSP90 co-chaperone protein hop/Stip1 may potentially decrease HSP90 activity (83). Although the potential role of SNO-HSP90 (or SNO-hop/Stip1) in neurodegeneration remains to be elucidated, these data raise the interesting possibility that SNO-HSP90 contributes to protein misfolding in NDD.

The chaperone VCP/p97 is a type II member of the AAA+ ATPase family that employs energy obtained from ATP hydrolysis to exert its activity. Specifically, VCP/p97 binds to ubiquitinated, misfolded proteins and remodels the targets to extract them from protein aggregates, chromatin complexes, the ER, mitochondria, or cell membranes, thus facilitating degradation of the misfolded proteins by the proteasome (84). Importantly, mutations in the *VCP/p97* gene trigger disease conditions known as IBMPFD (Paget's disease of bone and frontotemporal dementia) and MSP (multisystem proteinopathy); these conditions are manifest as inclusion body myopathy (IBM), Paget's disease of bone (PDB), frontotemporal dementia (FTD), sporadic and familial ALS, hereditary spastic paraplegia, and parkinsonism (84, 85). A recent study demonstrated that NO can S-nitrosylate yeast or plant orthologues of VCP/p97, CDC48 (86). S-Nitrosylation occurs at multiple sites (Cys110, Cys526, and Cys664) in CDC48. Among these SNO residues, Cys526 is evolutionarily conserved among VCP/p97/CDC48 families and localized in a domain responsible for ATP binding. As a consequence of S-nitrosylation, NO induces conformational changes near Cys526 and abolishes its ATPase activity. Further studies are needed to determine the possible role of SNO-VCP/p97 in protein misfolding and neurodegeneration.

Interestingly, using a colon cell line, a prior proteomic study identified a series of additional molecular chaperones that undergo S-nitrosylation (87). These SNO-chaperones include Hsp70 protein 4, Hsc71, calreticulin, endoplasmin, GRP78, and ORP150. Therefore, further investigation involving proteomic approaches should be performed to acquire a comprehensive list of S-nitrosylated chaperones that could affect protein misfolding in neurodegenerative and other systemic conditions.

S-NITROSYLATION AND THE UPS

NO has been shown to promote protein misfolding via S-nitrosylation of multiple cysteine residues on parkin, at RING-type ubiquitin E3 ligase (9, 10, 20). Mutations in the *parkin* gene (*PARK2*) have been associated with autosomal recessive juvenile PD and other rare forms of PD. Disruption of parkin activity, either by mutation or because of S-nitrosylation, causes a dysfunctional UPS, contributing to the accumulation of misfolded, neurotoxic proteins in both familial and sporadic PD. In addition, multiple cysteine residues in parkin can also undergo further oxidation due to reaction with ROS, resulting in dysfunctional E3 ligase activity and thus contributing to the pathogenesis of PD (88).

Recent evidence suggests that parkin participates in the process of mitophagy by which damaged mitochondria are eliminated by macroautophagy (discussed in detail later). Our group and others have demonstrated that S-nitrosylation and further oxidation of parkin result in a dysfunctional enzyme and disruption of UPS/mitophagy activity (9, 10, 20, 89). Initially, S-nitrosylation of parkin stimulates its ubiquitin E3 ligase activity, which may enhance the degradation of misfolded protein, representing a potential neuroprotective function of SNO. Subsequently, with time the E3 ligase activity of SNO-parkin decreases, resulting in UPS dysfunction that potentially contributes to Lewy body formation (10, 20). An increase in protein misfolding due to S-nitrosylation of parkin could also contribute to neuronal cell injury/death (9). We also found that nitrosative stress produces S-nitrosylation of parkin (forming SNO-parkin) in rodent models of PD and in brains of human patients with PD and the related α-synucleinopathy, diffuse Lewy body disease (DLBD), consistent with the notion that SNO-parkin may play a role in PD pathogenesis. Additionally, these findings raise the interesting possibility that nitrosative/oxidative stress, commonly found during normal aging, can mimic rare genetic causes of NDD by promoting SNO-mediated protein misfolding in sporadic cases (even in the absence of a genetic mutation of parkin in this instance). Although the effects of S-nitrosylation on protein misfolding have not yet been fully elucidated, this redox reaction influences the enzymatic function of a number of ubiquitin E3 ligases, including XIAP, pVHL, UBE3A, and RNFs (31, 90, 91). These findings suggest that this chemical process may be a common phenomenon contributing to protein misfolding under a variety of conditions.

In addition to the E3 ligases, NO can directly inhibit protein degradation via S-nitrosylation of the proteasome itself. NO can poly-S-nitrosylate at least 10 cysteine residues in the 20S catalytic core of the 26S proteasome, inhibiting its protease activity (92). Moreover, NO affects the ubiquitination of a variety of S-nitrosylated proteins. For instance, S-nitrosylation of PTEN, IRP2, Bcl-2, and FLIP regulates their ubiquitination and subsequent degradation via the UPS (93–97). Clearly, further studies are required to determine the pathophysiological relevance of these reactions in NDDs.

S-NITROSYLATION AND AUTOPHAGY

Concerning the link between S-nitrosylation of specific proteins and autophagy, recent work from the Rubinsztein laboratory has demonstrated that S-nitrosylation reactions can control autophagic processes in models of HD (98). These autophagy-related S-nitrosylated proteins include SNO-JNK1 and SNO-IKKβ. Prior studies had already shown that S-nitrosylation inhibits JNK1 and IKKβ activity (99, 100). In their report, Rubinsztein's group found that the generation of SNO-JNK1 and SNO-IKKβ results in decreased Beclin signaling, which is required for autophagosome formation, and increased mTOR complex 1 (mTORC1) activity, which is an inhibitor of autophagy. Along these lines, S-nitrosylation of TSC2 also leads to activation of the mTOR pathway (101). Collectively, these results suggest that S-nitrosylation inhibits autophagy in neurons, potentially contributing to the accumulation of misfolded proteins. However, another group reported that NO represses mTORC1 activity in an ATM-dependent fashion (102), which would lead to increased autophagy. Moreover, Filomeni et al. recently showed that genetic deletion of GSNO (S-nitrosoglutathione) reductase, which catalyzes many intracellular denitrosylation reactions, does not affect basal autophagy activity (103). Thus, these observations call attention to the need for further studies to fully understand the role of NO/S-nitrosylation in autophagy under neurodegenerative conditions.

Additionally, recent evidence suggests that parkin plays a critical role in mitophagy, an autophagic process that removes damaged mitochondria (104). In this scenario, damaged mitochondria activate the kinase PINK1, which recruits parkin to the damaged mitochondrial membrane (note that genetic mutation of *PINK1* underlies certain forms of familial PD). The translocated parkin ubiquitinates mitochondrial outer membrane proteins, marking the damaged mitochondria for mitophagic clearance. S-Nitrosylation can affect this mitophagic process, at least in part, through the formation of SNO-parkin. The resulting initial increase in E3 ligase activity upon S-nitrosylation upregulates mitophagy, whereas subsequent attenuation of parkin activity impedes mitophagy, resulting in the accumulation of unhealthy mitochondria (89).

In the past decade, extensive studies on the molecular mechanisms of autophagy have identified numerous autophagic regulators (103, 105). Interestingly, some of these regulators, including Atg4 (autophagy-related protein 4), PTEN, Akt, SIRT1, and HIF-1α, are known to be sensitive to S-nitrosylation or cysteine oxidation (94, 106–112). Thus, it is tempting to speculate that, when S-nitrosylated, these proteins can affect proteotoxicity through the regulation of autophagy. Future studies will be needed to test this hypothesis.

TYROSINE NITRATION AND PROTEIN MISFOLDING

As mentioned earlier in this chapter, NO· can form highly reactive peroxynitrite ($ONOO^-$) through reaction with superoxide anion ($O_2^{·-}$). Peroxynitrite can alter protein activity by facilitating disulfide formation or via another type of post-translational modification involving the nitration of tyrosine residues. This reaction results in nitrotyrosine formation, typically contributing to protein misfolding and cell death (113, 114). For example, α-syn can be nitrated on critical tyrosine residues (to form nitrotyrosine), leading to misfolding and aggregation (115). Nitration-induced aggregation of α-syn may result from the formation of dityrosine cross-linking (116). Moreover, nitration of human Aβ peptide at tyrosine 10 (Tyr10) accelerates its aggregation (117). Since Tyr10 is not present in mouse/rat Aβ, this finding may explain why mouse/rat Aβ is less prone to misfolding/aggregation compared to human Aβ. Furthermore, in the human AD brain, nitrated tau is found in the insoluble fraction (containing misfolded proteins), suggesting that NO/peroxynitrite promotes aggregation of tau as well (118, 119).

Nitration of HSP90 and Trx1 may also contribute to the accumulation of misfolded proteins in NDDs. For instance, akin to SNO-PDI formation, nitration of Trx1 inhibits its oxidoreductase activity (120). In addition, HSP90 undergoes nitration at Tyr33 and Try56, impairing its binding affinity to ATP and thus decreasing its ATPase/chaperone activity (121). Additionally, nitrated HSP90 stimulates cell death via activation of the P2X7/Fas pathway.

Despite these findings, routine and reliable experimental tools to study nitrated tyrosine residues are limited, and the mechanisms responsible for the nitration of specific tyrosine residues remain unclear. Thus, in order to demonstrate the biological relevance of tyrosine nitration, future studies are needed.

CONCLUSIONS

Sporadic forms of NDD share many common neuropathological signatures, including elevated generation of RNS/ROS, accumulation of misfolded/aggregated proteins, excitotoxic activation of NMDA-type glutamate receptors, mitochondrial dysfunction, synaptic impairment, and increased cell injury/death. In this chapter, we have delineated the pathophysiological role of severe nitrosative/oxidative stress in protein misfolding. Specifically, we have discussed how aberrant protein S-nitrosylation and further oxidation can contribute to malfunction of the quality control machinery in the nervous system, including molecular chaperones, the UPS, and autophagy. Further study of SNO-parkin, SNO-PDI, and many other SNO-proteins in NDD may provide new approaches to prevent not only protein misfolding, but also downstream pathological events such as mitochondrial dysfunction, synaptic loss, and neuronal cell death.

ACKNOWLEDGMENTS

This work was supported in part by NIH grants P30 NS076411, R01 NS086890, R01 ES017462, P01 HD029587, and R21 NS080799 (SAL), the Brain and Behavior Research Foundation (SAL), and the Michael J. Fox Foundation (SAL and TN).

REFERENCES

1. Ciechanover A, Brundin P (2003). The ubiquitin proteasome system in neurodegenerative diseases: sometimes the chicken, sometimes the egg. *Neuron* 40:427–446.
2. Arrasate M, Mitra S, Schweitzer ES, Segal MR, Finkbeiner S (2004). Inclusion body formation reduces levels of mutant huntingtin and the risk of neuronal death. *Nature* 431:805–810.
3. Benilova I, Karran E, De Strooper B (2012). The toxic Aβ oligomer and Alzheimer's disease: an emperor in need of clothes. *Nat Neurosci* 15:349–357.
4. Campioni S, et al. (2010). A causative link between the structure of aberrant protein oligomers and their toxicity. *Nat Chem Biol* 6:140–147.
5. Hess DT, Matsumoto A, Kim SO, Marshall HE, Stamler JS (2005). Protein S-nitrosylation: purview and parameters. *Nat Rev Mol Cell Biol* 6:150–166.
6. Nakamura T, et al. (2013) Aberrant protein S-nitrosylation in neurodegenerative diseases. *Neuron* 78:596–614.
7. Lei SZ, et al. (1992). Effect of nitric oxide production on the redox modulatory site of the NMDA receptor-channel complex. *Neuron* 8:1087–1099.
8. Lipton SA, et al. (1993). A redox-based mechanism for the neuroprotective and neurodestructive effects of nitric oxide and related nitroso-compounds. *Nature* 364:626–632.
9. Chung KK, et al. (2004). S-Nitrosylation of parkin regulates ubiquitination and compromises parkin's protective function. *Science* 304:1328–1331.
10. Yao D, et al. (2004). Nitrosative stress linked to sporadic Parkinson's disease: S-nitrosylation of parkin regulates its E3 ubiquitin ligase activity. *Proc Natl Acad Sci USA* 101:10810–10814.
11. Uehara T, et al. (2006). S-Nitrosylated protein-disulphide isomerase links protein misfolding to neurodegeneration. *Nature* 441:513–517.
12. Zhang K, Kaufman RJ (2006). The unfolded protein response: a stress signaling pathway critical for health and disease. *Neurology* 66:S102–S109.
13. Ross CA, Pickart CM (2004). The ubiquitin-proteasome pathway in Parkinson's disease and other neurodegenerative diseases. *Trends Cell Biol* 14:703–711.
14. Harris H, Rubinsztein DC (2012). Control of autophagy as a therapy for neurodegenerative disease. *Nat Rev Neurol* 8:108–117.
15. Muchowski PJ, Wacker JL (2005). Modulation of neurodegeneration by molecular chaperones. *Nat Rev Neurosci* 6:11–22.
16. Cookson MR (2005). The biochemistry of Parkinson's disease. *Annu Rev Biochem* 74:29–52.
17. McNaught KS, Perl DP, Brownell AL, Olanow CW (2004). Systemic exposure to proteasome inhibitors causes a progressive model of Parkinson's disease. *Ann Neurol* 56:149–162.
18. Auluck PK, Chan HY, Trojanowski JQ, Lee VM, Bonini NM (2002). Chaperone suppression of α-synuclein toxicity in a Drosophila model for Parkinson's disease. *Science* 295:865–868.
19. Isaacs AM, Senn DB, Yuan M, Shine JP, Yankner BA (2006). Acceleration of amyloid β-peptide aggregation by physiological concentrations of calcium. *J Biol Chem* 281:27916–27923.
20. Lipton SA, et al. (2005). Comment on "S-nitrosylation of parkin regulates ubiquitination and compromises parkin's protective function." *Science* 308:1870; author reply 1870.
21. Dawson VL, Dawson TM, London ED, Bredt DS, Snyder SH (1991). Nitric oxide mediates glutamate neurotoxicity in primary cortical cultures. *Proc Natl Acad Sci USA* 88:6368–6371.
22. Nisoli E, et al. (2003). Mitochondrial biogenesis in mammals: the role of endogenous nitric oxide. *Science* 299:896–899.
23. Garthwaite J, Charles SL, Chess-Williams R (1988). Endothelium-derived relaxing factor release on activation of NMDA receptors suggests role as intercellular messenger in the brain. *Nature* 336:385–388.

24. Stamler JS, Toone EJ, Lipton SA, Sucher NJ (1997). (S)NO signals: translocation, regulation, and a consensus motif. *Neuron* 18:691–696.

25. Mannick JB, et al. (1999). Fas-induced caspase denitrosylation. *Science* 284:651–654.

26. Gu Z, et al. (2002). S-Nitrosylation of matrix metalloproteinases: signaling pathway to neuronal cell death. *Science* 297:1186–1190.

27. Hara MR, et al. (2005). S-Nitrosylated GAPDH initiates apoptotic cell death by nuclear translocation following Siah1 binding. *Nat Cell Biol* 7:665–674.

28. Melino G, et al. (1997). S-Nitrosylation regulates apoptosis. *Nature* 388:432–433.

29. Shi ZQ, et al. (2013). S-Nitrosylated SHP-2 contributes to NMDA receptor-mediated excitotoxicity in acute ischemic stroke. *Proc Natl Acad Sci USA* 110:3137–3142.

30. Cho DH, et al. (2009). S-Nitrosylation of Drp1 mediates β-amyloid-related mitochondrial fission and neuronal injury. *Science* 324:102–105.

31. Nakamura T, et al. (2010). Transnitrosylation of XIAP regulates caspase-dependent neuronal cell death. *Mol Cell* 39:184–195.

32. Qu J, et al. (2011). S-Nitrosylation activates Cdk5 and contributes to synaptic spine loss induced by β-amyloid peptide. *Proc Natl Acad Sci USA*:14330–14335.

33. Benhar M, Forrester MT, Stamler JS (2009). Protein denitrosylation: enzymatic mechanisms and cellular functions. *Nat Rev Mol Cell Biol* 10:721–732.

34. Eaton P (2006). Protein thiol oxidation in health and disease: techniques for measuring disulfides and related modifications in complex protein mixtures. *Free Radic Biol Med* 40:1889–1899.

35. Papadia S, et al. (2008). Synaptic NMDA receptor activity boosts intrinsic antioxidant defenses. *Nat Neurosci* 11:476–487.

36. Okamoto SI, et al. (2009). Balance between synaptic versus extrasynaptic NMDA receptor activity influences inclusions and neurotoxicity of mutant huntingtin. *Nat Med* 15:1407–1413.

37. Molokanova E, et al. (2014). Differential effects of synaptic and extrasynaptic NMDA receptors on Aβ-induced nitric oxide production in cerebrocortical neurons. *J Neurosci* 34:5023–5028.

38. Talantova M, et al. (2013). Aβ induces astrocytic glutamate release, extrasynaptic NMDA receptor activation, and synaptic loss. *Proc Natl Acad Sci USA* 110:E2518–2527.

39. Betarbet R, et al. (2000). Chronic systemic pesticide exposure reproduces features of Parkinson's disease. *Nat Neurosci* 3:1301–1306.

40. Beal MF (2001). Experimental models of Parkinson's disease. *Nat Rev Neurosci* 2:325–334.

41. Beal MF (1998). Excitotoxicity and nitric oxide in Parkinson's disease pathogenesis. *Ann Neurol* 44:S110–114.

42. Liberatore GT, et al. (1999). Inducible nitric oxide synthase stimulates dopaminergic neurodegeneration in the MPTP model of Parkinson disease. *Nat Med* 5:1403–1409.

43. Schulz JB, Matthews RT, Muqit MM, Browne SE, Beal MF (1995). Inhibition of neuronal nitric oxide synthase by 7-nitroindazole protects against MPTP-induced neurotoxicity in mice. *J Neurochem* 64:936–939.

44. Hantraye P, et al. (1996). Inhibition of neuronal nitric oxide synthase prevents MPTP-induced parkinsonism in baboons. *Nat Med* 2:1017–1021.

45. Colton CA, et al. (2006). NO synthase 2 (NOS2) deletion promotes multiple pathologies in a mouse model of Alzheimer's disease. *Proc Natl Acad Sci USA* 103:12867–12872.

46. Wilcock DM, et al. (2008). Progression of amyloid pathology to Alzheimer's disease pathology in an amyloid precursor protein transgenic mouse model by removal of nitric oxide synthase 2. *J Neurosci* 28:1537–1545.

47. Nathan C, et al. (2005). Protection from Alzheimer's-like disease in the mouse by genetic ablation of inducible nitric oxide synthase. *J Exp Med* 202:1163–1169.

48. Medeiros R, et al. (2007). Connecting TNF-α signaling pathways to iNOS. expression in a mouse model of Alzheimer's disease: relevance for the behavioral and synaptic deficits induced by amyloid β protein. *J Neurosci* 27:5394–5404.

49. Lyles MM, Gilbert HF (1991). Catalysis of the oxidative folding of ribonuclease A by protein disulfide isomerase: dependence of the rate on the composition of the redox buffer. *Biochemistry* 30:613–619.

50. Andrews DW, Johnson AE (1996). The translocon: more than a hole in the ER membrane? *Trends Biochem Sci* 21:365–369.

51. Sidrauski C, Chapman R, Walter P (1998). The unfolded protein response: an intracellular signalling pathway with many surprising features. *Trends Cell Biol* 8:245–249.

52. Szegezdi E, Logue SE, Gorman AM, Samali A (2006). Mediators of endoplasmic reticulum stress-induced apoptosis. *EMBO Rep* 7:880–885.

53. Ellgaard L, Molinari M, Helenius A (1999). Setting the standards: quality control in the secretory pathway. *Science* 286:1882–1888.

54. Conn KJ, et al. (2004). Identification of the protein disulfide isomerase family member PDIp in experimental Parkinson's disease and Lewy body pathology. *Brain Res* 1022:164–172.

55. Tanaka S, Uehara T, Nomura Y (2000). Up-regulation of protein-disulfide isomerase in response to hypoxia/brain ischemia and its protective effect against apoptotic cell death. *J Biol Chem* 275:10388–10393.

56. Ko HS, Uehara T, Nomura Y (2002). Role of ubiquilin associated with protein-disulfide isomerase in the endoplasmic reticulum in stress-induced apoptotic cell death. *J Biol Chem* 277:35386–35392.

57. Hetz C, et al. (2005). The disulfide isomerase Grp58 is a protective factor against prion neurotoxicity. *J Neurosci* 25:2793–2802.

58. Hu BR, Martone ME, Jones YZ, Liu CL (2000). Protein aggregation after transient cerebral ischemia. *J Neurosci* 20:3191–3199.

59. Rao RV, Bredesen DE (2004). Misfolded proteins, endoplasmic reticulum stress and neurodegeneration. *Curr Opin Cell Biol* 16:653–662.

60. Atkin JD, et al. (2006). Induction of the unfolded protein response in familial amyotrophic lateral sclerosis and association of protein-disulfide isomerase with superoxide dismutase 1. *J Biol Chem* 281:30152–30165.

61. Benham AM (2012). The protein disulfide isomerase family: key players in health and disease. *Antioxid Redox Signal* 16:781–789.

62. Freedman RB, Klappa P, Ruddock LW (2002). Protein disulfide isomerases exploit synergy between catalytic and specific binding domains. *EMBO Rep* 3:136–140.

63. Edman JC, Ellis L, Blacher RW, Roth RA, Rutter WJ (1985). Sequence of protein disulphide isomerase and implications of its relationship to thioredoxin. *Nature* 317:267–270.

64. Vuori K, Pihlajaniemi T, Myllyla R, Kivirikko KI (1992). Site-directed mutagenesis of human protein disulphide isomerase: effect on the assembly, activity and endoplasmic reticulum retention of human prolyl 4-hydroxylase in Spodoptera frugiperda insect cells. *EMBO J* 11:4213–4217.

65. Ellgaard L, Ruddock LW (2005). The human protein disulphide isomerase family: substrate interactions and functional properties. *EMBO Rep* 6:28–32.

66. Gruber CW, Cemazar M, Heras B, Martin JL, Craik DJ (2006). Protein disulfide isomerase: the structure of oxidative folding. *Trends Biochem Sci* 31:455–464.

67. Tian R, et al. (2004). The acidic C-terminal domain stabilizes the chaperone function of protein disulfide isomerase. *J Biol Chem* 279:48830–48835.

68. Sun XX, Dai Y, Liu HP, Chen SM, Wang CC (2000). Contributions of protein disulfide isomerase domains to its chaperone activity. *Biochim Biophys Acta* 1481:45–54.

69. Gotoh T, Oyadomari S, Mori K, Mori M (2002). Nitric oxide-induced apoptosis in RAW 264.7 macrophages is mediated by endoplasmic reticulum stress pathway involving ATF6 and CHOP. *J Biol Chem* 277:12343–12350.

70. Oyadomari S, et al. (2001). Nitric oxide-induced apoptosis in pancreatic β cells is mediated by the endoplasmic reticulum stress pathway. *Proc Natl Acad Sci USA* 98:10845–10850.

71. Kabiraj P, Marin JE, Varela-Ramirez A, Zubia ES, Narayan M (2014). Ellagic acid mitigates SNO-PDI induced aggregation of Parkinsonian biomarkers. *ACS Chem Neurosci* 5:1209–1220.

72. Wu XF, et al. (2014). S-Nitrosylating protein disulphide isomerase mediates α-synuclein aggregation caused by methamphetamine exposure in PC12 cells. *Toxicol Lett* 230:19–27.

73. Xu B, et al. (2014). α-Synuclein oligomerization in manganese-induced nerve cell injury in brain slices: a role of NO-mediated S-nitrosylation of protein disulfide isomerase. *Mol Neurobiol* 50:1098–1110.

74. Chung KK, et al. (2001). Parkin ubiquitinates the α-synuclein-interacting protein, synphilin-1: implications for Lewy-body formation in Parkinson disease. *Nat Med* 7:1144–1150.

75. Jeon GS, et al. (2014). Potential effect of S-nitrosylated protein disulfide isomerase on mutant SOD1 aggregation and neuronal cell death in amyotrophic lateral sclerosis. *Mol Neurobiol* 49:796–807.

76. Walker AK, et al. (2010). Protein disulphide isomerase protects against protein aggregation and is S-nitrosylated in amyotrophic lateral sclerosis. *Brain* 133:105–116.

77. Chen X, et al. (2012). SOD1 aggregation in astrocytes following ischemia/reperfusion injury: a role of NO-mediated S-nitrosylation of protein disulfide isomerase (PDI). *J Neuroinflammation* 9:237.

78. Obukuro K, et al. (2013). Nitric oxide mediates selective degeneration of hypothalamic orexin neurons through dysfunction of protein disulfide isomerase. *J Neurosci* 33:12557–12568.

79. Mollapour M, Neckers L (2012). Post-translational modifications of Hsp90 and their contributions to chaperone regulation. *Biochim Biophys Acta* 1823:648–655.

80. Martinez-Ruiz A, et al. (2005). S-Nitrosylation of Hsp90 promotes the inhibition of its ATPase and endothelial nitric oxide synthase regulatory activities. *Proc Natl Acad Sci USA* 102:8525–8530.

81. Retzlaff M, et al. (2009). Hsp90 is regulated by a switch point in the C-terminal domain. *EMBO Rep* 10:1147–1153.

82. Qin Y, Dey A, Purayil HT, Daaka Y (2013). Maintenance of androgen receptor inactivation by S-nitrosylation. *Cancer Res* 73:6690–6699.

83. Marozkina NV, et al. (2010). Hsp 70/Hsp 90 organizing protein as a nitrosylation target in cystic fibrosis therapy. *Proc Natl Acad Sci USA* 107:11393–11398.

84. Meyer H, Bug M, Bremer S (2012). Emerging functions of the VCP/p97 AAA-ATPase in the ubiquitin system. *Nat Cell Biol* 14:117–123.

85. Kim NC, et al. (2013). VCP is essential for mitochondrial quality control by PINK1/Parkin and this function is impaired by VCP mutations. *Neuron* 78:65–80.

86. Astier J, et al. (2012). Nitric oxide inhibits the ATPase activity of the chaperone-like AAA+ ATPase CDC48, a target for S-nitrosylation in cryptogein signalling in tobacco cells. *Biochem J* 447:249–260.

87. Dall'Agnol M, Bernstein C, Bernstein H, Garewal H, Payne CM (2006). Identification of S-nitrosylated proteins after chronic exposure of colon epithelial cells to deoxycholate. *Proteomics* 6:1654–1662.

88. Meng F, et al. (2011). Oxidation of the cysteine-rich regions of parkin perturbs its E3 ligase activity and contributes to protein aggregation. *Mol Neurodegener* 6:34.

89. Ozawa K, et al. (2013). S-Nitrosylation regulates mitochondrial quality control via activation of parkin. *Scientific Rep* 3:2202.

90. Tsui AK, et al. (2011). Priming of hypoxia-inducible factor by neuronal nitric oxide synthase is essential for adaptive responses to severe anemia. *Proc Natl Acad Sci USA* 108:17544–17549.

91. Lee YI, et al. (2014). Protein microarray characterization of the S-nitrosoproteome. *Mol Cell Proteomics* 13:63–72.

92. Kapadia MR, Eng JW, Jiang Q, Stoyanovsky DA, Kibbe MR (2009). Nitric oxide regulates the 26S proteasome in vascular smooth muscle cells. *Nitric Oxide* 20:279–288.

93. Kwak YD, et al. (2010). NO signaling and S-nitrosylation regulate PTEN inhibition in neurodegeneration. *Mol Neurodegener* 5:49.

94. Numajiri N, et al. (2011). On-off system for PI3-kinase-Akt signaling through S-nitrosylation of phosphatase with sequence homology to tensin (PTEN). *Proc Nati Acad Sci USA* 108:10349–10354.

95. Kim S, Wing SS, Ponka P (2004). S-Nitrosylation of IRP2 regulates its stability via the ubiquitin-proteasome pathway. *Mol Cell Biol* 24:330–337.

96. Chanvorachote P, et al. (2006). Nitric oxide regulates cell sensitivity to cisplatin-induced apoptosis through S-nitrosylation and inhibition of Bcl-2 ubiquitination. *Cancer Res* 66:6353–6360.

97. Chanvorachote P, et al. (2005). Nitric oxide negatively regulates Fas CD95-induced apoptosis through inhibition of ubiquitin-proteasome-mediated degradation of FLICE inhibitory protein. *J Biol Chem* 280:42044–42050.

98. Sarkar S, et al. (2011). Complex inhibitory effects of nitric oxide on autophagy. *Mol Cell* 43:19–32.

99. Park HS, Huh SH, Kim MS, Lee SH, Choi EJ (2000). Nitric oxide negatively regulates c-Jun N-terminal kinase/stress-activated protein kinase by means of S-nitrosylation. *Proc Natl Acad Sci USA* 97:14382–14387.

100. Reynaert NL, et al. (2004). Nitric oxide represses inhibitory κB kinase through S-nitrosylation. *Proc Natl Acad Sci USA* 101:8945–8950.

101. Lopez-Rivera E, et al. (2014). Inducible nitric oxide synthase drives mTOR pathway activation and proliferation of human melanoma by reversible nitrosylation of TSC2. *Cancer Res* 74:1067–1078.

102. Tripathi DN, et al. (2013). Reactive nitrogen species regulate autophagy through ATM-AMPK-TSC2-mediated suppression of mTORC1. *Proc Natl Acad Sci USA* 110:E2950–2957.

103. Filomeni G, De Zio D, Cecconi F (2014). Oxidative stress and autophagy: the clash between damage and metabolic needs. *Cell Death Differ* 22:377–388.

104. Youle RJ van der Bliek AM (2012). Mitochondrial fission, fusion, and stress. *Science* 337: 1062–1065.

105. Lizama-Manibusan B, McLaughlin B (2013). Redox modification of proteins as essential mediators of CNS autophagy and mitophagy. *FEBS Lett* 587:2291–2298.

106. Li F, et al. (2007). Regulation of HIF-1α stability through S-nitrosylation. *Mol Cell* 26:63–74.

107. Cho H, Ahn DR, Park H, Yang EG (2007). Modulation of p300 binding by posttranslational modifications of the C-terminal activation domain of hypoxia-inducible factor-1α. *FEBS Lett* 581:1542–1548.

108. Sumbayev VV, Budde A, Zhou J, Brune B (2003). HIF-1α protein as a target for S-nitrosation. *FEBS Lett* 535:106–112.

109. Yasinska IM, Sumbayev VV (2003). S-Nitrosation of Cys-800 of HIF-1α protein activates its interaction with p300 and stimulates its transcriptional activity. *FEBS Lett* 549:105–109.

110. Yasukawa T, et al. (2005). S-Nitrosylation-dependent inactivation of Akt/protein kinase B in insulin resistance. *J Biol Chem* 280: 7511–7518.

111. Scherz-Shouval R, et al. (2007). Reactive oxygen species are essential for autophagy and specifically regulate the activity of Atg4. *EMBO J* 26:1749–1760.

112. Shinozaki S, et al. (2014). Inflammatory stimuli induce inhibitory S-nitrosylation of the deacetylase SIRT1 to increase acetylation and activation of p53 and p65. *Sci Signal* 7:ra106.

113. Ischiropoulos H, et al. (1992). Peroxynitrite-mediated tyrosine nitration catalyzed by superoxide dismutase. *Arch Biochem Biophysics* 298:431–437.

114. Franco MC, Estevez AG (2014). Tyrosine nitration as mediator of cell death. *Cell Mol Life Sci* 71:3939–3950.

115. Giasson BI, et al. (2000). Oxidative damage linked to neurodegeneration by selective α-synuclein nitration in synucleinopathy lesions. *Science* 290:985–989.

116. Souza JM, Giasson BI, Chen Q, Lee VM, Ischiropoulos H (2000). Dityrosine cross-linking promotes formation of stable α-synuclein polymers: implication of nitrative and oxidative stress in the pathogenesis of neurodegenerative synucleinopathies. *J Biol Chem* 275:18344–18349.

117. Kummer MP, et al. (2011). Nitration of tyrosine 10 critically enhances amyloid β aggregation and plaque formation. *Neuron* 71:833–844.

118. Horiguchi T, et al. (2003). Nitration of tau protein is linked to neurodegeneration in tauopathies. *Am J Pathol* 163:1021–1031.

119. Reyes JF, Fu Y, Vana L, Kanaan NM, Binder LI (2011). Tyrosine nitration within the proline-rich region of Tau in Alzheimer's disease. *Am J Pathol* 178:2275–2285.

120. Tao L, et al. (2006). Nitrative inactivation of thioredoxin-1 and its role in postischemic myocardial apoptosis. *Circulation* 114:1395–1402.

121. Franco MC, et al. (2013) Nitration of Hsp90 induces cell death. *Proc Natl Acad Sci USA* 110:E1102–1111.

3

Calcium Hypothesis of Neurodegeneration

The Case of Alzheimer's Disease and Huntington's Disease

DANIEL A. RYSKAMP, ELENA POPUGAEVA, AND ILYA BEZPROZVANNY

INTRODUCTION

Calcium (Ca^{2+}) signals orchestrate several neuronal functions including neurotransmission, signal transduction, synaptic plasticity, gene transcription, and energy production. Considering the vital importance of Ca^{2+} signals in the brain, it is not surprising that an extensive network of proteins tightly regulates Ca^{2+} fluxes spatially and temporally. Abnormalities in the function of Ca^{2+} handling proteins from polymorphisms, aging, injury, inflammation, oxidative stress, and so on, can evoke detrimental outcomes for neuronal function and survival. Despite distinct etiologies and symptoms, accumulating evidence implicates Ca^{2+} dysregulation as a common pathological feature of several neurodegenerative diseases, including Alzheimer's disease (AD), Huntington's disease (HD), Parkinson's disease (PD), spinocerebellar ataxia (SCA), and glaucoma. Understanding disease-specific mechanisms of Ca^{2+} dysregulation is therefore crucial to the treatment of neurodegenerative disorders. Accordingly, we review the current "Ca^{2+} hypothesis of neurodegeneration", focusing on AD and HD as examples to respectively illustrate concepts related to multifactorial versus monogenic neurodegenerative diseases.

The failure of treatments to prevent or delay neurodegenerative disease progression has fueled the search for key pathogenic mechanisms. As neuronal death represents the hallmark of neurodegenerative diseases, anti-apoptotic strategies have been developed in attempts to circumvent this endpoint. For example, deletion of the pro-apoptotic gene BAX in a mouse model of glaucoma preserves the neuron cell body, but fails to maintain other subcellular compartments required for vision (1). Because neuronal processes can be damaged separately from somata (2,3), keeping neurons alive or replacing them with neural stem cells might not be sufficient to restore neuronal

connectivity and functions. Although some neuronal functions might not require intricate wiring (4), others necessitate specific connections that last throughout life. Memories, for instance, are encoded and maintained by the strength of synaptic connections (5). Moreover, the far-reaching architecture of neuronal processes creates unique metabolic and technical challenges that make dendrites, axons, and synaptic elements susceptible to stressors related to aging and other factors contributing to disease. As inherently plastic structures, synaptic elements are highly prone to remodeling in disease. Synapse loss, often resulting from Ca^{2+} dysregulation, contributes to the initiation and progression of several neurodegenerative diseases (6–12). Therefore, we further focused this chapter on the role of synaptic Ca^{2+} dysregulation in neurodegenerative disease.

CALCIUM DYSREGULATION IN ALZHEIMER'S DISEASE

Alzheimer's disease (AD) is the most prevalent cause of elderly dementia. Advanced age represents the main risk factor for AD, but several polymorphisms (e.g., the APOE ε4 allele of apolipoprotein E) and life style factors can confer additional risk and rare mutations in genes encoding amyloid precursor protein (APP), presenilin 1 (PS1) and presenilin 2 (PS2) can cause familial AD (FAD) (13). Age-related changes in neurophysiology, risk alleles, and disease-causing mutations provide clues about the pathogenesis of AD, leading to several hypotheses about AD initiation and progression. As aging and several FAD mutations perturb Ca^{2+} signaling (14), which is widely implicated in synaptic instability and neuronal apoptosis (15), we focus here on the role of Ca^{2+} dysregulation in AD.

The Ca^{2+} hypothesis of AD was initially proposed by Zaven S. Khachaturian in the 1980s based on accumulating evidence associating age-related changes in neurons with alterations in Ca^{2+} homeostasis as well as evidence indicating that excessive NMDA receptor activity causes neuronal excitotoxicity (16,17). Since then, extensive research efforts have aimed to elucidate how Ca^{2+} signaling is dysregulated in AD. Abnormal Ca^{2+} signaling was observed in fibroblasts from patients with FAD, hinting at systemic alterations in cellular Ca^{2+} handling in FAD (18). More specifically, Ca^{2+} release from the endoplasmic reticulum was substantially enhanced (18). This phenomenon was recapitulated in a variety of AD models (19–24), but the mechanistic explanation for enhanced Ca^{2+} release in AD-afflicted neurons is under debate.

Growing evidence suggests that FAD-causing mutations in presenilins cause aberrant Ca^{2+} signaling. How do these mutations dysregulate neuronal Ca^{2+} homeostasis? Presenilins, together with nicastrin, APH-1, and PEN-2, form the γ-secretase complex. This protease complex is transported to the cell surface and endosomes, where it cleaves several substrates, including APP. Some FAD-causing mutations in APP or presenilins can alter the proteolytic cleavage of APP by γ-secretase, favoring higher levels of toxic Aβ42 peptides relative to nonpathogenic or neuroprotective Aβ40 peptides (25). An increased Aβ 42/Aβ40 ratio leads to formation of amyloid β (Aβ) oligomers and plaques, which are considered major driving factors of neuronal dysfunction and damage in AD (25). Therefore, the γ-secretase inhibitor semagacestat was very attractive as a potential AD therapeutic and advanced to clinical trials (26). However, this trial failed in phase III. Semagacestat-treated AD patients had significantly worsened functional ability, and they had higher incidents of cancer, infections, and inflammation in comparison to placebo-treated patients (26). This trial may have failed because APP is not the only substrate for γ-secretase (γ-secretase also cleaves Notch protein) and the γ-secretase has four variants (27) that probably have different substrate preferences (28). Prolonged inhibition of Notch signaling likely caused the main side effects (gastrointestinal problems, infection, and skin cancer) observed in semagacestat-treated patients (29).

Presenilins are cleaved after synthesis before functioning within the γ-secretase complex (30). We discovered that presenilin holoproteins have a unique function that is unrelated to the γ-secretase complex. We demonstrated that presenilins form passive, low-conductance endoplasmic

reticulum (ER) Ca^{2+} leak channels (31,32). Some but not all FAD-associated mutations in presenilins disrupt this function, leading to overfilling of the ER with Ca^{2+} (31–34). This increases the driving force for Ca^{2+} release, augmenting signals from other ER Ca^{2+} releasing channels, such as $InsP_3R1$ and RyanRs, which have also been implicated in the pathogenesis of AD. The "leak channel hypothesis" of presenilin function was initially received with skepticism (35), but was recently validated in independent studies (36,37). Mutant presenilins may also act by modulating the activity of $InsP_3R1$ (38), although this result most likely is due to changes in $InsP_3R1$ gating in response to elevated ER Ca^{2+} levels. Consistent with effects of presenilin mutations on ER Ca^{2+} levels, genetic reduction of $InsP_3R1$ expression by 50% normalizes ryanodine receptor function, CREB-dependent gene expression and hippocampal long-term potentiation (LTP) in PS1-M146V-KI mice (39). Increased expression of RyanR has been observed in FAD models and AD patients (34,40–43). Consequently, it has been proposed that upregulation of RyanRs at early stages of AD may be a compensatory mechanism for early Ca^{2+} dysregulation and synaptic failure (44). A number of studies administered dantrolene, an RyanR antagonist, to mouse models of AD and observed therapeutic effects (44–46). However, another study reported that long-term oral feeding of dantrolene induced plaque formation and resulted in loss of hippocampal synaptic markers (34). As dantrolene blocks RyanR1 (skeletal muscle expression), but not RyanR2 and RyanR3 (main isoforms in the brain) (47), we examined the importance of RyanR3 in the context of AD using knockout mice. We found that RyanR3 plays a protective role at early stages of AD pathology, but becomes detrimental at late stages of pathology (48). These results suggested that RyanR3 inhibitors are likely to be therapeutically useful at late stages, but not at early stages of the disease.

It is widely accepted that memory loss in AD results from synaptic failure (10,49–54). Mushroom spines are stable dendritic spines that form strong synapses and are therefore believed to be involved in memory storage (55). It was proposed that hippocampal neuron mushroom spines are preferentially eliminated in AD, causing cognitive decline (50,51,56). However, the biological mechanisms responsible for loss of mushroom spines in AD are poorly understood.

Upon stimulation, N-Methyl-D-aspartic acid receptors (NMDARs), α-amino-3-hydroxy-5-methyl-4-isoxazolepropionic acid receptors

(AMPARs), and voltage-gated Ca²⁺ channels (VGCCs) in postsynaptic compartments provide fast, pronounced Ca²⁺ signals subserving neurotransmission; however, mushroom spines appear to require additional Ca²⁺ signals for stability. Our laboratory recently uncovered a novel signaling pathway regulating the stability of mushroom spines (57). We observed that the M146V FAD mutation in PS1 causes ER Ca²⁺ overload from disruption of the ER Ca²⁺ leak function (31,32), thereby suppressing neuronal store-operated Ca²⁺ influx (nSOC) in spines (57). This results in a compensatory downregulation of the ER Ca²⁺ sensor/nSOC channel activator STIM2 as well as the loss of mushroom spines (Figure 3.1). STIM2 downregulation was also observed in the cortex of AD patients and this correlated with their MMSE scores (57). Overexpression of STIM2 rescued spine nSOC in hippocampal neurons from PS1-M146V-KI mice and prevented loss of mushroom spines *in vitro* and *in vivo*, whereas conditional deletion of STIM2 was sufficient to destabilize mushroom spines in WT hippocampal neurons *in vitro* and *in vivo* (57). Thus, STIM2-dependent Ca²⁺ entry via nSOC channels supports hippocampal mushroom spine stability through driving activity of Ca²⁺ effectors (Figure 3.1).

Ca²⁺/calmodulin-dependent protein kinase II (CaMKII) is a so-called memory molecule. Its activity is associated with the induction of LTP and it is highly expressed in dendritic spines (58). Sun et al. (57) observed that age-dependent decreases in CaMKII phosphorylation were prevented by STIM2 overexpression, whereas inhibition of nSOC decreased CaMKII phosphorylation. Thus, elevated ER Ca²⁺ levels and downregulation of nSOC may lead to reduced phosphorylation of CaMKII. This all coincides with other age-dependent changes in several Ca²⁺ handling proteins and their effectors. Aging precipitates increased ER Ca²⁺ release via InsP₃Rs and RyanRs, Ca²⁺ influx via VGCCs, and activation of Ca²⁺-dependent K⁺ channels as well as decreased Ca²⁺ buffering (59). This may lead to activation of the Ca²⁺-dependent calpain proteases that degrade signaling enzymes involved in learning and memory (60,61) and calcineurin (CaN), which is enhanced in aging neurons and plays an important role in LTD (62,63). Changes in synaptic strength and connectivity during aging and AD may ultimately depend on the "phosphorylation tone" of postsynaptic proteins set by the balance of CaMKII and CaN activity (64).

The amyloid hypothesis of AD posits that accumulation and aggregation of Aβ peptides and plaques drives neurotoxicity in AD. There is an abundance of evidence that soluble Aβ oligomers dysregulate Ca²⁺ and neuronal excitability (15,65). For example, *in vivo* Ca²⁺ imaging with Tg2567 mice revealed elevated cytosolic Ca²⁺ levels in neurites and spines directly apposed to Aβ plaques (66). Although the PS1-M146V-KI mice do not express human Aβ and do not mimic conditions of Aβ toxicity, the recently developed APP-KI mice serve as an amyloidogenic model of AD without artifacts associated with overexpression (67). Zhang et al. (68) examined the APP-KI mouse model and observed suppression of spine

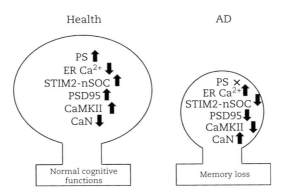

FIGURE 3.1. Ca²⁺ signaling and stability of postsynaptic mushroom spines in healthy neurons and in AD. In healthy neurons the STIM2-nSOC-CaMKII signaling pathway is functional and maintains the stability of mushroom spines, supporting normal cognitive functions of the brain. In FAD-afflicted neurons, the leak function of presenilins (PS) is disrupted, causing ER Ca²⁺ overload, downregulation of STIM2 protein expression, impaired nSOC influx, reduced CaMKII activity and increased CaN activity. Together, this causes elimination of mushroom spines and may underlie memory loss in AD.

nSOC, CaMKII hypophosphorylation, and loss of mushroom spines *in vitro* and *in vivo*. Similar to PS1-M146V-KI mice (57), STIM2 was downregulated in hippocampal cultures from APP-KI mice (68). In addition, Popugaeva et al. (69) applied Aβ42 oligomers to hippocampal cultures or injected them into the hippocampus of living mice and observed spine nSOC impairment, STIM2 downregulation, CaMKII hypophosphorylation, and mushroom spine loss. Interestingly, both studies demonstrated that STIM2 overexpression counteracts the effects of Aβ toxicity on spine nSOC levels, CaMKII activity, and mushroom spine stability. Thus, the STIM2-nSOC-CaMKII pathway constitutes an attractive target for potentially mitigating memory loss in AD.

As a multi-factorial disease, several pathways contribute to the pathogenesis and progression of AD and there is extensive synergy among them. Thus, it is important to consider the major hypotheses about AD as not mutually-exclusive; rather, the pathological cascades create a cacophonous symphony involving numerous interactions between Aβ42 toxicity, Ca^{2+} dysregulation, mitochondrial dysfunction, oxidative stress, glial reactivity, inflammation, tau hyperphosphorylation, and neurofibrillary tangles. Many of these interactions are bi-directional. For example, mutations in tau causing tangles promote Ca^{2+} influx via VGCCs (70). Conversely, excessive Ca^{2+} signals can lead to tau hyperphosphorylation and neurofibrillary tangles (71). Further complications arise from feedback loops that may also need to be broken to slow disease progression. For example, progressive physical restructuring of the brain from glial reactivity, synaptic remodeling, neuronal atrophy, and osmotic pressure may stimulate mechanosensitive ion channels that further contribute to excitotoxicity (72–75). Identification of a single node for therapeutic control of the entire pathogenic network of AD remains a daunting task; yet, accumulating preclinical evidence suggests that normalization of Ca^{2+} signaling may be sufficient to stabilize synaptic connections and prevent excitotoxicity. This approach could be complemented by other therapies that enhance cognitive function, bolster synaptic connections and reduce plaque load (76) to ensure the prevention of memory impairment.

CALCIUM DYSREGULATION IN HUNTINGTON'S DISEASE

Huntington's disease (HD) is an autosomal dominant neurodegenerative disorder characterized by motor, behavioral, and cognitive abnormalities that worsen until death, approximately 20 years following diagnosis (78). HD is caused by expansion of a CAG repeat tract in the N-terminal region of the huntingtin gene, encoding mutant Huntingtin (mHtt) protein with an expanded polyglutamine (polyQ) tract (>35 Qs) (80). Symptom onset is generally around 40 years of age, but varies due to the number of CAG repeats, environmental factors, and genetic modifiers (81,82). HD management is limited to symptomatic treatments and supportive care (83) because development of disease-modifying treatments requires a better understanding of early pathogenic events.

Atrophy of the striatum is the most pronounced neuropathological feature of HD (84). Synaptic dysfunction occurs early in HD patients (85–89) and animal models of HD (90–92), preceding overt neurodegeneration. More specifically, emerging evidence suggests that corticostriatal synaptic dysfunction and degradation precedes striatal neuron death and causes early HD symptoms (93–98). Dendritic spines in striatal medium spiny neurons (MSNs), the primary cell type affected in HD (96), start to weaken and disappear by 5 weeks in Q175 HD mice (99). Deletion of mHtt in both cortical and striatal neurons of BACHD mice completely rescues the HD phenotype (100), hinting at the importance of cell-cell interactions. Changes in cortical neuron activity may influence dendritic spine loss in striatal medium spiny neurons (MSNs) (101,102). Knowledge such as this hones the search for disease origins, but the mechanisms by which mHtt causes synaptic instability remain unclear.

Normal Htt preferentially localizes to pre- and postsynaptic elements of excitatory synapses. Htt associates with synaptic vesicles, promotes neurotransmitter release (103,104) and interacts with the postsynaptic scaffolding protein PSD95 (105,106). mHtt is generally thought to damage neurons through a toxic gain-of-function (107); however, loss of normal Htt functions, including apoptosis suppression (108) and synapse maturation (99), could also contribute to HD.

The toxic effects of mHtt expression in MSNs have motivated extensive research on therapeutic strategies aiming to knockdown mHtt. Some of the approaches do not discriminate between mHtt and normal Htt, which may fail to restore brain health (99). Although future innovations may lead to effective strategies for selectively targeting mHtt expression, optimal treatments will likely include therapeutic backups that counteract any potential toxicity from residual mHtt. The technical obstacles impeding HD cures warrant additional research on the toxic effects of mHtt.

Accumulating evidence suggests that mHtt induces synaptic dysfunction through interactions with cellular homeostatic and Ca^{2+} signaling mechanisms (93,94,96,109). Age-related failures of synaptic maintenance mechanisms may account for the onset of synaptic vulnerability and synergistically contribute to damage from the toxic insults related to mHtt expression (12). Extensive research has evaluated excitotoxicity and excessive Ca^{2+} signals as a trigger of MSN dendritic spine loss. Several Ca^{2+}-dependent enzymes and transcription factors are dysregulated in HD. For example, calpain activity is enhanced in the striatum of brains from HD patients and presymptomatic YAC128 HD mice (110–112). Excessive calpain function exacerbates striatal degeneration, possibly by degrading mHtt into more toxic fragments and/or activating pro-apoptotic cascades (113,114). Likewise, p38 MAPK is elevated in the striatum of YAC128 mice and may contribute to excitotoxicity (115). An HD model with limited MSN excitotoxicity features enhanced Ca^{2+} buffering with age, possibly accounting for its phenotypic resilience (116). A prominent mechanism by which mHtt dysregulated Ca^{2+} homeostasis is through direct and/ or indirect modulation of ion channel activity. Research on synaptotoxicity in HD has primarily focused on postsynaptic NMDAR, AMPAR, and VGCCs on the plasma membrane (117–121), whereas the role of endoplasmic reticulum (ER) Ca^{2+} stores remains largely uncharted. NMDA receptors may contribute to MSN excitotoxicity (94,121), with a potentially pathological role for extrasynaptic GluN2B (122). As NMDA currents require depolarization to remove the Mg^{2+} block, what mechanism of cation flux drives abnormal plasma membrane depolarization?

mHtt binds to the carboxy-terminal region of $InsP_3R1$, sensitizing it to $InsP_3$ (123) (Figure 3.2). The association of mHtt with $InsP_3R1$ was independently confirmed in an unbiased screen (124). Supranormal activity of $InsP_3R1$ contributes to mHtt-induced excitotoxicity of MSNs (109,124–127). Specifically disrupting the interaction between mHtt and $InsP_3R1$ with a peptide fragment of $InsP_3R1$ protects MSNs *in vitro* and *in vivo*, improving motor performance (128). polyQ-expanded ataxin 3 and ataxin 2 proteins also associate with the carboxy-terminal region of $InsP_3R1$ and increase its sensitivity to activation by $InsP_3$ (129–131). These results and others (132) support the "Ca^{2+} hypothesis of polyQ-expansion disorders" (109,127,133,134), assigning a key pathogenic role to $InsP_3R1$ hyperactivity. $InsP_3R1$ sensitization by mHtt tonically depletes ER Ca^{2+} and thereby increases neuronal store-operated Ca^{2+} (nSOC) entry in MSNs. In a

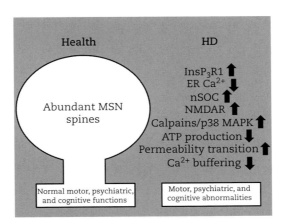

FIGURE 3.2. Ca^{2+} signaling and MSN spine loss in HD. Dendritic spines are abundant on MSNs under homeostatic conditions. However, mHtt directly sensitizes $InsP_3R1$, depleting ER Ca^{2+} and activating excessive STIM2-dependent nSOC. This presumably depolarizes MSNs and synergistically enhances cytosolic Ca^{2+} signals via NDMARs and VGCCs. Excessive Ca^{2+} signals drive abnormal activity of Ca^{2+} effectors such as calpains and p38 MAPK. Mitochondria become liable to depolarization, reduced ATP production, Ca^{2+} overloading and permeability transition pore opening. This and age-dependent reductions in the expression of Ca^{2+} buffering proteins further contributes to MSN vulnerability. These events culminate in early synapse dysfunction and loss, leading to clinical HD symptoms and progressive neurodegeneration.

phenotypic screen, we identified a class of quinazoline-derived compounds (e.g., EVP4593) that both delay the progression of motor symptoms in transgenic *Drosophila* HD flies and inhibit nSOC in mHtt-expressing neurons (135). Wu et al. (136) found that nSOC was preferentially enhanced by mHtt in MSN spines in corticostriatal co-cultures prepared from YAC128 HD mice. Either knockdown of InsP$_3$R1 or treatment with EVP4593 suppressed supranormal spine nSOC and prevented age-dependent loss of YAC128 MSN spines (136). STIM2 was upregulated in striatal lysates from YAC128 mice (136). STIM2 knockdown suppressed spine nSOC and prevented loss of YAC128 MSN spines, whereas STIM2 overexpression destabilized WT MSN spines (136). Intraventricular perfusion of EVP4593 over two months in aged YAC128 mice prevented MSN spine loss *in vivo* (136). These data indicate that InsP$_3$R1 hyperactivity elevates STIM2-dependent spine nSOC to synaptotoxic levels. This pathway represents an important lead for therapeutic development; however, the therapeutic window of nSOC inhibitors may be narrow due to their effects in other neurons. For example, nSOC suppression in hippocampal neurons causes mushroom spine loss. This necessitates the development of compounds that selectively modulate nSOC in specific populations of neurons to widen the therapeutic window.

In addition to driving excessive nSOC, supranormal InsP$_3$R1 activity at mitochondrial-associated membranes may disrupt cellular bioenergetics and/or open permeability transition pores. Energy production by mitochondria is important for synaptic function and maintenance (137). Like Ca^{2+} dysregulation, mitochondrial impairments are ubiquitous in neurodegenerative diseases (138). However, it is generally unclear whether mitochondria dysfunction is an early pathogenic event or secondary to other incidents such as Ca^{2+} dysregulation. In HD, striatal mitochondria preferentially exhibit impaired ATP production, abnormal Ca2+ handling, and increased susceptibility to permeability transition pore opening (139–141), an event that precipitates cellular demise. It is not clear how mitochondria become depolarized and reduce ATP production in the presence of mHtt, but it could involve Ca^{2+} overloading, oxidative stress, and/or impaired import of cytosolic proteins (127,142,143). Regardless of how mitochondria are impaired in HD, stabilization of these organelles remains important for buffering released Ca^{2+} and generating energy for synaptic activity.

Even though HD is a monogenic disease, several Ca^{2+}-handling proteins and organelles are directly and indirectly affected by mHtt. Secondary effects such as mitochondrial overloading could reflect common events in several neurodegenerative disorders, whereas other changes in Ca^{2+} regulation, such as sensitization of InsP$_3$R1 could be specific to polyglutamine expansion disorders. High-throughput *in vivo* testing with disease models (144) could accelerate the search for meaningful neuroprotective strategies that address the major complications in neurodegenerative disorders.

CONCLUSIONS

Despite extensive research, neurodegenerative diseases including AD, HD, PD, ALS, and SCA continue to pose colossal medical and societal problems. Treatments focus on symptoms and supportive care, whereas disease-modifying treatments and cures remain elusive because pathogenic mechanisms are poorly understood. Progress toward therapies largely stems from the identification of disease-causing mutations. This applies not only to monogenic diseases such as HD and SCAs, but to familial forms of AD, PD, and ALS. These discoveries have enabled the development of genetic disease models, providing a pathway to finding major causes of neurodegenerative diseases. Among pathogenic mechanisms, Ca^{2+} dysregulation has consistently emerged as a leading cause of early synapse loss and long-term neuronal damage. Ca^{2+} signaling pathways are dysregulated prior to the onset of symptoms in AD, HD, and other neurodegenerative diseases, contributing to disease initiation and progression (72,110–112,115,121,127,135,145,146). Albeit to a lesser degree, Ca^{2+} regulation may be similarly impaired by normal aging. Stabilization of Ca^{2+} regulation may therefore serve as an alternative and/or complementary therapeutic strategy to approaches that mitigate disease-specific ailments, such as Aβ accumulation in AD or mHtt expression in HD. Recent failures of trials inhibiting γ-secretase and the current technical challenges associated with suppression of mHtt expression have made the stabilization of Ca^{2+} homeostasis an appealing objective. This may be more easily achieved because many Ca^{2+} handling proteins, including ion channels, are druggable and the Ca^{2+} regulation network can be adjusted at several nodes. Thus, the elucidation of disease-specific malfunctions in Ca^{2+}-handling, as well as relevant targets to restore Ca^{2+} homeostasis, provides a diverse array of potential therapeutic options for treating neurodegenerative diseases. A better understanding of pathogenic Ca^{2+} signals may lead both to better biomarkers of early disease and to disease-modifying therapeutics.

OPEN QUESTIONS

- Does the STIM2-CaMKII-nSOC pathway regulate dendritic spine functions in other NDDs?
- What is the molecular identity of nSOC channels that regulates the stability of mushroom spines in AD?
- Are there specific enhancers of the STIM2-nSOC pathway?
- If there are effective modulators/activators of the STIM2-CaMKII-nSOC pathway, at what stage of AD should they be applied?
- How do changes in synaptic terminals relate to changes in dendritic spines and vice versa?
- Of the several reported mHtt-interacting proteins, which interactions directly affect function through mHtt binding?
- Which mechanisms of Ca^{2+} dysregulation extrapolate from somata to synaptic elements?
- What makes MSNs vulnerable to mHtt expression and other neurons resilient?
- Do specific Ca^{2+} signals and/or Ca^{2+} effectors account for selective vulnerability of specific neurons and circuits in NDDs?

DISCLOSURES

IB is a paid consultant to Ataxion and TEVA in the field of neurodegeneration. The other authors have no financial interests related to this work.

ACKNOWLEDGMENTS

We thank Leah Taylor and Polina Plotnikova for administrative assistance. IB is a holder of the Carl J. and Hortense M. Thomsen Chair in Alzheimer's Disease Research. This work was supported by the Dynasty Foundation grant DP–B–49/15 (EP), NIH grants R01NS056224 (IB), R01NS074376 (IB), R01NS080152 (IB), F32NS093786 (DR), and by the Russian Scientific Fund grant 14–25-00024 (IB, Alzheimer disease section).

REFERENCES

1. Libby, R. T., Li, Y., Savinova, O. V., Barter, J., Smith, R. S., Nickells, R. W., and John, S. W. (2005). Susceptibility to neurodegeneration in a glaucoma is modified by Bax gene dosage. *PLoS Genetics* **1**, e4.

2. Stevens, B., Allen, N. J., Vazquez, L. E., Howell, G. R., Christopherson, K. S., Nouri, N., Micheva, K. D., Mehalow, A. K., Huberman, A. D., and Stafford, B. (2007). The classical complement cascade mediates CNS synapse elimination. *Cell* **131**, 1164–1178.

3. Howell, G. R., Libby, R. T., Jakobs, T. C., Smith, R. S., Phalan, F. C., Barter, J. W., Barbay, J. M., Marchant, J. K., Mahesh, N., and Porciatti, V. (2007). Axons of retinal ganglion cells are insulted in the optic nerve early in DBA/2J glaucoma. *J Cell Biol* **179**, 1523–1537.

4. Baraban, S. C., Southwell, D. G., Estrada, R. C., Jones, D. L., Sebe, J. Y., Alfaro-Cervello, C., García-Verdugo, J. M., Rubenstein, J. L., and Alvarez-Buylla, A. (2009). Reduction of seizures by transplantation of cortical GABAergic interneuron precursors into Kv1. 1 mutant mice. *Proc Natl Acad Sci U S A* **106**, 15472–15477.

5. Yang, G., Pan, F., and Gan, W.-B. (2009). Stably maintained dendritic spines are associated with lifelong memories. *Nature* **462**, 920–924.

6. Spires, T. L., and Hyman, B. T. (2004). Neuronal structure is altered by amyloid plaques. *Rev Neurosci* **15**, 267–278.

7. Zaja-Milatovic, S., Milatovic, D., Schantz, A., Zhang, J., Montine, K., Samii, A., Deutch, A., and Montine, T. (2005). Dendritic degeneration in neostriatal medium spiny neurons in Parkinson disease. *Neurology* **64**, 545–547.

8. Zang, D. W., Lopes, E. C., and Cheema, S. S. (2005). Loss of synaptophysin-positive boutons on lumbar motor neurons innervating the medial gastrocnemius muscle of the SOD1G93A G1H transgenic mouse model of ALS. *J. Neurosci. Res.* **79**, 694–699.

9. Day, M., Wang, Z., Ding, J., An, X., Ingham, C. A., Shering, A. F., Wokosin, D., Ilijic, E., Sun, Z., and Sampson, A. R. (2006). Selective elimination of glutamatergic synapses on striatopallidal neurons in Parkinson disease models. *Nat. Neurosci.* **9**, 251–259.

10. Knobloch, M., and Mansuy, I. M. (2008). Dendritic spine loss and synaptic alterations in Alzheimer's disease. *Mol. Neurobiol.* **37**, 73–82.

11. Gillingwater, T., and Wishart, T. (2013). Mechanisms underlying synaptic vulnerability and degeneration in neurodegenerative disease. *Neuropathol Appl Neurobiol* **39**, 320–334.

12. Bezprozvanny, I., and Hiesinger, P. R. (2013). The synaptic maintenance problem: membrane recycling, Ca2+ homeostasis and late onset degeneration. *Mol Neurodegener* **8**, 23.

13. Gandy, S., and DeKosky, S. T. (2013). Toward the treatment and prevention of Alzheimer's disease: rational strategies and recent progress. *Annual Rev Med* **64**, 367.

14. Nelson, O., Tu, H., Lei, T., Bentahir, M., de Strooper, B., and Bezprozvanny, I. (2007). Familial Alzheimer disease-linked mutations specifically disrupt Ca2+ leak function of presenilin 1. *J Clin Invest* **117**, 1230–1239.

15. Bezprozvanny, I., and Mattson, M. P. (2008). Neuronal calcium mishandling and the pathogenesis of Alzheimer's disease. *Trends Neurosci* **31**, 454–463.

16. Khachaturian, Z. S. (1987). Hypothesis on the regulation of cytosol calcium concentration and the aging brain. *Neurobiol Aging* **8**, 345–346.

17. Khachaturian, Z. S. (1989). The role of calcium regulation in brain aging: reexamination of a hypothesis. *Aging Clin Exp Res* **1**, 17–34.

18. Ito, E., Oka, K., Etcheberrigaray, R., Nelson, T. J., McPhie, D. L., Tofel-Grehl, B., Gibson, G. E., and Alkon, D. L. (1994). Internal Ca2+ mobilization is altered in fibroblasts from patients with Alzheimer disease. *Proc Natl Acad Sci U S A* **91**, 534–538.

19. Leissring, M. A., Paul, B. A., Parker, I., Cotman, C. W., and LaFerla, F. M. (1999). Alzheimer's presenilin-1 mutation potentiates inositol 1,4,5-trisphosphate-mediated calcium signaling in Xenopus oocytes. *J Neurochem* **72**, 1061–1068.

20. Chan, S. L., Mayne, M., Holden, C. P., Geiger, J. D., and Mattson, M. P. (2000). Presenilin-1 mutations increase levels of ryanodine receptors and calcium release in PC12 cells and cortical neurons. *J Biol Chem* **275**, 18195–18200.

21. Stutzmann, G. E., Caccamo, A., LaFerla, F. M., and Parker, I. (2004). Dysregulated IP3 signaling in cortical neurons of knock-in mice expressing an Alzheimer's-linked mutation in presenilin1 results in exaggerated Ca2+ signals and altered membrane excitability. *J Neurosci* **24**, 508–513.

22. Smith, I. F., Hitt, B., Green, K. N., Oddo, S., and LaFerla, F. M. (2005). Enhanced caffeine-induced Ca2+ release in the 3xTg-AD mouse model of Alzheimer's disease. *J Neurochem* **94**, 1711–1718.

23. Tu, H., Nelson, O., Bezprozvanny, A., Wang, Z., Lee, S. F., Hao, Y. H., Serneels, L., De Strooper, B., Yu, G., and Bezprozvanny, I. (2006). Presenilins form ER Ca2+ leak channels, a function disrupted by familial Alzheimer's disease-linked mutations. *Cell* **126**, 981–993.

24. Sarasija, S., and Norman, K. R. (2015). A γ-Secretase Independent Role for Presenilin in Calcium Homeostasis Impacts Mitochondrial Function and Morphology in Caenorhabditis elegans. *Genetics* **201**, 1453–1466.

25. Kumar-Singh, S., Theuns, J., Van Broeck, B., Pirici, D., Vennekens, K. l., Corsmit, E., Cruts, M., Dermaut, B., Wang, R., and Van Broeckhoven, C. (2006). Mean age-of-onset of familial alzheimer disease caused by presenilin mutations correlates with both increased Aβ42 and decreased Aβ40. *Human Mutation* **27**, 686–695.

26. Doody, R. S., Raman, R., Farlow, M., Iwatsubo, T., Vellas, B., Joffe, S., Kieburtz, K., He, F., Sun, X., and Thomas, R. G. (2013). A phase 3 trial of semagacestat for treatment of Alzheimer's disease. *N Engl J Med* **369**, 341–350.

27. De Strooper, B. (2003). Aph-1, Pen-2, and nicastrin with presenilin generate an active γ-secretase complex. *Neuron* **38**, 9–12.

28. De Strooper, B. (2014). Lessons from a failed γ-secretase Alzheimer trial. *Cell* **159**, 721–726.

29. Henley, D. B., Sundell, K. L., Sethuraman, G., Dowsett, S. A., and May, P. C. (2014). Safety profile of semagacestat, a gamma-secretase inhibitor: IDENTITY trial findings. *Curr Med Res Opin* **30**, 2021–2032.

30. Tandon, A., and Fraser, P. (2002). The presenilins. *Genome Biol* **3**, 1–11.

31. Tu, H., Nelson, O., Bezprozvanny, A., Wang, Z., Lee, S.-F., Hao, Y.-H., Serneels, L., De Strooper, B., Yu, G., and Bezprozvanny, I. (2006). Presenilins form ER Ca2+ leak channels, a function disrupted by familial Alzheimer's disease-linked mutations. *Cell* **126**, 981–993.

32. Nelson, O., Supnet, C., Tolia, A., Horre, K., De Strooper, B., and Bezprozvanny, I. (2011). Mutagenesis mapping of the presenilin 1 calcium leak conductance pore. *J Biol Chem* **286**, 22339–22347.

33. Nelson, O., Supnet, C., Liu, H., and Bezprozvanny, I. (2010). Familial Alzheimer's disease mutations in presenilins: effects on endoplasmic reticulum calcium homeostasis and correlation with clinical phenotypes. *J. Alzheimers Dis.* **21**, 781–793.

34. Zhang, H., Sun, S., Herreman, A., De Strooper, B., and Bezprozvanny, I. (2010). Role of presenilins in neuronal calcium homeostasis. *J Neurosci* **30**, 8566–8580.

35. Shilling, D., Mak, D. O., Kang, D. E., and Foskett, J. K. (2012). Lack of evidence for presenilins as endoplasmic reticulum Ca2+ leak channels. *J Biol Chem* **287**, 10933–10944.

36. Bandara, S., Malmersjo, S., and Meyer, T. (2013). Regulators of Calcium Homeostasis Identified by Inference of Kinetic Model Parameters from Live Single Cells Perturbed by siRNA. *Sci Signal* **6**, ra56.

37. Bezprozvanny, I. (2013). Presenilins and calcium signaling-systems biology to the rescue. *Sci Signal* **6**, pe24.

38. Cheung, K.-H., Shineman, D., Müller, M., Cardenas, C., Mei, L., Yang, J., Tomita, T., Iwatsubo, T., Lee,

V. M.-Y., and Foskett, J. K. (2008). Mechanism of Ca2+ disruption in Alzheimer's disease by presenilin regulation of InsP 3 receptor channel gating. *Neuron* **58**, 871–883.

39. Shilling, D., Müller, M., Takano, H., Mak, D.-O. D., Abel, T., Coulter, D. A., and Foskett, J. K. (2014). Suppression of InsP3 receptor-mediated Ca2+ signaling alleviates mutant presenilin-linked familial Alzheimer's disease pathogenesis. *J Neurosci* **34**, 6910–6923.

40. Kelliher, M., Fastbom, J., Cowburn, R., Bonkale, W., Ohm, T., Ravid, R., Sorrentino, V., and O'Neill, C. (1999). Alterations in the ryanodine receptor calcium release channel correlate with Alzheimer's disease neurofibrillary and β-amyloid pathologies. *Neuroscience* **92**, 499–513.

41. Bruno, A. M., Huang, J. Y., Bennett, D. A., Marr, R. A., Hastings, M. L., and Stutzmann, G. E. (2012). Altered ryanodine receptor expression in mild cognitive impairment and Alzheimer's disease. *Neurobiol. Aging* **33**, 1001-e1.

42. Stutzmann, G. E., Smith, I., Caccamo, A., Oddo, S., LaFerla, F. M., and Parker, I. (2006). Enhanced ryanodine receptor recruitment contributes to Ca2+ disruptions in young, adult, and aged Alzheimer's disease mice. *J Neurosci* **26**, 5180–5189.

43. Chakroborty, S., Goussakov, I., Miller, M. B., and Stutzmann, G. E. (2009). Deviant ryanodine receptor-mediated calcium release resets synaptic homeostasis in presymptomatic 3xTg-AD mice. *J Neurosci* **29**, 9458–9470.

44. Chakroborty, S., Briggs, C., Miller, M. B., Goussakov, I., Schneider, C., Kim, J., Wicks, J., Richardson, J. C., Conklin, V., and Cameransi, B. G. (2012). Stabilizing ER Ca2+ channel function as an early preventative strategy for Alzheimer's disease. *PLoS One* **7**, e52056.

45. Peng, J., Liang, G., Inan, S., Wu, Z., Joseph, D. J., Meng, Q., Peng, Y., Eckenhoff, M. F., and Wei, H. (2012). Dantrolene ameliorates cognitive decline and neuropathology in Alzheimer triple transgenic mice. *Neurosci Lett* **516**, 274–279.

46. Oulès, B., Del Prete, D., Greco, B., Zhang, X., Lauritzen, I., Sevalle, J., Moreno, S., Paterlini-Bréchot, P., Trebak, M., and Checler, F. (2012). Ryanodine receptor blockade reduces amyloid-β load and memory impairments in Tg2576 mouse model of Alzheimer disease. *J Neurosci* **32**, 11820–11834.

47. Krause, T., Gerbershagen, M., Fiege, M., Weisshorn, R., and Wappler, F. (2004). Dantrolene: a review of its pharmacology, therapeutic use and new developments. *Anaesthesia* **59**, 364–373.

48. Liu, J., Supnet, C., Sun, S., Zhang, H., Good, L., Popugaeva, E., and Bezprozvanny, I. (2014). The role of ryanodine receptor type 3 in a mouse model of Alzheimer disease. *Channels* **8**, 230–242.

49. Selkoe, D. J. (2002). Alzheimer's disease is a synaptic failure. *Science* **298**, 789–791.

50. Tackenberg, C., Ghori, A., and Brandt, R. (2009). Thin, stubby or mushroom: spine pathology in Alzheimer's disease. *Curr Alzheimer Res* **6**, 261–268.

51. Luebke, J. I., Weaver, C. M., Rocher, A. B., Rodriguez, A., Crimins, J. L., Dickstein, D. L., Wearne, S. L., and Hof, P. R. (2010). Dendritic vulnerability in neurodegenerative disease: insights from analyses of cortical pyramidal neurons in transgenic mouse models. *Brain Struct Funct* **214**, 181–199.

52. Koffie, R. M., Hyman, B. T., and Spires-Jones, T. L. (2011). Alzheimer's disease: synapses gone cold. *Mol Neurodegener* **6**, 63–63.

53. Penzes, P., Cahill, M. E., Jones, K. A., VanLeeuwen, J.-E., and Woolfrey, K. M. (2011). Dendritic spine pathology in neuropsychiatric disorders. *Nat Neurosci* **14**, 285–293.

54. Wilcox, K. C., Lacor, P. N., Pitt, J., and Klein, W. L. (2011). Aβ oligomer-induced synapse degeneration in Alzheimer's disease. *Cell Mol Neurobiol* **31**, 939–948.

55. Bourne, J., and Harris, K. M. (2007). Do thin spines learn to be mushroom spines that remember? *Curr Opin Neurobiol* **17**, 381–386.

56. Popugaeva, E., Supnet, C., and Bezprozvanny, I. (2012). Presenilins, deranged calcium homeostasis, synaptic loss and dysfunction in Alzheimer's disease. *Messenger* **1**, 53–62.

57. Sun, S., Zhang, H., Liu, J., Popugaeva, E., Xu, N.-J., Feske, S., White, C. L., and Bezprozvanny, I. (2014). Reduced synaptic STIM2 expression and impaired store-operated calcium entry cause destabilization of mature spines in mutant presenilin mice. *Neuron* **82**, 79–93.

58. Lisman, J., Schulman, H., and Cline, H. (2002). The molecular basis of CaMKII function in synaptic and behavioural memory. *Nat Rev Neurosci* **3**, 175–190.

59. Bezprozvanny, I. (2009). Calcium signaling and neurodegenerative diseases. *Trends Mol Med* **15**, 89–100.

60. Vosler, P. S., Brennan, C. S., and Chen, J. (2008). Calpain-mediated signaling mechanisms in neuronal injury and neurodegeneration. *Mol Neurobiol* **38**, 78–100.

61. Trinchese, F., Fa, M., Liu, S., Zhang, H., Hidalgo, A., Schmidt, S. D., Yamaguchi, H., Yoshii, N., Mathews, P. M., Nixon, R. A., and Arancio, O. (2008). Inhibition of calpains improves memory and synaptic transmission in a mouse model of Alzheimer disease. *J Clin Invest* **118**, 2796–2807.

62. Foster, T. C., Sharrow, K. M., Masse, J. R., Norris, C. M., and Kumar, A. (2001). Calcineurin links Ca2+ dysregulation with brain aging. *J Neurosci* **21**, 4066–4073.

63. Jouvenceau, A., and Dutar, P. (2006). A role for the protein phosphatase 2B in altered hippocampal synaptic plasticity in the aged rat. *J Physiol Paris* **99**, 154–161.

64. Bezprozvanny, I., and Hiesinger, P. R. (2013). The synaptic maintenance problem: membrane recycling, Ca2+ homeostasis and late onset degeneration. *Mol Neurodegener* **8**, 23.

65. Bezprozvanny, I. (2009). Amyloid goes global. *Sci Signal* **2**, pe16.

66. Kuchibhotla, K. V., Goldman, S. T., Lattarulo, C. R., Wu, H. Y., Hyman, B. T., and Bacskai, B. J. (2008). Abeta plaques lead to aberrant regulation of calcium homeostasis in vivo resulting in structural and functional disruption of neuronal networks. *Neuron* **59**, 214–225.

67. Saito, T., Matsuba, Y., Mihira, N., Takano, J., Nilsson, P., Itohara, S., Iwata, N., and Saido, T. C. (2014). Single App knock-in mouse models of Alzheimer's disease. *Nat Neurosci* **17**, 661–663.

68. Zhang, H., Wu, L., Pchitskaya, E., Zaharova, O., Saito, T. Saido, T., and Bezprozvanny, I (2015). Neuronal store-operated calcium entry and mushroom spine loss in amyloid precursor protein knock-in mouse model of alzheimer's disease. *J Neurosci* **35**, 13275–13286.

69. Popugaeva, E., Pchitskaya, E., Zhang, H., Vlasova, O., and Bezprozvanny, I. (2015). STIM2 protects mushroom spines from amyloid synaptotoxicity. *Mol Neurodeger* **10**, 1–13.

70. Furukawa, K., Wang, Y., Yao, P. J., Fu, W., Mattson, M. P., Itoyama, Y., Onodera, H., D'Souza, I., Poorkaj, P. H., and Bird, T. D. (2003). Alteration in calcium channel properties is responsible for the neurotoxic action of a familial frontotemporal dementia tau mutation. *J Neurochem* **87**, 427–436.

71. Mattson, M. P. (1990). Antigenic changes similar to those seen in neurofibrillary tangles are elicited by glutamate and Ca2+ influx in cultured hippocampal neurons. *Neuron* **4**, 105–117.

72. Krizaj, D., Ryskamp, D. A., Tian, N., Tezel, G., Mitchell, C. H., Slepak, V. Z., and Shestopalov, V. I. (2013). From mechanosensitivity to inflammatory responses: new players in the pathology of glaucoma. *Cur Eye Res* **39**, 105–119.

73. Jo, A. O., Ryskamp, D. A., Phuong, T. T., Verkman, A. S., Yarishkin, O., MacAulay, N., and Križaj, D. (2015). TRPV4 and AQP4 channels synergistically regulate cell volume and calcium homeostasis in retinal müller glia. *J Neurosci* **35**, 13525–13537.

74. Ryskamp, D. A., Jo, A. O., Frye, A. M., Vazquez-Chona, F., MacAulay, N., Thoreson, W. B., and Križaj, D. (2014). Swelling and eicosanoid metabolites differentially gate TRPV4 channels in retinal neurons and glia. *J Neurosci* **34**, 15689–15700.

75. Ryskamp, D. A., Iuso, A., and Križaj, D. (2015). TRPV4 links inflammatory signaling and neuroglial swelling. *Channels* **9**, 70–72.

76. Fisher, A., Bezprozvanny, I., Wu, L., Ryskamp, D. A., Bar-Ner, N., Natan, N., Brandeis, R., Elkon, H., Nahum, V., and Gershonov, E. (2015). AF710B, a novel M1/σ1 agonist with therapeutic efficacy in animal models of Alzheimer's disease. *Neurodegen Dis.* **16**, 95–110.

77. Mattson, M. P. (2004). Pathways towards and away from Alzheimer's disease. *Nature* **430**, 631–639.

78. Foroud, T., Gray, J., Ivashina, J., and Conneally, P. M. (1999). Differences in duration of Huntington's disease based on age at onset. *J Neurol Neurosurg Psychiatry* **66**, 52–56.

79. Roos, R., Hermans, J., Vegter-Van Der Vlis, M., Van Ommen, G., and Bruyn, G. (1993). Duration of illness in Huntington's disease is not related to age at onset. *J Neurol Neurosurg Psychiatry* **56**, 98–100.

80. MacDonald, M. E., Ambrose, C. M., Duyao, M. P., Myers, R. H., Lin, C., Srinidhi, L., Barnes, G., Taylor, S. A., James, M., and Groot, N. (1993). A novel gene containing a trinucleotide repeat that is expanded and unstable on Huntington's disease chromosomes. *Cell* **72**, 971–983.

81. Wexler, N. S. (2004). Venezuelan kindreds reveal that genetic and environmental factors modulate Huntington's disease age of onset. *Proc Natl Acad Sci U S A* **101**, 3498–3503.

82. Kim, M. (2014). Pathogenic polyglutamine expansion length correlates with polarity of the flanking sequences. *Mol Neurodegener* **9**, 45.

83. Dayalu, P., and Albin, R. L. (2015). Huntington disease: pathogenesis and treatment. *Neurol Clin* **33**, 101–114.

84. Vonsattel, J.-P., Myers, R. H., Stevens, T. J., Ferrante, R. J., Bird, E. D., and Richardson Jr, E. P. (1985). Neuropathological classification of Huntington's disease. *J Neuropathol Exp Neurol* **44**, 559–577.

85. Graveland, G., Williams, R., and DiFiglia, M. (1985). Evidence for degenerative and regenerative changes in neostriatal spiny neurons in Huntington's disease. *Science* **227**, 770–773.

86. Ferrante, R., Kowall, N., and Richardson, E. (1991). Proliferative and degenerative changes in striatal spiny neurons in Huntington's disease: a combined study using the section-Golgi

method and calbindin D28k immunocytochemistry. *J Neurosci* **11**, 3877–3887.

87. Sotrel, A., Williams, R., Kaufmann, W., and Myers, R. (1993). Evidence for neuronal degeneration and dendritic plasticity in cortical pyramidal neurons of Huntington's disease a quantitative Golgi study. *Neurology* **43**, 2088–2096.

88. Paulsen, J., Langbehn, D., Stout, J., Aylward, E., Ross, C., Nance, M., Guttman, M., Johnson, S., MacDonald, M., and Beglinger, L. (2008). Detection of Huntington's disease decades before diagnosis: the Predict-HD study. *J Neurol Neurosurg Psychiatry* **79**, 874–880.

89. Orth, M., Schippling, S., Schneider, S. A., Bhatia, K. P., Talelli, P., Tabrizi, S. J., and Rothwell, J. C. (2010). Abnormal motor cortex plasticity in premanifest and very early manifest Huntington disease. *J Neurol Neurosurg Psychiatry* **81**, 267–270.

90. Murphy, K. P., Carter, R. J., Lione, L. A., Mangiarini, L., Mahal, A., Bates, G. P., Dunnett, S. B., and Morton, A. J. (2000). Abnormal synaptic plasticity and impaired spatial cognition in mice transgenic for exon 1 of the human Huntington's disease mutation. *J Neurosci* **20**, 5115–5123.

91. Guidetti, P., Charles, V., Chen, E.-Y., Reddy, P. H., Kordower, J. H., Whetsell, W. O., Schwarcz, R., and Tagle, D. A. (2001). Early degenerative changes in transgenic mice expressing mutant huntingtin involve dendritic abnormalities but no impairment of mitochondrial energy production. *Exp Neurol* **169**, 340–350.

92. Murmu, R. P., Li, W., Holtmaat, A., and Li, J.-Y. (2013). Dendritic spine instability leads to progressive neocortical spine loss in a mouse model of Huntington's disease. *The J Neurosci* **33**, 12997–13009.

93. Miller, B. R., and Bezprozvanny, I. (2010). Corticostriatal circuit dysfunction in Huntington's disease: intersection of glutamate, dopamine and calcium. *Future Neurol* **5**, 735–756.

94. Milnerwood, A. J., and Raymond, L. A. (2010). Early synaptic pathophysiology in neurodegeneration: insights from Huntington's disease. *Trends Neurosci* **33**, 513–523.

95. Crook, Z. R., and Housman, D. (2011). Huntington's disease: can mice lead the way to treatment? *Neuron* **69**, 423–435.

96. Eidelberg, D., and Surmeier, D. J. (2011). Brain networks in Huntington disease. *J Clin Invest* **121**, 484–492.

97. Raymond, L. A., André, V. M., Cepeda, C., Gladding, C. M., Milnerwood, A. J., and Levine, M. S. (2011). Pathophysiology of Huntington's disease: time-dependent alterations in synaptic and receptor function. *Neuroscience* **198**, 252–273.

98. Unschuld, P. G., Edden, R. A., Carass, A., Liu, X., Shanahan, M., Wang, X., Oishi, K., Brandt, J., Bassett, S. S., and Redgrave, G. W. (2012). Brain metabolite alterations and cognitive dysfunction in early Huntington's disease. *Mov. Disord.* **27**, 895–902.

99. McKinstry, S. U., Karadeniz, Y. B., Worthington, A. K., Hayrapetyan, V. Y., Ozlu, M. I., Serafin-Molina, K., Risher, W. C., Ustunkaya, T., Dragatsis, I., and Zeitlin, S. (2014). Huntingtin is required for normal excitatory synapse development in cortical and striatal circuits. *J Neurosci* **34**, 9455–9472.

100. Wang, N., Gray, M., Lu, X.-H., Cantle, J. P., Holley, S. M., Greiner, E., Gu, X., Shirasaki, D., Cepeda, C., and Li, Y. (2014). Neuronal targets for reducing mutant huntingtin expression to ameliorate disease in a mouse model of Huntington's disease. *Nat Med* **20**, 536–541.

101. Cepeda, C., Cummings, D. M., Andre, V. M., Holley, S. M., and Levine, M. S. (2010). Genetic mouse models of Huntington's disease: focus on electrophysiological mechanisms. *ASN Neuro* **2**, e00033.

102. Artamonov, D., Korzhova, V., Wu, J., Rybalchenko, P., Im, K., Krasnoborova, V., Vlasova, O., and Bezprozvanny, I. (2013). Characterization of synaptic dysfunction in an in vitro corticostriatal model system of Huntington's disease. *Biochemistry (Moscow)* **7**, 192–202.

103. DiFiglia, M., Sapp, E., Chase, K., Schwarz, C., Meloni, A., Young, C., Martin, E., Vonsattel, J.-P., Carraway, R., and Reeves, S. A. (1995). Huntingtin is a cytoplasmic protein associated with vesicles in human and rat brain neurons. *Neuron* **14**, 1075–1081.

104. Rozas, J. L., Gómez-Sánchez, L., Tomás-Zapico, C., Lucas, J. J., and Fernández-Chacón, R. (2011). Increased neurotransmitter release at the neuromuscular junction in a mouse model of polyglutamine disease. *J Neurosci.* **31**, 1106–1113.

105. Sun, Y., Savanenin, A., Reddy, P. H., and Liu, Y. F. (2001). Polyglutamine-expanded huntingtin promotes sensitization of N-methyl-D-aspartate receptors via post-synaptic density 95. *J Biol Chem* **276**, 24713–24718.

106. Marcora, E., and Kennedy, M. B. (2010). The Huntington's disease mutation impairs Huntingtin's role in the transport of NF-κB from the synapse to the nucleus. *Hum Mol Genet* **19**, 4373–4384.

107. Davies, S. W., Turmaine, M., Cozens, B. A., DiFiglia, M., Sharp, A. H., Ross, C. A., Scherzinger, E., Wanker, E. E., Mangiarini, L., and Bates, G. P. (1997). Formation of neuronal

38   NEURODEGENERATIVE DISEASES

intranuclear inclusions underlies the neurological dysfunction in mice transgenic for the HD mutation. *Cell* **90**, 537–548.

108. Dragatsis, I., Levine, M. S., and Zeitlin, S. (2000). Inactivation of Hdh in the brain and testis results in progressive neurodegeneration and sterility in mice. *Nat Genet* **26**, 300–306.

109. Bezprozvanny, I. (2011). Role of inositol 1, 4, 5-trishosphate receptors in pathogenesis of Huntington's disease and spinocerebellar ataxias. *Neurochem. Res.* **36**, 1186–1197.

110. Cowan, C. M., Fan, M. M., Fan, J., Shehadeh, J., Zhang, L. Y., Graham, R. K., Hayden, M. R., and Raymond, L. A. (2008). Polyglutamine-modulated striatal calpain activity in YAC transgenic huntington disease mouse model: impact on NMDA receptor function and toxicity. *J Neurosci* **28**, 12725–12735.

111. Gafni, J., and Ellerby, L. M. (2002). Calpain activation in Huntington's disease. *J Neurosci* **22**, 4842–4849.

112. Gladding, C. M., Sepers, M. D., Xu, J., Zhang, L. Y., Milnerwood, A. J., Lombroso, P. J., and Raymond, L. A. (2012). Calpain and STriatal-Enriched protein tyrosine phosphatase (STEP) activation contribute to extrasynaptic NMDA receptor localization in a Huntington's disease mouse model. *Hum Mol Genet* **21**, 3739–3752.

113. Kim, Y. J., Yi, Y., Sapp, E., Wang, Y., Cuiffo, B., Kegel, K. B., Qin, Z.-H., Aronin, N., and DiFiglia, M. (2001). Caspase 3-cleaved N-terminal fragments of wild-type and mutant huntingtin are present in normal and Huntington's disease brains, associate with membranes, and undergo calpain-dependent proteolysis. *Proc Natl Acad Sci U S A* **98**, 12784–12789.

114. Gafni, J., Hermel, E., Young, J. E., Wellington, C. L., Hayden, M. R., and Ellerby, L. M. (2004). Inhibition of calpain cleavage of huntingtin reduces toxicity accumulation of calpain/caspase fragments in the nucleus. *J Biol Chem* **279**, 20211–20220.

115. Fan, J., Gladding, C. M., Wang, L., Zhang, L. Y., Kaufman, A. M., Milnerwood, A. J., and Raymond, L. A. (2012) P38 MAPK is involved in enhanced NMDA receptor-dependent excitotoxicity in YAC transgenic mouse model of Huntington disease. *Neurobiol Dis* **45**, 999–1009.

116. Hansson, O., Guatteo, E., Mercuri, N. B., Bernardi, G., Li, X. J., Castilho, R. F., and Brundin, P. (2001). Resistance to NMDA toxicity correlates with appearance of nuclear inclusions, behavioural deficits and changes in calcium homeostasis in mice transgenic for exon 1 of the huntington gene. *Eur J Neurosci* **14**, 1492–1504.

117. Cepeda, C., Wu, N., Andre, V. M., Cummings, D. M., and Levine, M. S. (2007). The corticostriatal pathway in Huntington's disease. *Prog Neurobiol* **81**, 253–271.

118. Milnerwood, A. J., and Raymond, L. A. (2007). Corticostriatal synaptic function in mouse models of Huntington's disease: early effects of huntingtin repeat length and protein load. *J Physiol* **585**, 817–831.

119. Cummings, D. M., Andre, V. M., Uzgil, B. O., Gee, S. M., Fisher, Y. E., Cepeda, C., and Levine, M. S. (2009). Alterations in cortical excitation and inhibition in genetic mouse models of Huntington's disease. *J Neurosci* **29**, 10371–10386.

120. Okamoto, S., Pouladi, M. A., Talantova, M., Yao, D., Xia, P., Ehrnhoefer, D. E., Zaidi, R., Clemente, A., Kaul, M., Graham, R. K., Zhang, D., Vincent Chen, H. S., Tong, G., Hayden, M. R., and Lipton, S. A. (2009). Balance between synaptic versus extrasynaptic NMDA receptor activity influences inclusions and neurotoxicity of mutant huntingtin. *Nat Med* **15**, 1407–1413.

121. Milnerwood, A. J., Gladding, C. M., Pouladi, M. A., Kaufman, A. M., Hines, R. M., Boyd, J. D., Ko, R. W., Vasuta, O. C., Graham, R. K., and Hayden, M. R. (2010). Early increase in extrasynaptic NMDA receptor signaling and expression contributes to phenotype onset in Huntington's disease mice. *Neuron* **65**, 178–190.

122. Dau, A., Gladding, C. M., Sepers, M. D., and Raymond, L. A. (2014). Chronic blockade of extrasynaptic NMDA receptors ameliorates synaptic dysfunction and pro-death signaling in Huntington disease transgenic mice. *Neurobiol. Dis.* **62**, 533–542.

123. Tang, T. S., Tu, H., Chan, E. Y., Maximov, A., Wang, Z., Wellington, C. L., Hayden, M. R., and Bezprozvanny, I. (2003). Huntingtin and huntingtin-associated protein 1 influence neuronal calcium signaling mediated by inositol-(1,4,5) triphosphate receptor type 1. *Neuron* **39**, 227–239.

124. Kaltenbach, L. S., Romero, E., Becklin, R. R., Chettier, R., Bell, R., Phansalkar, A., Strand, A., Torcassi, C., Savage, J., and Hurlburt, A. (2007). Huntingtin interacting proteins are genetic modifiers of neurodegeneration. *PLoS genetics* **3**, e82.

125. Bezprozvanny, I., and Hayden, M. R. (2004). Deranged neuronal calcium signaling and Huntington disease. *Biochem Biophysical Res Comm* **322**, 1310–1317.

126. Tang, T. S., Slow, E., Lupu, V., Stavrovskaya, I. G., Sugimori, M., Llinas, R., Kristal, B. S., Hayden, M. R., and Bezprozvanny, I. (2005). Disturbed Ca2+ signaling and apoptosis of medium spiny

neurons in Huntington's disease. *Proc Natl Acad Sci U S A* **102**, 2602–2607.

127. Bezprozvanny, I. (2009). Calcium signaling and neurodegenerative diseases. *Trends Mol. Med.* **15**, 89–100.

128. Tang, T.-S., Guo, C., Wang, H., Chen, X., and Bezprozvanny, I. (2009). Neuroprotective effects of inositol 1, 4, 5-trisphosphate receptor C-terminal fragment in a Huntington's disease mouse model. *J Neurosci* **29**, 1257–1266.

129. Chen, X., Tang, T.-S., Tu, H., Nelson, O., Pook, M., Hammer, R., Nukina, N., and Bezprozvanny, I. (2008). Deranged calcium signaling and neurodegeneration in spinocerebellar ataxia type 3. *J Neurosci* **28**, 12713–12724.

130. Liu, J., Tang, T.-S., Tu, H., Nelson, O., Herndon, E., Huynh, D. P., Pulst, S. M., and Bezprozvanny, I. (2009). Deranged calcium signaling and neurodegeneration in spinocerebellar ataxia type 2. *J Neurosci* **29**, 9148–9162.

131. Zhemkov, V. A., Kulminskaya, A. A., Bezprozvanny, I. B., and Kim, M. (2016). The 2.2-Angstrom resolution crystal structure of the carboxy-terminal region of ataxin-3. *FEBS Open Bio* **6**, 168–178.

132. Schorge, S., van de Leemput, J., Singleton, A., Houlden, H., and Hardy, J. (2010). Human ataxias: a genetic dissection of inositol triphosphate receptor (ITPR1)-dependent signaling. *Trends Neurosci* **33**, 211–219.

133. Kasumu, A., and Bezprozvanny, I. (2012). Deranged Calcium Signaling in Purkinje Cells and Pathogenesis in Spinocerebellar Ataxia 2 (SCA2) and Other Ataxias. *Cerebellum (London, England)* **11**, 630–639.

134. Kasumu, A. W., Liang, X., Egorova, P., Vorontsova, D., and Bezprozvanny, I. (2012). Chronic suppression of inositol 1,4,5-triphosphate receptor-mediated calcium signaling in cerebellar purkinje cells alleviates pathological phenotype in spinocerebellar ataxia 2 mice. *J Neurosci* **32**, 12786–12796.

135. Wu, J., Shih, H.-P., Vigont, V., Hrdlicka, L., Diggins, L., Singh, C., Mahoney, M., Chesworth, R., Shapiro, G., and Zimina, O. (2011). Neuronal store-operated calcium entry pathway as a novel therapeutic target for Huntington's disease treatment. *Chem Biol* **18**, 777–793.

136. Wu, J., Ryskamp, D. A., Liang, X., Egorova, P., Zakharova, O., Hung, G., and Bezprozvanny, I. (2016). Enhanced Store-Operated Calcium Entry Leads to Striatal Synaptic Loss in a Huntington's Disease Mouse Model. *J Neurosci* **36**, 125–141.

137. Harris, J. J., Jolivet, R., and Attwell, D. (2012). Synaptic energy use and supply. *Neuron* **75**, 762–777.

138. Chaturvedi, R. K., and Beal, M. F. (2008). Mitochondrial approaches for neuroprotection. *Ann N Y Acad Sci* **1147**, 395–412.

139. Brustovetsky, N., Brustovetsky, T., Purl, K. J., Capano, M., Crompton, M., and Dubinsky, J. M. (2003). Increased susceptibility of striatal mitochondria to calcium-induced permeability transition. *J Neurosci* **23**, 4858–4867.

140. Reddy, P. H., and Shirendeb, U. P. (2012). Mutant huntingtin, abnormal mitochondrial dynamics, defective axonal transport of mitochondria, and selective synaptic degeneration in Huntington's disease. *BBA Mol Basis Dis* **1822**, 101–110.

141. Grünewald, T., and Beal, M. F. (1999). Bioenergetics in Huntington's disease. *Ann. N. Y. Acad. Sci.* **893**, 203–213.

142. Jonas, E. A. (2014) Impaired import: how huntingtin harms. *Nat. Neurosci.* **17**, 747–749.

143. Yano, H., Baranov, S. V., Baranova, O. V., Kim, J., Pan, Y., Yablonska, S., Carlisle, D. L., Ferrante, R. J., Kim, A. H., and Friedlander, R. M. (2014). Inhibition of mitochondrial protein import by mutant huntingtin. *Nat Neurosci* **17**, 822–831.

144. Liang, X., Wu, J., Egorova, P., and Bezprozvanny, I. (2014). An automated and quantitative method to evaluate progression of striatal pathology in Huntington's disease transgenic mice. *J Huntington's Dis* **3**, 343–350.

145. Zhang, H., Li, Q., Graham, R. K., Slow, E., Hayden, M. R., and Bezprozvanny, I. (2008). Full length mutant huntingtin is required for altered Ca2+ signaling and apoptosis of striatal neurons in the YAC mouse model of Huntington's disease. *Neurobiol Dis* **31**, 80–88.

146. Ryskamp, D. A., Witkovsky, P., Barabas, P., Huang, W., Koehler, C., Akimov, N. P., Lee, S. H., Chauhan, S., Xing, W., and Rentería, R. C. (2011). The polymodal ion channel transient receptor potential vanilloid 4 modulates calcium flux, spiking rate, and apoptosis of mouse retinal ganglion cells. *J Neurosci* **31**, 7089–7101.

4

Neuroinflammation and Neurodegenerative Diseases

TAYLOR R. JAY, SHANE M. BEMILLER, LEE E. NEILSON,
PAUL J. CHENG-HATHAWAY, AND BRUCE T. LAMB

INTRODUCTION

Mounting evidence suggests that neuroinflammation plays a critical role in modifying pathology in neurodegenerative diseases (NDDs). Understanding the mechanisms by which neuroinflammation contributes to NDD pathology promises to elucidate common biological processes underlying neurodegeneration and could provide novel targets for NDD therapeutics. In this chapter, we summarize the key concepts underlying neuroinflammation in NDDs, describing inflammation-related genetic and environmental NDD risk factors, mechanisms of how inflammation contributes to neurodegeneration, how the phenotype of immune cells is regulated by the unique brain microenvironment, and providing an overview of the preclinical and clinical research about neuroinflammation-related biomarkers and immunomodulatory NDD therapies.

IMMUNOLOGY, INFLAMMATION, AND NEUROINFLAMMATION OVERVIEW

Innate and adaptive immunity are the two major divisions of the immune system involved in defending the organism from pathogenic compromise. In brief, the *innate immune system* is the first line of defense, continually surveying the microenvironment for a broad range of potential pathogens. In contrast, the *adaptive immune system* (also commonly referred to as the *acquired immune system*) mounts a delayed, but specific response and maintains immunological memory. *Inflammation* is the local process by which the immune system responds to infection, from detection to clearance. In addition to responding to infection, the inflammatory response is also responsible for normal cell turnover throughout the life of the organism, clearing debris, and permitting remodeling and maintenance of healthy tissue. While the central nervous system (CNS) has historically been thought of as an immune-privileged site, extensive research has shown that *neuroinflammation* underlies many CNS disorders. While the neuroinflammatory response is important for protecting the organism from pathogens and cell damage, when the system becomes dysregulated, as occurs in the context of NDDs, it can also produce detrimental effects.

To establish a foundation for the remainder of the chapter, we will discuss how the inflammatory response is initiated in the periphery, signaling molecules that mediate this response, how cells hone and transmigrate to areas of infection or cell damage, mechanisms of pathogen clearance, and how the immune response is resolved. This section will conclude by connecting these processes to those involved in neuroinflammation and the relevant cell types that mediate normal and pathological functions of the immune system within the CNS.

Activation of the Innate Immune System

The innate immune system identifies extracellular pathogens and distinguishes between healthy and infected or damaged cells. Circulating pathogens express highly conserved pathogen associated molecular patterns (PAMPs), including polysaccharides, proteins, and dsRNA, which are not present on the organism's own cells. A wide variety of pattern recognition receptors (PRRs), expressed on immune surveillance cells, bind to PAMPs, initiating the release of inflammatory factors and immune-related signaling.[1] Toll-like receptors (TLRs) and soluble factors such as complement are well-characterized PRRs that, upon activation, facilitate phagocytosis, attract additional immune cells, and drive clearance of pathogenic debris.[2] The immune system can also recognize infected cells. During infection, self-antigens, which normally label an organism's own cells, are downregulated and replaced by epitopes that are recognized by circulating immune cells, which induce apoptosis and release of additional signaling molecules. These signals attract more immune cells and activate additional downstream immune responses. Finally, the immune system can recognize cells that have been damaged or stressed. These cells release or display on their cell surface damage associated molecular patterns (DAMPs), including membrane lipids, proteins, and intracellular components. These DAMPs can also serve as ligands for PRRs, stimulating release of inflammatory mediators, and further activating innate immune cells at the site of tissue damage.

Signaling Molecules in Innate Immunity and Cell Migration

There are several classes of important signaling components that mediate inflammatory responses. Cytokines are a diverse group of soluble signaling molecules that are released upon activation of the innate immune system. Interleukins (ILs) are a heterogeneous subset of cytokines that activate and stimulate proliferation of neighboring immune cells. ILs can also enhance the permeability of vascular cell walls, facilitating migration of immune cells from the bloodstream into the tissue. Chemokines are another group of cytokines that facilitate migration of peripheral immune cells into inflamed tissue.[3] Circulating immune cells that express chemokine receptors can respond to chemokine production in the affected tissue by upregulating cell surface components, which allows them to interact with proteins called selectins and integrins on vascular cell walls. Interaction with these vascular proteins allows these peripheral immune cells to migrate from the bloodstream into the affected tissue, and chemokines further guide these cells to the precise site of infection or damage.[6] Once these cells reach the site of infection, they can contribute to the inflammatory response. Together, these signaling molecules promote both the presence of immune cells at the site of injury and their activation.

Phagocytosis and Apoptosis

Upon reaching the site of pathology or damage, the immune cells must contain its spread to neighboring cells and tissue and clear dying cells and debris. This is accomplished by phagocytosis. This process begins with the resident tissue macrophage population, which are the first responders to tissue damage or infection. These cells are soon joined by neutrophils, which enter the tissue from circulation and phagocytose pathogens. Neutrophils are followed by monocytes, which differentiate into macrophages upon entering the tissue and also contribute to phagocytosis of pathogens and debris. Clearance of pathogens and dead or dying cells through phagocytosis is necessary for functional remodeling and restoration of homeostasis within tissue to begin.

Resolution of the Inflammatory Process and Clearance

Following these events, the inflammatory response needs to be resolved and homeostasis restored in order to prevent tissue damage. Debris needs to be cleared, immune cells that entered the inflamed tissue must exit, and the resident immune cells must revert to their resting phenotype. These effects are typically achieved through negative feedback mechanisms wherein stimulation of pro-inflammatory receptors on immune cells promote the downstream downregulation of cytokine production and cell activation. Further, anti-inflammatory cytokines help to downregulate the immune response to aid in restoring homeostasis. When the inflammatory stimulus is cleared and the immune cells are no longer activated, the chemokines that attracted peripheral immune cells are no longer produced, and infiltrating immune cells either drain out of the tissue through the lymphatic system or undergo programmed cell death.

In the context of chronic inflammation, these mechanisms are impaired or dysregulated. Continued exposure to an immune stimulus results in long-term activation of resident immune cells and continuous recruitment of new immune cells into the tissue. The perpetual activation of resident immune cells leads to senescence; they become unable to engage in beneficial immune functions such as debris clearance and tissue repair. Thus, chronic inflammation not only leads to tissue damage through promoting constant release of pro-inflammatory mediators, but also through impairing the beneficial functions of immune cells. A chronic inflammatory state is characteristic of neurodegenerative diseases, and the inability of chronically activated cells to resolve and clear inflammatory stimuli within the brain contributes to tissue damage and disease.

Adaptive Immunity

Unlike the innate immune system, the adaptive immune system mounts a robust yet highly specific response to pathogens. Foreign antigens are first detected and processed by antigen presenting cells such as macrophages and dendritic cells. These cells present and display these antigens on human leukocyte antigens (HLAs) in humans or major histocompatibility complexes (MHCs) in mice. T cells can interact with the antigen-HLA or antigen-MHC complexes and, if they express a receptor specific to that complex, can become activated. This activation also requires cytokines to be present in the microenvironment to induce T cell maturation. Depending on the specific antigen complex and the cytokines involved, T cells can mature to engage in different functions. First, CD8+ T cells can directly induce cell death in targeted cells. Second, CD4+ cells can instruct the release of antibodies specific to the antigen it recognizes by B cells, helping macrophages and other innate immune cells to target this antigen for phagocytosis. Finally, these T cells can also release cytokines that instruct other aspects of innate immune cell function.

Before T cells are released into the system, they undergo a maturation process to ensure that they do not recognize antigens that are expressed by the organism's own cells. In this negative selection process, T cells that recognize self-antigens undergo apoptosis. However, sometimes T cells that bind self-antigens are released into circulation. This can produce autoimmunity, where the self-antigen recognized by the T cell is then targeted for destruction by the body's immune system. As we will see later, multiple sclerosis is an autoimmune NDD in which T cells recognize an antigen expressed by oligodendrocytes, resulting in the death of these cells.

Parallels of Peripheral Inflammation to Neuroinflammation and Neurodegenerative Diseases

Until now, we have described the series of events that comprise the inflammatory response in the periphery. In healthy individuals, however, the cells of the peripheral immune system are effectively excluded from the CNS due to a blood–brain barrier (BBB) that tightly regulates entry of cells and macromolecules. While peripheral immune cells typically are not present in the CNS, the CNS does have its own immune cells that comprise a more limited central immune system. This system is comprised of microglia, a tissue resident macrophage population, as well as astrocytes, which can be induced to contribute to inflammatory processes when activated. The brain also has highly specialized macrophage populations associated with specific CNS compartments.[5] The relationship of these cells to their counterparts in the peripheral immune system will be discussed in detail in the following sections.

The Blood-Brain Barrier in Neuroinflammation

The blood–brain barrier is responsible for maintaining separation between the peripheral and central immune systems. This barrier is composed of vascular endothelial cells, connected by tight junctions that prevent unregulated passage of cells and other molecules between the periphery and the CNS. These endothelial cells are surrounded by pericytes and astrocytes, which further limit transport of cells into the CNS and regulate the function of the blood–brain barrier. In the context of disease, immune cells can undergo regulated trafficking to cross into the CNS through the BBB, similar to the extravasation process into other tissues as previously described. This requires expression of particular molecules on the cell surface of circulating immune cells, expression of corresponding factors on the endothelial cells of the BBB, and release of chemokines that promote migration of these cells into the brain parenchyma. Several of these factors are altered in the context of NDDs and contribute to aberrant entry of peripheral immune cells into the CNS.

Cell Types Involved in Neuroinflammation

The immune cells that contribute to neuroinflammation are diverse in both function and origin (Figure 4.1). One of the most prominent players in neuroinflammation are microglia, the primary brain resident macrophages. These cells serve important homeostatic functions by providing trophic support to surrounding neurons, clearing debris, and surveying and maintaining the extracellular environment in the brain. However, when activated, these cells can mediate neuroinflammation. The brain also has other resident macrophage populations, including meningeal macrophages, choroid plexus macrophages and perivascular macrophages in distinct specialized compartments. However, the function of these populations in health and disease is still under investigation.[5] Astrocytes are also brain-resident glial cells that can contribute to the inflammatory response. Both astrocytes and microglia can sense and respond to inflammatory stimuli, migrate to sites of injury or pathology, and release inflammatory cytokines and chemokines that recruit peripheral immune cells into the CNS.

Circulating monocytes from the peripheral blood can be recruited into the CNS by these chemokines. Once these monocytes enter the brain, they differentiate into macrophages and take on many characteristics of resident microglia. These monocyte-derived macrophages can also contribute to the release of pro-inflammatory mediators and debris clearance. However, in some disease contexts, resident and peripheral macrophages contribute to distinct aspects of the inflammatory response within the CNS. In addition to monocytes,

T cells can be recruited from the periphery. While the role of T cells in most neuroinflammatory contexts is not well understood, recruitment of these cells is especially important and well characterized in the context of multiple sclerosis (MS). In this neurodegenerative disorder, autoreactive T cells are important for mediating inflammation-induced damage of CNS cells. Other peripheral

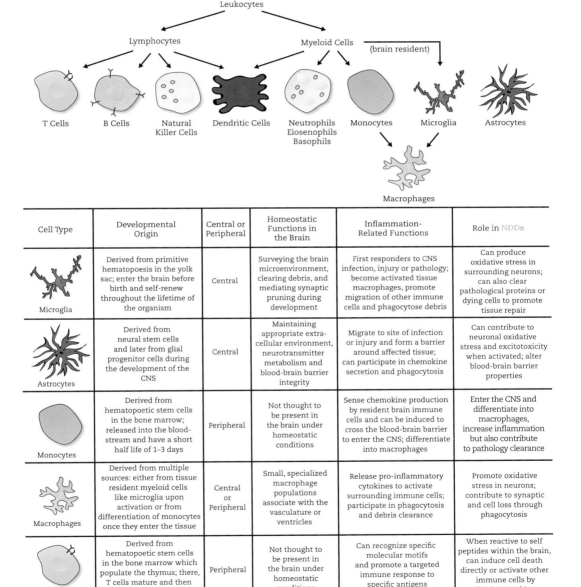

Cell Type	Developmental Origin	Central or Peripheral	Homeostatic Functions in the Brain	Inflammation-Related Functions	Role in NDDs
Microglia	Derived from primitive hematopoesis in the yolk sac; enter the brain before birth and self-renew throughout the lifetime of the organism	Central	Surveying the brain microenvironment, clearing debris, and mediating synaptic pruning during development	First responders to CNS infection, injury or pathology; become activated tissue macrophages, promote migration of other immune cells and phagocytose debris	Can produce oxidative stress in surrounding neurons; can also clear pathological proteins or dying cells to promote tissue repair
Astrocytes	Derived from neural stem cells and later from glial progenitor cells during the development of the CNS	Central	Maintaining appropriate extra-cellular environment, neurotransmitter metabolism and blood-brain barrier integrity	Migrate to site of infection or injury and form a barrier around affected tissue; can participate in chemokine secretion and phagocytosis	Can contribute to neuronal oxidative stress and excitotoxicity when activated; alter blood-brain barrier properties
Monocytes	Derived from hematopoetic stem cells in the bone marrow; released into the blood-stream and have a short half life of 1–3 days	Peripheral	Not thought to be present in the brain under homeostatic conditions	Sense chemokine production by resident brain immune cells and can be induced to cross the blood-brain barrier to enter the CNS; differentiate into macrophages	Enter the CNS and differentiate into macrophages, increase inflammation but also contribute to pathology clearance
Macrophages	Derived from multiple sources: either from tissue resident myeloid cells like microglia upon activation or from differentiation of monocytes once they enter the tissue	Central or Peripheral	Small, specialized macrophage populations associate with the vasculature or ventricles	Release pro-inflammatory cytokines to activate surrounding immune cells; participate in phagocytosis and debris clearance	Promote oxidative stress in neurons; contribute to synaptic and cell loss through phagocytosis
T Cells	Derived from hematopoetic stem cells in the bone marrow which populate the thymus; there, T cells mature and then are released into the blood	Peripheral	Not thought to be present in the brain under homeostatic conditions	Can recognize specific molecular motifs and promote a targeted immune response to specific antigens	When reactive to self peptides within the brain, can induce cell death directly or activate other immune cells by releasing cytokines

FIGURE 4.1. Cell types that contribute to neuroinflammation. Within the brain, several different cell types can contribute to the neuroinflammatory response. These cells have different developmental origins; some are part of the peripheral immune system and others reside within the central nervous system, and they have different functions in the brain in the contexts of health and disease. Together, the interactions among these different cell types within the brain mediate neuroinflammation.

immune cell subtypes, such as neutrophils, dendritic cells, and natural killer cells, have been proposed to enter the brain in various NDDs, though the exact roles of these cells are not yet clear. However, it is clear that, along with the resident cells of the central immune system, these peripheral immune cells are important mediators of neuroinflammation.

NEUROINFLAMMATION-RELATED RISK FACTORS FOR NEURODEGENERATIVE DISEASES

Genetic Risk Factors

It has long been known that neuroinflammation occurs in the context of neurodegenerative diseases. Over 100 years ago, at the same time Alois Alzheimer was establishing the fundamental characteristics of pathology in Alzheimer's disease (AD), he also documented the accumulation of activated glia. Since that time, much work has been done examining the role of neuroinflammation in AD and other neurodegenerative diseases. However, the question remains: Is neuroinflammation playing an active role in the pathogenesis of these NDDs, or is inflammation simply a secondary reaction to other primary pathologies?

In many neurodegenerative diseases, this question has been addressed by recent human genetic studies. These studies have used a variety of methods—genome-wide association studies (GWAS), gene-targeted approaches, and, more recently, whole exome sequencing—to identify genetic risk factors for NDDs that are involved in the immune response. Some of these genes encode proteins that are only expressed in immune cells. This wealth of genetic data makes clear that immune cells and neuroinflammation can modify risk for developing NDDs and strongly suggests that they play a central role in the disease process. Many groups are currently investigating the expression pattern and function of these genes to determine which specific immune cell subsets and functions are most important for modulating NDD pathologies. The following sections review examples of immune-related NDD genetic risk factors and discuss how identification of these risk factors has contributed to our understanding of the role of different immune cell components and pathways in NDDs.

Cytokine and Chemokine Genes

Cytokine and chemokine release results in altered inflammatory responses and the recruitment of additional immune cells to sites of infection or damage. As discussed later, this can lead to oxidative stress in surrounding neurons, potentially contributing to neuronal death in the context of NDDs. Several genetic studies have implicated genes that encode cytokines and chemokines in disease pathogenesis. Numerous genes associated with cytokine production, cytokine receptors, or activation of signaling pathways downstream of cytokine receptor activation have been identified in patients with multiple sclerosis (MS). Polymorphisms in genes that encode cytokine subsets, like the TNF family members and members of the JAK/STAT signaling pathway, have been identified as modifiers of MS risk. One member of the TNF family, TNF-α, has also been proposed to modify risk for developing Parkinson's disease (PD).[6] Polymorphisms in the genes encoding IL-1β and IL-6 have also been proposed to modify PD risk.

As mentioned earlier, cytokine release can promote the production of species that contribute to oxidative stress and cell death. There are several components within the cell to protect against damage from these species, including superoxide dismutase 1 (SOD1). Mutations in *Sod1* are the most prominent genetic risk factor for ALS, suggesting an important role for oxidative stress in disease pathogenesis. While this process is important within the neurons themselves, recent studies have also demonstrated that SOD1 function is important within microglia to prevent motor neuron death and maintain healthy motor function.[7] Microglia expressing mutant SOD1 had increased levels of cytokine production in culture, suggesting a mechanism by which increased cytokine production in microglia expressing mutant SOD1 increases oxidative stress within surrounding motor neurons.[8] Together, these genetic studies identify components of the cytokine pathways from ligand to downstream cellular functions in the etiology of NDDs.

Complement-Related Genes

Complement is a collection of proteins involved in the innate immune response. As discussed in detail later in the chapter, these different components underlie a variety of immune cell functions. In the context of neurodegeneration, complement proteins can facilitate aberrant stripping of synapses, potentially leading to the synaptic and neuronal dysfunction characteristic of neurodegenerative diseases. Alzheimer's disease and age-related macular degeneration (AMD) have complement-related genetic risk factors.

Complement receptor 1 (CR1) mediates complement-regulated phagocytosis, and variants in CR1 have been shown to increase risk for AD.[9] These variants result in altered expression of CR1 within the cell. AMD also has a strong complement-related genetic component. Genetic variants were identified in the complement component Factor H, which significantly increases risk for developing AMD.[10] Factor H is normally responsible for downregulating the complement cascade. This AMD risk variant in Factor H has been proposed to reduce Factor H binding to its targets,[11] thus leading to enhanced and prolonged activation of complement. These studies strongly indicate that overactivation of the complement system can play a causative role in neurodegeneration.

Genes Involved in the Control of Microglial Phenotype

There are also several genetic risk factors that modify other phenotypes and functions of immune cells. Holmans and colleagues[12] performed a meta-analysis of previous GWAS data comparing patients with Parkinson's disease to age-matched controls. They performed pathway analysis to assess common functional groups of genes that were altered in PD patients. They found that genetic networks related to regulation of leukocyte and lymphocyte activity and cytokine signaling were the functional groups that were most strongly associated with PD risk. Specifically, other studies have demonstrated that polymorphisms in the gene encoding TLR4 increase risk for developing PD.[13] TLR4 is important for the response of myeloid cells to inflammatory stimuli. Activation of TLR4 induces both cytokine production and phagocytosis. It is not clear how these PD-associated variants alter TLR4 function, but it is suggestive of an important role for myeloid cell inflammatory phenotypes in the disease process.

Other identified risk factors specifically modulate immune cell function by altering communication between myeloid cells and surrounding cell types. CD33 is an inhibitory receptor expressed on myeloid cells that, when bound to sialic acids on surrounding healthy neurons, results in suppression of microglial or macrophage activation. Recently, a single nucleotide polymorphism (SNP) near CD33 was shown to alter risk for developing AD by altering CD33 splicing.[14] Initial studies have shown that this alternative splicing of CD33 might be associated with Aß clearance, suggesting an important role for myeloid cell clearance of amyloid in the pathogenesis of AD.[15] CX3CR1 is a chemokine receptor also expressed on myeloid cells in the CNS. This receptor binds to its ligand CX3CL1 on neurons to reduce myeloid cell activation. Variants in the CX3CR1 gene do not affect risk for developing amyotrophic lateral sclerosis (ALS) but do modify the progression of ALS in patients with the disease.[16] Together, these genetic risk factors suggest an important role for intact communication between microglia and other cell types and the regulation of microglial phenotype by other cell types in the brain.

Another interesting risk factor that is involved in modifying myeloid cell phenotype is TREM2. Heterozygous variants in the *Trem2* gene were identified as strong risk factors for developing AD, and subsequent studies have further suggested that these *Trem2* variants could also confer risk for PD, frontotemporal dementia, and ALS.[17] Studies in AD mouse models have suggested that TREM2 might play a pro-inflammatory role in the disease process, promoting infiltration of peripheral macrophages into the CNS and promoting activation of these cells within the brain. While the effect of TREM2 on AD pathology is still controversial, the evidence so far points to an important role for peripherally derived immune cells in AD pathology.[18] Further studies will be required to determine whether this same mechanism contributes to the risk that *Trem2* variants confer for other neurodegenerative diseases. The function of normal and variants of *Trem2* are of particular interest in the field of neuroinflammation in NDDs because understanding their function might elucidate common mechanisms of phenotypic regulation of myeloid cells that are important across a wide range of neurodegenerative processes.

Genes Related to Adaptive Immunity

While innate immunity receives the most attention in the context of neurodegeneration, the role of the adaptive immune system has also been highlighted by human genetic studies. In MS, roughly half of the genetic risk factors identified thus far are variants in the HLA locus.[19] The genes encoded in this locus are HLA molecules, which are involved in a variety of immune functions, most notably presenting antigens to cells of the adaptive immune system. Polymorphisms were also identified in the HLA region, which increased risk for developing PD.[20] It is unclear whether these HLA polymorphisms identified in PD are directly impacting antigen presentation or whether they might be involved in other aspects of immune cell function. Further investigation will be required to understand which of these mechanisms is critical for modulating PD pathology. However, these studies strongly suggest that the cross-talk between innate and adaptive immune functions is important in the context of NDDs.

Additional genetic risk factors identified for MS suggest that the function of adaptive immune cells is also important in modifying disease risk. Outside the HLA locus, genetic risk factors have been identified that directly impact T cell function, stimulation, proliferation, and differentiation. Variants in the identified risk factor TYK2 are involved in altering T cell polarization.[21] This is important for determining whether T cells will promote or prohibit an autoimmune reaction to oligodendrocytes and subsequent demyelination. While the impact of T cells and other aspects of adaptive immunity are less well studied in other NDD contexts, these risk factors certainly suggest a central role for this system in the pathogenesis of MS.

ENVIRONMENTAL RISK FACTORS

In addition to known genetic risk factors for NDDs, there are also neuroinflammation-related environmental risk factors that confer disease risk. These risk factors are diverse. Some impact the immune response within the brain directly, like traumatic brain injury, while some primarily affect peripheral immune cell function, like infection. While the mechanisms underlying many of these environmental risk factors are not yet completely understood, many labs are currently investigating how they contribute to NDD risk. Many of these environmental risk factors are shared in common among diseases, suggesting that common immune-related mechanisms might underlie these diseases, despite their diverse pathological processes and clinical presentations. Following are a few examples of environmental risk factors that alter risk for NDD development.

Infection

Perhaps the most straightforward inflammation-related risk factor for neurodegenerative diseases is infection. The link between infection and NDDs has been extensively studied in the context of multiple sclerosis, the NDD with the best-established ties to peripheral immune system function. Epstein Barr virus (EBV) exposure, particularly later in life, can increase risk for developing MS.[22] This is thought to be due to the structural similarity between part of the EBV viral particle and a component of myelin. This molecular similarity can drive T cells, activated in response to EBV infection, to cross-react with self-myelin proteins. In addition to direct molecular mimicry between EBV and myelin, infection in general has been shown to be an important modifier of MS risk. It has been proposed that infections early in life can be protective against development of MS, whereas infections acquired later in life can promote MS development. In addition, viral infection in patients who have MS doubles the risk of a symptomatic relapse.[23] This suggests that perturbations to the immune system not only affect MS onset, but also modify its progression.

Even though the relationship between peripheral immune cell function in other neurodegenerative diseases has not been as well established, it has recently become a very active area of research. In the context of Parkinson's disease, certain encephalopathic viruses can cause similar pathological and clinical symptoms as sporadic PD,[24] suggesting that brain inflammation can induce PD symptoms. There is also evidence that inflammation-related changes outside the CNS can alter PD risk. Incidence of peripheral inflammatory disorders like Crohn's disease is increased in patients with PD.[25] Likewise, *H. pylori* infection increases risk for developing PD.[26] While the mechanism by which these infections result in enhanced risk for PD is not clear, these findings do suggest that systemic infections can be associated with PD development.

Interestingly, infection need not occur immediately prior to development of PD to be pathologically relevant. Recent studies suggest that maternal infection can result in dopaminergic neuron loss even during development *in utero*,[27] suggesting that even very early in development, infection might enhance risk for PD. More recent studies have found changes in lymphocyte composition and activation in PD patients—changes associated with infection.[8] While it is not clear whether this is a contributing factor to disease pathogenesis or a peripheral reaction to the central disease process, the evidence supports that changes in the peripheral immune system are related to disease state.

Vascular Disease

Vascular disease can result in changes to the brain vasculature, altering immune cell trafficking and leading to unregulated entry of immune cells from the periphery. Alzheimer's disease and vascular disease share several risk factors, including hypertension, alterations in cholesterol metabolism, and diabetes.[28] Indeed, AD patients are more likely to have atherosclerosis than age-matched controls. Additional evidence that vascular dysfunction can directly impact AD pathology comes from studies of AD patients following stroke. In these studies, small ischemic lesions exacerbate cognitive symptoms in AD patients,[29] causing cognitive decline much greater than that which occurred in individuals without AD who had similarly sized lesions. This suggests that intact and healthy vasculature is important to protect against AD progression. Atherosclerosis and inflammation of the vasculature have also been suggested to play a role in Parkinson's disease by allowing unregulated entry of peripheral immune cells into vulnerable brain regions. The role of immune cell trafficking and entry into the CNS in the context of NDDs is currently a very active research area.

Environmental Toxins and Protective Factors

Several other environmental components have been shown to modify risk for developing neurodegenerative diseases. Vitamin D and sun exposure are protective against the development of MS. Vitamin D is known to alter T cell function, and supplementation can reduce macrophage activation within the CNS.[30] Other environmental factors can exacerbate risk for neurodegenerative diseases through altering immune cell function. Cigarette smoke is known to increase the systemic inflammatory response. Smoking increases the risk for developing MS and can exacerbate MS symptoms in patients who already have the disease.[31] Cigarette smoke is also a risk factor for AMD.[32] This link has been mechanistically studied, and based on both patient data and mouse models of AMD, it seems that cigarette smoke activates the complement component C3.[33] This results in enhanced immune cell activation and increased oxidative stress due to resulting mitochondrial damage in retinal ganglion cells.[34] Interestingly, smoking is negatively correlated with risk of developing PD, suggesting that alterations to immune cell function could also be protective depending on the specific context.[35] While the exact pathways are still being worked out, several other environmental factors can modify NDD risk through inflammation-related mechanisms.

Traumatic Brain Injury

Repeated traumatic brain injury (TBI) can lead to the development of chronic traumatic encephalopathy (CTE). Similar to the other NDDs discussed here, CTE is characterized by neuronal death accompanied by cognitive decline, psychological changes, and motor symptoms. It is also characterized by neuroinflammation. It is thought that the acute inflammatory response in the CNS upon traumatic brain injury may promote a sustained increase in inflammation that eventually results in neurodegeneration. Indeed, mouse models of traumatic brain injury show long-term changes in myeloid cell activation and axonal dystrophy.

While TBI is the direct cause of CTE, it can also increase the risk of developing other neurodegenerative diseases. The most well-studied association is between TBI and AD.[36] Studies in which traumatic brain injury was administered to AD mouse models suggest that TBI does increase CNS inflammation and worsen AD-related pathologies. While this has been less well studied in PD, epidemiological data still indicate that TBI can increase risk for the development of PD pathology. However, because there are numerous interacting environmental and genetic risk factors for PD, it has been difficult to show that traumatic brain injury itself increases PD risk. Twin studies, used frequently to address the effect of a single variable among shared genetic and environmental risk factors, found that TBI does increase PD risk, independent of other factors.[37] Why individuals develop AD- or PD-related pathologies following TBI is still unclear. As with several of these environmental risk factors, the mechanism underlying their association with certain pathologies will need to be further examined. However, the current literature strongly suggests that environmental factors affecting inflammation or immune cell function can contribute to the development of NDDs.

MECHANISMS OF NEUROINFLAMMATION-MEDIATED NEURODEGENERATION

While it is clear that neuroinflammation can modulate NDD pathology, the question of how this occurs remains unresolved. This section describes a few mechanisms by which aberrant immune cell function can contribute to neurodegeneration (Figure 4.2). In the simplest case, factors released by immune cells within the CNS can directly lead to neuronal death. Microglia, astrocytes, and peripherally derived macrophages can release reactive oxygen and reactive nitrogen species that increase oxidative stress within neurons in the context of many NDDs. These immune cells can also release factors such as IL-1ß, which promote neuronal cell death through activation of the inflammasome, an

In ALS, macrophages produce ROS and RNS, contributing to neuronal oxidative stress. Astrocytes also become activated and downregulate glutamate transporters, promoting neuronal excitotoxicity. Together, these mechanisms can promote neurodegeneration of upper motor neurons in the motor cortex and spinal cord and peripheral lower motor neurons.

In MS, myelin-reactive T cells can directly mediate oligodendrocyte cell death and release cytokines that attract and activate other immune cells. Macrophages also release cytokines and contribute to axonal degeneration through phagocytosis. These mechanisms result in white matter lesions and neurodegeneration across the brain and spinal cord.

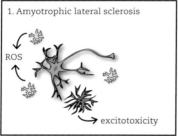

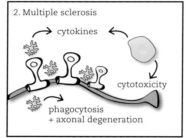

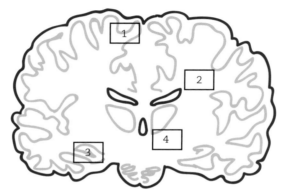

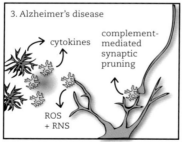

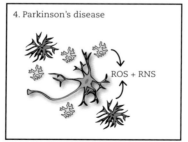

In AD, plaque-associated macrophages and astrocytes release cytokines as well as ROS and RNS, which contribute to degeneration of surrounding neurites. Macrophages can also engage in complement-mediated synaptic pruning, leading to synaptic loss. These mechanisms result in neurodegeneration across several brain regions, including the hippocampus, shown here.

In PD, macrophages and astrocytes contribute to already high levels of neuronal oxidative stress in the substantia nigra (SN) through release of ROS and RNS. The high density of macrophages within the SN might contribute to the particular susceptibility of this region to neuronal death in response to oxidative stress and immune cell activation.

FIGURE 4.2. Immune cell function in mechanisms of multiple neurodegenerative diseases. Multiple components of the neuroinflammatory response are involved in the mechanisms of neurodegeneration in different NDD pathologies. Here, we illustrate the interaction of immune cells with the CNS microenvironment in amyotrophic lateral sclerosis, multiple sclerosis, Alzheimer's disease, and Parkinson's disease. The areas of the brain that are impacted by these pathologies are highlighted in the representation of the coronal human brain section shown in the center panel.

immune-related apoptotic pathway. Myeloid cells and astrocytes can also cause neuronal damage through synaptic pruning. In this case, a pathway that is important in the normal refinement of neuronal circuits during development is reactivated, resulting in aberrant loss of synapses. In addition to pruning synapses, myeloid cells can engage in phagocytosis of neuronal cell bodies or axons. In most conditions, phagocytosis mediates the beneficial clearance of debris or pathological immune stimuli; in the context of neurodegeneration, it can result in inappropriate loss of neurons or other CNS cells. Finally, astrocytes and microglia contribute to maintaining the extracellular balance of ions and play important roles in neurotransmitter metabolism and clearance. In NDDs, the activation of astrocytes and myeloid cells impair these homeostatic functions, resulting in neuronal death through excitotoxic damage. While these are just a few examples of how immune cells and neuroinflammation can contribute to neurodegeneration, the topics in the following sections will discuss key general principles of how neuroinflammation can lead to neurodegeneration in different disease contexts.

Oxidative Stress and Neuroinflammation

Oxidative stress is associated with numerous neurodegenerative diseases. While this is discussed at length elsewhere, the following is a quick review of oxidative stress in neurodegeneration with a specific focus on how neuroinflammation contributes to oxidative stress in NDDs.

Oxidative stress is the cellular response to high levels of reactive oxygen species (ROS) within the cell. ROS are primarily created by mitochondrial activity. A small proportion of the electrons from the electron transport chain modify oxygen (O_2) or other oxygen-containing compounds, resulting in species with unpaired electrons. In addition to ROS, cells can also produce reactive nitrogen species (RNS), which contribute to nitrositive stress within cells. Nitric oxide (NO) is the most common RNS species and is continually produced in cells by nitric oxide synthase (NOS). NO production can also be increased through activation of the inducible NOS (iNOS) enzyme. In addition to these pathways, ROS and RNS can be produced through other cellular processes. Metal ions can react with these species to enhance levels of ROS or RNS, and damage to other cellular components can also increase levels of these compounds.

At low or moderate levels, ROS and RNS play important signaling roles within the cell. They can induce transcriptional programs that protect against oxidative damage. These transcriptional programs can promote proliferation and survival. However, at high levels, ROS and RNS can cause cellular damage. Because these species are so reactive, they can interact with DNA, proteins, and lipids within the cell and modify their structure so that they are unable to perform their normal functions. At high levels, these species can also induce signaling cascades that promote cell death. A balance in both the production and neutralization of ROS and RNS is necessary to maintain levels that promote normal cell signaling and function, while preventing cell damage and death.

Neurons are particularly susceptible to high levels of oxidative stress for several reasons. First, due to the high metabolic demands associated with neuronal structure and function, neurons produce high endogenous levels of ROS. Second, neurons rely on high levels of intracellular calcium to mediate signaling, and high levels of calcium enhance ROS production. Finally, neurons must survive for the lifetime of the organism and thus have a long time to accumulate ROS and RNS. Together, these factors make neurons vulnerable to perturbations in the production or clearance of ROS and RNS within the CNS. This susceptibility to oxidative stress explains why these reactive species are strong modifiers of NDDs.

Contribution of Macrophages to Neuronal Oxidative Stress

Macrophages and microglia have additional specialized mechanisms to produce ROS and RNS species. Macrophages express NADPH oxidase, which, when cells become activated by inflammatory stimuli, can induce a respiratory or oxidative burst associated with high levels of ROS production. This respiratory burst occurs in order to kill phagocytosed bacteria or surrounding pathogenic cells by inducing oxidative damage. However, in the context of the brain, this results in increased oxidative stress in surrounding neurons. Macrophages in the brain also express a specific isoform of iNOS, which is upregulated in response to inflammatory stimuli and cytokines. Upregulation of iNOS increases production of the primary RNS, NO. NO can damage surrounding cells directly by diffusing through cell membranes and reacting with constituents of the cell. It can also bind to other reactive molecules, like superoxide, to form more reactive and damaging species that can result in DNA fragmentation and other forms of cellular damage.

In addition to these mechanisms by which macrophages and other immune cells upregulate ROS and RNS, they can also release factors which induce production of reactive species within neurons. The cytokines IL-1ß, IL-6, TNF-α and IFN-γ have all been shown to induce a form of oxidative burst within other cell types, including neurons. Release of ROS from macrophages can also upregulate neuronal nitric oxide synthase (nNOS) expression within neurons. This results in enhanced endogenous production of ROS and RNS within neuronal cells.

Evidence for Macrophage Involvement in Oxidative Stress in Neurodegeneration

While it is known that oxidative stress occurs in most NDDs, the mechanisms of oxidative stress differ between the various disease processes. Mitochondrial stress and a cell-intrinsic loss of balance between ROS and RNS production and degradation pathways are sources of oxidative stress. Proteosomal stress due to accumulation of misfolded proteins within neurons is another contributor to oxidative stress within the cell. While these neuron-intrinsic mechanisms certainly contribute to the oxidative stress evident in NDDs, as discussed earlier, exogenous signals can also contribute to oxidative stress within cells. Evidence in several fields of neurodegeneration suggest that immune cells and their signaling mediators can contribute to the oxidative stress response within neurons and ultimately to cell death. The role of macrophage or astrocyte-mediated oxidative stress in neuronal death will be discussed in the following sections in the context of PD, ALS, and AD.

Parkinson's Disease

There is substantial evidence concerning oxidative stress in PD. Dopaminergic neurons in the substantia nigra (SN), the primary site of neurodegeneration in PD, have unusually high levels of oxidative stress at baseline. Levels of ROS and RNS are further increased in the SN of PD patients.[38,39] Recently, several studies have suggested that oxidative stress mediated by myeloid cells might be a primary contributor to the loss of dopaminergic neurons in PD.[40] When microglia or astrocytes are co-cultured with dopaminergic neurons or their secreted products, these cells upregulate inflammatory mediators like IL-6 and TNF-α and secrete nitric oxide .[41,42] In PD patients, levels of these cytokines are also increased. These reactive cells are clustered around the degenerating dopaminergic neurons in the brains of PD patients,[43] suggesting that these secreted products are in the right place to affect the degenerating cells.

While these cells are spatially and temporally poised to promote oxidative stress and degeneration within dopaminergic neurons, it has only recently been shown that they actively contribute to neuronal stress and degeneration.

Liberatore and colleagues[44] showed that administration of MPTP, a compound that selectively kills dopaminergic neurons, enhanced levels of immune cell activation and iNOS production in a mouse model of PD. Because iNOS is a form of nitric oxide synthase specific to myeloid cells, it was clear that this model of PD was specifically increasing RNS formation in myeloid cells, rather than in the neurons themselves. Mice lacking this myeloid-cell-specific NOS also had enhanced dopaminergic survival following MPTP administration. This suggests that RNS production by myeloid cells must normally contribute to neuronal cell death in this PD model. In other studies, they found that anti-inflammatory drugs resulted in improved dopaminergic cell survival in both the MPTP and 6-OHDA rodent models of PD.[45–47] This again suggests that inflammatory responses of immune cells are necessary for at least some of the dopamine-mediated cell death in PD models.

In studies by Herrera and colleagues[48] and Kim and colleagues,[49] the authors showed that microglial activation could also be sufficient for dopaminergic cell death to occur. In these studies, mice were injected with the inflammatory stimulus lipopolysaccharide (LPS) near the SN. LPS is known to promote activation of microglia and astrocytes, increasing production of ROS and RNS, and upregulating cytokines, which induce production of these species by surrounding cells. They found that activation of immune cells near the SN resulted in selective cell death of dopaminergic neurons within the SN, and recapitulated several aspects of well-established PD models. This led the field to consider that oxidative stress induced by immune cells might a key mediator of dopaminergic cell death in PD.

Amyotrophic Lateral Sclerosis

ALS is the neurodegenerative disease perhaps most strongly linked with oxidative stress because mutations in the oxidative-stress-related gene *Sod1* are the most common genetic cause of familial ALS. SOD1 is an enzymatic antioxidant that removes superoxide anions, protecting against oxidative stress. While mutations in *Sod1* were long thought to increase oxidative stress in neurons directly, recent evidence strongly suggests a role for microglia and macrophages in mediating the oxidative stress responses of neurons in ALS. It is known that there is increased microglial activation surrounding the upper and lower motor neurons that undergo degeneration in ALS. More recently, it has been shown that expression of mutant *Sod1* can contribute to this enhanced activation. Microglia cultured from adult mice expressing mutant *Sod1* had increased expression of TNF- α and IL-6 in response to LPS stimulation.[50] Thus *Sod1* mutations can generate pro-inflammatory cytokine production in activated microglia that ultimately leads to oxidative stress in surrounding motor neurons.

Mice that express mutant *Sod1*have also been used to show that myeloid cells can play a specific role in motor neuron degeneration and dysfunction. Mouse models suggest that expression of *Sod1* mutations in neurons alone are not sufficient to generate the neuronal death and motor dysfunction that comprise ALS pathology, suggesting that non-cell-autonomous mechanisms must contribute to oxidative stress and neuronal death.[51,52] This was further supported by studies that reduced mutant *Sod1* expression selectively in myeloid cells. This resulted in an increased life span in *Sod1* mutant mice.[53] The role of SOD1 in peripherally derived macrophages was also specifically assessed. *Sod1* mutant mice were irradiated and their bone marrow reconstituted with bone marrow from a mouse expressing WT SOD1. These mice also had increased life spans compared to non-transplanted controls, suggesting that mutant *Sod1* in bone-marrow-derived immune cells could also contribute to ALS pathogenesis. Together, these studies strongly suggest a role for microglial and peripheral macrophage dysfunction in contributing to oxidative stress and motor neuron death in ALS.

Alzheimer's Disease

In Alzheimer's disease, immune cell function is perhaps the most dichotomous, with clear detrimental and beneficial effects of inflammation in the disease process. IL-1ß, IL-6, and TNF-α are all upregulated in microglia derived from brains of AD patients,[54] which has been recapitulated in numerous AD mouse models. Increasing IL-1ß and IL-6 has been shown to reduce Aß plaque load in AD mouse models.[55,56] Enhancing microglial activation through inhibiting fracktalkine-mediated suppression of microglial activation also improved amyloid pathology.[57,58] However, these cytokines can also contribute to production of ROS and RNS species, resulting in neuronal damage. Indeed, in microglial cultures, adding Aß results in TNF-α-mediated increases in iNOS expression, which results in apoptosis in co-cultured neurons.[59] In humans, PET imaging studies that assessed microglial activation in AD patients demonstrated that the number of activated microglia correlated with worse cognitive

decline.[60] So, while inflammation and cytokine production can play beneficial roles in modulating AD pathologies, it also results in ROS and RNS production and potentially neurodegeneration, associated with cognitive decline.

In addition to the induction of ROS and RNS through cytokine production, there is also a well-documented role for an NADPH oxidase-mediated respiratory burst in myeloid cells in AD. In culture, Aß induces microglia to undergo a respiratory burst, increasing levels of NADPH oxidase and thus ROS.[61] This correlates well with the upregulation of NADPH oxidase that has been observed in the brains of AD patients.[62] Qin and colleagues[63] demonstrated a role for NADPH oxidase in microglia-mediated neuronal death in response to Aß. They showed that low levels of Aß applied to neurons in culture were not neurotoxic. However, when microglia were co-cultured with these neurons and the same concentration of Aß was applied, it resulted in neuronal death. When an NADPH oxidase inhibitor was added to the media, this neurotoxicity was ameliorated. This specific induction of respiratory burst activity certainly contributes to neuronal oxidative stress in AD and likely contributes to neuronal death in this NDD. However, the role of cytokine-induced inflammatory responses and oxidative stress is perhaps more complex than in the other NDDs discussed in this section.

COMPLEMENT-MEDIATED SYNAPTIC LOSS AND NEUROINFLAMMATION

As explained previously, complement is a collection of soluble proteins that underlie processes involved in inflammation and pathogen clearance in the peripheral immune system. Together, the proteins involved in the complement cascade can promote migration, lysis, and, important for our discussion, phagocytosis. In the latter case, binding of the complement component C1q to the surface of a pathogen results in a cascade of enzymatic reactions, eventually leading to C3b binding to C1q. C3b then interacts with complement receptors on phagocytic cells to promote the phagocytosis of the pathogen.

In the CNS, this system has been repurposed to promote phagocytosis of specific synapses during development. Stevens's group[64] and others have demonstrated that C1q and C3 localize to synapses during periods of synaptic refinement. Microglia prune these synapses through a C3 receptor-dependent mechanism. This microglial-mediated synaptic pruning seems to be largely restricted to specific developmental periods. However, it has been shown in several neurodegenerative diseases that complement components are highly upregulated, and it has been proposed that this might lead to aberrant synaptic pruning in the context of disease. This could underlie the synaptic and eventually neuronal loss that characterizes these disorders. While this is a relatively new mechanism to explain how immune cells and neuroinflammation might mediate neurodegeneration, it will no doubt be an area of research that rapidly expands in coming years. Thus far, the role of complement in NDDs has been best studied in the contexts of Alzheimer's disease and retinal degeneration, which we review in more detail in the following.

Alzheimer's Disease

Complement components are upregulated in the brains and CSF of AD patients.[65,66] As discussed earlier, recent identification of complement-related genes like CR1 as AD risk factors suggests an active role of complement in mediating AD pathogenesis.[67,68] Indeed, C1q-deficient AD mouse models show reduced synaptic loss and improved amyloid pathology, suggesting that alterations in complement can impact the pathological time course of AD, and specifically limit the synaptic loss seen in these mouse models.[69] However, increased pathology and neurodegeneration have been observed in C3-deficient AD mice.[70,71] These studies suggested that the complement pathway might also play an important role in amyloid clearance by microglia. While the exact mechanisms and detailed pathways underlying these changes remain to be elucidated, these data certainly provide a compelling case for the involvement of complement in AD.

Glaucoma and Age-Related Macular Degeneration

Complement components have also been implicated in two forms of retinal degeneration: glaucoma and AMD. In both of these diseases, C1q has been shown to be upregulated.[72] In mouse models of glaucoma, C1q was shown to increase at the same time synapses were lost, and C1q-deficient mice showed reduced degeneration of retinal ganglion cells.[73] In addition to upregulation of these complement proteins, both glaucoma and AMD also have concomitant decreases in negative regulators of the complement system like Factor H.[74,75] Together, these data suggest an important functional role for complement in these two diseases of retinal degeneration.

While AD, glaucoma, and AMD are the diseases where aberrant upregulation of complement has received the most attention, complement components have been shown to be upregulated in many NDDs. As the field moves forward, similar overpruning mechanisms will no doubt be investigated in other diseases as well.

PHAGOCYTOSIS AND NEUROINFLAMMATION

Phagocytosis is an important mechanism for clearance of pathogens and debris. Macrophages, neutrophils, dendritic cells, and even astrocytes can contribute to phagocytosis. These cells have receptors that interact with various components on phagocytic substrates that activate phagocytic machinery within these cells. These substrates can be components of microbes or apoptotic cells. But in the context of neurodegeneration, these phagocytic substrates are more often components of neurons or specific molecules, such as fibrillar Aß in AD or myelin components in MS. Just as the substrates are diverse, so are the receptors that interact with them. Complement receptors discussed earlier and Fc receptors that recognize immunoglobulins are two common phagocytic receptor subtypes. However, specific phagocytic substrates can also have their own receptor complexes. When the receptors interact with these substrates, cytoskeletal rearrangement causes membrane invagination and ingestion of the phagocytic substrate into a phagosome. This phagosome then fuses with a lysosome, and the acidified environment and lysosomal enzymes degrade the phagocytosed material. The hydrolyzed components of peptides and nucleotides are then released and recycled.

Cells can also engage in micro- or macropinocytosis, mechanisms that allow cells to take up smaller constituents from the extracellular space. Pinocytosis occurs through the formation of membrane ruffles which result in non-specific uptake of proteins from the surrounding microenvironment. Despite not being specific to a particular phagocytic substrate, micropinocytosis can still be a mechanism of clearance of soluble proteins from the interstitial fluid in the context of neurodegenerative disease. Macropinocytosis can also be regulated by many of the same mechanisms as phagocytosis, including receptor complexes specific to NDD-related proteins.

Within the CNS, microglia are the resident competent phagocytes. In the context of acute

CNS damage, microglia are important for the clearance of debris and dying cells. This clearance is necessary for regeneration following injury. However, in the context of NDDs in which there is a chronic inflammatory environment, the role of microglia in phagocytosis is less clear. In addition to dysfunctional clearance of aggregated proteins or dying cells from the brain, microglia can directly damage healthy cells and tissue through phagocytic mechanisms. It has also been proposed in different disease models that astrocytes and infiltrating macrophages play distinct and important roles in mediating disease-related phagocytosis. Here we discuss both the beneficial and detrimental roles of phagocytosis in the contexts of Alzheimer's disease and multiple sclerosis.

Alzheimer's Disease

In AD, myeloid cells play an important role in the clearance of Aß in both its soluble form through micropinocytosis[76] and its insoluble form through phagocytosis.[77] When the Aß peptide is present in high enough levels in the extracellular space, it is more likely to dimerize, oligomerize, and eventually deposit as insoluble fibrils in amyloid plaques. With the exception of rare mutations that result in familial forms of AD, it is not enhanced Aß production, but rather impaired Aß clearance that results in increased concentrations of Aß and its subsequent deposition into plaques. It has been appreciated for a long time that myeloid cells could clear Aß from the extracellular space and limit plaque deposition. This was first demonstrated by studies using electron microscopy, which showed Aß fibrils within lysosomal compartments of brain myeloid cells.[78] Wisniewski and colleagues[79] performed a similar study, but in the brain of an AD patient following a stroke. There, they found that cells they identified as peripherally derived macrophages but not resident microglia contained Aß fibrils. Others have shown that astrocytes are also active players in clearing Aß[70] and limiting amyloid accumulation.[80]

Since these first studies, it has remained controversial in the field which cells contribute to clearance of Aß and how effective these cells are at Aß phagocytosis. Bolmont and colleagues[81] performed *in vivo* imaging studies following migration of microglia to individual plaques in an AD mouse model. They found that microglia continue to migrate to plaques throughout disease progression and that these cells internalize Aß. They found that Aß was localized within lysosomal compartments in these cells, and suggested

that the cells were effectively engaging in Aß degradation. In contrast, others have shown that, while microglia can effectively take up Aß, they are not efficient at degrading the Aß species once the peptides are inside the lysosomal compartments.[82] Other studies suggest that myeloid cells do not actively contribute to Aß clearance at all. Studies that have used different methods to eliminate microglia from the brain altogether have found no change in amyloid plaque deposition within brains of AD mice.[83–85]

One possible explanation for these disparate findings is that the ability of microglia to engage in phagocytosis of Aß may be inhibited by the inflammatory environment. Yamamoto and colleagues[86] demonstrated that cytokines reduce the ability of myeloid cells to degrade Aß species *in vitro*. They also showed that microglia isolated from AD mice in which IFN-γ signaling was disrupted were able to degrade Aß species in culture, even after the application of cytokines. Others have recapitulated these findings *in vivo*, showing that treatment with anti-inflammatory agents can rescue the ability of myeloid cells to phagocytose Aß.[59] So, while myeloid cells may not always effectively phagocytose and clear Aß, this may be due to inhibition of this cellular function by the local microenvironment, rather than an intrinsic inability to clear Aß proteins. Several therapeutic strategies have been proposed for AD that involve altering the inflammatory state of brain macrophages to promote a more pro-phagocytic phenotype.

Multiple Sclerosis

Both resident microglia and peripherally derived macrophages contribute to phagocytosis in an MS mouse model, experimental autoimmune encephalomyelitis (EAE),[87] though it has been suggested that these different cell populations may contribute to phagocytosis at different stages in the disease process. Microglia are thought to phagocytose debris soon after lesion formation, while peripherally derived macrophages are involved later in the debris clearance process and may be especially important for remyelination to occur.

In the context of MS, phagocytosis is a double-edged sword. Phagocytosis is beneficial when it results in clearance of myelin and other debris, paving the way for regeneration.

However, it has also been shown that brain myeloid cells can phagocytose axonal or neuronal elements, promoting damage and degeneration within the MS lesion. Microglia isolated from autopsied MS patient brain tissue phagocytose both myelin debris and neurofilament antigens in culture.[88] *In vivo*, the involvement of myeloid cells in axonal damage is supported by evidence that axons can be damaged even in the absence of demyelination.[89] Phagocytosis of myelin can also increase activation of autoreactive T cells within the MS lesion, further promoting tissue damage.

While AD and MS are quite different in terms of their pathologies, both have dual roles of phagocytosis. On the one hand, phagocytosis is important to clear Aß or myelin debris; on the other hand, phagocytosis can result in loss of synapses, axons, or other neuronal elements, leading to neuronal degeneration. In addition, phagocytosis by these cells can result in the production of pro-inflammatory mediators, activating surrounding myeloid cells or reactive T cells within the CNS.

EXCITOTOXICITY AND NEUROINFLAMMATION

Excitotoxicity is the phenomenon of cellular damage from overstimulation. For neurons, this most often means prolonged glutamate signaling. Glutamate can signal through multiple receptor subtypes, but the most damaging to neurons involves signaling through NMDA receptors (NMDARs), which are calcium permeable. This increase in intracellular calcium activates a myriad of downstream signals, and results in dysregulation of ionic and molecular gradients, mitochondrial dysfunction, oxidative stress, and ultimately neuronal death.

While there are many cell-autonomous mechanisms of excitotoxicity, glial cells can also contribute to the excitatory balance in the context of NDDs. Astrocytes are normally responsible for buffering the neuronal microenvironment in the healthy brain. However, upon activation, astrocytic glutamate uptake is impaired, resulting in enhanced neuronal excitability and cell death through the excitotoxic mechanisms as described earlier.

In the healthy brain, microglia do not express the glutamate uptake transporter GLT-1, and do not substantially contribute to glutamate homeostasis. However, in NDDs, microglial expression of GLT-1 is induced.[90] Differential expression of glutamate modulation by microglia in different brain regions can directly impact neuronal survival following NMDAR activation.[91] Microglia can also contribute to glutamate dysregulation through affecting the expression and uptake activity of glutamate transporters on surrounding astrocytes. LPS injection into the CNS results in neuronal death, which can be prevented with NMDAR antagonists, suggesting an excitotoxic mechanism.[92] This results in increased expression of pro-inflammatory cytokines, which downregulate glutamate transporter expression.[93] While these cytokines can be produced by both microglia and astrocytes, the kinetics suggest that microglia induce downregulation of glutamate transporters on surrounding astrocytes. Therefore, both microglia and astrocytes contribute to glutamate dysregulation in the context of neuroinflammation and NDDs.

Amyotrophic Lateral Sclerosis

In ALS, motor neuron degeneration is associated with increased glutamate levels, which is thought to contribute to oxidative stress and neuronal death. This increase in glutamate has been shown to correlate with decreased expression of the glutamate transporter on glial cells in ALS patients.[94] There was reported to be a decrease in the glial glutamate transporter GLT-1 in a mouse model of ALS as well.[95] The reduction in transporter expression was shown to be functionally important in mediating pathology. Studies that increased GLT-1 expression within ALS mouse models showed pathological and functional improvements.[96] This suggests an important role for glial glutamate metabolism in the pathophysiology of ALS.

Conclusions

Taken together, these mechanisms represent some of the ways that immune cells and inflammation contribute to NDD pathology. The gamut of mechanisms is diverse. Some involve the specific targeting of neurons or neuronal components by immune cells through phagocytosis. Others are less targeted, such as glial-mediated increases in ROS and RNS and changes in glutamate metabolism. However, despite the differences among these mechanisms, there is a lot of cross-talk among them (Figure 4.3). Because all of these mechanisms are interrelated, perhaps it is not surprising that they contribute to multiple NDDs, despite their diverse pathophysiologies and clinical presentations. This commonality across diseases provides promise for neuroinflammation-directed diagnostics and therapeutics that could prove effective for multiple NDDs.

COMMUNICATION BETWEEN IMMUNE CELLS AND OTHER CNS CELL TYPES

Cell-to-cell communication in the healthy brain is critical in regulating many processes, including synaptic plasticity and debris clearance. The interaction between immune cells and other CNS cell types is also important to maintain homeostasis

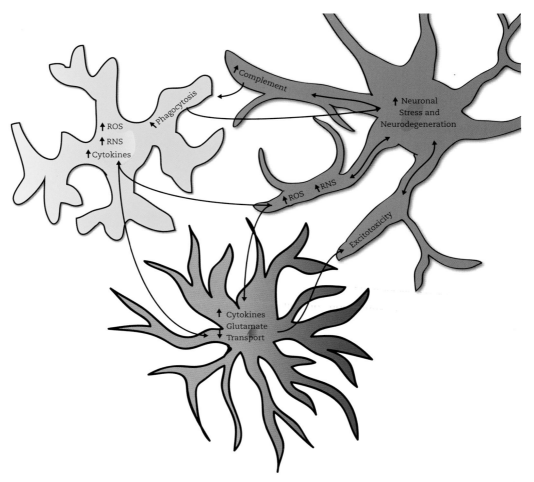

FIGURE 4.3. Interaction among mechanisms underlying neuroinflammation and neurodegeneration. While the mechanisms underlying the roles of neuroinflammation in NDDs were presented in this chapter in isolation, there are several points of interaction among these different mechanisms. Here we illustrate some of these interactions among key CNS cell types: macrophages (shown in yellow), astrocytes (shown in purple), and neurons (shown in blue).

and prevent activation of immune cell signaling pathways in homeostatic conditions (Figure 4.4). In response to a pathological insult, this cell-cell communication is disrupted and immune suppression released so the immune cells can respond to the insult and ultimately protect the tissue from damage. However, these signals can become chronically dysregulated, leading to persistently elevated immune cell activation. This can exacerbate pathological outcomes in many NDDs. The following sections will outline the major classes of molecules that regulate immune cell phenotypes in the CNS.

CYTOKINES AND CHEMOKINES

Cytokines are a class of small, soluble peptides released by immune cells that regulate immune responses, chemotaxis, and modulate blood-brain barrier (BBB) permeability. Microglia

and astrocytes are major producers of cytokines. Depending upon the pathological context, cytokine release can be helpful or harmful. For example, macrophages can produce the pro-inflammatory cytokine IL-1ß that acts on receptors on neurons, glia, and myeloid cells. Signaling through these receptors activates downstream signaling components that result in the production of increased pro-inflammatory effectors, including ROS and RNS species that cause oxidative damage. On the other hand, molecules such as IL-10, IL-4, and TGF-ß are anti-inflammatory molecules, acting to suppress immune responses.

It has been well documented that cytokine levels are elevated in a number of NDDs. Increased levels of IL-1β, IL-6, and TNF have been detected in the brains and CSF of AD and PD patients. Further, levels of the chemokine fractalkine are also increased in the CSF of AD patients compared to age-matched control subjects. Evidence for the involvement of cytokines and chemokines have been thoroughly investigated in numerous mouse models of disease. AD and MS are perhaps the best characterized examples. The following will outline some of the advances made in understanding the role of cytokines in NDDs.

Multiple Sclerosis

In MS and EAE, cytokines, and in particular chemokines, regulate leukocyte infiltration, which is a critical step in the clinical manifestation of autoimmune demyelination. As discussed in the introduction to this chapter, chemokines promote infiltration of cells into the brain parenchyma through the blood–brain barrier.[6] It was demonstrated that overexpression of IL-1ß in mice increased astrocyte expression of the chemokine CCL2, which is critical for recruiting CCR2+ monocytes into the CNS.[97] Likewise, Izikson and colleagues examined mice lacking expression of the chemokine receptor CCR2, and found that these mice were resistant to developing EAE.[98] Further studies revealed that deletion of CCL2 decreased inflammatory monocyte recruitment and decreased T cell activation, demonstrating a critical role for CCR2-CCL2 signaling in EAE pathogenesis.[99] Other chemokines have also been implicated in EAE pathogenesis. More recent studies have demonstrated that CD4+ T cells produce CXCL1 and CXCL2 in the brain, which are required for neutrophil infiltration and ultimately the development of BBB breakdown and EAE pathogenesis.[100] Taken together, these studies have helped pave the way for understanding the complexity of cytokine and chemokine signaling in EAE and have provided a basis for cytokine-directed drug targets in MS.

Alzheimer's Disease

Much of what is known about microglial involvement in CNS inflammation has been learned from studies outlining the role of the chemokine ligand-receptor pair CX3CL1-CX3CR1 (also known as fractalkine and the fractalkine receptor). Neurons can express soluble or membrane-bound CX3CL1, which interacts with CX3CR1 on microglia. Studies examining AD models of amyloid and tau pathology have demonstrated opposing roles of fractalkine signaling in modifying these two pathologies. Studies using fractalkine-deficient mice revealed increased inflammation, plaque-associated macrophage accumulation, and concomitant decreases in senile plaque size and

number in amyloid models of AD.[57] Subsequent studies revealed that elimination of the fractalkine receptor in a tau model of AD enhanced inflammation and exacerbated tau pathology.[101] These studies highlight the multifaceted role of chemokines and cytokines on different pathologies, even within the same disease. This exemplifies the difficulty in designing effective inflammation-directed therapeutics for NDDs, as modifying even the same pathway can have both beneficial and detrimental effects.

CD200/CD200R

Several ligand-receptor pairs expressed on microglia and neurons play important roles in regulating neuroinflammation and myeloid cell phenotype.[102] We previously reviewed the interaction between microglial CX3CR1 and neuronal CX3CL1 and the importance of this interaction in NDDs. Here, we discuss another ligand-receptor pair that is instrumental in regulating immune cell phenotype, CD200R and CD200. Neurons normally express CD200, but under certain inflammatory conditions, CD200 can be upregulated on astrocytes as well. This ligand communicates with its cognate myeloid cell-specific receptor CD200R. Targeted mutations were used to determine that the CD200-CD200R interaction is important in regulating the interaction between other cell surface ligand-receptor pairs.[103] Signaling through CD200R has been shown to downregulate microglial activation. Studies using CD200-null mice demonstrated an increase in CD45 and CD11b, markers associated with immune activation of myeloid cells.[104] Blocking the CD200 receptor in EAE models using a monoclonal antibody increases CNS levels of the pro-inflammatory cytokines IL-6, IFNγ,[105] and iNOS,[106] resulting in worse clinical scores.[107] CD200 and CD200R have also been studied in the context of AD pathology. *In vitro*, the addition of neurons into microglial culture reduces the inflammatory response to Aß. Blocking the interaction of these cells with a CD200 antibody eliminates this effect.[108]

SIGLECS/SIALIC ACIDS

Siglecs (sialic acid binding immunoglobulin-like lectins) are a subset of lectins that specifically recognize carbohydrates modified with sialic acid residues. The neuronal glycocalyx within the CNS is laden with sialic acid residues, which signal to neighboring cell types that these neurons are healthy and viable. Absence of this signaling leads to activation of microglia.[109]

In addition to their role in homeostasis, siglecs also have been shown to play an important role in neurodegenerative diseases. A number of siglecs have shown to modulate inflammation in AD, but CD33 is the best characterized. Binding of CD33 was shown to promote downregulation of myeloid cell activation in the periphery.[110] In the CNS, CD33 function is not yet clear. However, variants in CD33 have been identified as genetic risk factors for AD, and CD33 expression correlates with cognitive decline in AD patients.[111] Upregulation of CD33 *in vitro* has been shown to result in reduced Aβ phagocytosis. Conversely, primary microglial cultures from CD33-deficient mice demonstrate enhanced Aβ uptake.[112] The mechanisms underlying CD33 function in both the peripheral and the central immune responses remains to be fully elucidated, but these data suggest that siglec-mediated communication may play an important role in modifying NDDs.

MATRIX METALLOPROTEINASES

Matrix metalloproteinases (MMPs) and other molecules containing a disintegrin and metalloproteinase domain (ADAM) are produced in glial and myeloid cells. These molecules act to shed extracellular domains of certain proteins on the surface of the cell membrane. These cleavage products can act as signaling molecules in a variety of pathways. MMPs can also inhibit intercellular signaling. For example, ADAM10 and 17 cleave fractalkine, inhibiting microglial-neuronal signaling and promoting microglial migration and activation. Further actions of MMPs include increasing the permeability of the BBB by cleaving cellular matrix components and other adhesion molecules, allowing peripheral immune cells access to the CNS parenchyma. MMPs like ADAM10 can also shed extracellular growth factors,[113] altering cell proliferation and survival. Increases in the levels of numerous MMPs are detectable in various NDDs including AD, MS, PD, and Huntington's disease, highlighting the major role that MMPs may play in NDDs.

Alzheimer's Disease

MMPs are best known in the context of Alzheimer's disease for altering cleavage of the amyloid precursor protein, resulting in altered Aß production.[114] However, MMPs can also modify the inflammatory response in AD. Decreased activity of ADAM10 results in reduced cleavage of neuronal fractalkine, rendering microglia unable to mount an effective immune response. ADAM10 can also

cleave other immune related molecules such as TREM2, though the functional significance of this interaction is still under investigation.[115]

Multiple Sclerosis

As previously discussed, leukocyte recruitment into the CNS is a key event leading to the clinical manifestation of MS. MMPs facilitate this recruitment and infiltration of peripheral immune cells into the CNS parenchyma. In support of this, Maeda and Sobel[116] discovered that the macrophages within active MS lesions expressed MMPs-1, 2, 3, and 9 in both acute and chronic lesions. Cossins et al.[117] also detected upregulation of MMP7 and MMP9 within macrophages in active demyelinating lesions. In addition to their role in degrading tight junctions to mediate BBB breakdown, MMPs have been proposed to affect MS pathology through other mechanisms. MMPs can also degrade the extracellular matrix, which can directly lead to apoptosis of neurons.[118] So, MMPs can lead to neurodegeneration in MS directly or indirectly by altering BBB integrity.

Traumatic Brain Injury

As discussed previously, traumatic brain injury (TBI) can lead to chronic inflammation within the CNS, leading to development of chronic traumatic encephalopathy (CTE) and increasing risk for developing other neurodegenerative diseases. Rat models have been used to highlight the importance of MMPs in inflammation following TBI. Following administration of traumatic brain injury, MMP9 was increased in brain areas proximal to the lesion cavity.[119] Further studies demonstrated that MMP9 was actively involved in modifying tissue damage following TBI. MMP9-deficient mice had decreased neuronal loss and thus smaller lesion cavities after TBI administration.[120] Cell culture studies using a mechanical scratch paradigm demonstrated that astrocytes are the primary producers of MMP9 in response to cell damage. These studies also demonstrated that MMP2 is upregulated specifically in neurons post-injury in the same culture model.[121] Clinically, MMP2 and MMP9 increases have been detected in several models of injury.[122] Taken together, these studies demonstrate that MMP9 and MMP2 may induce tissue damage following TBI, perhaps through altering BBB permeability

EXOSOMAL COMMUNICATION

Exosomal transport has recently gained a significant amount of attention in the fields of neurodegeneration and inflammation. Exosomes are small, membrane-bound vesicles that contain proteins, RNA species, and other signaling mediators. Exosomes are constantly exchanged from cell to cell in a number of normal biological signaling processes. However, in the context of NDDs, exosomes can transmit pathogenic proteins from neuron to neuron, including AD-associated Aß[123] and tau[124] proteins and, at least in cell culture models, PD-associated α-synuclein.[125] Exosomes can also be released by macrophages and astrocytes within the CNS, and some studies suggest that when these cells are activated in the context of inflammation, their exosomal content changes. These studies demonstrate that the molecules contained in exosomes isolated from patients with neuroinflammatory diseases could functionally impair surrounding neurons.[126] While this is a relatively new area of study, this novel form of communication between immune cells and other CNS cells is currently under further investigation in the context of neuroinflammation in NDDs.

NEUROTROPHIC FACTORS AND NDDS

Neurotrophic factors support a wide range of developmental and regenerative processes. They can be categorized into three main superfamilies: neurotrophins, TGF-ß superfamily members, and neurotrophic cytokines. These factors have important roles in maintaining homeostasis. Reducing their expression, as occurs in the context of age or pathology, can adversely affect surrounding neurons. This was specifically demonstrated for microglial production of the neurotrophin BDNF. Parkhurst and colleagues[127] deleted the BDNF gene specifically from microglia and found that these mice had impaired learning and synapse formation, suggesting that microglial BDNF is important for mediating plasticity and memory. In addition to this role in normal brain function, BDNF and other neurotrophins also seem to play an important role in modulating NDDs such as Alzheimer's disease and multiple sclerosis, which are discussed further here.

Alzheimer's Disease

Neurotrophin signaling is reduced in AD, and this may contribute to both protein aggregation and synaptic and neuronal loss. BDNF and its receptor TrkB are reduced in brains of postmortem AD patients compared to healthy controls,[128] demonstrating an overall decrease in BDNF signaling. Decreases in BDNF and

other neurotrophic signaling components can enhance pathogenic protein accumulation. Interruption of NGF and BDNF signaling increases the production of Aß[129] and pathogenic modifications of the tau protein.[130] *In vivo* studies suggest that downregulation of these neurotrophins can be caused by inflammation. Injection of LPS and pro-inflammatory cytokines into mice rapidly reduce expression of BDNF as well as the other neurotophins NGF and NT-3.[131] While it is not yet understood how inflammation reduces neurotrophin levels, this reduction seems to contribute to protein aggregation and neurodegeneration in AD.

Multiple Sclerosis

Similar to what occurs in AD, neurotrophins are also reduced in multiple sclerosis. BDNF expression is decreased in postmortem MS patients.[132] Further evidence of BDNF involvement in MS pathogenesis comes from studies that examined mice haploinsufficient for the BDNF gene. When these haploinsufficient mice are induced to develop EAE, they exhibit dramatically slower remyelination.[133] NGF signaling is also thought to play a protective role in EAE. NGF stimulation suppresses peripheral immune cell inflammation and ameliorates pathological phenotypes in EAE models.[134] Neurotrophin signaling seems to play important roles, both limiting initial tissue damage and promoting tissue regeneration in MS.

Other Neurodegenerative Diseases

Glial-derived neurotrophic factor (GDNF) produced by astrocytes and oligodendrocytes has a neuroprotective effect in multiple NDDs. Studies that transplanted human neural progenitors overexpressing GDNF into a rat model of PD demonstrated decreased dopaminergic neuron loss.[135] In a model of Huntington's disease, viral-mediated overexpression of GDNF rescued neuronal loss in the striatum and improved behavioral deficits,[136] further highlighting the neuroprotective effects of GDNF. Taken together, these studies suggest that loss of neurotrophic signaling reduces synaptic integrity, decreases neuronal viability, and limits regenerative processes in multiple NDD models.

INFLAMMATION-RELATED BIOMARKERS FOR EARLY DETECTION OF NDDS

Early detection and diagnosis of NDDs is critical to provide the best course of treatment, and

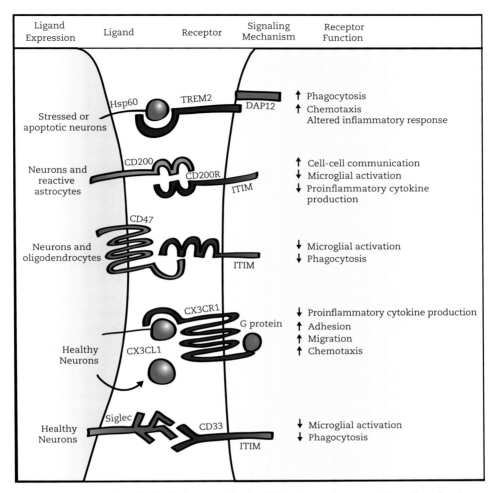

FIGURE 4.4. Regulation of myeloid cell phenotype by the CNS microenvironment. Several mechanisms govern the regulation of microglial phenotype. Ligands expressed on or by other CNS resident cells such as neurons, astrocytes, and oligodendrocytes can interact with receptors on the microglial cell surface to suppress microglial activation and maintain low levels of inflammation within the CNS in homeostatic conditions. However, several of these interactions are lost in the context of neuroinflammation in NDDs, resulting in enhanced microglial activation and ultimately neurodegeneration.

to evaluate the efficacy of new therapeutic interventions aimed at preventing disease onset or progression in early stages of pathology. However, definitive diagnostic tools are still limited in many NDDs, with many still requiring a postmortem diagnosis. While neuroimaging has been used in several NDDs and its capacities continually improve, its expense is limiting as a routine diagnostic tool. Imaging can also lack the sensitivity needed to detect changes that occur in the earliest stages of pathology. Thus, there is tremendous interest in identifying early and robust NDD biomarkers. Since reliability and reproducibility are paramount, panels of biomarkers may prove to be the best strategy.

Multiple body fluids can be sampled, each with their own drawbacks. Cerebrospinal fluid (CSF) gives the best representation of changes that occur within the CNS, and is therefore heavily targeted in research efforts. However, CSF draws are somewhat invasive, so other efforts have been focused on biomarkers in blood plasma. The following sections will outline detection strategies and inflammation-related biomarker candidates for several NDDs.

Multiple Sclerosis
Multiple sclerosis is a heterogeneous disease, and patients with MS can present with a wide range of clinical symptoms. This often leads to a delayed

diagnosis. While MRI is important for following lesion progression and resolution, imaging often does not correlate with clinical findings, and is used only as supportive evidence. There is a long history of evaluating changes in CSF in MS patients. In the 1920s, differences in CSF were first observed between MS patients and healthy individuals.[137] By the 1950s, electrophoresis was used to detect the presence of oligoclonal bands (OCBs) in the CSF,[138,139] which identified the immunoglobulins secreted by pathologically modified T and B cells in MS patients. In 1983, these tests were first incorporated alongside clinical measures to improve diagnostic accuracy.[140] While not required for the diagnosis of MS, OCB presence is a strong indicator of neurodegeneration when present.[141]

In addition, elevated ratios of immunoglobulins in the CSF compared to the blood are detected in approximately 70%–90% of MS patients with positive OCB associations. However, this is not the case in patients without positive OCB, and thus is used as a confirmatory marker, but not a biomarker, of disease.[137] Therefore additional markers have been investigated, which include the soluble cell adhesion molecule-1 (sVCAM-1) and neuron specific 24S-hydroxycholestrol,[142] which are both increased intrathecally in MS patients.[143] Finally, levels of CSF neurofilaments are being investigated in MS, as well as a number of other neurodegenerative disorders.[144] While these biomarkers have improved our ability to make early and accurate diagnoses for MS, they still have limitations. Some have proposed using analysis of single cells, such as T cells in MS patients, to assess changes in expression within the specific cells that underlie the disease process.

Parkinson's Disease

Parkinson's disease, like MS, is a disorder that is typically diagnosed well into the neurodegenerative process. Current CSF biomarkers for PD include α-synuclein, the primary constituent of the Lewy bodies that characterize PD pathology.[145] Interestingly, AD-related proteins tau and Aß are also used as PD biomarkers.[146] In addition to directly measuring these pathology-associated protein species, inflammation-related biomarkers have also been proposed for PD. DJ-1 is present on reactive astrocytes and has anti-inflammatory and antioxidant properties, and mutations in DJ-1 have been found to cause autosomal recessive PD.[147] A small study correlated levels of CSF DJ-1 and tau, which improved discrimination of PD from multiple systems atrophy. This again

highlights the utility of analyzing multiple biomarkers. Biomarkers have also been examined that are involved in the phagolysomal system. Lysosomal dysfunction has been implicated in the impaired clearance and degradation of α-synuclein. Proteins involved in regulating phagolysosomal processes such as GCase have been examined as potential CSF biomarkers for PD. These studies found that GCase was significantly reduced in PD patients compared with healthy controls.[148] Finally, efforts are underway to unify the field of PD biomarker discovery in order to identify prodromal biomarkers, risk biomarkers, and motor stage biomarkers in order to establish the most relevant and effective treatment plans throughout each respective disease state.

Alzheimer's Disease

The classical biomarkers for AD are CSF levels of Aβ and tau, the two proteins that deposit within the parenchyma of AD patients. Consistent increases in levels of total tau have been detected in AD patients compared to healthy control subjects in a large number of studies within different populations.[149] However, tau elevation is a nonspecific marker, as it is also observed in a number of other disease states including PD, as described earlier. Because tau contains over 30 phosphorylation sites, which have been posited to be modified in different combinations in different pathological states, measuring specific phosphorylated forms of tau has been proposed to provide better disease specificity. Phosphorylation of many of these sites can be modified by inflammation within the CNS, and thus measuring these specific tau phosphorylation sites might, in part, reflect disease-specific inflammatory signatures. Aβ has also been used as a biomarker for AD.[150] The Aß42 species is the most prone to aggregate, and when phagocytic cells are not able to effectively clear and break down these aggregates, levels of soluble Aß42 decrease. Indeed, AD patients have a lower concentration of Aß42 in their CSF.[150] Taken together, reduced CSF Aβ levels, along with increased CSF total tau levels, have led to a diagnostic accuracy of 94%.[151] While these protein species are not solely inflammation-related, inflammation and phagocytosis can alter their abundance within the CSF.

Other inflammation-related biomarkers have also been proposed for AD. Similar to PD, phagolysosomal dysfunction is implicated in AD pathogenesis and phagolysosome-related components have also been proposed as AD biomarkers. In a study of a number of lysosomal degradation molecules in CSF, significantly higher levels of EEA1, LAMP-1, LAMP-2, LC3, Rab3, and Rab4 were detected in patients diagnosed with AD compared to healthy controls.[152] Blood biomarkers are also of interest in AD, as recent studies suggest involvement of peripheral immune cells in AD pathogenesis.[18] Recently, one group studying plasma concentrations of various proteins in AD patients and healthy controls identified 18 proteins that were significantly altered in AD patients.[153] In concert with the work of several other groups, these findings provide evidence for potential diagnostic targets in the blood.[154]

CURRENT THERAPEUTIC APPROACHES TO NDDS

Immune-based therapies are an attractive treatment modality for NDDs because of the important role that inflammation plays in neurodegeneration, coupled with rapidly advancing technologies for manipulating the immune response. One of the major limitations to this approach, however, is the potential for undesirable off-target effects. Enhancing the immune response can lead to tissue damage, and even a small amount of tissue damage in the CNS is problematic. Alternatively, suppressing the immune response greatly increases the risk of infections, particularly in the elderly population, who are overrepresented in this group and may be partially immunocompromised for other reasons.

Though some NDDs have well understood pathophysiologic mechanisms and clear targets for therapeutic intervention, we still have much more to learn about the role of inflammation in these diseases. As such, multiple strategies have been attempted in the development of inflammation-related therapeutics for NDDs. Here we discuss some of these strategies in the context of multiple NDDs.

Multiple Sclerosis

In consideration of the multiple potential immune targets in multiple sclerosis, disease-modifying therapies (DMTs) have been designed to employ different strategies: modulating the immune system into a more anti-inflammatory state, preventing the entry of autoreactive immune cells into the CNS, eliminating specific immune cell populations, and generalized immunosuppression. The first published treatment for MS was adrenocorticoptrophic hormone (ACTH), used somewhat unsuccessfully in modulation of the chronic course[155] but more successfully in acute MS flares.[156] Along with the acceptance of high-dose

corticosteroids as the standard of care came the presumption that the efficacy of ACTH came from its corticotropic effects. This was borne out in later trials, which showed that corticosteroids were equally efficacious in a direct comparison with ACTH.[157,158] Oral administration has more recently gained favor as a practical and less expensive option.[159,160] The efficacy of these treatments suggests that general immunosuppression can improve MS, at least acutely.

However, an ideal therapy would also alter the chronic time course of MS pathology. The most common form of MS is the relapsing remitting form, where pathological flares occur, but patients often return to baseline throughout the disease course. However, as more relapses occur, disease may progress to the point where patients are no longer able to return to baseline function. Thus, it becomes important to prevent those relapses and hopefully prevent or delay progression. The FDA approved interferon ß-1b as the first DMT in 1993, with other interferons (IFNs) being approved in 1996 (ß-1a), 2002 (ß-1a), and 2009 (ß-1b). Their efficacy was shown in several landmark trials.[161–163]

Disruption of the BBB at sites of active lesions permits the migration of peripheral immune cells into the CNS. These immune cells secrete proinflammatory mediators, which are ultimately myelinotoxic. Thus, therapies that reduce inflammation within these cells could provide therapeutic benefit. IFNß-1a has been shown to enhance the production of anti-inflammatory cytokines. In an *ex vivo* study by Kozovska et al.,[164] production of the anti-inflammatory cytokine IL-10 was significantly enhanced in IFNß-1a treated cultures. The same was shown in immune cells isolated from human blood.[165] Two clinical studies of patients treated with IFNß-1a showed an increased production of CD56bright NK cells, producers of IL-10 and other anti-inflammatory cytokines.[166–167] Other studies have shown a decrease in production of the pro-inflammatory IL-17[168] and TNF-α.[169] Taken together, there seems to be no specific target responsible for the therapeutic benefit of IFNß-1a, but rather a reduction in several inflammation-related pathways.

More recently, an interferon with a polyethylene glycol (PEG) molecule attached has been shown to be efficacious.[170] The PEGylated form extends the biological activity of the compound and thus allows patients to decrease the frequency of administration to biweekly.[171]

While attempting to generate synthetic polypeptides with a similar amino acid structure to myelin basic protein (MBP) in order to induce experimental autoimmune encephalomyelities (EAE), Teitelbaum and colleagues serendipitously created Copolymer 1, a composite of L-alanine, L-lysine, L-glutamic acid, and L-tyrosine, which instead improved EAE outcomes.[172] It was later formulated as glatiramer acetate (GA), and once proven efficacious in the REGARD and BEYOND trials,[173,174] was marketed for patient use.

In vitro studies of antigen presenting cells (APCs) in human and murine models showed that GA binds preferentially with MHC class II molecules, even displacing other binding partners. This competitive activity prevents the presentation of other antigens and blocks subsequent T-cell activation.[175] This generates an anti-inflammatory response, as demonstrated by Vieira and colleagues,[176] which showed that APCs from GA-treated MS patients produced less TNF-α, IL-12, and IL-10 compared to untreated controls. GA treatment might also reduce T cell activation through upregulating an anti-inflammatory T cell subset called Tregs. Pretreatment of mice with GA, before EAE induction, results in increased Treg numbers that are more efficacious at delaying EAE induction compared to Tregs isolated from untreated mice.[177]

Natalizumab (Tysabri) was proven efficacious with the AFFIRM[178] and SENTINEL[179] trials. It is a humanized monoclonal antibody that selectively targets the α4 subunit of the cell adhesion molecule very late antigen 4 (VLA4) expressed on the surface of lymphocytes and monocytes.[180] It prevents the interaction between the VLA4 integrin and its ligand vascular cell adhesion molecule-1 (VCAM-1) on the brain vascular endothelium. This interaction is necessary for the transmigration of immune cells across the BBB. Thus, treatment with natalizumab prevents circulating peripheral immune cells from entering the CNS and triggering acute MS lesions.

Alemtuzumab (Lemtrada) is the most recently approved DMT, approved in 2014 after the CARE-MS I[181] and CARE-MS II[181] trials showed efficacy. It is also a humanized monoclonal antibody that binds to CD52, a cell surface glycoprotein present on all T and B lymphocytes, monocytes, and eosinophils. B cell numbers recover within 3 months, though the proportion of memory B cells are significantly depleted.[182] In contrast, T cells are suppressed for 20 months or longer.[183] Without a significant T cell population, they are unable to induce significant damage.

Fingolimod (Gilenya) was approved in 2010 after the TRANSFORMS,[184] FREEDOMS,[185] and FREEDOMS II[170] trials. It is a sphingosine-1-phosphate (S1P) functional antagonist, binding to four of the five S1P receptor subtypes. Fingolimod interferes with a key S1P mechanism that lymphocytes use to exit lymph nodes.[186] Once trapped in the lymph nodes, they are unable to enter the CNS to induce MS lesions. Since they are effectively removed from the circulation, mild lymphopenia is the chief side effect.

Teriflunomide (Aubagio) was approved in 2012 after success in the TEMSO[187] trial. It is an inhibitor of dihydroorotate dehydrogenase, an enzyme required for de novo pyrimidine synthesis in proliferating cells. This resource-limited state means that lymphocytes cannot effectively proliferate and promote disease progression.[188]

Dimethyl fumarate (Tecfidera) was approved in 2013 after the DEFINE[189] and CONFIRM[181] trials showed efficacy. Though the mechanism is unclear, it is believed that it gets hydrolyzed into monomethyl fumarate in the gut and activates the nuclear-related factor 2 transcriptional pathway, downstream of which is a reduction in oxidative cell stress, and modulates nuclear factor κB, which could have generalized anti-inflammatory effects.[190,191]

Other neuroinflammation-related drugs are under clinical investigation for multiple sclerosis. Daclizumab and ocrelizumab are presently in late stage III clinical trials. Daclizumab, a humanized monoclonal antibody that binds to CD25, the alpha subunit of the IL-2 receptor as monotherapy has shown efficacy in reducing annualized relapse rate compared to both placebo[192] and IFNß-1a.[193] Though a discrete mechanism is yet to be elucidated, it is interesting to note that one of the proposed pathways is the proliferation and enhanced function of CD56bright NK cells, similar to that of its comparator, IFNß-1a.[194] Ocrelizumab, a CD20 inhibitor, has shown some efficacy and safety in phase two trials and is currently under phase three investigation.[195] B cells are potent activators of proinflammatory T cells and producers of proinflammatory cytokines. By a complement-dependent lysis or apoptosis via cross-linking of CD20, the phosphoprotein selectively expressed on B lymphocytes, ocrelizumab may deplete this immunogenic population thereby reducing inflammation and disease progression.[196]

Although conceptually attractive because of the promise that two mechanistically distinct therapies may have greater efficacy than either alone, there have been few successful large trials using combination therapies. The largest and longest duration combination therapy study, CombiRx, compared IFNß-1a plus placebo injections and GA plus placebo injections. Combination IFN+GA was not superior to the better of the single agents (GA) in risk of relapse. Both the combination therapy and GA were significantly better than IFN in reducing the risk of relapse.[197] Though trials are continuing with multiple DMTs, or with adjuvants like statins or other immuno-modulators like intravenous immunoglobulin or corticosteroids, current practice is best described as sequential monotherapy.

Alzheimer's Disease

While DMTs exist for MS, few options are available for other NDDs. However, neuroinflammation-based therapeutics could be good candidates. Some of the drug targets address the neuroin-flammatory pathways discussed earlier. These therapies include NSAIDs, which dampen the inflammatory response in both central and peripheral arms of the immune system, and nuclear receptor agonists, which modify myeloid cell phenotypes. Some of these drugs instead take advantage of the immune system and its ability to target and clear immune stimuli from the brain and body. These therapeutic strategies involve active vaccination against or monoclonal antibodies that recognize disease-related epitopes. Together, these immune-targeted therapies represent novel therapeutic strategies for many of the neurodegenerative diseases discussed in this chapter and may provide benefit in multiple disease contexts.

NSAIDs

Epidemiological data provided the first clue that NSAIDs might be useful AD therapeutics. Patients who reported long-term NSAID use were less likely to develop AD, and if they did develop the disease, had slower disease progression.[198] It is known that NSAIDs reduce inflammation in the periphery through inhibition of COX-1 and COX-2 activity and enhancing PPAR-γ activation. Further preclinical data showed that, in addition to reducing inflammation in peripheral immune cells, NSAID administration to AD mouse models reduces microglial activation.[199] It is this central modification in microglial phenotype that is proposed to underlie beneficial effects of NSAIDs in AD.

Since then, several prospective clinical trials have been designed to assess the efficacy of NSAIDs in treating AD. The non-selective NSAIDs, indomethacin and ibuprofen, were both shown to decrease Aß in AD mouse models.[200] Indomethacin was found to be protective against cognitive decline in a small cohort of patients with mild to moderate AD.[201] Ibuprofen is currently in a phase III trial for patients with mild AD. However, no significant improvements were seen in clinical trials with the COX-selective NSAIDs rofecoxib and naproxen.[202] An important caveat is that these studies enrolled patients with mild to moderate AD, and it has since been suggested that reducing inflammation could be of greater benefit in patients who are presymptomatic.

The ADAPT study was designed to address that hypothesis, treating patients before the development of AD symptoms and assessing the ability of NSAIDs to prevent AD development.[203] Presymptomatic patients were treated with the COX-selective naproxen and the COX-2 selective celecoxib. Unfortunately, the trial had to be discontinued due to adverse events related to cardiovascular toxicity of these drugs. It has also since been shown that NSAID efficacy in preclinical models is not dependent on how potently they inhibit COX-1 or COX-2. Thus, perhaps treatment with less selective NSAIDs would reduce the likelihood of these adverse events and, based on preclinical models, would be more likely to provide clinical benefits.

Nuclear Receptor Agonists

Nuclear receptors are intracellular receptors that, when bound to their ligand, alter transcriptional programs within the cell. Several of these receptor families—PPARs, LXRs, and RXRs—have transcriptional targets that are involved in the regulation of myeloid cell phenotypes. In preclinical models, agonists to these receptors reduce production of inflammatory cytokines and promote phagocytosis.[204] As discussed earlier, the PPAR-γ receptor is also targeted by non-selective NSAIDs, and some have posited that NSAID action on this nuclear receptor may be responsible for some of its beneficial effects. Specific nuclear receptor agonists have also been studied in clinical trials. The PPAR-γ agonist pioglitazone is currently in clinical trials for patients with mild to moderate AD. LXR agonists are also promising candidates to move into clinical trials based on reduced inflammatory responses and improved pathology and performance in cognitive and memory-related behavioral tasks upon agonist treatment of AD mouse models. The RXR agonist bexarotene activates both the PPAR and LXR pathways and is another promising candidate currently in clinical trials.

Statins

Statins are a widely used class of drugs for the treatment of cardiovascular disease. They have also been shown to reduce antigen presentation by myeloid cells, decrease leukocyte trafficking across the BBB, and reduce pro-inflammatory cytokine production.[205] While these properties have been best studied in preclinical models of MS, many of these actions would also be relevant to AD pathology. Epidemiological studies show that use of statins in older individuals is correlated with a decrease in AD prevalence.[206] A small, prospective trial using atorvastatin showed some protection against cognitive decline in patients with mild to moderate AD, and large, phase III trials are now ongoing to assess the effectiveness of atorvastatin and simvastatin for AD treatment. There is also an ongoing phase IV trial with a combination therapy of lovastatin and ibuprofen.

Vaccines

Instead of altering immune cell function, some drugs can be used to co-opt immune cells to ameliorate pathology. The first strategy that was used to do this were vaccinations against the Aß peptide. Aß-targeted vaccines proved very successful at plaque clearance and prevention of plaque development in AD mouse models.[207] The first clinical trial of Aß vaccination resulted in meningoencephalitis in some immunized patients and was stopped prematurely.[208] However, responders to the vaccine did show reduced amyloid pathology at autopsy, suggesting that the vaccine may have had some efficacy.[209] The adverse events in this trial were thought to be mediated by T cells, so future iterations of Aß vaccines are being developed against epitopes selective for B cells to reduce possible adverse events. Currently there is a plaque-specific Aß-directed antibody with encouraging phase I results in clinical trials. New strategies are also being developed to target tau epitopes in novel vaccination therapy designs.

Aß-Directed Monoclonal Antibodies

An alternative solution to active immunization is passive immunization through the administration of Aß-directed monoclonal antibodies. The first Aß-directed monoclonal antibodies developed were N-terminus directed, like its vaccine precursors. One of these antibodies, bapineuzamab, was shown *in vitro* to bind Aß monomers as well as multimeric and fibrillar species.[210] However, due to significant edema, the dosage was decreased for phase III clinical trials. Despite this lower dose, patients administered bapineuzemab still had significant reductions in amyloid by PET imaging and a reduction in aggregation-prone hyperphosphorylated tau species in their CSF. However, there was no significant cognitive improvement in these patients. To circumvent the safety concerns with induction of edema at higher dosing concentrations, antibodies are currently being developed that have lower affinity IgG components in hope that a weaker interaction between the antibody and effector cells might reduce unwanted side effects. Potential success remains unclear, as using a weaker IgG effector subtype has been shown to decrease Aß clearance in response to monoclonal antibody administration in AD mouse models.[211]

The second Aß-directed monoclonal antibody designed was solanezumab, which is directed toward residues in the middle of the Aß peptide and was shown to primarily bind monomeric Aß species. The difference in affinity for different Aß species resulted in no vascular edema, so it could be given at a substantially higher dose than the previous monoclonal antibodies. In phase III trials, solanezumab administration resulted in a significant reduction in the rate of cognitive decline in patients with mild AD, but provided no benefit to patients with moderate AD. Solanezumab is currently being used in a large trial enrolling patients only with mild AD and is being given to asymptomatic individuals who harbor genetic mutations that cause or confer high risk for developing AD in prevention trials. The hope is that earlier administration of the drug will provide greater benefit for preventing or slowing progression of the disease.

Monoclonal antibodies have also been designed that target the C-terminus of Aß. In mouse models, these antibodies were shown to selectively bind to a low-abundance modified form of Aß called pyroGlu Aß. Previous studies have shown that this species can act as a strong seed for aggregation of other Aß species. So, while these antibodies would not promote Aß clearance as globally as those directed against the N-terminus or middle of the Aß peptide, it might prevent these species from aggregating within the brain. Indeed, this antibody has been shown to decrease Aß levels in an AD mouse model.[212]

Alzheimer's Disease Genetics and Novel Therapeutic Targets

Several of the recently identified risk factors for Alzheimer's disease have been genes involved in immune-related pathways.[213] These genetic studies have demonstrated that altered function of these immune-related risk factors can modify disease pathogenesis. Thus, genetic risk factors such as TREM2, CD33, and CR1 have provided novel therapeutic targets. Studies have also suggested that some of these targets, including TREM2 and CD33, might play important roles in peripheral immune cell populations.[18,214] This means that therapeutics targeting these receptors may not need to cross the BBB, a major impediment to development of many AD therapeutics. While inhibitors and activators of these different cellular components are being developed, we need to expand our basic knowledge of the function of these new genetic risk factors and how they contribute to different aspects of AD pathology. However, these may provide important and specific neuroinflammation-related targets for the next generation of AD therapeutics.

Huntington's Disease

Semaphorins are a family of transmembrane proteins that influence many downstream effects, including the immune response.[215]. Semaphorin 4D (SEMA4D) is expressed on infiltrating immune cells, while its receptors are expressed on resident CNS cell types.[216] Agonism leads to immune cell activation and migration. Thus, an antibody against SEMA4D could suppress the immune response. This could be particularly useful in Huntington's disease where SEMA4D expression is elevated in the cortex of HD brains.[217] In the YAC128 mouse model of HD, anti-SEMA4D monoclonal antibodies were injected weekly from 6 weeks of age and were evaluated at 6 and 12 month time points. Ultimately, treatment minimized cortical atrophy and improved cognitive deficits, but had no effect on motor function.

Another well-established pathogenic mechanism underlying HD is the overactivation of the innate immune system by mHTT, mediated through NFκB.[218,219] Laquinimod has been shown to mitigate NFκB activation in astrocytes[220] and may prove useful.

Lastly, CB2 cannabinoid receptors are anti-inflammatory receptors expressed in microglia and peripheral immune cells that have been implicated in HD pathology. CB2 levels are increased in postmortem HD brains. Treatment with an agonist, GW405833, ameliorated pathology and prolonged survival in mice, whereas treatment with an antagonist reversed those effects.[221]

Amyotrophic Lateral Sclerosis

Riluzole is the only approved therapy for ALS, acting by dampening glutamate excitotoxicity, though the benefit is marginal. Immune-based therapies may prove more effective. With the discovery of *Sod1* as the primary mutation found in familial ALS, therapeutic development has been largely targeted against that gene. Though *Sod1* mutations represent only 10% of all familial ALS cases, SOD1 function has also been implicated in sporadic cases,[222] suggesting that it may be a more broadly applicable therapeutic target.

Oxidative stress and the progressive accumulation of reactive oxygen species, as a consequence of *Sod1* mutations, are major contributing factors to the progression of ALS. It stands to reason, then, that targeting this enzyme could be protective. A mouse monoclonal antibody against SOD1, infused intracerebroventricularly, was shown to reduce the levels of toxic SOD1 species in the spinal cord and extended the life span of ALS model mice.[223]

Other immunomodulators have been tried recently, but stalled when attempting to translate to clinical trials. These include minocycline, a tetracycline antibiotic, which decreases the ability of T cells to contact microglia and subsequently impairs their production of cytokines;[224] thalidomide and lenalidomide, which modulate the production of inflammatory cytokines TNF- α, Il-1, IL-6, IL10, and IL-12;[225,226] celecoxib, an NSAID which, as described earlier, results in reduced production of inflammatory prostaglandins;[227] and the anti-diabetic drug pioglitazone, which also decreases production of pro-inflammatory cytokines.[228] While these drugs have not made it into clinical trials, there are certainly many immunomodulatory candidates for future ALS therapeutics.

Parkinson's Disease

PD is a chronic, progressive disease characterized by significant pathological change prior to symptom onset. Several studies have failed to show efficacy in human trials, likely because of the extensive pathologic burden at time of diagnosis. As biomarkers of early disease are discovered and more immune pathways are elucidated, DMTs may prove to be beneficial.

The most straightforward and promising target for PD is α-synuclein (α-syn), the toxic accumulation of which is the pathologic hallmark of PD. Passive immunization with anti-α-syn antibodies in mouse models has been investigated. In mice expressing human α-syn, administration of an anti-α-synuclein antibody improves behavioral performance and promoted degradation of accumulated α-synuclein.[229,230] Clearance of α-synuclein is thought to occur via uptake by surrounding microglia. A second monoclonal antibody has also been shown to block the intercellular transmission of α-syn pathology and resulted in decreased levels of α-syn, preserved dopaminergic cell numbers, and improved motor function.[231]

Active immunization is an alternative approach.[232] A vaccine composed of short immunogenic peptides that mimic the C-terminus of α-syn (PD01A) with adjuvant was injected into two different transgenic PD mouse models. Vaccination yielded high antibody titers in CSF and plasma, decreased accumulation of α-syn oligomers, and improved motor and memory deficits.

Glatiramer acetate, the copolymer used in the treatment of MS, has also been tried as a PD therapeutic. Adoptive transfer of T cells from GA-immunized mice has been shown to reduce cell death in MPTP models of PD.[233] The adoptively transferred T cells accumulate in the substantia nigra and suppress microglial activation.[234] This suggests that suppression of T cell and ultimately myeloid cell activation could have neuroprotective benefits in PD.

CONCLUSION

In this chapter, we have presented a case for the involvement of neuroinflammation in the pathogenesis of NDDs. An important role of inflammation in disease pathology has been illustrated by the increasing number of inflammation-related risk factors, both genetic and environmental, for NDDs. The roles that neuroinflammation plays in mediating neurodegeneration are diverse, ranging from increasing oxidative stress, to aberrant phagocytosis, to promoting neuronal excitotoxicity. We discussed several of the mechanisms involved in communication between immune cells and other cells in the CNS. These interactions are important in the healthy brain and, when dysregulated in the context of NDDs, can cause altered activation of immune cells and neuronal death. We know that these mechanisms and cells are important in NDDs because inflammation-related biomarkers can be used to identify NDD patients, and inflammation-directed drugs have been shown to provide therapeutic benefit. In the coming chapters, you will see how these different immune-related mechanisms interact with other systems and pathways to alter the pathology and neurodegeneration of NDDs.

REFERENCES

1. Akira, S., Uematsu, S. & Takeuchi, O. Pathogen recognition and innate immunity. *Cell* **124**, 783–801, doi:10.1016/j.cell.2006.02.015 (2006).

2. Janeway, C. A., Jr., & Medzhitov, R. Innate immune recognition. *Annual Review of Immunology* **20**, 197–216, doi:10.1146/annurev.immunol.20.083001.084359 (2002).

3. Charo, I.F. & Ransohoff, R.M. Mechanisms of disease – the many roles of chemokines and cytokine receptors in inflammation. *New England Journal of Medicine* **354**, 610–621, doi:10.1056/NEJMra052723 (2006).

4. Ley, K., Laudanna, C., Cybulsky, M.I., & Nourshargh, S. Getting to the site of inflammation: the leukocyte adhesion cascade updated. *Nature Reviews Immunology* **7**, 678–689, doi:10.1038/nri2156 (2007).

5. Prinz, M. & Priller, J. Microglia and brain macrophages in the molecular age: from origin to neuropsychiatric disease. *Nature Reviews Neuroscience* **15**, 300–312, doi:10.1038/nrn3722 (2014).

6. Hirsch, E. C., & Hunot, S. Neuroinflammation in Parkinson's disease: a target for neuroprotection? *Lancet Neurol* **8**, 382–397, doi:10.1016/s1474-4422(09)70062-6 (2009).

7. Boillee, S. et al. Onset and progression in inherited ALS determined by motor neurons and microglia. *Science* **312**, 1389–1392, doi:10.1126/science.1123511 (2006).

8. Dimayuga, F.O. et al. SOD1 overexpression alters ROS production and reduces neurotoxic inflammatory signaling in microglial cells. *Journal of Neuroimmunology* **182**, 89–99, doi:10.1016/j.jneruoim.2006.10.003 (2007).

9. Crehan, H. et al. Complement receptor 1 (CR1) and Alzheimer's disease. *Immunobiology* **217**, 244–250, doi:10.1016/j.jimbio.2011.07.017 (2012).

10. Hecker, L. A., et al. Genetic control of the alternative pathway of complement in humans and age-related macular degeneration. *Human Molecular Genetics* **19**, 209–215, doi:10.1093/hmg/ddp472 (2010).

11. Day, A. J., Clark, S. J., & Bishop, P. N. Understanding the molecular basis of age-related macular degeneration and how the identification of new mechanisms may aid the development of novel therapies. *Expert Review of Ophthalmology* **6**, 123–128, doi:10.1586/eop.11.10 (2011).

12. Holmans, P., et al. A pathway-based analysis provides additional support for an immune-related genetic susceptibility to Parkinson's disease. *Human Molecular Genetics* **22**, 1039–1049, doi:10.1093/hmg/dds492 (2013).

13. Zhao, J., et al. Association of TLR4 gene polymorphisms with sporadic Parkinson's disease in a Han Chinese population. *Neurological Sciences: Official Journal of the Italian Neurological Society and of the Italian Society of Clinical Neurophysiology*

36, 1659–1665, doi:10.1007/s10072–015-2227–9 (2015).

14. Malik, M., et al. CD33 Alzheimer's risk-altering polymorphism, CD33 expression, and exon 2 splicing. *Journal of Neuroscience* **33**, 13320–13325, doi:10.1523/jneurosci.1224–13.2013 (2013).

15. Jiang, T. et al. CD33 in Alzheimer's Disease. *Molecular Neurobiology* **49**, 529–535, doi:10.1007/s12035–013-8536–1 (2014).

16. Lopez-Lopez, A., et al. CX3CR1 is a modifying gene of survival and progression in amyotrophic lateral sclerosis. *PloS One* **9**, e96528, doi:10.1371/journal.pone.0096528 (2014).

17. Lill, C.M. et al. The role of TREM2 R47H as a risk factor for Alzheimer's disease, Frontotemporal lobar dementia, Amyotrophic lateral sclerosis and Parkinson's disease. *Alzheimer's and Dementia* **11**, 1407–1416, doi:10.1016/j.jalz.2014.12.009 (2015).

18. Jay, T. R., et al. TREM2 deficiency eliminates TREM2+ inflammatory macrophages and ameliorates pathology in Alzheimer's disease mouse models. *The Journal of Experimental Medicine* **212**, 287–295, doi:10.1084/jem.20142322 (2015).

19. Bashinskaya, V. V., Kulakova, O. G., Boyko, A. N., Favorov, A. V., & Favorova, O. O. A review of genome-wide association studies for multiple sclerosis: classical and hypothesis-driven approaches. *Human Genetics* **134**, 1143–1162, doi:10.1007/s00439–015-1601–2 (2015).

20. Hamza, T. H., et al. Common genetic variation in the HLA region is associated with late-onset sporadic Parkinson's disease. *Nature Genetics* **42**, 781–785, doi:10.1038/ng.642 (2010).

21. Ban, M. et al. Replication analysis identified TKY2 as a multiple sclerosis suceptibility factor. *European Journal of Human Genetics* **17**, 1309–1313, doi:10.1038/ejhg.2009.41 (2009).

22. Levin, L. I., et al. Multiple sclerosis and Epstein-Barr virus. *Journal of the American Medical Association* **289**, 1533–1536, doi:10.1001/jama.289.12.1533 (2003).

23. Buljevac, D., et al. Prospective study on the relationship between infections and multiple sclerosis exacerbations. *Brain: A Journal of Neurology* **125**, 952–960 (2002).

24. Shoji, H., Watanabe, M., Itoh, S., Kuwahara, H., & Hattori, F. Japanese encephalitis and parkinsonism. *Journal of Neurology* **240**, 59–60 (1993).

25. Bialecka, M., et al. Polymorphisms of catechol-0-methyltransferase (COMT), monoamine oxidase B (MAOB), N-acetyltransferase 2 (NAT2) and cytochrome P450 2D6 (CYP2D6) gene in patients with early onset of Parkinson's disease. *Parkinsonism & Related Disorders* **13**, 224–229, doi:10.1016/j.parkreldis.2006.10.006 (2007).

26. Dobbs, R. J., Charlett, A., Dobbs, S. M., Weller, C., & Peterson, D. W. Parkinsonism: differential age-trend in Helicobacter pylori antibody. *Alimentary Pharmacology & Therapeutics* **14**, 1199–1205 (2000).

27. Ling, Z., et al. In utero bacterial endotoxin exposure causes loss of tyrosine hydroxylase neurons in the postnatal rat midbrain. *Movement Disorders: Official Journal of the Movement Disorder Society* **17**, 116–124 (2002).

28. de la Torre, J. C. Alzheimer disease as a vascular disorder: nosological evidence. *Stroke: A Journal of Cerebral Circulation* **33**, 1152–1162 (2002).

29. Snowdon, D. A. Healthy aging and dementia: findings from the Nun Study. *Annals of Internal Medicine* **139**, 450–454 (2003).

30. Hayes, C. E., Nashold, F. E., Spach, K. M., & Pedersen, L. B. The immunological functions of the vitamin D endocrine system. *Cellular and Molecular Biology (Noisy-le-Grand, France)* **49**, 277–300 (2003).

31. Ghadirian, P., Dadgostar, B., Azani, R., & Maisonneuve, P. A case-control study of the association between socio-demographic, lifestyle and medical history factors and multiple sclerosis. *Canadian Journal of Public Health / Revue canadienne de sante publique* **92**, 281–285 (2001).

32. Khan, J. C., et al. Smoking and age related macular degeneration: the number of pack years of cigarette smoking is a major determinant of risk for both geographic atrophy and choroidal neovascularisation. *The British Journal of Ophthalmology* **90**, 75–80, doi:10.1136/bjo.2005.073643 (2006).

33. Kew, R. R., Ghebrehiwet, B., & Janoff, A. Cigarette smoke can activate the alternative pathway of complement in vitro by modifying the third component of complement. *Journal of Clinical Investigation* **75**, 1000–1007, doi:10.1172/jci111760 (1985).

34. Wang, A. L., et al. Changes in retinal pigment epithelium related to cigarette smoke: possible relevance to smoking as a risk factor for age-related macular degeneration. *PloS One* **4**, e5304, doi:10.1371/journal.pone.0005304 (2009).

35. Baron, J. A. Cigarette smoking and Parkinson's disease. *Neurology* **36**, 1490–1496 (1986).

36. Van Den Heuvel, C., Thornton, E., & Vink, R. Traumatic brain injury and Alzheimer's disease: a review. *Progress in Brain Research* **161**, 303–316, doi:10.1016/s0079–6123(06)61021–2 (2007).

37. Goldman, S. M., et al. Head injury and Parkinson's disease risk in twins. *Annals of Neurology* **60**, 65–72, doi:10.1002/ana.20882 (2006).

38. Prigione, A., et al. Oxidative stress in peripheral blood mononuclear cells from patients with Parkinson's disease: negative correlation with

levodopa dosage. *Neurobiology of Disease* **23**, 36–43, doi:10.1016/j.nbd.2006.01.013 (2006).

39. Hunot, S., et al. Nitric oxide synthase and neuronal vulnerability in Parkinson's disease. *Neuroscience* **72**, 355–363 (1996).

40. Peterson, L. J., & Flood, P. M. Oxidative stress and microglial cells in Parkinson's disease. *Mediators of Inflammation* **2012**, 401264, doi:10.1155/2012/401264 (2012).

41. Wilms, H., et al. Activation of microglia by human neuromelanin is NF-kappaB dependent and involves p38 mitogen-activated protein kinase: implications for Parkinson's disease. *FASEB Journal: Official Publication of the Federation of American Societies for Experimental Biology* **17**, 500–502, doi:10.1096/fj.02–0314fje (2003).

42. Zecca, L., et al. Human neuromelanin induces neuroinflammation and neurodegeneration in the rat substantia nigra: implications for Parkinson's disease. *Acta Neuropathologica* **116**, 47–55, doi:10.1007/s00401–008-0361–7 (2008).

43. McGeer, P. L., & McGeer, E. G. Glial cell reactions in neurodegenerative diseases: pathophysiology and therapeutic interventions. *Alzheimer Disease and Associated Disorders* **12 Suppl 2**, S1–6 (1998).

44. Liberatore, G. T., et al. Inducible nitric oxide synthase stimulates dopaminergic neurodegeneration in the MPTP model of Parkinson disease. *Nature Medicine* **5**, 1403–1409, doi:10.1038/70978 (1999).

45. Kurkowska-Jastrzebska, I., et al. Dexamethasone protects against dopaminergic neurons damage in a mouse model of Parkinson's disease. *International Immunopharmacology* **4**, 1307–1318, doi:10.1016/j.intimp.2004.05.006 (2004).

46. Carrasco, E., & Werner, P. Selective destruction of dopaminergic neurons by low concentrations of 6-OHDA and MPP+: protection by acetylsalicylic acid aspirin. *Parkinsonism & Related Disorders* **8**, 407–411 (2002).

47. Wu, D. C., et al. Blockade of microglial activation is neuroprotective in the 1-methyl-4-phenyl-1,2,3,6-tetrahydropyridine mouse model of Parkinson disease. *Journal of Neuroscience* **22**, 1763–1771 (2002).

48. Herrera, A. J., Castano, A., Venero, J. L., Cano, J., & Machado, A. The single intranigral injection of LPS as a new model for studying the selective effects of inflammatory reactions on dopaminergic system. *Neurobiology of Disease* **7**, 429–447, doi:10.1006/nbdi.2000.0289 (2000).

49. Kim, W. G., et al. Regional difference in susceptibility to lipopolysaccharide-induced neurotoxicity in the rat brain: role of microglia. *Journal of Neuroscience* **20**, 6309–6316 (2000).

50. Weydt, P., Yuen, E. C., Ransom, B. R., & Moller, T. Increased cytotoxic potential of microglia from ALS-transgenic mice. *Glia* **48**, 179–182, doi:10.1002/glia.20062 (2004).

51. Lino, M. M., Schneider, C., & Caroni, P. Accumulation of SOD1 mutants in postnatal motoneurons does not cause motoneuron pathology or motoneuron disease. *Journal of Neuroscience* **22**, 4825–4832 (2002).

52. Pramatarova, A., Laganiere, J., Roussel, J., Brisebois, K., & Rouleau, G. A. Neuron-specific expression of mutant superoxide dismutase 1 in transgenic mice does not lead to motor impairment. *Journal of Neuroscience* **21**, 3369–3374 (2001).

53. Beers, D. R., et al. Wild-type microglia extend survival in PU.1 knockout mice with familial amyotrophic lateral sclerosis. *Proceedings of the National Academy of Sciences of the United States of America* **103**, 16021–16026, doi:10.1073/pnas.0607423103 (2006).

54. Lue, L.F. et al. Inflammatory repertoire of Alzheimer's disease and nondemented elderly microglia in vitro. *Glia* **35**, 72–79, doi:10.1002/glia.1072 (2001).

55. Shaftel, S. S., et al. Chronic interleukin-1beta expression in mouse brain leads to leukocyte infiltration and neutrophil-independent blood brain barrier permeability without overt neurodegeneration. *Journal of Neuroscience* **27**, 9301–9309, doi:10.1523/jneurosci.1418–07.2007 (2007).

56. Chakrabarty, P., et al. Massive gliosis induced by interleukin-6 suppresses Abeta deposition in vivo: evidence against inflammation as a driving force for amyloid deposition. *FASEB Journal: Official Publication of the Federation of American Societies for Experimental Biology* **24**, 548–559, doi:10.1096/fj.09–141754 (2010).

57. Lee, S., et al. CX3CR1 deficiency alters microglial activation and reduces beta-amyloid deposition in two Alzheimer's disease mouse models. *The American Journal of Pathology* **177**, 2549–2562, doi:10.2353/ajpath.2010.100265 (2010).

58. Lee, S., et al. Opposing effects of membrane-anchored CX3CL1 on amyloid and tau pathologies via the p38 MAPK pathway. *Journal of Neuroscience* **34**, 12538–12546, doi:10.1523/JNEUROSCI.0853–14.2014 (2014).

59. Combs, C. K., Bates, P., Karlo, J. C., & Landreth, G. E. Regulation of beta-amyloid stimulated proinflammatory responses by peroxisome proliferator-activated receptor alpha.

Neurochemistry International **39**, 449–457 (2001).

60. Edison, P., et al. Microglia, amyloid, and cognition in Alzheimer's disease: an [11C](R)PK11195-PET and [11C]PIB-PET study. *Neurobiology of Disease* **32**, 412–419, doi:10.1016/j.nbd.2008.08.001 (2008).

61. Bianca, V. D., Dusi, S., Bianchini, E., Dal Pra, I., & Rossi, F. beta-amyloid activates the O-2 forming NADPH oxidase in microglia, monocytes, and neutrophils: a possible inflammatory mechanism of neuronal damage in Alzheimer's disease. *The Journal of Biological Chemistry* **274**, 15493–15499 (1999).

62. Shimohama, S., et al. Activation of NADPH oxidase in Alzheimer's disease brains. *Biochemical and Biophysical Research Communications* **273**, 5–9, doi:10.1006/bbrc.2000.2897 (2000).

63. Qin, L., et al. Microglia enhance beta-amyloid peptide-induced toxicity in cortical and mesencephalic neurons by producing reactive oxygen species. *Journal of Neurochemistry* **83**, 973–983 (2002).

64. Schafer, D. P., & Stevens, B. Phagocytic glial cells: sculpting synaptic circuits in the developing nervous system. *Current Opinion in Neurobiology* **23**, 1034–1040, doi:10.1016/j.conb.2013.09.012 (2013).

65. Yasojima, K., Schwab, C., McGeer, E. G., & McGeer, P. L. Up-regulated production and activation of the complement system in Alzheimer's disease brain. *The American Journal of Pathology* **154**, 927–936, doi:10.1016/s0002-9440(10)65340-0 (1999).

66. Ringman, J. M., et al. Proteomic changes in cerebrospinal fluid of presymptomatic and affected persons carrying familial Alzheimer disease mutations. *Archives of Neurology* **69**, 96–104, doi:10.1001/archneurol.2011.642 (2012).

67. Jun, G., et al. Meta-analysis confirms CR1, CLU, and PICALM as alzheimer disease risk loci and reveals interactions with APOE genotypes. *Archives of Neurology* **67**, 1473–1484, doi:10.1001/archneurol.2010.201 (2010).

68. Chibnik, L. B., et al. CR1 is associated with amyloid plaque burden and age-related cognitive decline. *Annals of Neurology* **69**, 560–569, doi:10.1002/ana.22277 (2011).

69. Fonseca, M. I., Zhou, J., Botto, M., & Tenner, A. J. Absence of C1q leads to less neuropathology in transgenic mouse models of Alzheimer's disease. *Journal of Neuroscience* **24**, 6457–6465, doi:10.1523/jneurosci.0901–04.2004 (2004).

70. Wyss-Coray, T., et al. Prominent neurodegeneration and increased plaque formation in complement-inhibited Alzheimer's mice. *Proceedings of the National Academy of Sciences of the United States of America* **99**, 10837–10842, doi:10.1073/pnas.162350199 (2002).

71. Maier, M., et al. Complement C3 deficiency leads to accelerated amyloid beta plaque deposition and neurodegeneration and modulation of the microglia/macrophage phenotype in amyloid precursor protein transgenic mice. *Journal of Neuroscience* **28**, 6333–6341, doi:10.1523/jneurosci.0829–08.2008 (2008).

72. Stevens, B., et al. The classical complement cascade mediates CNS synapse elimination. *Cell* **131**, 1164–1178, doi:10.1016/j.cell.2007.10.036 (2007).

73. Howell, G. R., et al. Molecular clustering identifies complement and endothelin induction as early events in a mouse model of glaucoma. *Journal of Clinical Investigation* **121**, 1429–1444, doi:10.1172/jci44646 (2011).

74. Lukiw, W. J., Zhao, Y., & Cui, J. G. An NF-kappaB-sensitive micro RNA-146a-mediated inflammatory circuit in Alzheimer disease and in stressed human brain cells. *The Journal of Biological Chemistry* **283**, 31315–31322, doi:10.1074/jbc.M805371200 (2008).

75. Lukiw, W. J., Surjyadipta, B., Dua, P., & Alexandrov, P. N. Common micro RNAs (miRNAs) target complement factor H (CFH) regulation in Alzheimer's disease (AD) and in age-related macular degeneration (AMD). *International Journal of Biochemistry and Molecular Biology* **3**, 105–116 (2012).

76. Mandrekar, S., et al. Microglia mediate the clearance of soluble Abeta through fluid phase macropinocytosis. *Journal of Neuroscience* **29**, 4252–4262, doi:10.1523/jneurosci.5572–08.2009 (2009).

77. Koenigsknecht, J., & Landreth, G. Microglial phagocytosis of fibrillar beta-amyloid through a beta1 integrin-dependent mechanism. *Journal of Neuroscience* **24**, 9838–9846, doi:10.1523/jneurosci.2557–04.2004 (2004).

78. Frackowiak, J., et al. Ultrastructure of the microglia that phagocytose amyloid and the microglia that produce beta-amyloid fibrils. *Acta Neuropathologica* **84**, 225–233 (1992).

79. Wisniewski, H. M., Barcikowska, M., & Kida, E. Phagocytosis of beta/A4 amyloid fibrils of the neuritic neocortical plaques. *Acta Neuropathologica* **81**, 588–590 (1991).

80. Wilhelmsson, U., et al. Absence of glial fibrillary acidic protein and vimentin prevents hypertrophy of astrocytic processes and improves post-traumatic regeneration. *Journal of Neuroscience* **24**, 5016–5021, doi:10.1523/JNEUROSCI.0820–04.2004 (2004).

81. Bolmont, T., et al. Dynamics of the microglial/amyloid interaction indicate a role in plaque maintenance. *Journal of Neuroscience* **28**, 4283–4292, doi:10.1523/jneurosci.4814-07.2008 (2008).

82. Paresce, D. M., Chung, H., & Maxfield, F. R. Slow degradation of aggregates of the Alzheimer's disease amyloid beta-protein by microglial cells. *The Journal of Biological Chemistry* **272**, 29390–29397 (1997).

83. Grathwohl, S. A., et al. Formation and maintenance of Alzheimer's disease beta-amyloid plaques in the absence of microglia. *Nature Neuroscience* **12**, 1361–1363, doi:10.1038/nn.2432 (2009).

84. Varvel, N. H., et al. Replacement of brain-resident myeloid cells does not alter cerebral amyloid-beta deposition in mouse models of Alzheimer's disease. *The Journal of Experimental Medicine* **212**, 1803–1809, doi:10.1084/jem.20150478 (2015).

85. Prokop, S., et al. Impact of peripheral myeloid cells on amyloid-beta pathology in Alzheimer's disease-like mice. *The Journal of Experimental Medicine* **212**, 1811–1818, doi:10.1084/jem.20150479 (2015).

86. Yamamoto, M., et al. Interferon-gamma and tumor necrosis factor-alpha regulate amyloid-beta plaque deposition and beta-secretase expression in Swedish mutant APP transgenic mice. *The American Journal of Pathology* **170**, 680–692, doi:10.2353/ajpath.2007.060378 (2007).

87. Rinner, W. A., Bauer, J., Schmidts, M., Lassmann, H., & Hickey, W. F. Resident microglia and hematogenous macrophages as phagocytes in adoptively transferred experimental autoimmune encephalomyelitis: an investigation using rat radiation bone marrow chimeras. *Glia* **14**, 257–266, doi:10.1002/glia.440140403 (1995).

88. Huizinga, R., et al. Phagocytosis of neuronal debris by microglia is associated with neuronal damage in multiple sclerosis. *Glia* **60**, 422–431, doi:10.1002/glia.22276 (2012).

89. Nikic, I., et al. A reversible form of axon damage in experimental autoimmune encephalomyelitis and multiple sclerosis. *Nature Medicine* **17**, 495–499, doi:10.1038/nm.2324 (2011).

90. Persson, M., Brantefjord, M., Hansson, E., & Ronnback, L. Lipopolysaccharide increases microglial GLT-1 expression and glutamate uptake capacity in vitro by a mechanism dependent on TNF-alpha. *Glia* **51**, 111–120, doi:10.1002/glia.20191 (2005).

91. van Weering, H.R. et al. CXCL10/CXCR3 signaling in glia cells differentially affects NMDA-induced cell death in CA and DG neurons of the mouse hippocampus. *Hippocampus* **21**, 220–232, doi:10.1002/hipo.20742 (2011).

92. Willard, L. B., Hauss-Wegrzyniak, B., Danysz, W., & Wenk, G. L. The cytotoxicity of chronic neuroinflammation upon basal forebrain cholinergic neurons of rats can be attenuated by glutamatergic antagonism or cyclooxygenase-2 inhibition. *Experimental Brain Research* **134**, 58–65 (2000).

93. Fine, S. M., et al. Tumor necrosis factor alpha inhibits glutamate uptake by primary human astrocytes. Implications for pathogenesis of HIV-1 dementia. *The Journal of Biological Chemistry* **271**, 15303–15306 (1996).

94. Rothstein, J. D., Van Kammen, M., Levey, A. I., Martin, L. J., & Kuncl, R. W. Selective loss of glial glutamate transporter GLT-1 in amyotrophic lateral sclerosis. *Annals of Neurology* **38**, 73–84, doi:10.1002/ana.410380114 (1995).

95. Bruijn, L. I., et al. ALS-linked SOD1 mutant G85R mediates damage to astrocytes and promotes rapidly progressive disease with SOD1-containing inclusions. *Neuron* **18**, 327–338 (1997).

96. Guo, H., et al. Increased expression of the glial glutamate transporter EAAT2 modulates excitotoxicity and delays the onset but not the outcome of ALS in mice. *Human Molecular Genetics* **12**, 2519–2532, doi:10.1093/hmg/ddg267 (2003).

97. Shaftel, S. S., et al. Sustained hippocampal IL-1 beta overexpression mediates chronic neuroinflammation and ameliorates Alzheimer plaque pathology. *Journal of Clinical Investigation* **117**, 1595–1604, doi:10.1172/jci31450 (2007).

98. Izikson, L., Klein, R. S., Charo, I. F., Weiner, H. L., & Luster, A. D. Resistance to experimental autoimmune encephalomyelitis in mice lacking the CC chemokine receptor (CCR)2. *The Journal of Experimental Medicine* **192**, 1075–1080 (2000).

99. Huang, D. R., Wang, J., Kivisakk, P., Rollins, B. J., & Ransohoff, R. M. Absence of monocyte chemoattractant protein 1 in mice leads to decreased local macrophage recruitment and antigen-specific T helper cell type 1 immune response in experimental autoimmune encephalomyelitis. *The Journal of Experimental Medicine* **193**, 713–726 (2001).

100. Carlson, T., Kroenke, M., Rao, P., Lane, T. E., & Segal, B. The Th17-ELR+ CXC chemokine pathway is essential for the development of central nervous system autoimmune disease. *The Journal of Experimental Medicine* **205**, 811–823, doi:10.1084/jem.20072404 (2008).

101. Bhaskar, K., et al. Regulation of tau pathology by the microglial fractalkine receptor. *Neuron* **68**, 19–31, doi:10.1016/j.neuron.2010.08.023 (2010).

102. Malm, T.M., Jay, T.R. & Landreth, G.E. The evolving biology of microglia in Alzheimer's disease. *Neurotherapeutics* **12**, 81–93, doi:10.1007/s13311-014-0316-8 (2015).

103. Koning, N., Swaab, D.F., Hoek, R.M. & Huitinga, I. Distribution of the immune inhibitory molecules CD200 and CD200R in the normal central nervous system and multiple sclerosis lesions suggests neuron-glia and glia-glia interactions. *Journal of Neuropathology and Experimental Neurology* **68**, 159–167, doi:10.1097/NEN.0b013e3181964113 (2009).

104. Hoek, R.M. et al. Down-regulation of the macrophage lineage through interaction with OX2 (CD200). *Science* **290**, 1768–1771, doi:10.1126/science.290.5497.1768 (2000).

105. Meuth, S.G., et al. CNS inflammation and neuronal degeneration is aggravated by impaired CD200-CD200R-mediated macrophage silencing. *Journal of Neuroimmunology* **194**, 62–69, doi:10.1016/j.neuroim.2007.11.013 (2008).

106. Wright, G.J., et al. Characterization of the CD200 receptor family in mice and humans and their interactions with CD200. *Journal of Immunology* **171**, 3034–3046, doi:10.4049/jimmunol.171.6.3034 (2003).

107. Walker, D.G., Dalsing-Hernandez, J.E., Campbell, N.A. & Lue, L.F. Decreased expression of CD200 and CD200 receptor in Alzheimer's disease: a potential mechanism leading to chronic inflammation. *Experimental Neurology* **215**, 5–19, doi:10.1016/j.expneurol.2008.09.003 (2009).

108. Lyons, A., et al. CD200 ligand receptor interaction modulates microglial activation in vivo and in vitro: a role for IL4. *Journal of Neuroscience* **27**, 8309–8313, doi:10.1523/jneurosci.1781-07.2007 (2007).

109. Linnartz, B., & Neumann, H. Microglial activatory (immunoreceptor tyrosine-based activation motif)-signaling receptors for recognition of the neuronal glycocalyx. *Glia* **61**, 37–46, doi: 10.1002/glia.22359 (2013).

110. Paul, S.P., Taylor, L.S., Stansbury, E.K., & McVicar, D.W. Myeloid specific human CD33 is an inhibitory receptor with differential ITIM function in recruiting the phosphatases SHP-1 and SHP-2. *Blood* **96**, 483–490 (2000).

111. Karch, C.M., et al. Expression of novel Alzheimer's disease risk genes in control and Alzheimer's disease brains. *PLoS One* **7**, e50976, doi:10.1371/journal.pone.0050976 (2012).

112. Griciuc, A., et al. Alzheimer's disease risk gene CD33 inhibits microglial uptake of amyloid beta. *Neuron* **78**, 631–643, doi:10.1016/j.neuron.2013.04.014 (2013).

113. Arduise, C., et al. Tetraspanins regulate ADAM10-mediated cleavage of TNF-alpha and epidermal growth factor. *Journal of Immunology (Baltimore, Md.: 1950)* **181**, 7002–7013 (2008).

114. Kim, M., et al. Potential late-onset Alzheimer's disease-associated mutations in the ADAM10 gene attenuate {alpha}-secretase activity. *Human Molecular Genetics* **18**, 3987–3996, doi:10.1093/hmg/ddp323 (2009).

115. Kleinberger, G., et al. TREM2 mutations implicated in neurodegeneration impair cell surface transport and phagocytosis. *Science Translational Medicine* **6**, 243ra86, doi:10.1126/scitranlmed.3009093 (2014).

116. Maeda, A., & Sobel, R. A. Matrix metalloproteinases in the normal human central nervous system, microglial nodules, and multiple sclerosis lesions. *Journal of Neuropathology and Experimental Neurology* **55**, 300–309 (1996).

117. Cossins, J. A., et al. Enhanced expression of MMP-7 and MMP-9 in demyelinating multiple sclerosis lesions. *Acta Neuropathologica* **94**, 590–598 (1997).

118. Brkic, M., Balusu, S., Libert, C., & Vandenbroucke, R. E. Friends or foes: matrix metalloproteinases and their multifaceted roles in neurodegenerative diseases. *Mediators of Inflammation* **2015**, 620581, doi:10.1155/2015/620581 (2015).

119. Shigemori, Y., Katayama, Y., Mori, T., Maeda, T. & Kawamata, T. Matrix metalloproteinase-9 is associated with blood-brain barrier opening and brain edema formation after cortical contusion in rats. *Acta Neurochirurgica. Supplement* **96**, 130–133 (2006).

120. Hadass, O., et al. Selective inhibition of matrix metalloproteinase-9 attenuates secondary damage resulting from severe traumatic brain injury. *PloS One* **8**, e76904, doi:10.1371/journal.pone.0076904 (2013).

121. Wang, X., Mori, T., Jung, J. C., Fini, M. E., & Lo, E. H. Secretion of matrix metalloproteinase-2 and -9 after mechanical trauma injury in rat cortical cultures and involvement of MAP kinase. *Journal of Neurotrauma* **19**, 615–625, doi:10.1089/089771502753754082 (2002).

122. Vilalta, A., et al. Brain contusions induce a strong local overexpression of MMP-9. Results of a pilot study. *Acta Neurochirurgica. Supplement* **102**, 415–419 (2008).

123. Dinkins, M. B., Dasgupta, S., Wang, G., Zhu, G., & Bieberich, E. Exosome reduction in vivo is associated with lower amyloid plaque load in the 5XFAD mouse model of Alzheimer's disease. *Neurobiology of Aging* **35**, 1792–1800, doi:10.1016/j.neurobiolaging.2014.02.012 (2014).

124. de Calignon, A., et al. Propagation of tau pathology in a model of early Alzheimer's disease. *Neuron* **73**, 685–697, doi:10.1016/j.neuron.2011.11.033 (2012).

125. Emmanouilidou, E., et al. Cell-produced α-synuclein is secreted in a calcium-dependent manner by exosomes and impacts neuronal survival. *Journal of Neuroscience* **30**, 6838–6851, doi:10.1523/jneurosci.5699–09.2010 (2010).

126. Gupta, A., & Pulliam, L. Exosomes as mediators of neuroinflammation. *Journal of Neuroinflammation* **11**, doi:Artn 6810.1186/1742-2094-11-68 (2014).

127. Parkhurst, Christopher N., et al. Microglia promote learning-dependent synapse formation through brain-derived neurotrophic factor. *Cell* **155**, 1596–1609, doi:10.106/j.cell.2013.11.030 (2013).

128. Phillips, H. S., et al. BDNF mRNA is decreased in the hippocampus of individuals with Alzheimer's disease. *Neuron* **7**, 695–702 (1991).

129. Matrone, C., Ciotti, M. T., Mercanti, D., Marolda, R., & Calissano, P. NGF and BDNF signaling control amyloidogenic route and Abeta production in hippocampal neurons. *Proceedings of the National Academy of Sciences of the United States of America* **105**, 13139–13144, doi:10.1073/pnas.0806133105 (2008).

130. Elliott, E., Atlas, R., Lange, A., & Ginzburg, I. Brain-derived neurotrophic factor induces a rapid dephosphorylation of tau protein through a PI-3 Kinase signalling mechanism. *The European Journal of Neuroscience* **22**, 1081–1089, doi:10.1111/j.1460–9568.2005.04290.x (2005).

131. Lapchak, P. A., Araujo, D. M., & Hefti, F. Systemic interleukin-1 beta decreases brain-derived neurotrophic factor messenger RNA expression in the rat hippocampal formation. *Neuroscience* **53**, 297–301 (1993).

132. Sarchielli, P., Greco, L., Stipa, A., Floridi, A., & Gallai, V. Brain-derived neurotrophic factor in patients with multiple sclerosis. *Journal of Neuroimmunology* **132**, 180–188 (2002).

133. VonDran, M. W., Singh, H., Honeywell, J. Z., & Dreyfus, C. F. Levels of BDNF impact oligodendrocyte lineage cells following a cuprizone lesion. *Journal of Neuroscience* **31**, 14182–14190, doi:10.1523/jneurosci.6595–10.2011 (2011).

134. Villoslada, P., & Genain, C. P. Role of nerve growth factor and other trophic factors in brain inflammation. *Progress in Brain Research* **146**, 403–414, doi:10.1016/s0079–6123(03)46025–1 (2004).

135. Deng, X., et al. Co-transplantation of GDNF-overexpressing neural stem cells and fetal dopaminergic neurons mitigates motor symptoms in a rat model of Parkinson's disease. *PloS One* **8**, e80880, doi:10.1371/journal.pone.0080880 (2013).

136. McBride, J. L., et al. Viral delivery of glial cell line-derived neurotrophic factor improves behavior and protects striatal neurons in a mouse model of Huntington's disease. *Proceedings of the National Academy of Sciences of the United States of America* **103**, 9345–9350, doi:10.1073/pnas.0508875103 (2006).

137. Awad, A., et al. Analyses of cerebrospinal fluid in the diagnosis and monitoring of multiple sclerosis. *Journal of Neuroimmunology* **219**, 1–7, doi:10.1016/j.jneuroim.2009.09.002 (2010).

138. Laterre, E. C., Callewaert, A., Heremans, J. F., & Sfaello, Z. Electrophoretic morphology of gamma globulins in cerebrospinal fluid of multiple sclerosis and other diseases of the nervous system. *Neurology* **20**, 982–990 (1970).

139. Link, H., & Huang, Y. M. Oligoclonal bands in multiple sclerosis cerebrospinal fluid: an update on methodology and clinical usefulness. *Journal of Neuroimmunology* **180**, 17–28, doi:10.1016/j.jneuroim.2006.07.006 (2006).

140. Poser, C. M., et al. New diagnostic criteria for multiple sclerosis: guidelines for research protocols. *Annals of Neurology* **13**, 227–231, doi:10.1002/ana.410130302 (1983).

141. Tumani, H., et al. Cerebrospinal fluid biomarkers in multiple sclerosis. *Neurobiology of Disease* **35**, 117–127, doi:10.1016/j.nbd.2009.04.010 (2009).

142. Leoni, V. Oxysterols as markers of neurological disease: a review. *Scandinavian Journal of Clinical and Laboratory Investigation* **69**, 22–25, doi:10.1080/00365510802651858 (2009).

143. Leoni, V., et al. Changes in human plasma levels of the brain specific oxysterol 24S-hydroxycholesterol during progression of multiple sclerosis. *Neuroscience Letters* **331**, 163–166 (2002).

144. Kuhle, J., et al. Neurofilament light and heavy subunits compared as therapeutic biomarkers in multiple sclerosis. *Acta Neurologica Scandinavica* **128**, e33–36, doi:10.1111/ane.12151 (2013).

145. Vekrellis, K., Xilouri, M., Emmanouilidou, E., Rideout, H. J., & Stefanis, L. Pathological roles of alpha-synuclein in neurological disorders. *Lancet Neurology* **10**, 1015–1025, doi:10.1016/s1474–4422(11)70213–7 (2011).

146. Parnetti, L., et al. Cerebrospinal fluid biomarkers in Parkinson disease. *Nature Reviews Neurology* **9**, 131–140, doi:10.1038/nrneurol.2013.10 (2013).

147. Kilarski, L. L., et al. Systematic review and UK-based study of PARK2 (parkin), PINK1, PARK7 (DJ-1) and LRRK2 in early-onset Parkinson's disease. *Movement Disorders* **27**, 1522–1529, doi:10.1002/mds.25132 (2012).

148. Parnetti, L., et al. Cerebrospinal fluid beta-glucocerebrosidase activity is reduced in dementia with Lewy bodies. *Neurobiology of Disease* **34**, 484–486, doi:10.1016/j.nbd.2009.03.002 (2009).

149. Rosen, C., Hansson, O., Blennow, K., & Zetterberg, H. Fluid biomarkers in Alzheimer's disease: current concepts. *Molecular Neurodegeneration* **8**, 20, doi:10.1186/1750–1326-8–20 (2013).

150. Zetterberg, H., Blennow, K., & Hanse, E. Amyloid beta and APP as biomarkers for Alzheimer's disease. *Experimental Gerontology* **45**, 23–29, doi:10.1016/j.exger.2009.08.002 (2010).

151. Maddalena, A., et al. Biochemical diagnosis of Alzheimer disease by measuring the cerebrospinal fluid ratio of phosphorylated tau protein to beta-amyloid peptide42. *Archives of Neurology* **60**, 1202–1206, doi:10.1001/archneur.60.9.1202 (2003).

152. Armstrong, A., et al. Lysosomal network proteins as potential novel CSF biomarkers for Alzheimer's disease. *Neuromolecular Medicine* **16**, 150–160, doi:10.1007/s12017–013-8269–3 (2014).

153. Ray, S., et al. Classification and prediction of clinical Alzheimer's diagnosis based on plasma signaling proteins. *Nature Medicine* **13**, 1359–1362, doi:10.1038/nm1653 (2007).

154. Henriksen, K., et al. The future of blood-based biomarkers for Alzheimer's disease. *Alzheimers & Dementia* **10**, 115–131, doi:10.1016/j.jalz.2013.01.013 (2014).

155. Glaser, G. H., & Merritt, H. H. Effects of corticotropin (ACTH) and cortisone on disorders of the nervous system. *Journal of the American Medical Association* **148**, 898–904 (1952).

156. Miller, H. G., & Gibbons, J. L. Acute disseminated encephalomyelitis and acute disseminated sclerosis: results of treatment with A.C.T.H. *British Medical Journal* **2**, 1345–1348 (1953).

157. Thompson, A. J., et al. Relative efficacy of intravenous methylprednisolone and ACTH in the treatment of acute relapse in MS. *Neurology* **39**, 969–971 (1989).

158. Barnes, M. P., et al. Intravenous methylprednisolone for multiple sclerosis in relapse. *Journal of Neurology, Neurosurgery, and Psychiatry* **48**, 157–159 (1985).

159. Alam, S.M., Kyriakides, T., Lawden, M. & Newman, P.K. Methylprednisolone in multiple sclerosis – a comparison of oral with intravenous therapy at an equivalent dose. *Journal of Neurology Neurosurgery and Psychiatry* **56**, 1219–1220, doi:10.1136/jnnp.56.11.1219 (1993).

160. Le Page, E., et al. Oral versus intravenous high-dose methylprednisolone for treatment of relapses in patients with multiple sclerosis (COPOUSEP): a randomized, controlled, double-blind, non-inferiority trial. *Lancet* **386**, 974–981, doi:10.1016/S0140–6736(15)61137–0 (2015).

161. Jacobs, L. D., et al. Intramuscular interferon beta-1a for disease progression in relapsing multiple sclerosis. The Multiple Sclerosis Collaborative Research Group (MSCRG). *Annals of Neurology* **39**, 285–294, doi:10.1002/ana.410390304 (1996).

162. PRISMS. Randomised double-blind placebo-controlled study of interferon beta-1a in relapsing/remitting multiple sclerosis. PRISMS (Prevention of Relapses and Disability by Interferon beta-1a Subcutaneously in Multiple Sclerosis) Study Group. *Lancet (London, England)* **352**, 1498–1504 (1998).

163. Kappos, L., et al. Effect of early versus delayed interferon beta-1b treatment on disability after a first clinical event suggestive of multiple sclerosis: a 3-year follow-up analysis of the BENEFIT study. *Lancet (London, England)* **370**, 389–397, doi:10.1016/s0140–6736(07)61194–5 (2007).

164. Kozovska, M. E., et al. Interferon beta induces T-helper 2 immune deviation in MS. *Neurology* **53**, 1692–1697 (1999).

165. Liu, Z., Pelfrey, C. M., Cotleur, A., Lee, J. C., & Rudick, R. A. Immunomodulatory effects of interferon beta-1a in multiple sclerosis. *Journal of Neuroimmunology* **112**, 153–162 (2001).

166. Saraste, M., Irjala, H., & Airas, L. Expansion of CD56Bright natural killer cells in the peripheral blood of multiple sclerosis patients treated with interferon-beta. *Neurological Sciences: Official Journal of the Italian Neurological Society and of the Italian Society of Clinical Neurophysiology* **28**, 121–126, doi:10.1007/s10072–007-0803–3 (2007).

167. Vandenbark, A. A., et al. Interferon-beta-1a treatment increases CD56bright natural killer cells and CD4+CD25+ Foxp3 expression in subjects with multiple sclerosis. *Journal of Neuroimmunology* **215**, 125–128, doi:10.1016/j.jneuroim.2009.08.007 (2009).

168. Chen, M., et al. Regulatory effects of IFN-beta on production of osteopontin and IL-17 by CD4+ T Cells in MS. *European Journal of Immunology* **39**, 2525–2536, doi:10.1002/eji.200838879 (2009).

169. Salama, H. H., Kolar, O. J., Zang, Y. C., & Zhang, J. Effects of combination therapy of

beta-interferon 1a and prednisone on serum immunologic markers in patients with multiple sclerosis. *Multiple Sclerosis (Houndmills, Basingstoke, England)* **9**, 28–31 (2003).

170. Calabresi, P. A., et al. Pegylated interferon beta-1a for relapsing-remitting multiple sclerosis (ADVANCE): a randomised, phase 3, double-blind study. *Lancet Neurology* **13**, 657–665, doi:10.1016/s1474–4422(14)70068–7 (2014).

171. Kieseier, B. C., & Calabresi, P. A. PEGylation of interferon-beta-1a: a promising strategy in multiple sclerosis. *CNS Drugs* **26**, 205–214, doi:10.2165/11596970–000000000–00000 (2012).

172. Teitelbaum, D., Meshorer, A., Hirshfeld, T., Arnon, R., & Sela, M. Suppression of experimental allergic encephalomyelitis by a synthetic polypeptide. *European Journal of Immunology* **1**, 242–248, doi:10.1002/eji.1830010406 (1971).

173. Johnson, K. P., et al. Copolymer 1 reduces relapse rate and improves disability in relapsing-remitting multiple sclerosis: results of a phase III multicenter, double-blind placebo-controlled trial. The Copolymer 1 Multiple Sclerosis Study Group. *Neurology* **45**, 1268–1276 (1995).

174. Mikol, D. D., et al. Comparison of subcutaneous interferon beta-1a with glatiramer acetate in patients with relapsing multiple sclerosis (the REbif vs Glatiramer Acetate in Relapsing MS Disease [REGARD] study): a multicentre, randomised, parallel, open-label trial. *Lancet Neurology* **7**, 903–914, doi:10.1016/s1474–4422(08)70200-x (2008).

175. Fridkis-Hareli, M., et al. Direct binding of myelin basic protein and synthetic copolymer 1 to class II major histocompatibility complex molecules on living antigen-presenting cells--specificity and promiscuity. *Proceedings of the National Academy of Sciences of the United States of America* **91**, 4872–4876 (1994).

176. Vieira, P. L., Heystek, H. C., Wormmeester, J., Wierenga, E. A., & Kapsenberg, M. L. Glatiramer acetate (copolymer-1, copaxone) promotes Th2 cell development and increased IL-10 production through modulation of dendritic cells. *Journal of Immunology (Baltimore, Md.: 1950)* **170**, 4483–4488 (2003).

177. Jee, Y., et al. CD4(+)CD25(+) regulatory T cells contribute to the therapeutic effects of glatiramer acetate in experimental autoimmune encephalomyelitis. *Clinical Immunology (Orlando, Fla.)* **125**, 34–42, doi:10.1016/j.clim.2007.05.020 (2007).

178. Polman, C. H., et al. A randomized, placebo-controlled trial of natalizumab for relapsing multiple sclerosis. *The New England Journal of Medicine* **354**, 899–910, doi:10.1056/NEJMoa044397 (2006).

179. Rudick, R. A., et al. Natalizumab plus interferon beta-1a for relapsing multiple sclerosis. *The New England Journal of Medicine* **354**, 911–923, doi:10.1056/NEJMoa044396 (2006).

180. Ransohoff, R. M. Natalizumab for multiple sclerosis. *The New England Journal of Medicine* **356**, 2622–2629, doi:10.1056/NEJMct071462 (2007).

181. Cohen, J. A., et al. Alemtuzumab versus interferon beta 1a as first-line treatment for patients with relapsing-remitting multiple sclerosis: a randomised controlled phase 3 trial. *Lancet (London, England)* **380**, 1819–1828, doi:10.1016/s0140–6736(12)61769–3 (2012).

182. Thompson, S. A., Jones, J. L., Cox, A. L., Compston, D. A., & Coles, A. J. B-cell reconstitution and BAFF after alemtuzumab (Campath-1H) treatment of multiple sclerosis. *Journal of Clinical Immunology* **30**, 99–105, doi:10.1007/s10875–009-9327–3 (2010).

183. Hill-Cawthorne, G. A., et al. Long term lymphocyte reconstitution after alemtuzumab treatment of multiple sclerosis. *Journal of Neurology, Neurosurgery, and Psychiatry* **83**, 298–304, doi:10.1136/jnnp-2011–300826 (2012).

184. Cohen, J. A., et al. Oral fingolimod or intramuscular interferon for relapsing multiple sclerosis. *The New England Journal of Medicine* **362**, 402–415, doi:10.1056/NEJMoa0907839 (2010).

185. Kappos, L., et al. A placebo-controlled trial of oral fingolimod in relapsing multiple sclerosis. *The New England Journal of Medicine* **362**, 387–401, doi:10.1056/NEJMoa0909494 (2010).

186. Chun, J., & Hartung, H. P. Mechanism of action of oral fingolimod (FTY720) in multiple sclerosis. *Clinical Neuropharmacology* **33**, 91–101, doi:10.1097/WNF.0b013e3181cbf825 (2010).

187. O'Connor, P., et al. Randomized trial of oral teriflunomide for relapsing multiple sclerosis. *The New England Journal of Medicine* **365**, 1293–1303, doi:10.1056/NEJMoa1014656 (2011).

188. Bar-Or, A., Pachner, A., Menguy-Vacheron, F., Kaplan, J., & Wiendl, H. Teriflunomide and its mechanism of action in multiple sclerosis. *Drugs* **74**, 659–674, doi:10.1007/s40265–014-0212-x (2014).

189. Gold, R., et al. Placebo-controlled phase 3 study of oral BG-12 for relapsing multiple sclerosis. *The New England Journal of Medicine* **367**, 1098–1107, doi:10.1056/NEJMoa1114287 (2012).

190. Linker, R. A., et al. Fumaric acid esters exert neuroprotective effects in neuroinflammation via activation of the Nrf2 antioxidant pathway. *Brain: A Journal of Neurology* **134**, 678–692, doi:10.1093/brain/awq386 (2011).

191. Albrecht, P., et al. Effects of dimethyl fumarate on neuroprotection and immunomodulation. *Journal of Neuroinflammation* **9**, 163, doi:10.1186/1742–2094-9-163 (2012).

192. Gold, R., et al. Daclizumab high-yield process in relapsing-remitting multiple sclerosis (SELECT): a randomised, double-blind, placebo-controlled trial. *Lancet* **381**, 2167–2175, doi: 10.1016/S0140–6736(12)62190–4 (2013).

193. Kappos, L., et al. Daclizumab HYP versus Interferon Beta-1a in Relapsing Multiple Sclerosis. *New England Journal of Medicine* **373**, 1418–1428, doi: 10.1056/NEJMoa1501481 (2015).

194. Wiendl, H. & Gross, C.C. Modulation of IL-2Rα with daclizumab for treatment of multiple sclerosis. *Nature Reviews Neurology* **9**, 394–404, doi: 10.1038/nrneurol.2013.95 (2013).

195. Kappos, L., et al. Ocrelizumab in relapsing-remitting multiple sclerosis: a phase 2, randomised, placebo-controlled, multicentre trial. *Lancet* **378**, 1779–1787, doi: 10.1016/S0140–6736(11)61649–8 (2011).

196. Sorensen, P.S. & Blinkenberg, M. The potential role for ocrelizumab in the treatment of multiple sclerosis: current evidence and future prospects. *Therapeutic Advances in Neurological Disorders* **9**, 44–52, doi: 10.1177/1756285615601933 (2016).

197. Lublin, F. D., et al. Randomized study combining interferon and glatiramer acetate in multiple sclerosis. *Annals of Neurology* **73**, 327–340, doi:10.1002/ana.23863 (2013).

198. Etminan, M., Gill, S. & Samii, A. Effect of non-steroidal anti-inflammatory drugs on risk of Alzheimer's disease: systematic review and meta-analysis of observational studies. *BMJ (Clinical Research Ed.)* **327**, 128, doi:10.1136/bmj.327.7407.128 (2003).

198. Netland, E. E., Newton, J. L., Majocha, R. E., & Tate, B. A. Indomethacin reverses the microglial response to amyloid beta-protein. *Neurobiology of Aging* **19**, 201–204 (1998).

200. Lim, G. P., et al. Ibuprofen suppresses plaque pathology and inflammation in a mouse model for Alzheimer's disease. *Journal of Neuroscience* **20**, 5709–5714 (2000).

201. Rogers, J., et al. Clinical trial of indomethacin in Alzheimer's disease. *Neurology* **43**, 1609–1611 (1993).

202. Aisen, P. S., et al. Effects of rofecoxib or naproxen vs placebo on Alzheimer disease progression: a randomized controlled trial. *Journal of the American Medical Association* **289**, 2819–2826, doi:10.1001/jama.289.21.2819 (2003).

203. Martin, B.K. Breitner, J.C.S., Evans, D., Lyetsos, C.G., & Meinert, C.L. Cardiovascular and cerebrovascular events in the randomized, controlled Alzheimer's disease anti-inflammatory prevention trial (ADAPT). *PLoS Clinical Trials* **1**, e33, doi:10.1371/journal.ptcr.0010033 (2006).

204. Mandrekar-Colucci, S., & Landreth, G.E. Nuclear receptors as therapeutic targets for Alzheimer's disease. *Expert Opinion on Therapeutic Targets* **15**, 1085–1097, doi:10.1517/14728222.2011.594043 (2011).

205. DiPaolo, G., & Kim, T.W. Linking lipids to Alzheimer's disease: cholesterol and beyond. *Nature Reviews Neuroscience* **12**, 284–296, doi:10.1038/nrn3012 (2011).

206. Jick, H., Zornberg, G.L., Jick, S.S., Seshadri, S., & Drachman, D.A. Statins and the risk of dementia. *Lancet* **356**, 1627–1631, doi:10.1016/S0140–6736(00)03155-X (2000).

207. Schenk, D., et al. Immunization with amyloid-beta attenuates Alzheimer-disease-like pathology in the PDAPP mouse. *Nature* **400**, 173–177, doi:10.1038/22124 (1999).

208. Nicoll, J. A., et al. Neuropathology of human Alzheimer disease after immunization with amyloid-beta peptide: a case report. *Nature Medicine* **9**, 448–452, doi:10.1038/nm840 (2003).

209. Holmes, C., et al. Long-term effects of Abeta42 immunisation in Alzheimer's disease: follow-up of a randomised, placebo-controlled phase I trial. *Lancet (London, England)* **372**, 216–223, doi:10.1016/s0140–6736(08)61075–2 (2008).

210. Sperling, R., et al. Amyloid-related imaging abnormalities in patients with Alzheimer's disease treated with bapineuzumab: a retrospective analysis. *Lancet Neurology* **11**, 241–249, doi:10.1016/s1474–4422(12)70015–7 (2012).

211. Demattos, R. B., et al. A plaque-specific antibody clears existing beta-amyloid plaques in Alzheimer's disease mice. *Neuron* **76**, 908–920, doi:10.1016/j.neuron.2012.10.029 (2012).

212. Frost, J. L., et al. Passive immunization against pyroglutamate-3 amyloid-beta reduces plaque burden in Alzheimer-like transgenic mice: a pilot study. *Neuro-degenerative Diseases* **10**, 265–270, doi:10.1159/000335913 (2012).

213. Karch, C. M., & Goate, A. M. Alzheimer's disease risk genes and mechanisms of disease pathogenesis. *Biological Psychiatry* **77**, 43–51, doi:10.1016/j.biopsych.2014.05.006 (2015).

214. Chan, G., et al. CD33 modulates TREM2: convergence of Alzheimer loci. *Nature Neuroscience* **18**, 1556–1558, doi:10.1038/nn.4126 (2015).

215. Suzuki, K., Kumanogoh, A., & Kikutani, H. Semaphorins and their receptors in immune cell interactions. *Nature Immunology* **9**, 17–23, doi:10.1038/ni1553 (2008).

216. Okuno, T., et al. Roles of Sema4D-plexin-B1 interactions in the central nervous system for pathogenesis of experimental autoimmune

encephalomyelitis. *Journal of Immunology (Baltimore, Md.: 1950)* **184**, 1499–1506, doi:10.4049/jimmunol.0903302 (2010).

217. Hodges, A., et al. Regional and cellular gene expression changes in human Huntington's disease brain. *Human Molecular Genetics* **15**, 965–977, doi:10.1093/hmg/ddl013 (2006).

218. Bjorkqvist, M., et al. A novel pathogenic pathway of immune activation detectable before clinical onset in Huntington's disease. *The Journal of Experimental Medicine* **205**, 1869–1877, doi:10.1084/jem.20080178 (2008).

219. Trager, U., et al. HTT-lowering reverses Huntington's disease immune dysfunction caused by NFkappaB pathway dysregulation. *Brain: A Journal of Neurology* **137**, 819–833, doi:10.1093/brain/awt355 (2014).

220. Bruck, W., et al. Reduced astrocytic NF-kappaB activation by laquinimod protects from cuprizone-induced demyelination. *Acta Neuropathologica* **124**, 411–424, doi:10.1007/s00401–012-1009–1 (2012).

221. Bouchard, J., et al. Cannabinoid receptor 2 signaling in peripheral immune cells modulates disease onset and severity in mouse models of Huntington's disease. *Journal of Neuroscience* **32**, 18259–18268, doi:10.1523/jneurosci.4008–12.2012 (2012).

222. Gagliardi, S., et al. SOD1 mRNA expression in sporadic amyotrophic lateral sclerosis. *Neurobiology of Disease* **39**, 198–203, doi:10.1016/j.nbd.2010.04.008 (2010).

223. Gros-Louis, F., Soucy, G., Lariviere, R., & Julien, J. P. Intracerebroventricular infusion of monoclonal antibody or its derived Fab fragment against misfolded forms of SOD1 mutant delays mortality in a mouse model of ALS. *Journal of Neurochemistry* **113**, 1188–1199, doi:10.1111/j.1471–4159.2010.06683.x (2010).

224. Kriz, J., Nguyen, M. D., & Julien, J. P. Minocycline slows disease progression in a mouse model of amyotrophic lateral sclerosis. *Neurobiology of Disease* **10**, 268–278 (2002).

225. Kiaei, M., et al. Thalidomide and lenalidomide extend survival in a transgenic mouse model of amyotrophic lateral sclerosis. *Journal of Neuroscience* **26**, 2467–2473, doi:10.1523/jneurosci.5253–05.2006 (2006).

226. Neymotin, A., et al. Lenalidomide (Revlimid) administration at symptom onset is neuroprotective in a mouse model of amyotrophic lateral sclerosis. *Experimental Neurology* **220**, 191–197, doi:10.1016/j.expneurol.2009.08.028 (2009).

227. Drachman, D. B., et al. Cyclooxygenase 2 inhibition protects motor neurons and prolongs survival in a transgenic mouse model of ALS. *Annals of Neurology* **52**, 771–778, doi:10.1002/ana.10374 (2002).

228. Kiaei, M., Kipiani, K., Chen, J., Calingasan, N. Y., & Beal, M. F. Peroxisome proliferator-activated receptor-gamma agonist extends survival in transgenic mouse model of amyotrophic lateral sclerosis. *Experimental Neurology* **191**, 331–336, doi:10.1016/j.expneurol.2004.10.007 (2005).

229. Masliah, E., et al. Effects of alpha-synuclein immunization in a mouse model of Parkinson's disease. *Neuron* **46**, 857–868, doi:10.1016/j.neuron.2005.05.010 (2005).

230. Masliah, E., et al. Passive immunization reduces behavioral and neuropathological deficits in an alpha-synuclein transgenic model of Lewy body disease. *PLoS One* **6**, e19338, doi:10.1371/journal.pone.0019338 (2011).

231. Tran, H. T., et al. Alpha-synuclein immunotherapy blocks uptake and templated propagation of misfolded alpha-synuclein and neurodegeneration. *Cell Reports* **7**, 2054–2065, doi:10.1016/j.celrep.2014.05.033 (2014).

232. Mandler, M., et al. Next-generation active immunization approach for synucleinopathies: implications for Parkinson's disease clinical trials. *Acta Neuropathologica* **127**, 861–879, doi:10.1007/s00401-014-1256-4 (2014).

233. Reynolds, A. D., et al. Regulatory T cells attenuate Th17 cell-mediated nigrostriatal dopaminergic neurodegeneration in a model of Parkinson's disease. *Journal of Immunology (Baltimore, Md.: 1950)* **184**, 2261–2271, doi:10.4049/jimmunol.0901852 (2010).

234. Benner, E. J., et al. Therapeutic immunization protects dopaminergic neurons in a mouse model of Parkinson's disease. *Proceedings of the National Academy of Sciences of the United States of America* **101**, 9435–9440, doi:10.1073/pnas.0400569101 (2004).

5

Prion Paradigm of Human Neurodegenerative Diseases Caused by Protein Misfolding

JIRI G. SAFAR

ORIGIN AND MECHANISM OF PROPAGATION OF HUMAN PRIONS

A rising number of neurodegenerative diseases, including Alzheimer's disease (AD), Creutzfeldt-Jakob disease (CJD), Parkinson's disease (PD), frontotemporal dementias (FTD), and amyotrophic lateral sclerosis (ALS), share four fundamental characteristics. First, the most significant risk factor for their development is age. Second, more than 80% of cases are sporadic. Third, pathogenic mutations in different proteins have established the link of the cause of each disease to the specific protein and to its structural transformation into a pathogenic (misfolded) form (1–4). Fourth, the strong protective effect of the amyloid precursor protein (APP) A673T substitution against cognitive decline and Alzheimer's disease (5), and the recently discovered protective prion protein (PrP) V127 polymorphism against CJD and kuru (6), provide further evidence for a causative role of protein processing and specifically misfolding in both diseases. Even though the pathogenic mutations are present from early embryogenesis, the genetic forms of these disorders have an onset at a later age (7, 8). This aspect indicates that some event occurring in later age renders the disease-specific proteins pathogenic, likely involving a stochastic refolding of the etiologic protein into an alternatively folded, self-propagating conformational state, or a failure of the defensive clearance mechanisms. This new self-replicating conformational state was originally discovered in laboratory experiments with a prototypical transmissible neurodegenerative disease—scrapie—and was termed *prion* (1).

Prion diseases are invariably fatal neurodegenerative disorders that affect humans and animals. The annual incidence of human forms peaks at ~6 cases per million between the ages of 65–74, accounting for approximately 1 in 10,000 deaths (9). Despite their rarity, human prion diseases have gained considerable importance due to their unique features: they display characteristics of neurodegenerative diseases but are infectious; the infectious agent is highly resistant to inactivation; they display marked heterogeneity of their clinical and histopathological phenotypes; and a single pathologic process may present as a sporadic, genetic, or infectious disease. These unique aspects have posed unprecedented and challenging problems to studies of their pathogenesis, as well as to disease control and public health, as they can spread not only between humans but also from animals to humans. Human prion diseases include sporadic Creutzfeldt-Jakob disease (sCJD), fatal insomnia, and variably protease-sensitive prionopathy (VPSPr); autosomal dominant genetic forms include familial CJD, fatal familial insomnia (FFI), and Gerstmann-Sträussler-Scheinker disease (GSS); infectious forms are kuru, variant CJD (zoonosis transmitted by meat from cows infected with bovine spongiform encephalopathy—BSE), and iatrogenic CJD transmitted from patients incubating prion diseases with tissue transplants or by contaminated instruments (9). Originally described as transmissible spongiform encephalopathy (TSEs) (10, 11), the most common form of human prion disease is sCJD, accounting for ~90% of cases. It was shown to be transmissible to non-human primates 48 years ago (10, 11), and now the generally accepted model posits that the infectious pathogen responsible for TSEs is a misfolded protein, designated pathogenic prion protein (PrP^Sc), where superscript "Sc" stands for the prototypical disease—scrapie (1). This protein is a structural isoform of the normal cellular prion protein, PrP^C (12–16), that is encoded by the host's prion protein gene (*PRNP*) and expressed at different levels in all mammalian cells (17). The discovery that misfolded proteins may be infectious represents a new biological paradigm, and this protein-only model is now supported by many lines of evidence from biochemical, genetic, and animal studies (15, 16, 18–21), including recent success in generating synthetic infectious prions in vitro (22–28). The amyloid-forming PrP^{Sc} state with predominantly beta sheet secondary structure is believed to self-replicate by binding to monomers of PrP^{C} that have a predominantly alpha-helical secondary structure; this causes the protein to convert to the new molecule of PrP^{Sc}. However, the exact structural intermediate steps of this process remain poorly understood (29, 30), and a high resolution structure of prions is not known. The low-resolution spectroscopic studies indicate that compared to PrP^{C}, the beta-sheet secondary structure of brain-derived PrP^{Sc} increases from ~3% to ~45%, and this conformational transition leads to its insolubility in non-denaturing detergents and resistance to proteolysis (12, 14). Consequently, the half-life of the protein increases in the brains of affected mice from physiological ~18 hours for PrP^{C} to 36 hours for PrP^{Sc} (31), leading to the progressive accumulation of PrP^{Sc}. The replication of the PrP^{Sc} conformer is one of the fundamental problems of biology that remains to be solved.

STRAINS OF HUMAN PRIONS

Human prion diseases are one of, if not the most, diverse neurodegenerative disorders, as evidenced by their neuropathologic and clinical characteristics. The broad phenotypic spectrum of sCJD (9) is currently understood as a complex interplay between polymorphisms in codon 129 of the PRNP gene, translated to either methionine (M) or valine (V), and different PrP^{Sc} conformers coding for distinct strains of prions (9, 32). On serial passages in the same host, distinct prion strains propagate and replicate unique phenotypes of the disease with remarkable reproducibility, including major molecular characteristics of PrP^{Sc}, incubation time, symptoms, and targeting of different anatomical brain structures (32, 33). Variations within the same species of prion, which cause remarkably different disease phenotypes in the same host, are referred to as prion strains (32, 33). Subsequently, rapid progress in the past decade has produced multiple lines of evidence convincingly demonstrating that prion strain characteristics are encoded in the unique self-replicating conformation of PrP^{Sc} (34–37). Additionally, experiments in transgenic mice expressing PrP^{C} of different species led to the conclusion that the species of prion is dictated by the amino acid sequence of the host's prion protein, and the mismatch between amino acid sequences of the infecting prion and host PrP^{C} is responsible for the so-called species barrier, which may restrict prion replication and cause a change in prion characteristics (32).

MECHANISMS CONTROLLING PRION REPLICATION, ADAPTATION, AND EVOLUTION

In experiments with yeast prions, the critical determinant of the prion replication speed is the susceptibility of prions to fragmentation, which exposes new sites for normal precursor attachment, with the less stable structure corresponding to the faster strain (38). Even though there are no known mammalian homologs of the disaggregating chaperone HsP104, which seems to be responsible for this effect in yeast, the general hypothesis that less stable prions are more virulent has been adopted in the field of mammalian prions, and this model appears to be supported by studies in vivo with some rodent prion strains (39–41), but not by others (42, 43). Recent structural studies in our laboratory with hydrogen/deuterium exchange followed by mass spectroscopy (HX MS) addresses this apparent conundrum. Substantial differences were identified between the molecular organization of MM1 and MM2 sCJD prions, both at the level of the polypeptide backbone as well as the quaternary packing arrangements (44). Based on these experiments, it appears that it is not the conformational stability per se that controls the replication rate of human prions. Instead, the data strongly suggest that distinct replication rates of MM1 and MM2 sCJD prions are dictated by specific structural features of corresponding prion particles, features that control the intrinsic growth rate of these aggregates (i.e., the rate of templated conformational conversion of the PrP^{C} substrate). Cumulatively, the balance of factors controlling the strain-specific replication tempo of human prions appears to be diametrically different from that described for yeast prions. In contrast, the faster replicating strain of sCJD prion is characterized by higher conformational stability, implying that, in this case, the dominant factor in controlling the replication tempo is the conformational structure of prions controlling the intrinsic growth rate, and that the impact on the prion stability is a secondary outcome of this primordial aspect (44).

Changes in the biological characteristics of prions observed upon crossing from one species to another, and in experiments with subcloned cell lines, indicate that prions may undergo evolution and adaptation, even though no informative nucleic acid is present. The exact molecular mechanism of this effect has remained speculative (37, 45, 46), but recent experiments indicate that under favorable conditions with compatible PrP^C substrate, the mixture of human PrP^{Sc} conformers may undergo an evolution that selects a subset with the highest replication rate, likely due to the lowest stability. Notably, the adaptation phase and prion strain evolution inferred from experiments with cloned cells (37) and transgenic mice (45, 47) have been shown in experiments to be a conformational process (48). Thus, the selection of a relatively narrow population of conformers with similar conformational stability during passage in experimental animals or cells, together with high activation energy barriers preventing conversion to different prion strains, is likely responsible for the exceptional stability of the biological characteristics of laboratory prion strains, as long as they are propagated in the same host or cells. Moreover, the evolutionary conformational selection mechanism of PrP^{Sc} may explain the recently observed drug-induced evolution of mammalian prions (49). In these experiments, Oelschlegel and Weissmann exposed different prion-infected cell sub-lines to a drug (Swainsonine), and observed not only drug-resistant, but also drug-dependent prion populations, which propagated more rapidly in the presence rather than the absence of the drug. Their data demonstrated that new, initially drug-dependent prions became new stable prion variants after drug withdrawal. These prion adaptations are most likely driven by the conformational selection mechanism observed in experiments *in vitro* and calls for the re-evaluation of different therapeutic strategies that target amyloid-forming aggregates of PrP^{Sc} (48). High-resolution structural tools and research into the role of PrP^{Sc} ligands must address the apparent conformational plasticity of PrP^{Sc}, which is likely responsible for the coexistent spectrum of prion conformers, and enables the prion evolution that results in extensive phenotypic diversity (32, 33, 48).

PRION PARADIGM OF ALZHEIMER'S DISEASE

The advanced understanding of clinicopathological heterogeneity and pathogenesis of late-onset AD, PD, ALS, and other diseases caused by depositions of misfolded proteins, demands identifying biological factors that lead to a spectrum of different phenotypes and different progression rates. The predominant form of dementia is late-onset (> 65 years of age) AD (50). The main pathological features of both early- and late-onset forms are amyloid β peptides (Aβ) plaques, and intra-neuronal tangles of hyperphosphorylated forms of microtubule associated protein tau (MAPT) (51). The causal mutations in the amyloid precursor protein gene (APP), Presenilin 1 (*PSEN1*), and Presenilin 2 (*PSEN2*) genes, which have been identified in early-onset forms, and protective polymorphism in the APP gene, established the central role of Aβ and its processing in AD (8, 52, 53). A major determinant in the risk of late-onset AD is the polymorphism of the apolipoprotein E gene (*APOE*), in which a single e4 allele increases the risk by a factor of 4, and two e4 alleles increase the risk by a factor of 13. Additional polymorphisms in several recently added genes may also moderately increase the risk of disease (53–55).

While these genetic and environmental factors linked to the risk of developing AD are well recognized, the currently identified risk genes can explain only ~25% of phenotypic variance of late-onset AD (54). Further extending the phenotypic spectrum of AD, the Prion Surveillance Centers in the United States and Europe, independently, described a novel subgroup of patients who have a rapidly progressive malignant form of dementia that clinically imitates prion diseases, and which, after a detailed neuropathological investigation, was concluded to be rapidly progressive late-onset sporadic AD (rpAD) (56–61). These data uniformly demonstrate the absence of a positive family history or comorbidity, an absent link to mutations or significant polymorphism in *PRNP* and *PSEN 1, 2* genes, the presence of distinctive clinical characteristics, and a frequency of e4 alleles in the *APOE* gene that corresponds to the general population.

Since the classical neuropathology, comorbidity, or known genetic risk factors did not explain the rapid clinical decline of these patients, we decided to investigate the structural species of Aβ in the brains of these cases. Although genetics established the central role of Aβ in the pathogenesis of early onset AD, the loose correlations between amyloid plaque load and severity of sporadic late-onset AD (62) have generated a controversy, and have led to the questioning of its role in the pathogenesis (63). The discrepancies, together with structural plasticity of synthetic Aβ peptide observed in experiments *in vitro*, called for improved understanding of the structure of Aβ in brain tissue. To fill this gap, we decided to determine the domain display and the stability of Aβ using techniques derived from conformation-dependent immunoassay (CDI) (64), which allowed us to compare different conformational structures formed by the same protein or peptide. If the structures are made from the same protein or peptide and have the same amino acid sequence, then the difference in the domain display and the susceptibility to denaturation (stability) is a reliable indicator of a distinct native conformation in brain tissue (64, 65). We have extensively validated these techniques previously for differentiation of human and animal prions strains, and they are used in prion laboratories worldwide (66–69). Determining the stability of the protein using CDI allows for the comparison of the protein structures directly in the brain tissue, over a concentration range of five orders of magnitude, with sensitivity ~4pg/ml; as a result, the procedure yields highly reproducible data for distinct strains of prions (32, 64).

The recent data obtained with CDI techniques and rapid sedimentation velocity separation by a high-speed centrifugation in sucrose gradient provide evidence of at least three discrete populations of brain Aβ42 (human amyloid β with amino acid sequence 1–42) conformers with varying structures. Despite the extensive conformational variability of Aβ42 in all 48 AD cases examined, a distinct pattern with significantly more conformers that were less stable at 3.5 and 5.5 M of denaturant in rapidly progressive cases has emerged from these experiments (61). In contrast to the more abundant and very stable conformers at ≥7M Guanidine hydrochloride (Gdn HCl), the generally lower stability of these Aβ42 structures suggests that they constitute a unique set of conformers. Cumulatively, the extraordinary structural diversity of brain Aβ42 in rpAD is remarkable, and far exceeds the structural heterogeneity of human prions (61, 70, 71).

Toxic subspecies of Aβ assemblies were posited previously to explain the discrepancy between amyloid load and the onset of clinical symptoms in AD (62, 72). However, there is an ongoing debate over which, if any, of the toxic oligomers observed *in vitro* and in transgenic models of AD exist in the brains of AD patients, and what role they play in AD pathogenesis (73, 74). Our recent experiments performed under non-denaturing conditions provide direct evidence for a broad spectrum of Aβ42 particles in the AD brain, with three particle populations composed of ~30, ~100, and >3,000 monomers (61). These native

particles feature differently exposed N- and C-terminal domains of Aβ42, suggesting that they represent distinct structures. Surprisingly, Aβ40 (human amyloid β with amino acid sequence 1–40) did not form a major particle of discernible size at all and did not participate in the formation of the major Aβ42 particles, and is present uniformly as a monomeric peptide. The Aβ42 particles composed of >3,000 monomers were present in both rapidly and slowly progressive cases, and shared similar levels and domain displays. In contrast, rapidly progressive AD cases accumulated fewer ~30-mers and more ~100-mers, with more exposed N- and C-terminal domains. The demonstration that even identically sized particles may have different conformations suggests differences in the structure of the monomeric Aβ42 building block, or the way the monomers are assembled (quaternary structure), but the prevailing view is that both these aspects must be thermodynamically and kinetically linked (75, 76).

These recent data, obtained with a tandem of advanced biophysical techniques, convincingly demonstrate that especially malignant forms of AD with rapid progression are linked to different polymorphisms in the *APOE* gene and distinct conformational characteristics of the Aβ42 (61). Thus far, the findings argue for the paradigm that emerged in investigations of human prion diseases, where the synergy between polymorphisms in the *PRNP* and variable conformational characteristics of the pathogenic prion protein leads to vastly different disease phenotypes (9, 32, 33). To determine if polymorphisms in genes may be contributing to the rapidly progressive AD phenotype, in parallel with additional external disease modifiers, such as early life environment, education, occupation, and toxic exposures, it will be necessary to analyze, prospectively, detailed endophenotypic characteristics using advanced genetic techniques. However, the highest priority is establishing detailed characteristics of different conformational subsets of brain Aβ42 using advanced tools such as solid state nuclear magnetic resonance (SSNMR) (77).

CONCLUDING REMARKS AND IMPLICATIONS FOR OTHER NEURODEGENERATIVE DISEASES

The recent progress in the investigation of the cellular biology of PD, FTD, and ALS suggests that the prion-like aggregates generated from α-synuclein, tau, and superoxide dismutase may accelerate the pathogenesis in transgenic disease models (4, 78–80). Although these seminal findings are exciting and prove in principle prion-like mechanisms, and in some cases prion-like strains, whether such strains exist in the brains of patients with PD, FTD, and ALS and are responsible for the phenotypic variability still remains to be established. Such studies will require new biophysical methods that are able to differentiate distinct structures formed by the same protein. The data obtained on AD, with distinctly different phenotypes and rate of progression, validate this approach and represent the first step for a systematic investigation of the genetics and molecular pathology of Aβ and tau in patients, which should lead to the identification of biological factors responsible for the variable progression rates of AD. These findings will be crucial in developing new therapeutic targets for AD, for molecular probes targeting disease-causing proteins, and for individualized therapeutic approaches (50). Investigating the conformational structure of brain Aβ and tau is critical for deciphering their role in the variable progression rates and phenotypes of AD.

Several therapeutic trials targeting amyloid deposits in AD have failed. These disappointing results triggered a re-examination of the pathogenetic assumptions that led to their development, and exposed a critical need for new therapeutic targets and earlier diagnostic detection of the disease (63). This goal is especially challenging in light of investigations of prion adaptation and evolution, which imply that misfolded proteins, including those causing AD and PD, may evolve, and thus gain resistance to the therapeutic ligand that originally targeted them (32, 48, 81). Transgenic mice expressing target proteins inoculated with distinct isolates of Aβ and tau should provide a better model for AD in the search for therapeutics designed for delaying or slowing down the progression of the disease. However, it is equally important to advance our understanding of the phenotypic heterogeneity of AD, and the essential requirement for the identification of conformational proteomic markers that would differentiate distinct subgroups of patients, who may respond differently to administered therapeutics.

ACKNOWLEDGMENTS

The authors are grateful to the patient's families, the CJD Foundation, and all the members of the National Prion Disease Pathology Surveillance Center. This work was supported by grants from NIH (NS074317), CDC (UR8/CCU515004), Spitz Fund, and the Charles S. Britton Fund.

REFERENCES

1. Prusiner SB. Novel proteinaceous infectious particles cause scrapie. *Science*. 1982;216:136–144.
2. Glenner GG. On causative theories in Alzheimer's disease. *Hum Pathol*. 1985;16:433–435.
3. Grundke-Iqbal I, Iqbal K, Tung Y-C, Quinlan M, Wisniewski HM, Binder LI. Abnormal phosphorylation of the microtubule-associated protein (tau) in Alzheimer cytoskeletal pathology. *Proc Natl Acad Sci USA*. 1986;83:4913–4917.
4. Prusiner SB. Biology and genetics of prions causing neurodegeneration. *Annu Rev Genet*. 2013;47:601–623.
5. Jonsson T, Atwal JK, Steinberg S, Snaedal J, Jonsson PV, Bjornsson S, et al. A mutation in APP protects against Alzheimer's disease and age-related cognitive decline. Nature. 2012;488 (7409):96–99.
6. Asante EA, Smidak M, Grimshaw A, Houghton R, Tomlinson A, Jeelani A, et al. A naturally occurring variant of the human prion protein completely prevents prion disease. *Nature*. 2015.
7. Kong Q, Surewicz WK, Petersen RB, Zou W, Chen SG, Gambetti P, et al. Inherited prion diseases. In: Prusiner SB, ed. *Prion Biology and Diseases*. 2nd ed. Cold Spring Harbor: Cold Spring Harbor Laboratory Press; 2004: 673–775.
8. Hardy J. Has the amyloid cascade hypothesis for Alzheimer's disease been proved? *Curr Alzheimer Res*. 2006;3(1):71–73.
9. Puoti G, Bizzi A, Forloni G, Safar JG, Tagliavini F, Gambetti P. Sporadic human prion diseases: molecular insights and diagnosis. *Lancet Neurol*. 2012;11(7):618–628.
10. Gibbs CJ, Jr., Gajdusek DC, Asher DM, Alpers MP, Beck E, Daniel PM, et al. Creutzfeldt-Jakob disease (spongiform encephalopathy): transmission to the chimpanzee. *Science*. 1968;161:388–389.
11. Brown P, Gibbs CJ, Jr, Rodgers-Johnson P, Asher DM, Sulima MP, Bacote A, et al. Human spongiform encephalopathy: the National Institutes of Health series of 300 cases of experimentally transmitted disease. *Ann Neurol*. 1994;35:513–529.
12. Caughey BW, Dong A, Bhat KS, Ernst D, Hayes SF, Caughey WS. Secondary structure analysis of the scrapie-associated protein PrP 27–30 in water by infrared spectroscopy. *Biochemistry*. 1991;30:7672–7680.
13. Pan K-M, Baldwin M, Nguyen J, Gasset M, Serban A, Groth D, et al. Conversion of a-helices into b-sheets features in the formation of the scrapie prion proteins. *Proc Natl Acad Sci USA*. 1993;90:10962–1096.
14. Safar J, Roller PP, Gajdusek DC, Gibbs CJ, Jr. Conformational transitions, dissociation, and unfolding of scrapie amyloid (prion) protein. *J Biol Chem*. 1993;268:20276–20284.

15. Prusiner SB. Prions. *Proc Natl Acad Sci USA*. 1998;95:13363–13383.

16. Prusiner SB, ed. *Prion Biology and Diseases*. 2nd ed. Cold Spring Harbor: Cold Spring Harbor Laboratory Press; 2004.

17. Oesch B, Westaway D, Wälchli M, McKinley MP, Kent SBH, Aebersold R, et al. A cellular gene encodes scrapie PrP 27–30 protein. *Cell*. 1985;40:735–746.

18. Collinge J, Clarke AR. A general model of prion strains and their pathogenicity. *Science*. 2007;318(5852):930–936.

19. Morales R, Abid K, Soto C. The prion strain phenomenon: molecular basis and unprecedented features. *Biochim Biophys Acta*. 2007;1772(6): 681–691.

20. Caughey B, Baron GS, Chesebro B, Jeffrey M. Getting a grip on prions: oligomers, amyloids, and pathological membrane interactions. *Annu Rev Biochem*. 2009;78:177–204.

21. Cobb NJ, Surewicz WK. Prion diseases and their biochemical mechanisms. *Biochemistry*. 2009;48(12):2574–2585.

22. Legname G, Baskakov IV, Nguyen H-OB, Riesner D, Cohen FE, DeArmond SJ, et al. Synthetic mammalian prions. *Science*. 2004;305:673–676.

23. Castilla J, Saa P, Hetz C, Soto C. In vitro generation of infectious scrapie prions. *Cell*. 2005;121:195–206.

24. Deleault NR, Harris BT, Rees JR, Supattapone S. Formation of native prions from minimal components in vitro. *Proc Natl Acad Sci USA*. 2007;104:9741–9746.

25. Barria MA, Mukherjee A, Gonzalez-Romero D, Morales R, Soto C. De novo generation of infectious prions in vitro produces a new disease phenotype. *PLoS Pathog*. 2009;5(5):e1000421.

26. Geoghegan JC, Miller MB, Kwak AH, Harris BT, Supattapone S. Trans-dominant inhibition of prion propagation in vitro is not mediated by an accessory cofactor. *PLoS Pathog*. 2009;5(7):e1000535.

27. Kim JI, Cali I, Surewicz K, Kong Q, Raymond GJ, Atarashi R, et al. Mammalian prions generated from bacterially expressed prion protein in the absence of any mammalian cofactors. *J Biol Chem*. 2010;285(19):14083–14087.

28. Wang F, Wang X, Yuan CG, Ma J. Generating a prion with bacterially expressed recombinant prion protein. *Science*. 2010;327(5969): 1132–1135.

29. Kocisko DA, Come JH, Priola SA, Chesebro B, Raymond GJ, Lansbury PT, Jr, et al. Cell-free formation of protease-resistant prion protein. *Nature*. 1994;370:471–474.

30. Prusiner SB. Prion diseases and the BSE crisis. *Science*. 1997;278:245–251.

31. Safar JG, DeArmond SJ, Kociuba K, Deering C, Didorenko S, Bouzamondo-Bernstein E, et al. Prion clearance in bigenic mice. *J Gen Virol*. 2005;86:2913–2923.

32. Safar JG. Molecular mechanisms encoding quantitative and qualitative traits of prion strains. In: Gambetti P, ed. *Prions and Diseases*. New York: Springer Verlag; 2012; 161–179.

33. Safar JG. Molecular pathogenesis of sporadic prion diseases in man. *Prion*. 2012;6(2).

34. Bessen RA, Marsh RF. Distinct PrP properties suggest the molecular basis of strain variation in transmissible mink encephalopathy. *J Virol*. 1994;68:7859–7868.

35. Telling GC, Parchi P, DeArmond SJ, Cortelli P, Montagna P, Gabizon R, et al. Evidence for the conformation of the pathologic isoform of the prion protein enciphering and propagating prion diversity. *Science*. 1996;274:2079–2082.

36. Safar J, Prusiner SB. Molecular studies of prion diseases. *Prog Brain Res*. 1998;117:421–434.

37. Li J, Browning S, Mahal SP, Oelschlegel AM, Weissmann C. Darwinian evolution of prions in cell culture. *Science*. 2010;327(5967):869–872.

38. Tanaka M, Collins SR, Toyama BH, Weissman JS. The physical basis of how prion conformations determine strain phenotypes. *Nature*. 2006;442: 585–589.

39. Legname G, Nguyen H-OB, Peretz D, Cohen FE, DeArmond SJ, Prusiner SB. Continuum of prion protein structures enciphers a multitude of prion isolate-specified phenotypes. *Proc Natl Acad Sci USA*. 2006;103:19105–19110.

40. Colby DW, Prusiner SB. Prions. *Cold Spring Harb Perspect Biol*. 2011;3(1):a006833.

41. Bett C, Joshi-Barr S, Lucero M, Trejo M, Liberski P, Kelly JW, et al. Biochemical properties of highly neuroinvasive prion strains. *PLoS Pathog*. 2012;8(2):e1002522.

42. Peretz D, Scott M, Groth D, Williamson A, Burton D, Cohen FE, et al. Strain-specified relative conformational stability of the scrapie prion protein. *Protein Sci*. 2001;10:854–863.

43. Ayers JI, Schutt CR, Shikiya RA, Aguzzi A, Kincaid AE, Bartz JC. The strain-encoded relationship between PrP replication, stability and processing in neurons is predictive of the incubation period of disease. *PLoS Pathog*. 2011;7(3): e1001317.

44. Safar JG, Xiao X, Kabir ME, Chen S, Kim C, Haldiman T, et al. Structural determinants of phenotypic diversity and replication rate of human prions. *PLoS Pathog*. 2015;11(4):e1004832.

45. Scott M, Peretz D, Ridley RM, Baker HF, DeArmond SJ, Prusiner SB. Transgenetic investigations of the species barrier and prion strains. In: Prusiner SB, ed. *Prion Biology and Diseases*.

2nd ed. Cold Spring Harbor: Cold Spring Harbor Laboratory Press; 2004: 435–482.

46. Mahal SP, Baker CA, Demczyk CA, Smith EW, Julius C, Weissmann C. Prion strain discrimination in cell culture: the cell panel assay. *Proc Natl Acad Sci USA.* 2007;104(52):20908–20913.

47. Scott MR, Peretz D, Nguyen H-OB, DeArmond SJ, Prusiner SB. Transmission barriers for bovine, ovine, and human prions in transgenic mice. *J Virol.* 2005;79:5259–5271.

48. Haldiman T, Kim C, Cohen Y, Chen W, Blevins J, Qing L, et al. Coexistence of distinct prion types enables conformational evolution of human prpsc by competitive selection. *J Biol Chem.* 2013; 288(41): 29846–61.

49. Oelschlegel AM, Weissmann C. Acquisition of drug resistance and dependence by prions. *PLoS Pathog.* 2013;9(2):e1003158.

50. Cummings JL. Biomarkers in Alzheimer's disease drug development. *Alzheimers Dement.* 2011;7(3): e13–44.

51. Braak H, Thal DR, Ghebremedhin E, Del Tredici K. Stages of the pathologic process in Alzheimer disease: age categories from 1 to 100 years. *J Neuropathol Exp Neurol.* 2011;70(11):960–996.

52. Ridge PG, Mukherjee S, Crane PK, Kauwe JS, Alzheimer's Disease Genetics C. Alzheimer's disease: analyzing the missing heritability. *PLoS One.* 2013;8(11):e79771.

53. Naj AC, Jun G, Reitz C, Kunkle BW, Perry W, Park YS, et al. Effects of multiple genetic loci on age at onset in late-onset alzheimer disease: a genome-wide association study. *JAMA Neurol.* 2014; 71(11):1457.

54. Schellenberg GD, Montine TJ. The genetics and neuropathology of Alzheimer's disease. *Acta Neuropathol.* 2012;124(3):305–323.

55. Lambert JC, Ibrahim-Verbaas CA, Harold D, Naj AC, Sims R, Bellenguez C, et al. Meta-analysis of 74,046 individuals identifies 11 new susceptibility loci for Alzheimer's disease. *Nat Genet.* 2013;45(12):1452–1458.

56. Schmidt C, Redyk K, Meissner B, Krack L, von Ahsen N, Roeber S, et al. Clinical features of rapidly progressive Alzheimer's disease. *Dement Geriatr Cogn Disord.* 2010;29(4):371–378.

57. Chitravas N, Jung RS, Kofskey DM, Blevins JE, Gambetti P, Leigh RJ, et al. Treatable neurological disorders misdiagnosed as Creutzfeldt-Jakob disease. *Ann Neurol.* 2011;70(3):437–444.

58. Schmidt C, Wolff M, Weitz M, Bartlau T, Korth C, Zerr I. Rapidly progressive Alzheimer disease. *Arch Neurol.* 2011;68(9):1124–1130.

59. Schmidt C, Haik S, Satoh K, Rabano A, Martinez-Martin P, Roeber S, et al. Rapidly progressive Alzheimer's disease: a multicenter update. *J Alzheimers Dis.* 2012;30(4):751–756.

60. Schmidt C, Artjomova S, Hoeschel M, Zerr I. CSF prion protein concentration and cognition in patients with Alzheimer disease. *Prion.* 2013;7(3).

61. Cohen ML, Kim C, Haldiman T, ElHag M, Mehndiratta P, Pichet T, et al. Rapidly progressive Alzheimer's disease features distinct structures of amyloid-beta. *Brain.* 2015; 138(Pt 4):1009–22.

62. Masters CL, Selkoe DJ. Biochemistry of amyloid beta-protein and amyloid deposits in Alzheimer disease. *Cold Spring Harb Perspect Med.* 2012;2(6): a006262.

63. Colom LV, Perry G, Kuljis RO. Tackling the elusive challenges relevant to conquering the 100-plus year old problem of Alzheimer's disease. *Curr Alzheimer Res.* 2013;10(1):108–116.

64. Safar J, Wille H, Itri V, Groth D, Serban H, Torchia M, et al. Eight prion strains have PrPSc molecules with different conformations. *Nat Med.* 1998;4: 1157–1165.

65. Shirley BA, ed. *Protein Stability and Folding: Theory and Practice.* Totowa, NJ: Humana Press; 1995.

66. Peretz D, Williamson RA, Legname G, Matsunaga Y, Vergara J, Burton D, et al. A change in the conformation of prions accompanies the emergence of a new prion strain. *Neuron.* 2002;34:921–932.

67. Colby DW, Wain R, Baskakov IV, Legname G, Palmer CG, Nguyen HO, et al. Protease-sensitive synthetic prions. *PLoS Pathog.* 2010;6(1): e1000736.

68. Choi YP, Peden AH, Groner A, Ironside JW, Head MW. Distinct stability states of disease-associated human prion protein identified by conformation-dependent immunoassay. *J Virol.* 2011;84(22):12030–12038.

69. Pirisinu L, Di Bari M, Marcon S, Vaccari G, D'Agostino C, Fazzi P, et al. A new method for the characterization of strain-specific conformational stability of protease-sensitive and protease-resistant PrP. *PLoS One.* 2011;5(9): e12723.

70. Kim C, Haldiman T, Cohen Y, Chen W, Blevins J, Sy MS, et al. Protease-sensitive conformers in broad spectrum of distinct prp structures in sporadic Creutzfeldt-Jakob Disease are indicator of progression rate. *PLoS Pathog.* 2011;7(9):e1002242.

71. Kim C, Haldiman T, Surewicz K, Cohen Y, Chen W, Blevins J, et al. Small Protease sensitive oligomers of PrP(Sc) in distinct human prions determine conversion rate of PrP(C). *PLoS Pathog.* 2012;8(8):e1002835.

72. Lesne SE, Sherman MA, Grant M, Kuskowski M, Schneider JA, Bennett DA, et al. Brain amyloid-beta oligomers in ageing and Alzheimer's disease. *Brain.* 2013;136(Pt 5):1383–1398.

73. Benilova I, Karran E, De Strooper B. The toxic Abeta oligomer and Alzheimer's disease: an

emperor in need of clothes. *Nat Neurosci.* 2012;15(3):349–357.

74. Hayden EY, Teplow DB. Amyloid beta-protein oligomers and Alzheimer's disease. *Alzheimers Res Ther.* 2013;5(6):60.

75. Tycko R. Molecular structure of amyloid fibrils: insights from solid-state NMR. *Q Rev Biophys.* 2006; 39(1):1–55.

76. Paravastu AK, Leapman RD, Yau WM, Tycko R. Molecular structural basis for polymorphism in Alzheimer's beta-amyloid fibrils. *Proc Natl Acad Sci USA.* 2008;105(47):18349–18354.

77. Lu JX, Qiang W, Yau WM, Schwieters CD, Meredith SC, Tycko R. Molecular structure of beta-amyloid fibrils in Alzheimer's disease brain tissue. *Cell.* 2013;154(6):1257–1268.

78. Guo JL, Covell DJ, Daniels JP, Iba M, Stieber A, Zhang B, et al. Distinct alpha-synuclein strains differentially promote tau inclusions in neurons. *Cell.* 2013;154(1):103–117.

79. Guo JL, Lee VM. Neurofibrillary tangle-like tau pathology induced by synthetic tau fibrils in primary neurons over-expressing mutant tau. *FEBS Lett.* 2013;587(6):717–723.

80. Jucker M, Walker LC. Self-propagation of pathogenic protein aggregates in neurodegenerative diseases. *Nature.* 2013;501(7465):45–51.

81. Kabir ME, Safar JG. Implications of prion adaptation and evolution paradigm for human neurodegenerative diseases. *Prion.* 2014;8(1).

6

Neuropsychiatric Features Across Neurodegenerative Diseases

CLAUDIA R. PADILLA AND MARIO F. MENDEZ

INTRODUCTION

It has been more than 100 years since Alois Alzheimer first presented his patient, Auguste Deter, a 51-year-old woman with agitation, anxiety, delusions, and hallucinations, who proved to have the neuropathology of Alzheimer's disease (AD) [1]. Since then, we have a greater understanding of how neuropsychiatric symptoms (NPS) are related to neurodegeneration. NPS, also known as behavioral and psychological symptoms of dementia (BPSD), are the range of psychiatric symptoms and behaviors associated with neurodegenerative diseases (see Table 6.1) [2]. These non-cognitive symptoms affect up to 90% of all dementia patients over the course of their illness and are often the most debilitating manifestations of neurodegenerative disorders [3]. The most common NPS, with approximate overall prevalences, include apathy in 65%, delusions in 60%, outbursts (especially verbal) in 33%, hallucinations (especially visual) in 20%, and, as the diseases progress, frequent agitation, aggression, aberrant motor activity, and appetite and sleep changes [3–5]. An additional important category of NPS from neurodegenerative disorders are pervasive changes in personality and social behavior, including disinhibition [6].

There are several basic facts about NPS. First, the occurrence of NPS can diverge from cognitive and other neurological symptoms, indicating that they are more directly related to the neurobiological processes themselves. Although NPS are related to the stage and severity of the disorder and can be worsened by other impairments, most are not directly explained by cognitive or functional decline. Second, despite the fact that many of these NPS are disease-specific, they have overlapping features that suggest common, shared underlying neurobiological processes, including patterns of involvement of neural tracts and neural networks. Some of these overlapping features are also shared

with non-degenerative conditions, such as strokes, tumors, or infections. Third, the genetic aspects of NPS are a rapidly expanding area of research. One recent and intriguing example is the relationship between the frontotemporal dementia (FTD)–related chromosome 9 open reduction frame 72 (*C9orf72*) mutation and the development of paranoid or persecutory delusions and psychosis [7]. Finally, secondary factors such as context and psychological reactions to disease undoubtedly play a causal role in NPS. Nevertheless, current neuroscience indicates changes in specific neuronal structures, neural networks, and neurotransmitters in each NPS, even after other factors are taken into consideration.

This chapter summarizes the major NPS in neurodegenerative diseases, defined clinically and by neuropsychiatric scales, followed by a brief discussion of neural tract and network involvement. The most commonly used scale for NPS is the Neuropsychiatric Inventory (NPI), a semi-structured caregiver interview that retrospectively assesses 12 symptoms [8]. The most important neurodegenerative disorders with NPS are AD, behavioral variant frontotemporal dementia (bvFTD), Huntington's disease (HD), dementia with Lewy bodies (DLB), Parkinson's disease (PD), and the atypical parkinsonian disorders of progressive supranuclear palsy (PSP) and corticobasal syndrome (CBS). Additionally, this chapter will review the common neurobiological correlates of the major NPS, emphasizing regional pathology or dysfunction, involvement of neural networks, and neurotransmitter systems.

APATHY

Apathy, the most common behavioral symptom in neurodegenerative diseases, is a disorder of motivation with cognitive, behavioral, and affective features such as lack of interest, decreased behavioral initiation, and emotional blunting

TABLE 6.1. MOST COMMON NPS IN THE MAJOR
NEURODEGENERATIVE DISEASES

Alzheimer's disease	Apathy, delusions (paranoid, content-specific, misidentifications), depression, anxiety, hallucinations, depression, agitation / aggression, appetite and sleep changes
Behavioral variant frontotemporal dementia	Apathy, disinhibition, repetitive and obsessive-compulsive behaviors, euphoria/eutonia, other personality and social behavior changes; psychosis in subgroups with specific genetic mutations or associated motor neuron disease
Semantic dementia	Personality changes with rigidity and obsessive-compulsive behavior, dietary fads, depression, suicidal ideation
Dementia with Lewy bodies	Visual hallucinations (from pareidolias to complex animate hallucinations), auditory or tactile hallucinations, apathy, delusions, depression, sleep disorders, anxiety, agitation/aggression
Huntington's disease	Apathy, depression, mania, irritability and agitation, personality changes sometimes with antisocial behavior, suicidal and homicidal ideation, obsessive-compulsive symptoms
Parkinson's disease	Frequent depression, anxiety, visual hallucinations, occasional delusions or mania especially after dopaminergic therapy, rigid personality traits, obsessive-compulsive symptoms
Corticobasal syndrome and progressive supranuclear palsy	Depression, apathy, irritability and agitation, delusions, may have disinhibition or obsessive-compulsive symptoms

[9]. While apathy is overtly similar to depression, it is distinguishable by a lack of endorsement of decreased mood or anhedonia. Like depression, patients with apathy may be impaired in their ability to perform basic and instrumental activities of daily living and may appear disengaged from others [10, 11]. The prevalence rates in AD range from 55% to 80%, and its presence is predictive of a more rapid cognitive decline than those patients without apathy [12]. In bvFTD, apathy is a core diagnostic criterion present in 62%–89% of patients [13]. Whether apathy is more cognitive, behavioral, or affective varies among different neurodegenerative disorders [14]. Apathy in AD may be more affective, with dysphoric mood, than in bvFTD [15], whereas apathy in bvFTD may have more of a diminished motor activity or lack of behavioral initiation than in AD [16].

In neurodegenerative disorders, apathy is most commonly attributed to mesial frontal disease or its frontosubcortical connections. In AD, neuroimaging studies associate apathy with hypoperfusion and hypometabolism in the anterior cingulate cortex (ACC), proximal ventromedial prefrontal cortex (vmPFC), and orbitofrontal cortex (OFC) [10, 17]. In vascular dementia (VaD), a related non-neurodegenerative condition, there is disruption of deep white matter pathways in frontal regions, as well as decreased metabolic activity in the frontal subcortical regions [10]. In bvFTD, apathy is associated with disease in the ACC and vmPFC, the right caudate nucleus, and the left frontal operculum-anterior insula (AI) region [10, 18], and extensive dorsolateral frontal cortex (DLFC) disease can lead to a prominent dysexecutive state with apathetic features. Lower cholinergic receptor binding in the left frontal cortex has been associated with the motor and mood changes of apathy in AD, whereas lower dopamine transporter binding is associated with decreased initiative [19, 20]. In sum, the specific mechanism of apathy in neurodegenerative diseases is unknown, but studies suggest disturbance of the frontal cortical-basal ganglia circuits, which play an important role in impairing motivation and goal-oriented behavior.

DELUSIONS

Many patients with neurodegenerative diseases experience some kind of delusional symptom during the progression of their illness. In AD, the prevalence of delusions varies greatly from as low as 15% to as high as 76% [21]. There are a number of common delusional themes and subclasses within those themes. The most common are persecutory delusions, which make up 10%–53% of all delusional beliefs in dementia [21]. The most frequently reported persecutory delusion is the delusion of theft, in which the patients believe that others are stealing their property. Other common persecutory delusions include the belief that a patient's spouse is unfaithful (infidelity), a stranger is living in the home (phantom boarder), or the patient has been abandoned by a caretaker (abandonment).

Content-specific delusions are a common type of delusion seen in neurodegenerative diseases in mild or moderate stages; the most common subclass are the misidentification syndromes, in which a patient consistently misidentifies persons, places, objects, or events [22]. The misidentification syndromes occur in 15.8% of patients with AD, 16.6% of patients with DLB, and 8.3% of patients with semantic dementia (SD; a syndromic variant related to bvFTD, characterized by loss of the meaning of words and objects) [22, 23]. The misidentification syndromes initially included the syndromes of Capgras, Frégoli, intermetamorphosis, and subjective doubles [24], but now they extend to many other false beliefs with a specific content. The Capgras syndrome is one of the most dramatic content-specific misidentification delusions: the patient, despite recognizing familiar faces, such as a spouse or sibling, concludes that they have been replaced by a malevolent double. In contrast, patients with Frégoli syndrome misidentify unfamiliar people and places as familiar ones. Other misidentification syndromes frequently seen in neurodegenerative disorders are reduplicative paramnesia, such as confusing an unfamiliar place with a familiar one, intermetamorphosis, such as transferring the identity of one familiar individual to another familiar one, and the "mirror sign," or the inability to recognize oneself in a mirror.

Grandiose, religious, somatic, and erotomanic delusions are less common, but also occur from neurodegenerative diseases. There are AD patients with erotomania, also known as de Clerambault's syndrome, in which patients were convinced that another person loves them [25, 26], and somatic delusions such as the belief that their stomach is hemorrhaging, they have wandering vaginal polyps, and they are pregnant or blind [27]. Somatic delusions and Cotard's syndrome, the belief of physical deterioration or actually being dead, may be particularly associated with SD [28].

Frontal and temporal neurodegeneration is most commonly implicated with delusions, especially right hemisphere lesions with misidentification syndromes [21]. Investigations with SPECT and PET yield a variety of results involving bilateral hypoperfusion of frontal and superior and inferior temporal lobes. One important study of content-specific delusions in AD found hypometabolism in the right prefrontal cortex, the superior dorsolateral area, and the inferior frontal pole [29]. Others report a correlation between delusional severity in patients with AD and hypoperfusion in the right AI area [30]. The mechanism of misidentification syndromes is memory impairment, and these "paramnestic" delusions often involve an alteration or displacement of the sense of familiarity for a person, place, or event [31]. For example, patients with Capgras delusions may recognize a face but fail to receive a confirmatory feeling of familiarity, so that the joint information representing face recognition and affective response does not match a stored representation of that person [22]. Lack of right frontal "reality monitoring," coupled with this memory impairment, may be the second component that facilitates the emergence of various content-specific delusions and misidentification syndromes.

Most studies implicate dysfunction of the frontal and temporal lobe circuitry, especially the right hemisphere, as the source of delusions in neurodegenerative diseases. Misidentification syndromes may be linked to right hemisphere lesions due to specific disruption of the connections of the fusiform gyrus [22]. Farber et al. (2009) showed a higher neurofibrillary tangle burden in these regions among AD patients with psychosis [32], and a later study, confirmed by Ferman et al., found the same [33], while the converse has been shown in DLB [34]. In bvFTD, hallucinations and delusions have been associated with ubiquitin positive, transactive response DNA-binding protein (TDP-43) and fused in sarcoma (FUS) pathology [7, 13, 35]. Genetic models of AD with psychosis show that there is a familial link and the risk for psychosis is transmitted in families [36]. Studies have been mixed regarding an association of apolipoprotein E (APOE) epsilon 4 allele with AD and psychosis, although a recent study that looked at a large cohort of AD patients found no association [37].

AFFECTIVE SYMPTOMS, INCLUDING DEPRESSION

Depression with mood swings, emotional lability, sadness, crying, hopelessness, low self-esteem, and guilt occurs in 40%–50% of individuals with neurodegenerative diseases over the course of their illness [38, 39]. Depression in AD is more commonly characterized by motivational symptoms, such as fatigue, psychomotor slowing, and apathy, while depression in the cognitively normal elderly population is often characterized by mood symptoms such as dysphoria, anxiety, suicidality, sleep disturbances, and appetite changes [40]. Among AD patients, 40% or more have symptoms of dysthymia and depression, such as sad affect and feelings of hopelessness and helplessness, and show overt clinical depression within 5 years of onset [12, 27]. AD patients with depression, compared to those without, have worse clinical outcomes [41] but can have fluctuations with spontaneous remissions [39]. The relationship between depression and dementia is complex, with depression reported as both a risk factor and a prodrome for AD and other dementias [42] and as qualitatively different from depression in the cognitively normal elderly [40]. Depression is infrequent in bvFTD, possibly because of the lack of insight, but SD patients pose a special risk for suicidal behavior, possibly because of impaired self-concepts due to loss of semantic autobiographical memory [43]. Finally, in parkinsonian conditions, depressive symptoms are part of the disorder and are associated with decreased dopaminergic functions [44–46].

Most studies of depression implicate abnormalities in the frontal and limbic regions with increased neuropathology and neurotransmitter deficits. One PET study exhibited bilateral hypometabolism in the ACC and superior temporal lobes [47]. Other PET studies have shown bilateral superior frontal hypometabolism [48, 49]. Kataoka et al. (2010) showed that compared to non-depressed AD patients, those with depression exhibited hypoperfusion in the left frontal lobe on SPECT imaging [50]. In contrast, Bozeat et al. (2000) found depression present in 45% of his bvFTD patients with predominant temporal involvement, versus only 7% of those with predominant frontal involvement [51]. Neuropathological studies have indicated that a previous history of depression and comorbid depression are associated with more severe AD pathologic changes, with higher accumulation of amyloid plaques and neurofibrillary tangles in the hippocampus of depressed patients with AD [52]. Noradrenergic deficits are associated with depression in dementias. Depression in AD is associated with serotonergic markers in the hippocampus and loss of 5-HT1A receptors [53]. Serotonergic dysfunction has also been seen in FTD; studies have shown a decrease in serotonergic receptors in the temporal and frontal cortices, as well as a decrease in 5-HT2A and 5-HT1A receptors in the vmPFC, OFC, and ACC and a decrease in raphe nucleus neurons [54]. Overall, studies suggest that depression is connected with changes in the frontolimbic brain circuitry and altered associations between emotion-processing regions, including evidence of serotonergic and noradrenergic receptor deficits.

In addition to depression, a euphoric mood can occur in neurodegenerative diseases. In bvFTD, it is fairly common, with prevalence rates ranging between 30% and 36% [55]. Some patients with bvFTD will develop childish, frivolous, and silly behavior, and this is thought to occur more with right temporal and probable adjacent OFC involvement [56].

ANXIETY

Anxiety is one of the most common neuropsychiatric symptoms experienced by patients with dementia, with the prevalence rates ranging from 38% to 72% [57]. Anxiety is often difficult to distinguish from other neuropsychiatric symptoms such as agitation and depression, and therefore can be difficult to assess in patients with AD, bvFTD, and other neurodegenerative disorders [58, 59]. In AD, anxiety, which is often associated with sleep disturbances [27], manifests as a worried appearance, fearfulness, tension, restlessness, and fidgeting [60]. In PD, anxiety has a prevalence of 25%–49% [59]. It was found to be less common in Parkinson's disease dementia (PDD) patients when compared to PD patients with depression, and more common in patients with motor fluctuations, particularly in the off condition [61, 62]. Some studies have shown a high frequency of anxiety in bvFTD [63, 64]; however, other studies indicate lower rates [65, 66].

Anxiety in neurodegenerative diseases is a result of multiple contributing factors, including severity of cognitive and functional decline, environment, level of insight and awareness, and underlying brain disease. In AD, anxiety may be associated with hypometabolism in the bilateral entorhinal cortex, amygdala, anterior parahippocampal gyrus, left superior temporal gyrus, and AI [67]. In bvFTD, anxiety, if present, may be associated with temporal hypometabolism [56, 65]. In a study to identify markers of non-motor function in PD, anxiety is associated with caudate hypometabolism [68]. In sum, the anatomical correlates of anxiety in neurodegenerative diseases are challenging to define; most studies implicate aberrant limbic connections between emotion-generating structures like the amygdala and AI.

HALLUCINATIONS

Hallucinations in AD can occur in any sensory modality, though the most commonly reported type is visual. In a cohort of 55 AD patients, 76.4% of patients experienced visual hallucinations, with the most common themes reported as a deceased person, unfamiliar human, or animal [27]. Typically associated later in the disease course, visual hallucinations in AD often correlate with severity of cognitive impairment, with more impaired patients being at risk for hallucinations [69]. Furthermore, one must consider a superimposed delirium, medication effect, or vision loss as a cause associated in the development of visual hallucinations in AD patients. In comparison to AD, hallucinations are rare occurrences in bvFTD but can occur in subgroups with the progranulin or *C9orf72* genes [7, 35].

Vivid and complex hallucinations are particularly common in the parkinsonian disorders of DLB and PD [70]. In the current consensus criteria, recurrent visual hallucinations are among the core features suggestive of DLB [71], and they are commonly seen early in the disease course, even before the development of motor symptoms. DLB patients may be involved in their hallucinatory experience and thus are affected by what they see [72]. The hallucinations, which may be due to release phenomena or rapid eye-movement (REM) breakthrough, may range from pareidolia, or vague shapes or patterns in the periphery, or complex hallucinations of small people or living things, typically referred to as Lilliputian hallucinations [73]. In PD, 75% of patients develop visual hallucinations usually as a non-medication-induced inherent feature of the disorder, with typically complex hallucinations of people and animals [74, 75]. PD patients can also experience passage hallucinations, in which they have brief perceptions of animals or people in their peripheral visual field [76], and presence hallucinations,

also referred to as "extracampine hallucinations, where they sense the presence of somebody either somewhere in the room, or less often, behind them" [77, 78]. In PDD, recurrent visual hallucinations are a diagnostic feature and may signify disease progression [79]. Additionally, dopaminergic medications can precipitate or exacerbate visual hallucinations in parkinsonian disorders.

Specific mechanisms may be involved in the formation of hallucinations in neurodegenerative diseases. In a large cohort of AD patients, Donovan et al. found reduced supramarginal cortical thickness predictive of increasing hallucinations over time [80], and histopathologic studies indicate a cholinergic and serotonergic imbalance as an etiology of hallucinations in AD [81]. Other studies show selective reduction in gray matter volume of the lingual gyrus and superior parietal lobe, indicating dysfunction of the visual associative cortex [76]. In addition to involvement of visual association areas of the brain, in parkinsonian synucleinopathies there may be additional dysfunction of the limbic and ventral striatum [76]. DLB and PD patients with hallucinations have gray matter loss in the right inferior frontal lobe [82], and similar to AD patients, hallucinations are correlated with hypometabolism in the right frontal cortex [83]. Other investigators have shown a heavier limbic Lewy body burden related to the development of visual hallucinations with a strong association with the ACC [33]. In summary, the mechanism of hallucinations is complex and no single mechanism has been identified; studies indicate that hallucinations occur as a result of disruption of the visual association cortex and other mesial temporal limbic structures, as well as important central neurotransmitter deficits.

AGITATION, AGGRESSION, AND ABERRANT MOTOR BEHAVIOR

Commonly observed in patients with dementia, agitation, aggression, and aberrant motor behavior describe a range of behaviors including physically aggressive acts, verbal agitation, irritability, repetitive actions, wandering, walking aimlessly, sleep disturbance, and repetitive dressing/undressing. A recent work group formed by the International Psychogeriatric Association proposed a consensus definition of agitation in patients with cognitive disorders [84]. Table 6.2 shows the immense variety of behaviors suggested as part of a definition of agitation. Agitation is common in patients with moderate to severe AD and correlates with cognitive decline and

TABLE 6.2. RANGE OF BEHAVIORS INCLUDED IN A DEFINITION OF AGITATION

Physically aggressive	Physically non-aggressive	Verbally agitated
Tearing things or destroying property	General restlessness	Verbal aggression
Hitting others	Pacing	Screaming
Hitting self	Resistiveness	Shouting
Throwing things	Aimless wandering	Constant unwarranted requests for attention or help
Pushing people	Trying to get to a different place (e.g., out of the room or building)	Cursing
Hurting self	Slamming doors intentionally	Making strange noises (weird laughter or crying)
Hurting others	Performing repetitious mannerisms	Repetitive questions
Kicking furniture	Spitting at meals	Repetitive sentences
Biting	Handling things inappropriately	Making verbal sexual advances
Grabbing people	Intentional falling	Negativism
Scratching	Eating/drinking inappropriate substances	Complaining
Making physical sexual advances	Hiding things Hoarding things	Stubbornness

Note: Table modified and categorized by the three subtypes of agitation [84, 85].

loss of independence [12]. While it may include aggressive behaviors, agitation is not the same as aggression; Cohen-Mansfield et al. (1989) identified three subtypes of agitation: (a) physically nonaggressive behavior, (b) physically aggressive behavior, and (c) verbally agitated behavior [85]. Physically nonaggressive behavior includes, for example, wandering or trespassing in inappropriate places, whereas physically aggressive behavior includes actions such as hitting, kicking, biting, spitting, and throwing objects [86]. Verbally agitated behavior, or verbal outbursts such as cursing and shouting, is the most common subtype identified in dementia patients and is commonly thought to be due to the patient's physical or psychological discomfort [87].

In AD, the prevalence of agitation or aggression increases with increased burden of neurofibrillary tangles in the OFC and with neuronal loss in the locus ceruleus [88, 89]. Evidence suggests that agitation and aggression in AD may be related to cholinergic deficits as well as an increase in the D2/D3 receptors in the striatum [90, 91]. In contrast, in bvFTD, irritability and aggressive behavior are variously associated with right temporal involvement [92], or left more than right temporal predominant bvFTD [93]. In conclusion, studies have found dysfunction of the frontal, temporal, and limbic regions involved in the pathogenesis of agitation and aggression.

Various repetitive behaviors occur in patients with dementia, particularly the majority of those with bvFTD [94–96]. A repetitive behavior can include a simple repetitive act such as lip smacking, hand rubbing or clapping, counting aloud, and humming, or complex repetitive acts such as counting, checking, cleaning, and obsessive hoarding and collecting [55]. Repetitive behaviors are reported in 60% of AD patients, with verbal repetition being the most common type [97, 98]. This can include repeating phrases, words, questions, or actions, and telling a story multiple times in the same conversation [95, 99]. Repetitive behavior may be related to prefrontal cortical dysfunction, and positron emission tomography studies show that repetitive behaviors in bvFTD correlate with hypometabolism in the right OFC [100, 101].

APPETITE AND SLEEP CHANGES

Neurodegenerative diseases can produce pronounced changes in appetite and eating behaviors, particularly among those with bvFTD or SD [102]. Patients with bvFTD develop craving for sweets and carbohydrates, and those with SD favor obsessions with particular foods and dietary fads. In some cases with bitemporal involvement, patients place non-food items in their mouths, or exhibit hyperorality, characteristic of the Klüver-Bucy syndrome [103, 104]. The orbitofrontal-insular-striatal brain network is associated with the dietary and eating behavioral disturbances in bvFTD patients [105]. In addition, Piguet et al. found that bvFTD patients with severe eating disturbances exhibited significant atrophy of the hypothalamus, specifically the posterior area [106].

Sleep disturbances are common in patients with dementia, particularly hypersomnia, insomnia, sleep-wake cycle reversal, fragmented sleep, and rapid eye movement (REM) sleep behavior disorder [3]. REM sleep behavior disorder is particularly associated with parkinsonian conditions and occurs in 50%–80% of DLB patients and 46%–58% of PD patients [44, 107]. REM sleep behavior disorder in these conditions is linked to degeneration of the brainstem nuclei [107].

PERSONALITY AND SOCIAL BEHAVIOR CHANGES

Personality and social behavior changes are common occurrences in neurodegenerative diseases, especially in FTD. Patients with bvFTD will have problems with impulse control, self-monitoring, and emotional regulation, which in social settings leads to disruptions of social norms and boundaries. Disinhibited behavior, a core diagnostic criteria of bvFTD [108], includes social, sexual, and physiologic disinhibition. BvFTD patients can act impulsively without considering how others may perceive their behavior. For example, they may laugh at a funeral or make offensive jokes. Sexual disinhibition in bvFTD can include compulsive masturbation, self-exposure of genitalia, or inappropriate sexual advances and touching [109]. They can sometimes have physiologic disinhibition where they have difficulty controlling their bladder or bowel function. Furthermore, bvFTD patients can develop a certain unique proclivity to engage in antisocial and criminal behaviors like theft, traffic violations, trespassing, and public urination, which can lead to unfortunate legal consequences [110, 111]. Other personality changes seen in bvFTD patients may include an inability to empathize with others, and families often report that the individual has become distant and detached in his or her relationships.

Neuroimaging studies with bvFTD patients have consistently implicated the vmPFC, subgenual ACC, AI, OFC, and anterior temporal lobe (aTL), on the right more than the left, with the personality and social behavioral changes in bvFTD [112–115].

NEURAL NETWORK CONNECTIONS

Neural Circuitry Dysfunction

NPS in neurodegenerative diseases are associated with neural circuitry dysfunction involving three frontosubcortical circuits, the dorsolateral prefrontal, OFC, and ACC, which originate in the prefrontal cortex and complete a loop involving the basal ganglia and thalamus [116]. The dorsolateral prefrontal circuit, associated with executive function, is important in planning, organization, goal selection, and monitoring; the OFC circuit and its limbic connections are involved in impulse control and conformity with social norms [117]; and the ACC circuit is engaged in controlling motivational behavior.

Dysfunction in the prefrontal cortex and basal ganglia can disrupt any three of the main frontosubcortical circuits, leading to apathy, disinhibition, or impaired executive function, best exemplified in bvFTD. Apathy results from lesions in the ACC and other cortical areas involved in the circuit. Behavioral disinhibition, emotional lability, lack of judgment and social tact, and impulsivity are particularly consequent to OFC involvement [115]. Executive dysfunction results in difficulty with goal selection, planning, and monitoring, and occurs in parkinsonian and other disorders affecting the dorsolateral prefrontal cortex and its frontosubcortical connections. All neurodegenerative diseases involve changes in social and emotional processes that are linked to the frontosubcortical brain circuits, which have provided models for better understanding behavioral changes in dementia.

Functional Connectivity Alterations and Network Dysfunction

Distinctive large-scale structural and functional networks are linked to specific neurodegenerative diseases, and NPS can result from alterations in the function and interrelationships of the default mode network (DMN) and the salience network (SN). AD is specifically associated with the disruption of the DMN consisting of the posterior cingulate cortex (PCC), precuneus, vmPFC, and hippocampal formation [118]. The DMN is

TABLE 6.3. SUMMARY OF MAJOR NEUROBIOLOGICAL CORRELATES
OF NEUROPSYCHIATRIC SYMPTOMS IN NEURODEGENERATIVE DISEASES

Apathy	Cholinergic and dopaminergic deficits	Anterior cingulate cortex, ventromedial prefrontal cortex and orbitofrontal cortex, frontosubcortical-basal ganglia circuits
Delusions	Serotonergic and dopaminergic receptor dysfunction	Frontal and temporal cortex, especially right hemisphere, fusiform gyrus with misidentification syndromes
Depression	Serotonergic and noradrenergic deficits	Frontal and anterior cingulate cortex, possibly especially on the left, frontolimbic circuits; increased default mode network
Anxiety	Serotonergic imbalance	Frontal with aberrant limbic connections; temporal cortex including the amygdalae and hippocampal region; increased salience network
Hallucinations	Serotinergic and cholinergic imbalance, D2/D3 receptor dysfunction	Visual association cortex, frontal cortex (possibly more on right), mesotemporal limbic regions and ventral striatum, supramarginal gyrus
Agitation/Aggression	Cholinergic deficits and increased D2/D3 receptors	Right hemisphere: frontal (especially OFC) and temporal, locus ceruleus, increased salience network
Appetite and sleep changes	Serotonergic system	Orbitofrontal-insular-striatal network and hypothalamus; brain stem nuclei for sleep
Personality/Social behavior changes	Dopaminergic and serotonergic systems	vmPFC, subgenual ACC, anterior insulae, OFC, and aTL, on the right more than the left; abnormal salience network

active at rest and in internal orientation and self-referential thought and deactivates in response to diverse cognitive tasks such as episodic memory retrieval, mental state attribution, and visual imagery. In contrast, bvFTD specifically targets the SN, consisting of the bilateral ventral and dorsal AI, ACC, ventral striatum, thalamus, central nucleus of the amygdala, hypothalamus, and brainstem [119]. The SN activates in response to emotionally significant internal and external stimuli, especially those involved in social behavior [118, 120].

Studies are increasingly focusing on the association between major neuropsychiatric symptoms and specific neural network changes in neurodegenerative diseases. Zhou et al. (2010) showed that an overactive SN connectivity is associated with reduced connectivity throughout the DMN, and possibly could explain worsening anxiety and agitation with advancing AD [120]. Increased connectivity between the amygdala, AI, and ACC of the SN is associated with anxiety disorders [121–124]; and agitation, disinhibition, irritability, euphoria, and aberrant motor behavior or a "hyperactivity

syndrome" may be associated with enhanced connectivity in the AI and ACC, the key nodes of the SN [125]. The development of depressive symptoms is linked to changes in the DMN and increased connectivity in the subgenual ACC and thalamus [126, 127], and Blanc et al. (2014) associated hallucinations with dysfunction in the right predominant anterior-posterior network, implicating the AI as the core region [128], suggesting possible dysfunction of the SN. Furthermore, dysfunction of the SN is also implicated in the development of symptoms of apathy (see Table 6.3).

CONCLUSION

NPS are characteristic and frequent in neurodegenerative diseases, with complex underlying factors, pathophysiology, and involvement of different neural mechanisms. They are consequent to the underlying neurodegenerative process, including alterations in critical frontolimbic structures, such as the ACC and AI, frontosubcortical circuits and related neural networks such as the salience and default mode networks. Behavioral, cognitive, and emotional dysfunction can occur when these specific brain regions and their neurochemical associations are disturbed. Although there has been considerable progress understanding the brain regions and neural circuitry involved, further studies with structural and functional imaging are necessary to continue to clarify the mechanisms linking NPS with neurodegenerative diseases.

REFERENCES

1. Finkel, S. I., and A. Burns. Behavioral and Psychological Symptoms of Dementia (BPSD): A Clinical and Reasearch Update Introduction. *International Psychogeriatrics*, 2000. 12(S1): 9–12.
2. Cerejeira, J., L. Lagarto, and E. B. Mukaetova-Ladinska. Behavioral and psychological symptoms of dementia. *Front Neurol*, 2012. 3: 73.
3. Miyoshi, K., and Y. Morimura. "Clinical manifestations of neuropsychiatric disorders." *Neuropsychiatric Disorders*. Eds. K. Miyoshi, et al., Japan: Springer, 2010. 3–15.
4. *International Psychogeriatric Association BPSD: Introduction to Behavioral and Psychological Symptoms of Dementia*. The IPA Complete Guides to Behavioral and Psychological Symptoms of Dementia, 2010.
5. Dillon, C., et al. Behavioral symptoms related to cognitive impairment. *Neuropsychiatr Dis Treat*, 2013. 9: 1443–1455.
6. Maurer, K., S. Volk, and H. Gerbaldo. Auguste D and Alzheimer's disease. *The Lancet*, 1997. 349(9064): 1546–1549.
7. Shinagawa, S., et al. Psychosis in frontotemporal dementia. *J Alzheimer's Dis*, 2014. 42(2): 485–499.
8. Cummings, J. L., et al. The Neuropsychiatric Inventory comprehensive assessment of psychopathology in dementia. *Neurology*, 1994. 44(12): 2308–2308.
9. Marin, R. S. Apathy: a neuropsychiatric syndrome. *J Neuropsychiatry Clin Neurosci*, 1991. 3(3): 243–254.
10. Cipriani, G., et al. Apathy and dementia. Nosology, assessment and management. *J Nerv Ment Dis*, 2014. 202(10): 718–724.
11. Zawacki, T. M., et al. Behavioral problems as predictors of functional abilities of vascular dementia patients. *J Neuropsychiatry Clin Neurosci*, 2002. 14(3): 296–302.
12. Li, X. L., et al. Behavioral and psychological symptoms in Alzheimer's disease. *Biomed Res Int*, 2014. 2014: 927804.
13. Mendez, M. F., et al. Psychotic symptoms in frontotemporal dementia: prevalence and review. *Dement Geriatr CognDisord*, 2008. 25(3): 206–211.
14. Levenson, R. W., V. E. Sturm, and C. M. Haase. Emotional and behavioral symptoms in neurodegenerative disease: a model for studying the neural bases of psychopathology. *Annu Rev Clin Psychol*, 2014. 10: 581–606.
15. Chow, T. W., et al. Apathy symptom profile and behavioral associations in frontotemporal dementia vs dementia of Alzheimer type. *Arch Neurol*, 2009. 66(7): 888–893.
16. Shinagawa, S., et al. Initial symptoms in frontotemporal dementia and semantic dementia compared with Alzheimer's disease. *Dement Geriatr Cogn Disord*, 2006. 21(2): 74–80.
17. Theleritis, C., et al. A review of neuroimaging findings of apathy in Alzheimer's disease. *Int Psychogeriatr*, 2014. 26(2): 195–207.
18. Eslinger, P. J., et al. Apathy in frontotemporal dementia: behavioral and neuroimaging correlates. *Behav Neurol*, 2012. 25(2): 127–136.
19. Sultzer, D. L., Melrose, R., Campa, O. R., Achamallah, N., Harwood, D., Brody, A., et al. Cholinergic receptor imaging in Alzheimer's disease: method and early results, in Annual Meeting of the American Association for Geriatric Psychiatry. *Am J Geriatr Psychiatry*, 2010. 18: S71–72.
20. David, R., et al. Striatal dopamine transporter levels correlate with apathy in neurodegenerative diseases: a SPECT study with partial volume effect correction. *Clinical Neurol Neurosurg*, 2008. 110(1): 19–24.
21. Cipriani, G., et al. Understanding delusion in dementia: a review. *Geriatr Gerontol Int*, 2014. 14(1): 32–39.
22. Cipriani, G., et al. Delusional misidentification syndromes and dementia: a border zone between neurology and psychiatry. *Am J Alzheimers Dis Other Demen*, 2013. 28(7): 671–678.
23. Christodoulou, G. N. The delusional misidentification syndromes. *Br J Psychiatry Suppl*, 1991. 14: 65–69.
24. Harciarek, M., and A. Kertesz. The prevalence of misidentification syndromes in neurodegenerative diseases. *Alzheimer Dis Assoc Disord*, 2008. 22(2): 163–169.
25. Cipriani, G., C. Logi, and A. Di Fiorino. A romantic delusion: de Clerambault's syndrome in dementia. *Geriatr Gerontol Int*, 2012. 12(3): 383–387.
26. Brüne, M., and S. G. Schröder. Erotomania variants in dementia. *J Geriatr Psychiatry Neurol*, 2003. 16(4): 232–234.
27. Mendez, M. F., et al. Psychiatric symptoms associated with Alzheimer's disease. *J Neuropsychiatry Clin Neurosci*, 1990. 2(1): 28–33.
28. Mendez, M. F., and J. Ramírez-Bermúdez. Cotard syndrome in semantic dementia. *Psychosomatics*, 2011. 52(6): 571.
29. Sultzer, D. L., et al. Delusional thoughts and regional frontal/temporal cortex metabolism

in Alzheimer's disease. *Am J Psychiatry*, 2003. 160(2): 341–349.

30. Matsuoka, T., et al. Insular hypoperfusion correlates with the severity of delusions in individuals with Alzheimer's disease. *Dement Geriatr Cogn Disord*, 2010. 29(4): 287–293.

31. Pick, A. Clinical studies. *Brain*, 1903. 26(2): 242–267.

32. Farber, N. B., et al. Increased neocortical neurofibrillary tangle density in subjects with Alzheimer disease and psychosis. *Arch Gen Psychiatry*, 2000. 57(12): 1165–1173.

33. Ferman, T., et al. Pathology and temporal onset of visual hallucinations, misperceptions and family misidentification distinguishes dementia with Lewy bodies from Alzheimer's disease. *Parkinsonism Relat Disord*, 2013. 19(2): 227–231.

34. Ballard, C. G., et al. Neuropathological substrates of psychiatric symptoms in prospectively studied patients with autopsy-confirmed dementia with Lewy bodies. *Am J Psychiatry*, 2004. 161(5): 843–849.

35. Kertesz, A., et al., Psychosis and hallucinations in frontotemporal dementia with the C9ORF72 mutation: a detailed clinical cohort. *Cogn Behav Neurology*, 26(3): 146–154.

36. Murray, P. S., et al. Psychosis in Alzheimer's disease. *Biol Psychiatry*, 2014. 75(7): 542–552.

37. DeMichele-Sweet, M. A. A., O. L. Lopez, and R. A. Sweet. Psychosis in Alzheimer's disease in the national Alzheimer's disease coordinating center uniform data set: clinical correlates and association with apolipoprotein e. *Int J Alzheimers Dis*, 2011. 2011: 926597.

38. Ford, A. H. Neuropsychiatric aspects of dementia. *Maturitas*, 2014. 79(2): 209–215.

39. Milano, W., C. Saturnino, and A. Capasso. Behavioural and psychological symptoms of dementia: an overview. *Curr Neurobiol*, 4(1–2): 31–34.

40. Hsiao, J. J., and E. Teng. Depressive symptoms in clinical and incipient Alzheimer's disease. *Neurodegener Dis Manag*, 2013. 3(2): 147–155.

41. Zahodne, L. B., et al. Longitudinal relationships between Alzheimer disease progression and psychosis, depressed mood, and agitation/aggression. *Am J Geriatr Psychiatry*, 2015. 23(2): 130–140. .

42. Bennett, S., and A. J. Thomas. Depression and dementia: cause, consequence or coincidence? *Maturitas*, 2014. 79(2): 184–190.

43. Sabodash, V., et al. Suicidal behavior in dementia: a special risk in semantic dementia. dementias *Am J Azheimers Dis Other Demen*, 2010. 28(6): 592–599.

44. Aarsland, D., J. P. Taylor, and D. Weintraub. Psychiatric issues in cognitive impairment. *Mov Disord*, 2014. 29(5): 651–662.

45. Bruns, M. B., and K. A. Josephs. Neuropsychiatry of corticobasal degeneration and progressive supranuclear palsy. *Int Rev Psychiatry*, 2013. 25(2): 197–209.

46. Litvan, I., J. L. Cummings, and M. Mega. Neuropsychiatric features of corticobasal degeneration. *J Neurol Neurosurg Psychiatry*, 1998. 65(5): 717–721.

47. Lopez, O. L., et al., Psychiatric symptoms associated with cortical-subcortical dysfunction in Alzheimer's disease. *J Neuropsychiat Clin Neurosci*, 2001. 13(1): 56–60.

48. Levy-Cooperman, N., et al. Frontal lobe hypoperfusion and depressive symptoms in Alzheimer disease. *J Psychiatry Neurosci*, 2008. 33(3): 218.

49. Hirono, N., et al. Frontal lobe hypometabolism and depression in Alzheimer's disease. *Neurology*, 1998. 50(2): 380–383.

50. Kataoka, K., et al. Frontal hypoperfusion in depressed patients with dementia of Alzheimer type demonstrated on 3DSRT. *Psychiatry Clin Neurosci*, 2010. 64(3): 293–298.

51. Bozeat, S., et al. Which neuropsychiatric and behavioural features distinguish frontal and temporal variants of frontotemporal dementia from Alzheimer's disease? *J Neurol Neurosurg Psychiatry*, 2000. 69(2): 178–186.

52. Rapp, M. A., et al. Increased hippocampal plaques and tangles in patients with Alzheimer disease with a lifetime history of major depression. *Arch Gen Psychiatry*, 2006. 63(2): 161–167.

53. Lai, M. K., et al. Differential involvement of hippocampal serotonin1A receptors and re-uptake sites in non-cognitive behaviors of Alzheimer's disease. *Psychopharmacology*, 2011. 213(2–3): 431–439.

54. Yang, Y., and H. P. Schmitt, Frontotemporal dementia: evidence for impairment of ascending serotoninergic but not noradrenergic innervation. *Acta Neuropathologica*, 2001. 101(3): 256–270.

55. Mendez, M., E. Lauterbach, and S. Sampson. An evidence-based review of the psychopathology of frontotemporal dementia: a report of the ANPA Committee on Research. *J Neuropsychiatry Clin Neurosci*, 2008. 20(2): 130–149.

56. Mendez, M. F., et al. Functional neuroimaging and presenting psychiatric features in frontotemporal dementia. *J Neurol Neurosurg Psychiatry*, 2006. 77(1): 4–7.

57. Badrakalimuthu, V. R., and A. F. Tarbuck. Anxiety: a hidden element in dementia. *Adv Psychiatric Treat*, 2012. 18(2): 119–128.

58. Seignourel, P. J., et al. Anxiety in dementia: a critical review. *Clin Psychol Rev*, 2008. 28(7): 1071–1082.

59. Kano, O., et al. Neurobiology of depression and anxiety in Parkinson's disease. Parkinson's disease. 2011, 2011: 143547.

60. Ferretti, L., et al. Anxiety and Alzheimer's disease. *J Geriatr Psychiatry Neurol*, 2001. 14(1): 52–58.

61. Riedel, O., et al. Frequency of dementia, depression, and other neuropsychiatric symptoms in 1,449 outpatients with Parkinson's disease. *JNeurol*, 2010. 257(7): 1073–1082.
62. Chen, J. J., and L. Marsh. Anxiety in Parkinson's disease: identification and management. *Ther Adv Neurol Disord*, 2014. 7(1): 52–59.
63. Lopez, O. L., et al. Symptoms of depression and psychosis in Alzheimer's disease and frontotemporal dementia: exploration of underlying mechanisms. *Cogn Behav Neurology*, 1996. 9(3): 154–161.
64. Porter, V. R., et al. Frequency and characteristics of anxiety among patients with Alzheimer's disease and related dementias. *J Neuropsychiat Clin Neurosci*, 2003. 15(2): 180–186.
65. Liu, W., et al. Behavioral disorders in the frontal and temporal variants of frontotemporal dementia. *Neurology*, 2004. 62(5): 742–748.
66. de Vugt, M. E., et al. Impact of behavioural problems on spousal caregivers: a comparison between Alzheimer's disease and frontotemporal dementia. *Dement Geriatr Cogn Disord*, 2006. 22(1): 35–41.
67. Hashimoto, H., et al. Anxiety and regional cortical glucose metabolism in patients with Alzheimer's disease. *J Neuropsychiat Clin Neurosci*, 2006. 18(4): 521–528.
68. Huang, C., et al. Neuroimaging markers of motor and nonmotor features of Parkinson's disease: an [18f] fluorodeoxyglucose positron emission computed tomography study. *Dement Geriatr Cogn Disord*. 2013. 35(3–4): 183–196.
69. Papapetropoulos, S., and B. K. Scanlon. "Visual hallucinations in neurodegenerative disorders." *Neuropsychiatric Disorders*. Eds. K. Miyoshi, et al., Japan: Springer, 2010. 51–64.
70. Pelak, V. S. Visual hallucinations and higher cortical visual dysfunction. *Continuum*, 2009. 15(4, Neuro-Ophthalmology): 93–105.
71. Burghaus, L., et al. Hallucinations in neurodegenerative diseases. *CNS Neurosci Ther*, 2012. 18(2): 149–159.
72. McKeith, I. G., et al. Diagnosis and management of dementia with Lewy bodies: third report of the DLB Consortium. *Neurology*, 2005. 65(12): 1863–1872.
73. Mosimann, U. P., et al. Visual perception in Parkinson disease dementia and dementia with Lewy bodies. *Neurology*, 2004. 63(11): 2091–2096.
74. Leroy, R., and Rd., Fursac. Les hallucinations liliputiennes. *Ann Médico-Psychologiques*, 1909. 67: 278–289.
75. Diederich, N. J., et al. Hallucinations in Parkinson disease. *Nat Rev Neurol*, 2009. 5(6): 331–342.
76. Onofrj, M., et al. Visual hallucinations in PD and Lewy body dementias: old and new hypotheses. *Behav Neurol*, 2013. 27(4): 479–493.
77. Chan, D., and M. N. Rossor. "—but who is that on the other side of you?": Extracampine hallucinations revisited. *The Lancet*, 2002. 360(9350): 2064–2066.
78. Fenelon G., F. Mahieux, R. Huon, and M. Ziegler. Hallucinations in Parkinson's disease: prevalence, phenomenology and risk factors. *Brain*, 2000. 123: 733–745.
79. Emre, M., et al. Clinical diagnostic criteria for dementia associated with Parkinson's disease. *Mov Disord*, 2007. 22(12): 1689–1707; quiz 1837.
80. Donovan, N. J., et al. Regional cortical thinning predicts worsening apathy and hallucinations across the Alzheimer disease spectrum. *Am J Geriatr Psychiatry*, 2014. 22(11): 1168–1179.
81. Garcia-Alloza, M. N., et al. Cholinergic-serotonergic imbalance contributes to cognitive and behavioral symptoms in Alzheimer's disease. *Neuropsychologia*, 2005. 43(3): 442–449.
82. Sanchez-Castaneda, C., et al. Frontal and associative visual areas related to visual hallucinations in dementia with Lewy bodies and Parkinson's disease with dementia. *Mov Disord*, 2010. 25(5): 615–622.
83. Sultzer, D. L., et al. The relationship between psychiatric symptoms and regional cortical metabolism in Alzheimer's disease. *J Neuropsychiat Clin Neurosci*, 1995. 7(4): 476–484.
84. Cummings, J., et al. Agitation in cognitive disorders: International Psychogeriatric Association provisional consensus clinical and research definition. *Int Psychogeriatr*, 2014. 27(1): 7–17.
85. Cohen-Mansfield, J., M. S. Marx, and A. S. Rosenthal. A description of agitation in a nursing home. *J Gerontol*, 1989. 44(3): M77–M84.
86. Cohen-Mansfield, J. Agitated behaviors in the elderly: II. Preliminary results in the cognitively deteriorated. *J Am Geriatr Soc*, 1986. 34(10): 722–727.
87. Lemay, M., and P. Landreville. Review: verbal agitation in dementia: the role of discomfort. *Am J Alzheimers Dis Other Demen*, 2010. 25(3): 193–201.
88. Tekin, S., et al. Orbitofrontal and anterior cingulate cortex neurofibrillary tangle burden is associated with agitation in Alzheimer disease. *Ann Neurology*, 2001. 49(3): 355–361.
89. Matthews, K. L., et al. Noradrenergic changes, aggressive behavior, and cognition in patients with dementia. *Biol Psychiatry*, 2002. 51(5): 407–416.
90. Pinto, T., K. L. Lanctôt, and N. Herrmann. Revisiting the cholinergic hypothesis of behavioral and psychological symptoms in dementia of the Alzheimer's type. *Ageing Res Rev*, 2011. 10(4): 404–412.
91. Nowrangi, M. A., C. G. Lyketsos, and P. B. Rosenberg. Principles and management of neuropsychiatric symptoms in Alzheimer's dementia. *Alzheimers Res Ther*, 2015. 7(1): 1–10.

92. Edwards-Lee, T., et al. The temporal variant of frontotemporal dementia. *Brain*, 1997. 120(6): 1027–1040.

93. Thompson, S. A., K. Patterson, and J. R. Hodges. Left/right asymmetry of atrophy in semantic dementia: behavioral-cognitive implications. *Neurology*, 2003. 61(9): 1196–1203.

94. Ready, R. E., B. R. Ott, and J. Grace. Amnestic behavior in dementia: symptoms to assist in early detection and diagnosis. *J Am Geriatr Soc*, 2003. 51(1): 32–37.

95. Cipriani, G., et al. Repetitive and stereotypic phenomena and dementia. *Am J Alzheimers Dis Other Demen*, 2013. 28(3): 223–227.

96. Quinn, B., and M. Mahler. Frontal dementia: repetitive and compulsive behaviour in frontal lobe degenerations. *J Neuropsychiat Clin Neurosci*, 1994. 6: 100–113.

97. Hwang, J.-P., et al. Repetitive phenomena in dementia. *Int J Psychiat Med*, 2000. 30(2): 165–172.

98. Poletti, M., et al. Cognitive correlates of negative symptoms in behavioral variant frontotemporal dementia: implications for the frontal lobe syndrome. *Neurol Sci*, 2013. 34(11): 1893–1896.

99. Cohen-Mansfield, J., and A. Libin. Assessment of agitation in elderly patients with dementia: correlations between informant rating and direct observation. *Int J Geriatr Psychiatry*, 2004. 19(9): 881–891.

100. Casasanto, D. J., et al. Neural correlates of successful and unsuccessful verbal memory encoding. *Brain Language*, 2002. 80(3): 287–295.

101. Sarazin, M., et al. Metabolic correlates of behavioral and affective disturbances in frontal lobe pathologies. *J Neurology*, 2003. 250(7): 827–833.

102. Diehl-Schmid, J., et al. Behavioral disturbances in the course of frontotemporal dementia. *Demen Geriatr Cogn Disord*, 2006. 22(4): 352–357.

103. Gustafson, L., A. Brun, and U. Passant. Frontal lobe degeneration of non-Alzheimer type. *Bailliere's Clin Neurol*, 1992. 1(3): 559–582.

104. Mendez, M., and D. Foti. Lethal hyperoral behaviour from the Klüver-Bucy syndrome. *J Neurol Neurosurg Psychiatry*, 1997. 62(3): 293.

105. Piguet, O. Eating disturbance in behavioural-variant frontotemporal dementia. *J Molec Neurosci*, 45(3): 589–593.

106. Piguet, O., et al. Eating and hypothalamus changes in behavioral variant frontotemporal dementia. *Ann Neurology*, 2011. 69(2): 312–319.

107. Boeve, B., et al. Pathophysiology of REM sleep behaviour disorder and relevance to neurodegenerative disease. *Brain*, 2007. 130(11): 2770–2788.

108. Neary, D., et al. Frontotemporal lobar degeneration A consensus on clinical diagnostic criteria. *Neurology*, 1998. 51(6): 1546–1554.

109. Miller, B. L., and B. F. Boeve. *The Behavioral Neurology of Dementia*. Cambridge: Cambridge University Press, 2009.

110. Liljegren, M., et al. Criminal behavior in frontotemporal dementia and Alzheimer disease. *JAMA Neurology*, 2015. 72(3): 295–300.

111. Mendez, M. F. The unique predisposition to criminal violations in frontotemporal dementia. *J Am Acad Psychiatry*, 2010. 38(3): 318–323.

112. Rosen, H. J., et al. Neuroanatomical correlates of behavioural disorders in dementia. *Brain*, 2005. 128(11): 2612–2625.

113. Hornberger, M., et al. Orbitofrontal dysfunction discriminates behavioral variant frontotemporal dementia from Alzheimer's disease. *Demen Geriatr Cogn Disord*, 2010. 30(6): 547.

114. Massimo, L., et al. Neuroanatomy of apathy and disinhibition in frontotemporal lobar degeneration. *Demen Geriatr Cogn Disord*, 2009. 27(1): 96.

115. Bonelli, R. M., and J. L. Cummings. Frontal-subcortical circuitry and behavior. *Dialogues Clin Neurosci*, 2007. 9(2): 141.

116. Cummings, J. L. Frontal-subcortical circuits and human behavior. *Arch Neurology*, 1993. 50(8): 873–880.

117. Lichter, D. G., and J. L. Cummings. *Frontal-subcortical circuits in psychiatric and neurological disorders*. : Guilford Press, 2001.

118. Zhou, J., and W. W. Seeley. Network dysfunction in Alzheimer's disease and frontotemporal dementia: implications for psychiatry. *Biol Psychiatry*, 2014. 75(7): 565–573.

119. Seeley, W. W., et al. Dissociable intrinsic connectivity networks for salience processing and executive control. *J Neuroscience*, 2007. 27(9): 2349–2356.

120. Zhou, J., et al. Divergent network connectivity changes in behavioural variant frontotemporal dementia and Alzheime's disease. *Brain*, 2010. 133(Pt 5): 1352–1367.

121. Menon, V. Large-scale brain networks and psychopathology: a unifying triple network model. *Trends Cogn Sciences*, 2011. 15(10): 483–506.

122. Stein, M., et al. Increased amygdala and insula activation during emotion processing in anxiety-prone subjects. *Am J Psychiatry*, 2007. 164(2): 318–327.

123. Paulus, M. P., and M. B. Stein. An insular view of anxiety. *Biol Psychiatry*, 2006. 60(4): 383–387.

124. Pannekoek, J. N., et al. Resting-state functional connectivity abnormalities in limbic and salience networks in social anxiety disorder without comorbidity. *Eur Neuropsychopharmacology*, 2013. 23(3): 186–195.

125. Balthazar, M. L., et al. Neuropsychiatric symptoms in Alzheimer's disease are related to functional connectivity alterations in the

salience network. *Human Brain Mapping*, 2014. 35(4): 1237–1246.

126. Greicius, M.D., et al, Resting-state functional connectivity in major depression: abnormally increased contributions from subgenual cingulate cortex and thalamus. *Biol Psychiatry*, 2007. 62(5): 429–437.

127. Sambataro, F., et al. Default mode network in depression: a pathway to impaired affective cognition. *Clin Neuropsychiatry*, 2013. 10(5): 212–216.

128. Blanc, F.D.R., et al. Right anterior insula: core region of hallucinations in cognitive neurodegenerative diseases. *PLoS One*. 2014. 9(12): e114774.

7

Brain Circuits

Neurodegenerative Diseases

JUAN ZHOU AND WILLIAM W. SEELEY

INTRODUCTION

Selective Vulnerability and Clinico-Pathological Features in Neurodegenerative Disease

Selective vulnerability defines the neurodegenerative diseases, which are united by the gradual and anatomically targeted spread of pathological inclusions, gliosis, and synaptic and neuronal loss. The prototypical patterns of regional spread give rise to distinctive clinical syndromes. Table 7.1 summarizes the selective vulnerability patterns seen in several major neurodegenerative disease syndromes. Each syndrome is defined by selectively vulnerable neurons, regions, networks, and functions, as well as genetic risk factors. This chapter focuses on two common forms of dementia: Alzheimer's disease (AD) and frontotemporal dementia (FTD), illustrating class-wide principles whenever possible.

AD is the most prevalent neurodegenerative disorder overall and the most common cause of dementia in older adults. Typical AD-type dementia begins with episodic memory loss due to medial temporal lobe neurofibrillary pathology (1) before progressing to language and visuospatial impairment as degeneration spreads to posterior cingulate/precuneus and lateral temporoparietal neocortex (2, 3). AD is related to an extra-cellular brain accumulation of beta-amyloid (Aß) and intraneuronal tangles, composed of hyperphosphorylated tau, that affect cortical networks related to memory, language, visuospatial, and executive functions (4).

FTD, in contrast, describes a group of clinical syndromes, including a behavioral variant (bvFTD), semantic variant primary progressive aphasia (PPA), and non-fluent/agrammatic PPA (5, 6). BvFTD features prominent social conduct and emotion-processing deficits associated with anterior cingulate, frontoinsular, ventral striatal, and variably dorsolateral frontal or temporopolar degeneration (7–9). Semantic variant PPA begins with loss of word and object meaning, accompanied by left-predominant temporal pole and amygdala involvement, or loss of emotional meaning and attachment due to a mirror-image right temporal-predominant degeneration (10–12). Nonfluent/agrammatic PPA presents with non-fluent, effortful, and agrammatic speech associated with left frontal opercular, dorsal anterior insular, precentral gyrus, and dorsal striatal atrophy (10, 13, 14).

Alzheimer-type dementia, the clinical syndrome, strongly predicts underlying AD neuropathology. Possession of an apolipoprotein E (APOE) ε4 allele is the strongest genetic risk factor for sporadic AD (15). FTD syndromes, in contrast, result from a group of distinct underlying molecular pathological entities referred to collectively as frontotemporal lobar degeneration (FTLD). FTLD is further divided into three major molecular classes, including tau (FTLD-tau), transactive response DNA-binding protein of 43 kDA (TDP-43, FTLD-TDP), and, least commonly, fused in sarcoma (FUS) protein (FTLD-FUS) (16), based on the protein composition of neuronal and glial inclusions. Although most patients have sporadic disease, several autosomal dominant culprit genes have been identified, with mutations in the genes encoding microtubule-associated protein tau (*MAPT*), progranulin (*GRN*), and *C9orf72* accounting for the majority of known genetic causes (17).

Network-Based Neurodegeneration: Historical Notes

The myriad neuronal types of the adult human brain exhibit differential vulnerability to each neurodegenerative disease. Early on, misfolded

TABLE 7.1. SELECTIVE VULNERABILITY IN NEURODEGENERATIVE DEMENTIA

Syndrome	Early Symptom(s)	Early Neuron	Early Regions	Affected network	Proteins	Genes*
AD	Episodic memory loss	ERC Layer II pyramidal neurons	Medial temporal-posterior cingulate-precuneus-ANG	Default mode	Aβ42 Tau	APP PS1, PS2
FTD						
bvFTD	Apathy, disinhibition, compulsivity	Von Economo neurons, Fork cells	ACC-frontoinsular cortex	Salience	Tau = TDP-43 >> FUS	MAPT GRN C9ORF72
svPPA	Anomia, loss of word meaning, emotional detachment	Unknown	Temporal pole-amygdala-ventral striatum-orbitofrontal	Semantic-appraisal	TDP-43 >> Tau	Rarely genetic
nfvPPA	Nonfluent aphasia	Unknown	Dominant perisylvian cortex	Motor speech/language	Tau > TDP-43	GRN
ALS	Motor weakness, spasticity	Upper and lower motor neurons	Primary motor cortex and spinal cord anterior horn	Sensorimotor	TDP-43	C9ORF72 TARDBP SOD-1** FUS
CBS	Asymmetric bradykinesia-rigidity, dystonia, myoclonus	Unknown	Perirolandic cortex	Sensorimotor association	Tau >> TDP-43	MAPT GRN
PSP-S	Falls, executive dysfunction	Unknown	Rostral midbrain tegmentum, dentate nucleus, STN, pallidum	Oculomotor control	Tau	MAPT
DLB	RBD, arousal fluctuations, VH, parkinsonism	Aminergic projection neurons	DMNX, LC, PPTN	Long-range brainstem projection systems	α-synuclein	Rarely genetic
MSA-P	Autonomic insufficiency; parkinsonism	Preganglionic sympathetic neurons, DA & MSP neurons	Brainstem, spinal cord (IML), S. Nigra, putamen	Lower sympathetic control, nigrostriatal circuit	α-synuclein	Rarely genetic
MSA-C	Autonomic insufficiency; ataxia	Preganglionic sympathetic neurons, olivopontine & Purkinje neurons	Brainstem, spinal cord (IML), inferior olive, pontine nuclei, cerebellum	Lower sympathetic control, cerebellar circuits	α-synuclein	Rarely genetic
HD	Chorea, depression, executive dysfunction	MSP neurons	Dorsal caudate	Dorsal frontal-striatal-thalamic circuit	Huntingtin	IT15
CJD	Variable	Unknown	Variable	Variable	PrPsc	PRNP

* Only the most common associations with autosomal dominant inheritance are listed. ** SOD-1 mutations are associated with ubiquitin-positive, TDP-43-negative intraneuronal inclusions (Mackenzie et al., 2007).

disease proteins aggregate within small, exquisitely vulnerable neuron populations that reside in specific brain regions (1, 18 19). Synaptic and neuronal loss then appears in new regions, accompanied by worsening clinical deficits (20). The established patterns of early selectivity and subsequent expansion have long stimulated researchers to link neuronal networks to the relentless clinical and anatomical progression observed in patients (2, 21–23). Despite these seminal perspectives, for decades oversimplifications dominated the clinical literature, which often divided neurodegenerative disorders into focal versus diffuse or subcortical versus cortical. The notion that each disorder represents a network-based degeneration flows naturally, however, from the cross-sectional postmortem neuropathological data (2, 3, 22, 24). The dawn of human brain mapping, made possible by unbiased brain-wide, voxel-wise statistical methods and network-sensitive imaging approaches, provided a means to image human network degeneration in living patients. Complementary *in vitro* and animal model studies have begun to clarify key mechanisms of network-based dysfunction and spread, which may be most parsimoniously explained by the prion-like spread of misfolded disease protein conformers within and between neurons and across synapses (25–28). Structural, molecular, and functional neuroimaging studies have largely replicated the stereotyped spread of AD pathological markers (29–31).

Mapping Brain Circuits: Structural and Functional Magnetic Resonance Imaging

The introduction of new network-sensitive neuroimaging methods has made it possible to test hypotheses about network degeneration in living humans (32–36). Structural and functional connectivity analyses provide noninvasive methods for mapping large-scale networks in the healthy living human brain (Figure 7.1) (37–40) and for detecting early network-level alterations in disease (33, 41). Using these methods, Seeley and others directly tested the notion that neurodegenerative syndromes reflect large-scale network degeneration. They showed that five different syndromes cause circumscribed atrophy (Figure 7.2A) within five distinct healthy human intrinsic connectivity networks (Figure 7.2B). Moreover, a direct link between intrinsic connectivity and gray matter structure was found, specifically that nodes within each functional network also exhibit tightly correlated gray matter volumes across healthy individuals (Figure 7.2C) (35). These findings suggested

that human neural networks can be defined by synchronous baseline activity and a unified corticotrophic fate and can serve as anatomical templates for neurodegenerative illness. The following paragraphs provide a brief overview of the main structural and functional MR-based network-sensitive neuroimaging methods.

Intrinsic Connectivity

With task-free functional magnetic resonance imaging (tf-fMRI), researchers can now identify functional intrinsic connectivity networks (ICNs) derived from temporally synchronous, spatially distributed, spontaneous low frequency (<0.1 Hz) blood-oxygen level-dependent signal fluctuations (39, 42–44) (Figure 7.1C). ICNs represent a highly conserved and robust form of organized macroscopic brain activity. Comparable networks are observed in distinct species such as mice, monkeys, and humans (45), in distinct developmental stages including after preterm birth and in infancy, childhood, adulthood, and old age (46), and during diverse stages of awareness from sleep to conscious goal-directed behavior (47). Compared to conventional task-based fMRI studies, tf-fMRI is free of performance confounds, making it easier to apply and interpret in cognitively impaired populations. To derive ICNs, seed-based analysis uses correlations of tf-fMRI spontaneous low-frequency fluctuations between a seed region and the rest of the brain (42). Alternative approaches such as independent component analysis and clustering methods take advantage of multiple simultaneous brain interactions to pull apart coherent brain networks (48, 49). Future work will include characterizing temporal dynamics of ICNs and elucidating the possible causal relationships (see reviews 50 and 51). Synchronization across neuronal assemblies can likewise be computed from task-free EEG or MEG data.

Structural Covariance

Coordinated variations in brain morphology (e.g., gray-matter volume or cortical thickness) across subjects have been used as measures of structural association between regions to construct large-scale structural covariance networks (Figure 7.1A) (35, 52–54). This approach relies on the hypothesis that connectivity confers a mutually trophic effect on the growth of connected regions. Based on this principle, the mean gray matter volume or thickness of a region of interest is used to conduct a whole-brain voxel-wise regression across subjects to identify those voxels

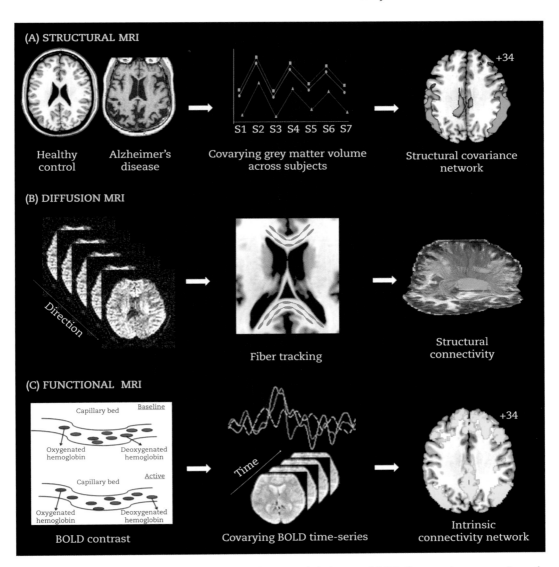

FIGURE 7.1. Network-sensitive neuroimaging techniques. (A). Structural MRI. By covarying grey matter volume (or cortical thickness) of each region of interest across subjects, structural covariance networks (in green) can be constructed for a group of subjects. (B). Diffusion MRI: Based on the principle that water diffusion is restricted by tissue structure, fiber tracking can be performed to infer the white matter pathways linking multiple brain regions within or between networks, i.e., structural connectivity. (C). Task-free fMRI: Functional intrinsic connectivity networks (ICNs, in yellow) can be derived from temporally synchronous, spatially distributed, spontaneous low frequency (<0.1 Hz) blood-oxygen level-dependent signal fluctuations recorded in task-free fMRI.

(or regions or vertices) whose magnitude is correlated with the region-of-interest.

Structural Connectivity

The term *structural connectivity* refers to the interconnection between neurons or brain regions by nerve fibers. Although axonal connectivity remains beyond the resolution of

current techniques, the integrity of medium- to large-fiber tracts can be assessed *in vivo* using diffusion-weighted imaging (DWI) techniques, which map the diffusion of water molecules and rely on the principle that diffusion is restricted by tissue structure (55). A tensor model is estimated that can be represented as an ellipsoid with three principal axes, the length of which reflects

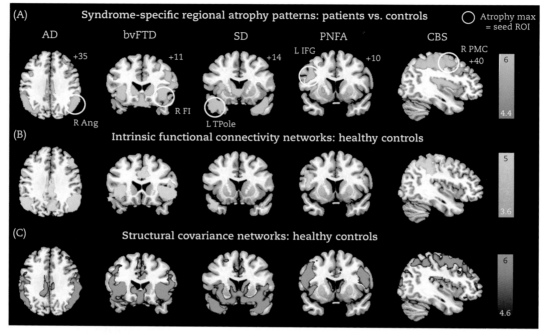

FIGURE 7.2. Convergent syndromic atrophy, healthy intrinsic connectivity network (ICN), and healthy structural covariance network (SCN) patterns. (A) Five distinct clinical syndromes showed dissociable atrophy patterns, whose cortical atrophy maxima (circled) provided seed regions of interest (ROIs) for ICN and SCN analyses. **(B)** ICN mapping experiments identified five distinct networks anchored by the five syndromic atrophy seeds. **(C)** Healthy subjects further showed grey matter volume covariance patterns that recapitulated results shown in **(A)** and **(B)**.[35] Results are displayed on representative sections of the MNI template brain. In coronal and axial images, the left side of the image corresponds to the left side of the brain. ANG = angular gyrus; FI = frontoinsula; IFGoper = inferior frontal gyrus, pars operculum; PMC = premotor cortex; TPole = temporal pole.

the diffusion tendency along each direction (λ_1, λ_2, λ_3). Scalar tissue integrity measures characterizing the shape of the ellipsoid include fractional anisotropy and mean diffusivity (56). Region of interest analysis or data-driven voxel-based analysis allows estimation of group differences in fiber tract integrity or associations with cognitive functioning (Figure 7.1B). Fiber tracking can further be performed based on the shape and principal direction of the ellipsoid (57, 58).

Finally, the term *connectome* refers to a comprehensive map of the brain's neural connections (59), whether the connections are defined based on structural (MRI, DWI) or functional (fMRI, EEG, MEG) grounds. By modeling networks as graphs (brain regions as nodes and node-to-node connections as edges), graph theoretical analyses offer a flexible and quantitative approach for characterizing brain network topology. Several graph theoretical metrics quantify brain network "hubs," that is, regions with high degree centrality (60–64), while other metrics, such as clustering

coefficient and path length, emphasize modularity or efficiency of communication.

Neurodegenerative Disease: Unifying Anatomical Principles

When discussing the neuroanatomy of neurodegenerative conditions, it is critical to disambiguate terms that refer to the clinical syndrome from terms that describe the underlying neuropathological entity giving rise to that syndrome. Throughout this chapter, we use "syndrome" when describing a recognizable pattern of symptoms and deficits. Examples include "behavioral variant frontotemporal dementia" or "AD-type dementia" or "corticobasal syndrome." In contrast, we use "disease" to refer to the histopathological entities found at autopsy in patients exhibiting a dementia syndrome during life. Examples include frontotemporal lobar degeneration with TDP-43 immunoreactive inclusions (FTLD-TDP), Alzheimer's disease, or corticobasal degeneration (a subtype of FTLD with tau immunoreactive inclusions

[FTLD-tau]). In short, syndromes reflect *where* the damaging pathological process is, whereas disease terms describe *what* the pathological process is.

In this section, we briefly introduce the key concepts of neurodegenerative disease onset and progression. In our view, these concepts encapsulate the most critical unanswered questions for neurodegenerative disease research. In addition, we introduce two interrelated observations about neurodegenerative disease: clinico-anatomical convergence and phenotypic heterogeneity. Any comprehensive model of disease onset and spread must also account for these observations, which cut across this class of human illness.

Onset

Patients with each neurodegenerative syndrome emerge from an incipient preclinical stage during which the patient's symptoms remain absent or subtle and the lesion remains restricted to just one or few brain regions and only the most susceptible cells and microcircuits within the affected regions. This focal onset manifests as targeted misfolded disease protein aggregation, followed by quantifiable neuronal dropout (1, 18, 19). For example, the cortical stage of AD begins with focal neurofibrillary tangle formation within stellate projection neurons of the Layer 2 entorhinal cortex islands, followed by the loss of associated synapses and neurons that gives rise to episodic memory dysfunction (1–3). Recent cross-sectional postmortem studies have refined our understanding of the anatomical site of AD onset, revealing that tau deposition within the brainstem locus ceruleus and dorsal raphe likely anticipate tangle formation in entorhinal cortex (65, 66).

Progression

A relentless spatiotemporal progression characterizes every neurodegenerative disease. What anatomical principles govern this downhill march? Postmortem and in vivo neuroimaging studies suggest that the pattern of regional injury reflects a network-based landscape, arguing against the notion that disease spreads across the cortical mantle via spatial contiguity (2, 3, 22, 24, 27, 32, 33, 35). But what factors govern how disease spreads from the onset node(s) to downstream regions within and beyond the target network? We will consider three possible scenarios (Figure 7.3, bottom panel):

1. *Unifocal (or simultaneous oligofocal) onset with connectional spread.* In this scenario, the later-affected regions are determined entirely by the axonal connections of the most vulnerable cells within the onset region(s).

2. *Staggered multifocal onset without connectional spread.* Here, anatomical progression reflects independent, temporally staggered eruption of disease within multiple (not necessarily interconnected) regions. In this way, progression is connectivity-independent and is generated by a graded hierarchy of regional and/or cellular vulnerabilities.

3. *Combined unifocal and staggered multifocal onset with connectional spread.* In this model, which blends aspects of the previous two, disease progression reflects not only the connectivity of the initial onset regions but also the emergence of later but independent onset sites and the connections of affected neurons within those sites. For example, amyotrophic lateral sclerosis (ALS) and behavioral variant frontotemporal dementia (bvFTD) often co-occur in an individual patient (67). This scenario may represent at least two distinct (simultaneous or staggered) sites of onset: one within the salience network that participates in behavioral guidance and another within the pyramidal motor network responsible for voluntary movement (68–70). Progression then may reflect the propagation of disease from these two distinct brain systems.

Clinico-anatomical Convergence

We use *clinico-anatomical convergence* to refer to the observation that most clinical syndromes can be caused by diverse underlying pathological entities. For example, patients with bvFTD may be found to have one of at least 15 different underlying pathological diagnoses, spanning three FTLD major molecular classes (FTLD with tau, TDP-43, or FUS immunoreactive inclusions) and AD. The key question is whether convergence occurs at the clinical, regional, or neuronal level (Figure 7.4). In other words, distinct proteinopathies could converge at the clinical/network level by targeting disease-specific nodes within the same syndrome-relevant network. In this scenario, neuroimaging studies might help discriminate between diseases causing the same syndrome by virtue of differing regional atrophy patterns across the pathological causes of that syndrome. Alternatively, convergence could occur at the regional or even neuronal level, in which case anatomically based methods, such as structural and functional imaging, would

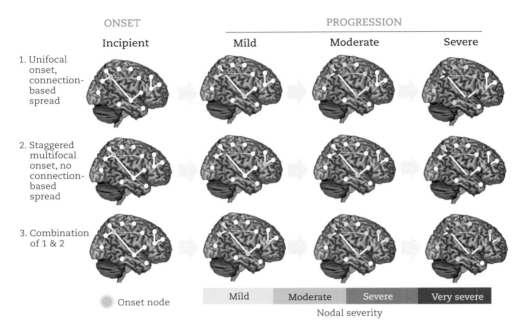

FIGURE 7.3. Principles of disease onset and progression. Here we offer three possible scenarios to explain the spatial patterning of neurodegenerative disease. In all scenarios, for ease of comparison the disease begins focally within a single region. In scenario 1, progression is connectivity-dependent and mediated by spread. In scenario 2, progression is due to connectivity-independent emergence of disease within autonomous onset sites without true spreading. In scenario 3, both mechanisms of progression are at work.

fail to discriminate between diseases within a given syndrome, and alternative approaches, such as molecular imaging or fluid biomarkers, more closely linked to the disease proteins themselves, would be required. Further work is needed to determine at which level clinico-anatomical convergence occurs, but credible models of onset and progression must somehow account for this important observation.

Phenotypic Diversity

We use *phenotypic diversity* to refer to the observation that the same histopathological entity (disease) may be associated with several distinct clinical syndromes, reflecting distinct patterns of regional involvement. For example, Pick's disease, a subtype of FTLD-tau, may present with bvFTD, semantic variant primary progressive aphasia (svPPA), nonfluent variant primary progressive aphasia (nfvPPA), or corticobasal syndrome, based on the targeted epicenter and its network-based affiliations. This observation suggests either that each disease protein maintains a certain non-random variability with regard to where it first aggregates in an individual brain, or that neuropathological taxonomy remains inadequately

specified and that further characterization (i.e., "splitting") of the tau protein found in Pick's disease will, extending the example, reveal different forms of post-translationally modified or misfolded tau in each of the syndromic presentations of Pick's disease.

Based on the unifying principle of network-based neurodegeneration, the next section will discuss disease onset in more detail. Then the subsequent section will review neuroimaging data as it informs competing models of disease progression, and the final section will touch on the most important frontiers in the field of network-based neurodegeneration.

MODELING ONSET: WHERE DOES EACH DISEASE BEGIN?

Evidence to Date

The most mysterious aspect of neurodegenerative disease regards how each disease selects its initial target or targets. Merely identifying those initial targets has proved challenging enough. For AD and Parkinson's disease (PD), this process has relied on cross-sectional postmortem studies that included patients at all stages of the disease process,

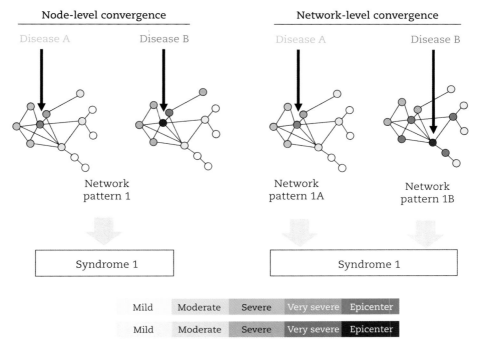

FIGURE 7.4. Potential models to explain clinico-anatomical convergence. Clinico-anatomical convergence describes the observation that multiple distinct histopathological entities can produce the same (or a similar) clinical syndrome. The anatomical convergence could occur at the nodal or network levels. Node-level convergence predicts highly similar spatial patterns based on connectional spread. Network-level convergence predicts subtle differences in spatial patterns based on differing onset sites. These subtle anatomical differences may manifest with the same syndrome or two (or more) syndromes that have yet to be sufficiently disambiguated.

from asymptomatic to prodromal to full-blown symptomatic and even end-stage disease (71, 72). This approach has helped identify not only specific vulnerable areas but even neuronal subtypes. Generally, regional-level insights derived with this approach have been well-supported by longitudinal studies in living individuals. For example, studies following older individuals from health to mild memory impairment and later AD-type dementia show early involvement of the entorhinal cortex (73–75), consistent with classical post-mortem studies (2, 71). On the other hand, *in vivo* brain imaging lacks the subnuclear and neuronal subtype resolution required to provide a complete picture. This limitation is exemplified by AD and PD, in which the earliest brain protein aggregates are now understood to emerge in brainstem nuclei difficult to resolve with conventional brain MRI: the locus coeruleus and dorsal raphe in AD (66, 76, 77) and the dorsal motor nucleus of the vagus nerve in PD (78). For less common diseases, like FTLD, early neuronal subtype selectivity has been even more difficult to define, owing to the diversity of FTD syndromes and the scarcity of postmortem materials from patients with asymptomatic or prodromal

disease. The few laudable attempts to derive distinct stages using cross-sectional materials have suffered from the lack of early-stage cases (79, 80). Furthermore, because each FTLD pathological subtype produces diverse clinical phenotypes, it would be difficult to interpret materials from presymptomatic FTLD even if they became available.

How can brain imaging studies in symptomatic patients inform our understanding of disease onset? Regions showing greatest atrophy during symptomatic disease may or may not represent the sites of initial injury, but recent neuroimaging studies support an emerging model for understanding where each syndrome begins before it spreads. To pursue these issues, it was first critical to demonstrate that each neurodegenerative syndrome is linked to a specific network. To evaluate this possibility, Seeley and colleagues identified the most atrophied cortical region in each of five clinical syndromic patient groups (Figure 7.2) and used these regions of interest (ROIs) to seed ICN mapping in tf-fMRI data from a group of healthy controls. As predicted, the healthy ICN maps, though generated from isolated cortical seed ROIs, closely mirrored the distinct atrophy patterns seen in the five neurodegenerative syndromes. Building on this work, Zhou and coworkers showed that each syndrome-associated brain network contains a vulnerable "epicenter" (or epicenters), whose connectivity in health closely mirrors—and may template—the spatial patterning of each syndrome (Figure 7.5) (36). These epicenters bear close relationships to the early clinical and neuronal deficits that define each syndrome. For instance, in bvFTD the identified epicenters in the right frontoinsula and pregenual anterior cingulate cortex are known for their

co-activation during salience processing (81), and both regions harbor a unique class of large, bipolar projection neurons, called von Economo neurons, targeted in early-stage bvFTD (19, 82). Identifying an epicenter, as defined above, does not prove that this epicenter represents the site of initial injury; nonetheless, there is a striking overlap between the regions of peak atrophy (35) and those that serve as epicenters (36). To determine sites of regional onset more definitively requires research on presymptomatic at-risk individuals, as discussed in the following.

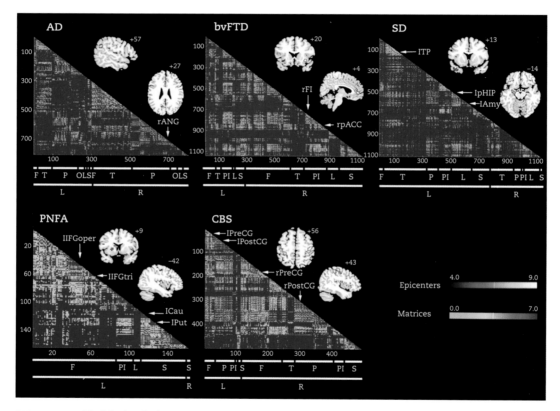

FIGURE 7.5. Healthy intrinsic connectivity matrices and network epicenters for each of five neurodegenerative syndrome atrophy patterns.[36] Regions anchoring healthy ICNs that corresponded to each of the five atrophy maps were identified as epicenters, shown here superimposed on the MNI template brain. The red-orange color bar represents the t-scores associated with the group-level significance of the epicenter-seeded network goodness-of-fit scores. Matrices representing the group-level node pair-wise connectivity strengths were organized from left to right (and top to bottom) in the order of frontal (F), temporal (T), parietal (P), occipital (O), paralimbic (Pl), limbic (L), and subcortical (S) regions. The blue-red color bar represents the intrinsic connectivity between each node pair, defined as the t-score from the thresholded group-level one-sample t-test. Subthreshold node pair connectivity strengths were colored dark blue and omitted from the matrices. Abbreviations: AD: Alzheimer's disease; bvFTD: behavioral variant frontotemporal dementia; SD: semantic dementia; PNFA: progressive non-fluent aphasia; CBS: corticobasal syndrome; ANG: angular gyrus; FI: frontoinsula; pACC: pregenual anterior cingulate cortex; TP: temporal pole; pHIP: posterior hippocampus; Amy: amygdala; IFGoper: inferior frontal gyrus operculum; IFGtri: inferior frontal gyrus triangular; Cau: caudate nucleus; Put: putamen; PreCG: precentral gyrus; PostCG: postcentral gyrus; l: left; r: right.

Prodromal Stages of AD

Accumulating evidence suggests that DMN connectivity may emerge during the presymptomatic phase of AD, as assessed in individuals who harbor imaging evidence of cortical amyloid pathology (83, 84) or an APOE-e4 positive genotype, a major genetic risk factor for late onset AD (85–87).

Combining PiB-PET (i.e., Pittsburgh Compound B PET) to detect *in vivo* amyloid-β deposition with tf-fMRI to assess intrinsic functional connectivity, Drzezga and colleagues found that asymptomatic and mildly impaired elderly with higher amyloid plaque load showed greater reductions in parietal cortex global centrality, a measure of functional connectivity with all other voxels of the brain (88). Whether amyloid deposition was driving the connectivity disruption remains unknown. In parallel, DTI studies have shown converging patterns of white matter microstructural changes, including the fornix, uncinate fasciculus, and posterior and parahippocampal fibers of the cingulum in healthy subjects showing biomarker evidence of amyloid and tau pathology (89–95).

In healthy young APOE-e4 carriers, increased medial temporal lobe functional connectivity and task-based recruitment was found within the DMN (96). In contrast, healthy APOE-e4+ elders showed DMN connectivity reductions across several temporal regions (86). In MCI subjects, the functional isolation of the posterior cingulate from its main interaction sites in the medial temporal lobe and the medial prefrontal cortex was associated with worsening episodic memory function (97). Posterior cingulate cortex showed reduced connectivity in MCI, even in the absence of gray matter atrophy, which was only detectable in patients with fully developed AD-type dementia (98). Recent DTI studies have focused on asymptomatic at-risk populations, such as healthy subjects carrying AD susceptibility genes (most notably the APOE-e4 allele) (99–104). Together, the findings converge on a pattern of microstructural white matter changes in AD-type dementia that begin and are most severe in limbic tracts, including the fornix, uncinate fasciculus, and posterior and parahippocampal fibers of the cingulum. Microstructural alterations of the limbic tracts were detectable even in presymptomatic subjects, years before they developed cognitive deficits and at a time when gray matter volume was widely preserved (102, 105, 106). Finally, combined assessment of structural and functional abnormalities in asymptomatic young adult and middle-aged APOE4 carriers indicated that abnormalities in functional network communication may precede the breakdown of structural white matter connections in the pathogenesis of AD (107, 108). However, other studies in asymptomatic APOE-e4 carriers have found parallel decreases in functional and structural connectivity (109) or even more pronounced structural network changes (110). These diverse and at times conflicting findings suggest that further work is needed to determine the possible genetic and age-dependent and multifocal brain structural and functional alternations in AD onset.

Prodromal Stage of FTD

As in AD, in FTD structural and functional connectivity changes emerge before first symptoms arise. This claim rests on observations from asymptomatic carriers of FTD-causing genes. In the largest study of this kind, 39 asymptomatic carriers of microtubule-associated protein tau (*MAPT*) or progranulin (*GRN*) mutations showed fractional anisotropy reductions in the right uncinate fasciculus and decreased functional connectivity between key salience network hubs, anterior mid-cingulate cortex, and fronto-insula, compared with non-carriers (111). More recently, using region-of-interest-based structural MRI, researchers have identified sites presumed to reflect incipient atrophy in each of the three major FTD-causing genetic mutations (*MAPT, GRN*, and *C9orf72*) (112). These studies share a methodological limitation, however, that in presymptomatic FTD gene carriers we have no way to predict which of the several associated clinical syndromes will later emerge; in this way, group-level results are likely distorted by the anticipated blending of preclinical syndromes, as well as the anatomical heterogeneity within each syndrome.

Relationship to Clinico-anatomical Convergence and Phenotypical Diversity

Does clinico-anatomical convergence reflect onset within the same vulnerable neuron population, or within different neuronal constituents of the same region or network? To address this question requires that we study all relevant levels in a single syndrome as caused by multiple diseases. For example, does bvFTD begin in the von Economo neurons whether the syndrome is caused by FTLD-tau, TDP-43, or FUS? Emerging data from autopsy series suggest that convergence may occur at least at the regional level, with diverse proteinopathies converging on the anterior insula, but whether this site represents the starting point for each patient's disease remains doubtful and unexamined at the level of single syndromes. At the neuronal level, some studies have provided clues toward cell type convergence (19, 82), but the studies needed to resolve the issue have yet to be performed and remain difficult to imagine considering the late stage at which most patients come to autopsy.

Phenotypic diversity issues are similarly important to relate to the concept of disease onset. For example, although most patients with underlying AD present with early memory loss, a significant minority presents with a non-amnestic syndrome (Figure 7.3, phenotypic diversity). Patients with non-familial early-onset AD (EOAD, defined as onset < 65 years in most studies) show a mix of cognitive deficits, often beginning with attentional or executive impairment (113, 114). Focal syndromes such as posterior cortical atrophy (PCA), characterized by predominant visuospatial and visuoperceptual deficits (115) and the logopenic variant of primary progressive aphasia (lvPPA), a progressive disorder of language (116), are also most commonly caused by AD pathology. Indeed, up to 15% of patients with AD seen in dementia centers have non-amnestic presentations (117). The factors driving this phenotypic diversity are not well understood, but the clinico-anatomical variation between patients could reflect an internal hierarchy or "pecking order" of vulnerability that differs between individual patients based on their genetic backgrounds, life experiences, or region-specific stressors (trauma, seizures, vascular malformations, etc.) or developmental anomalies (118). Alternatively, the process could reflect some randomness in the locality of the onset site; this account seems unlikely, however, given the relatively finite range of clinical presentations caused by AD. A related question concerns whether protein misfolding and aggregation tend to occur only in a finite group of cell types/brain regions or, alternatively, are ongoing throughout the aging brain but remain homeostatically controlled in all but that protein's short list of onset cells/regions, which are somehow ill-equipped to manage the quality-control process for that protein.

Lingering Questions and Uncertainties

Many key questions remain within the general concept of disease onset. How many cell types and/or brain regions undergo independent (sometimes referred to as *cell autonomous*) onsets? What is the pecking order of neuron-type vulnerabilities

to each disease? Does this order vary across individuals? Does onset occur within neurons, glia, or both? Can cells undergo a "reversible onset," such as protein aggregation and dysfunction, but then revert to a healthy state?

MODELING PROGRESSION: HOW DOES DISEASE MOVE BEYOND THE CELLS AND REGIONS WHERE IT BEGINS?

Evidence to Date

That each neurodegenerative syndrome reflects a large-scale network breakdown has been established, as discussed above, through a variety of convergent approaches. But what do we know about how disease progresses to create a network-related spatial pattern? At least four hypotheses have been put forth and are summarized in Figure 7.6:

1. *Nodal stress*, in which regions subject to heavy network traffic (i.e., "hubs") undergo activity-related "wear and tear" that gives rise to or worsens disease (119, 120) (Figure 7.7);
2. *Transneuronal spread*, in which some toxic agent propagates along network connections, perhaps through "prion-like" templated conformational change (25, 121–127);
3. *Trophic failure*, in which network connectivity disruption undermines inter-nodal trophic factor support, accelerating disease within nodes lacking collateral trophic sources (128, 129); and
4. *Shared vulnerability*, in which networked regions feature a common gene or protein expression signature (130) that confers disease-specific susceptibility, evenly distributed throughout the network.

These non-mutually exclusive candidate network degeneration mechanisms make competing predictions about how healthy network architecture should influence disease-associated regional vulnerability. Notably, although "network degeneration" is often understood to mean "network-based spread," only the "transneuronal spread" model proposes that progression represents the physical spreading of a pathological process along axons connecting individual neurons.

The ideal approach for examining disease progression and predicting neurodegeneration from

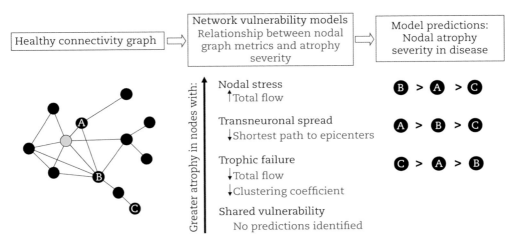

FIGURE 7.6. Predictions made by network-based degeneration models: effects of healthy intrinsic connectivity graph metrics on atrophy severity in disease.[36] A simplified healthy connectivity graph is shown (far left) for illustration purposes only; circles represent nodes (brain regions), lines represent edges (a connection between two nodes), and edge lengths represent the connectivity strength between nodes, with shorter edges representing stronger connections. The orange node represents an epicenter. Three nodes, labeled as 'A', 'B', and 'C', feature contrasting graph theoretical properties to illustrate predictions made by the network-based vulnerability models (far right). Listed in the center column are the relationships predicted by each model. For example, the transneuronal spread model predicts that nodes with shorter (↓) paths to the epicenter in health will be associated with greater (↑) atrophy severity in disease.

brain connectivity would be to follow individuals from health to disease, exploring connectivity-vulnerability interactions within single subjects. Although this approach may prove challenging for the FTD syndromes, longitudinal analyses of this type are beginning to be pursued for AD-type dementia through large, ongoing, collaborative longitudinal studies. To date, efforts to investigate disease progression mechanisms have mainly relied on cross-sectional data. As discussed in relation to disease onset, for each of five syndromes Zhou and coworkers identified critical network epicenters whose normal connectivity profiles most resemble the syndrome-associated atrophy patterns. Graph theoretical analyses in healthy subjects revealed that regions with higher total connectional flow and, more consistently, shorter functional paths to the epicenters, showed greater syndrome-associated vulnerability (Figure 7.8) (36). Across all five syndromes, network nodes subject to greater intra-network total information flow were found to undergo greater atrophy.

This observation raised the possibility that activity-dependent mechanisms, such as oxidative stress, local extracellular milieu fluctuations, or glia-dependent phenomena, influence regional vulnerability; this influence might be a key factor in determining sites of initial onset or secondary

onset (i.e., progression). Second, nodes with shorter connectional paths to an epicenter showed greater vulnerability, suggesting that transneuronal spread represents one of the key factors driving early target network degeneration, most likely by physical transmission of toxic disease proteins or other agents along axons. In other words, epicenter infiltration by disease may provide privileged but graded access across the network that determines where the disease will arrive next. Although trophic factor insufficiency or a shared gene or protein expression profile may help to determine sites of onset, the findings of this study were difficult to reconcile with predictions made by these models regarding the graded vulnerability seen within the target networks. To extend the anatomical scope of the analyses, the authors further examined connectivity-vulnerability relationships within the "off-target" networks to determine how nodal characteristics influence downstream vulnerability. Here, overwhelmingly, the evidence supported the transneuronal spread model. In summary, the findings best fit a model in which initial vulnerability may reflect a node's centrality (i.e., "hubness") within the target network, whereas downstream vulnerability was more closely related to a node's connectional proximity to the most vulnerable "epicenter" regions.

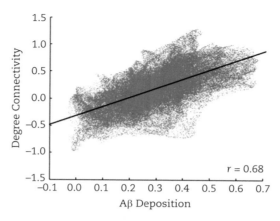

FIGURE 7.7. Direct comparison of cortical hubs and amyloid-β deposition. Shown is the high voxel-by-voxel correlation between the cortical "hubness" and estimated amyloid-beta deposition.[60] A consensus map of cortical hubs, based on intrinsic functional connectivity degree, was derived by pooling fMRI data from 127 participants. The pattern of Aβ deposition in Alzheimer's disease (AD) was measured using PiB–PET imaging. High amyloid-β deposition in the locations of cortical hubs is consistent with the possibility that hubs, while acting as critical way stations for information processing, may also augment amyloid deposition in AD.

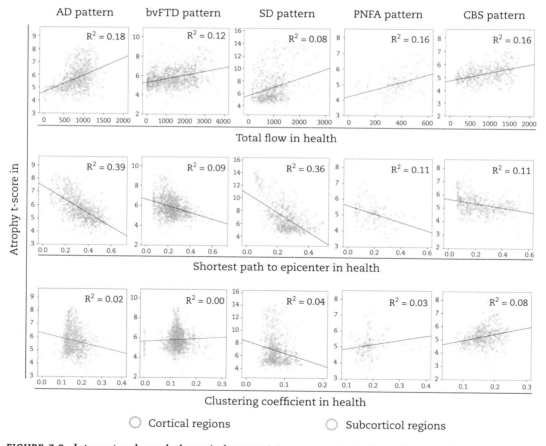

FIGURE 7.8. Intra-network graph theoretical connectivity measures in health predict atrophy severity in disease.[36] Regions with high total connectional flow (Row 1) and shorter functional paths to the epicenters (Row 2) showed significantly greater disease vulnerability ($p < 0.05$ family-wise-error corrected for multiple comparisons in AD, bvFTD, SD, PNFA, and CBS), whereas inconsistent weaker or non-significant relationships were observed between clustering coefficient and atrophy (Row 3). Cortical regions = blue circles; subcortical regions = orange circles.

In AD, a region's overall strength of functional connections (i.e., "hubness") in the healthy brain was shown to predict the amount of regional amyloid deposition as measured with amyloid-sensitive PET imaging (60, 131). To test the hypothesis that hub regions interconnecting distinct, functionally specialized systems might play a role in augmenting metabolic cascades relevant to AD, Buckner and colleagues identified regions with a high degree of functional connectivity, estimated from tf-fMRI and task-based fMRI, in the healthy human cerebral cortex. Prominent hubs were mainly located within DMN, including regions such as posterior cingulate, lateral temporal, lateral parietal, and medial/lateral prefrontal cortices. Intriguingly, regions with high Aβ deposition in AD were associated with greater functional degree centrality (i.e., "hubness") in the healthy brain. One step further, based on a within-patient design, spatial patterns of Aβ deposition (measured by Pittsburgh compound B positron emission tomography) and intrinsic functional connectivity (measured by tf-fMRI) in patients with prodromal Alzheimer's disease were compared via spatial correlations in intrinsic networks covering frontoparietal heteromodal cortices. At the global network level, Aβ and intrinsic connectivity patterns were positively correlated in the default mode and several frontoparietal attention networks, confirming that Aβ aggregates in areas of high intrinsic connectivity on a within-network basis. After accounting for this globally positive correlation, local Aβ deposition in regions of high connectivity covaried negatively with intrinsic connectivity, indicating that Aβ pathology reduces connectivity anywhere in an affected network as a function of local Aβ deposition (60, 131). Taken together, those hubs or regions with high connectional flow, acting as critical waystations for information processing, may augment the underlying pathological cascade in AD. In related work, an "epidemic-spreading model" that considered axonal propagation of amyloid proteins along the healthy structural connectome in combination with regional clearance mechanisms was able to explain approximately 50% of the variance in real amyloid deposition patterns as observed by amyloid PET (132) (Figure 7.9). Thus, this model supports the hypothesis that regional amyloid deposition likelihood is explained to a large extent by the connectional distance from specific outbreak regions estimated to lie in the anterior and posterior cingulate cortex.

Collectively, the studies cited in the preceding provide the first evidence in humans for hypotheses on molecular disease mechanisms derived from preclinical studies, including increased vulnerability of highly connected network hubs due to increased amyloid accumulation and oxidative stress (133, 134) or prion-like spread of pathogenic protein conformations (such as misfolded tau and amyloid proteins) along synaptic connections (25, 65, 135, 136).

Relationship to Clinico-anatomical Convergence and Phenotypic Diversity

How do emerging principles of disease progression relate to the observation that multiple histopathological diseases can converge on the same set of neurons, regions, or networks to produce a given clinical syndrome? If progression is driven by spread of disease across brain connections, then convergence could be merely the reflection of a shared population of onset neurons. Alternatively, distinct onset sites within the same network could, via connectional spread, produce convergent involvement of the overall network. In other words, there may be alternative anatomical pathways to the same syndrome. A particularly clear example of this notion comes from bvFTD. In a subset of patients who carry the *C9orf72* hexanucleotide repeat expansion, large-scale "salience network" dysfunction resembles that seen in sporadic bvFTD, but the loss of network integrity relates to a strategic lesion of the medial pulvinar thalamus (137), in contrast to bvFTD, where network dysfunction results from damage to the anterior cingulate and frontoinsular cortices.

The phenotypic diversity produced by AD naturally raises the question of whether each clinical AD variant can be linked to a distinct large-scale network. A recent study tested this hypothesis by assessing intrinsic functional connectivity in healthy subjects, seeding regions commonly or specifically atrophied in EOAD, lvPPA, or posterior cortical atrophy (138). The authors found that the connectivity maps derived from commonly atrophied regions of interest resembled the default mode network, which was affected in all AD variants, whereas seeding regions specifically atrophied in each AD variant revealed distinct, syndrome-specific connectivity patterns in the healthy brain. EOAD was associated with anterior salience and right executive-control networks; lvPPA was associated with the language network; and PCA was associated with the high-level visual network (Figure 7.10). These findings indicated that the syndrome-specific neurodegenerative patterns in AD variants are driven by the involvement

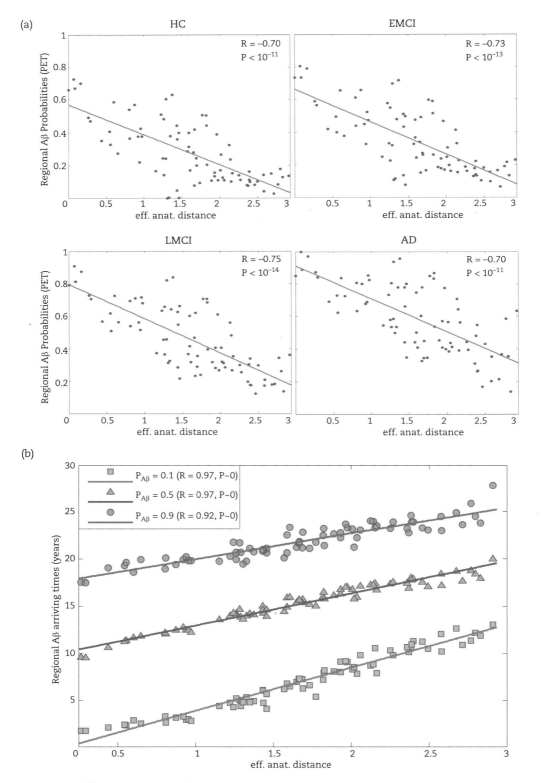

FIGURE 7.9. Effective anatomical distance to outbreak regions modulates the amyloid-ß propagation processes. (a) PET-based regional Aß deposition probabilities for the different groups versus effective anatomical distances. (b) Regional Aß arriving times versus effective anatomical distances, for different Aß probability thresholds (i.e. 0.1, 0.5 and 0.9). In (a) and (b), note the co-linearity between different clinical states or Aß probability thresholds, with more advanced disease states corresponding to higher deposition and propagation times.[132]

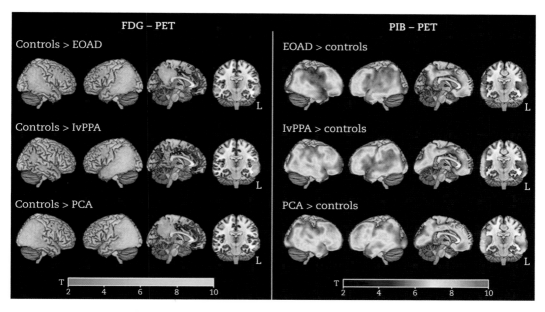

FIGURE 7.10. Patterns of FDG and PIB binding in early-onset Alzheimer's disease (EOAD), logopenic variant PPA (lvPPA) and posterior cortical atrophy (PCA) compared with healthy controls. All three Alzheimer's disease-associated clinical subgroups showed syndrome-specific patterns of glucose hypometabolism (FDG). In contrast, compared with control subjects, all three groups showed diffuse patterns of PIB uptake across the cortex symmetrically in both hemispheres, with some sparing of the sensorimotor strip, parts of the striate cortex and the medial temporal lobes.[138] Shown are T-maps after correction for multiple comparisons (FWE at $P < 0.05$) rendered on the MNI template brain. Blue in the FDG maps indicates significantly lower FDG uptake in the patient groups compared with controls, whereas warmer colors in the PIB maps indicate significantly greater PIB binding in the patient groups.

of specific networks outside the DMN. As a working model, we predict that spread into these distinct networks reflects differences in the precise localization of onset in the three variants; where exactly (in which regions and neuronal subtypes) these syndromes begin remains uncertain.

Lingering Questions and Uncertainties

Moving forward, several exciting but challenging questions remain within the general concept of disease progression. Considering the three disease-spread scenarios (Figure 7.3), what is the balance between connection-based spread versus secondary sites of onset? Does spread within the local microcircuitry occur via contiguity, or is it governed by axo-dendritic or dendro-dendritic synapses? What better predicts disease progression: a patient's current connectome or a normative connectome? How do genetic risk factors interact with the connectome to influence disease progression? Resolving these questions may help to facilitate the development of individualized treatment and prevention trials.

FUTURE DIRECTIONS

Network-based principles have begun to shed light on group-level changes across a host of neurodegenerative disease syndromes (139). To aid in the search for treatments, however, connectivity methods will need to be developed for use in tracking single subjects over time. More refined and comprehensive models of spread may aid in this process. In the subsections that follow, we outline important priorities for future research.

Disease Monitoring

To date, most evidence supporting the feasibility of tracking disease severity with connectivity-based metrics has come from cross-sectional correlations with disease severity. By examining patients with mild, moderate, or severe AD-type dementia with task-free fMRI, Zhang et al. found that all patients showed disrupted intrinsic functional connectivity between posterior cingulate cortex and DMN regions, which worsened with increasing AD severity (140). Similarly, in bvFTD, clinical severity correlated with loss of right frontoinsular salience network (SN) connectivity and enhancement of parietal DMN connectivity, suggesting that functional connectivity reductions and enhancements both carry the potential to track disease progression (41). This capacity provides an advantage over structural MRI methods and may prove more relevant when we seek to detect early changes in brain circuits before symptoms arise.

Despite these group-level, cross-sectional findings, to characterize the real-world onset and progression of neurodegenerative disease will require longitudinal studies in individuals. One longitudinal study showed decreased intrinsic connectivity in the posterior DMN and increased connectivity in the anterior and ventral DMN subnetworks in AD compared to healthy controls at baseline. At follow-up, patients showed worsening connectivity across all default mode subsystems (141), in keeping with a network-based neurodegeneration model in which disease spreads from hot spots or "epicenters" to interconnected nodes within the target and, ultimately, off-target systems (36). Atrophy progression mapping in early-onset and late-onset AD over one year also suggested that atrophy eventually progressed along the same DMN regions in both groups, although it mainly involved different lateral neocortical or medial temporal hubs at baseline (142). In parallel, longitudinal studies differentiated stable from progressive mild cognitive impairment based on the baseline DMN functional connectivity (143, 144). Moreover, one recent multimodal longitudinal neuroimaging study in AD indicated that amyloid accumulation in remote but functionally connected brain regions (defined by tf-fMRI) may contribute to the longitudinally evolving hypometabolism in brain regions not strongly affected by local amyloid pathology, supporting the network-degeneration hypothesis (145). Longitudinal studies of connectivity and other candidate biomarkers are needed for FTD and other dementia subtypes (146), and efforts are under way to organize large-collaborative networks inspired by the AD model.

Whether network integrity metrics can predict clinical outcome has yet to be widely explored. Regional diffusion measures of white matter integrity, most notably within the fornix, posterior cingulum, and parahippocampal white matter, have shown promising accuracies between 77% and 95% for the prediction of conversion from MCI to AD dementia over clinical follow-up times of 2 to 3 years (147–150). Preliminary findings further suggest that mean diffusivity may be of higher predictive value compared to fractional anisotropy (147), and that diffusion metrics may be generally better predictors of conversion than volumetric measurements on structural MRI (149, 151), particularly for the prediction of future cognitive impairments in cognitively normal elderly (105, 106). These single-center studies were limited by relatively small sample sizes, and diagnostic and prognostic findings within the highly controlled experimental conditions of these studies, such as uniform image acquisition protocols and selected patient populations, will make it difficult to translate seamlessly into the broader clinical context. Moving forward, resolving these issues will help to determine the role of imaging metrics in the selection or stratification of individuals enrolled in clinical prevention or treatment trials geared toward specific molecular pathogenic mechanisms.

Network Degeneration Mechanisms

Although network degeneration mechanistic hypotheses are based on the assumption that networks constrain and determine the anatomical disease pattern, apparent network-based spread could emerge, in a network-independent manner, if individual nodes within each target network possessed differential vulnerability to the disease process, leading those nodes to succumb sequentially according to their vulnerability. These mechanistic considerations raise the question of whether neurodegenerative diseases should be deemed primary diseases of networks. Alternatively, networks might be damaged and disrupted in these illnesses without representing the most relevant primary target. Longitudinal multimodal neuroimaging studies will enable researchers to more formally test the predictions made by these various disease progression models and determine their prognostic value in individual patients.

Technical Considerations: Validation Across Sites, Sequences, and Cohorts

The systematic collection and analysis of multicenter multimodal imaging data, including biomarkers of functional and structural connectivity, are an indispensable requirement for the future assessment of the diagnostic, prognostic, monitoring, and therapeutic response value of these markers, both for clinical trials as well as for healthcare applications. This validation process also involves the analysis of the robustness or vulnerability of the markers to degraded image quality or varying numbers of available imaging modalities. Systematic studies need to explore the minimum image quality and data dimensions that still yield diagnostically useful information for an individual subject.

Additional methods development will also fuel new discoveries. Sub-millimeter resolution human brain imaging provides a means to examine structure—and perhaps someday structural connectivity patterns—at the level of specific cortical layers (152). Ultra-high resolution diffusion tensor imaging allows for estimation of increasingly fine white matter tracts (153). Simultaneous multi-slice imaging has dramatically reduced scan time for fMRI and DTI, increasing the feasibility of real-time applications in clinical settings (154) and providing opportunities to model causal networks with greater confidence. These advances create tremendous opportunities to further refine the human brain connectome and exploit this knowledge in the search for new neurological and psychiatric disease treatments.

REFERENCES

1. Hyman, B. T., Damasio, A. R., Van Hoesen, G. W., and Barnes, C. L. (1984). Alzheimer's disease: cell-specific pathology isolates the hippocampal formation. *Science 298*, 83–95.
2. Braak, H., and Braak, E. (1991). Neuropathological staging of Alzheimer-related changes. *Acta Neuropathol 82*, 239–259.
3. Brun, A., and Gustafson, L. (1978). Limbic lobe involvement in presenile dementia. *Arch Psychiatr Nervenkr 226*, 79–93.
4. Pievani, M., de Haan, W., Wu, T., Seeley, W. W., and Frisoni, G. B. (2011). Functional network disruption in the degenerative dementias. *Lancet Neurol 10*, 829–843.
5. Gorno-Tempini, M. L., Hillis, A. E., Weintraub, S., Kertesz, A., Mendez, M., Cappa, S. F., Ogar, J. M., Rohrer, J. D., Black, S., Boeve, B. F., et al. (2011). Classification of primary progressive aphasia and its variants. *Neurology 76*, 1006–1014.
6. Rascovsky, K., Hodges, J. R., Knopman, D., Mendez, M. F., Kramer, J. H., Neuhaus, J., van Swieten, J. C., Seelaar, H., Dopper, E. G., Onyike, C. U., et al. (2011). Sensitivity of revised diagnostic criteria for the behavioural variant of frontotemporal dementia. *Brain 134*, 2456–2477.
7. Rosen, H. J., Gorno-Tempini, M. L., Goldman, W. P., Perry, R. J., Schuff, N., Weiner, M., Feiwell, R., Kramer, J. H., and Miller, B. L. (2002). Patterns of brain atrophy in frontotemporal dementia and semantic dementia. *Neurology 58*, 198–208.
8. Seeley, W. W., Crawford, R., Rascovsky, K., Kramer, J. H., Weiner, M., Miller, B. L., and Gorno-Tempini, M. L. (2008). Frontal paralimbic network atrophy in very mild behavioral variant frontotemporal dementia. *Arch Neurol 65*, 249–255.
9. Whitwell, J. L., Przybelski, S. A., Weigand, S. D., Ivnik, R. J., Vemuri, P., Gunter, J. L., Senjem, M. L., Shiung, M. M., Boeve, B. F., Knopman, D. S., et al. (2009). Distinct anatomical subtypes of the behavioural variant of frontotemporal dementia: a cluster analysis study. *Brain 132*, 2932–2946.
10. Gorno-Tempini, M. L., Dronkers, N. F., Rankin, K. P., Ogar, J. M., Phengrasamy, L., Rosen, H. J., Johnson, J. K., Weiner, M. W., and Miller, B. L. (2004). Cognition and anatomy in three variants of primary progressive aphasia. *Ann Neurol 55*, 335–346.
11. Seeley, W. W., Bauer, A. M., Miller, B. L., Gorno-Tempini, M. L., Kramer, J. H., Weiner, M., and Rosen, H. J. (2005). The natural history of temporal variant frontotemporal dementia. *Neurology 64*, 1384–1390.
12. Thompson, S. A., Patterson, K., and Hodges, J. R. (2003). Left/right asymmetry of atrophy in semantic dementia: behavioral-cognitive implications. *Neurology 61*, 1196–1203.
13. Cabeza, B., Santos, C. G., Hernangomez, S., Serrano, A., Ruiz, E. S., and Santos, S. (2013). [Aspiration of a foreign body.]. *Anales de pediatria 79*, 52–53.
14. Rohrer, J. D., Warren, J. D., Modat, M., Ridgway, G. R., Douiri, A., Rossor, M. N., Ourselin, S., and Fox, N. C. (2009). Patterns of cortical thinning in the language variants of frontotemporal lobar degeneration. *Neurology 72*, 1562–1569.
15. Dubois, B., Feldman, H. H., Jacova, C., Dekosky, S. T., Barberger-Gateau, P., Cummings, J., Delacourte, A., Galasko, D., Gauthier, S., Jicha, G., et al. (2007). Research criteria for the diagnosis of Alzheimer's disease: revising the NINCDS-ADRDA criteria. *Lancet Neurol 6*, 734–746.
16. Mackenzie, I. R., Neumann, M., Bigio, E. H., Cairns, N. J., Alafuzoff, I., Kril, J., Kovacs, G. G., Ghetti, B., Halliday, G., Holm, I. E., et al. (2010). Nomenclature and nosology for neuropathologic subtypes of frontotemporal lobar degeneration: an update. *Acta Neuropathol 119*, 1–4.
17. Loy, C. T., Schofield, P. R., Turner, A. M., and Kwok, J. B. (2014). Genetics of dementia. *Lancet 383*, 828–840.
18. Graveland, G. A., Williams, R. S., and DiFiglia, M. (1985). Evidence for degenerative and regenerative changes in neostriatal spiny neurons in Huntington's disease. *Science 227*, 770–773.
19. Seeley, W. W., Carlin, D. A., Allman, J. M., Macedo, M. N., Bush, C., Miller, B. L., and Dearmond, S. J. (2006). Early frontotemporal dementia targets neurons unique to apes and humans. *Ann Neurol 60*, 660–667.

20. Selkoe, D. J. (2002). Alzheimer's disease is a synaptic failure. *Science 298*, 789–791.

21. Pearson, R. C., Esiri, M. M., Hiorns, R. W., Wilcock, G. K., and Powell, T. P. (1985). Anatomical correlates of the distribution of the pathological changes in the neocortex in Alzheimer disease. *Proc Natl Acad Sci U S A 82*, 4531–4534.

22. Saper, C. B., Wainer, B. H., and German, D. C. (1987). Axonal and transneuronal transport in the transmission of neurological disease: potential role in system degenerations, including Alzheimer's disease. *Neuroscience 23*, 389–398.

23. Weintraub, S., and Mesulam, M.-M. (1996). From neuronal networks to dementia: four clinical profiles. In *La demence: Pourquoi?*, Foret F., Christen Y., and Boller F., eds. Paris: Foundation Nationale de Gerontologie, pp. 75–97.

24. Steele, J. C., Richardson, J. C., and Olszewski, J. (1964). Progressive Supranuclear Palsy. *Arch Neurol 10*, 333–360.

25. Frost, B., and Diamond, M. I. (2010). Prion-like mechanisms in neurodegenerative diseases. *Nat Rev Neurosci 11*, 155–159.

26. Goedert, M., Clavaguera, F., and Tolnay, M. (2010). The propagation of prion-like protein inclusions in neurodegenerative diseases. *Trends Neurosci 33*, 317–325.

27. Palop, J. J., Chin, J., Roberson, E. D., Wang, J., Thwin, M. T., Bien-Ly, N., Yoo, J., Ho, K. O., Yu, G.-Q., Kreitzer, A., et al. (2007). Aberrant excitatory neuronal activity and compensatory remodeling of inhibitory hippocampal circuits in mouse models of Alzheimer's disease. *Neuron 55*, 697–711.

28. Prusiner, S. B. (2012). Cell biology: a unifying role for prions in neurodegenerative diseases. *Science 336*, 1511–1513.

29. Choo, I. H., Lee, D. Y., Youn, J. C., Jhoo, J. H., Kim, K. W., Lee, D. S., Lee, J. S., and Woo, J. I. (2007). Topographic patterns of brain functional impairment progression according to clinical severity staging in 116 Alzheimer disease patients: FDG-PET study. *Alzheimer Dis Assoc Disord 21*, 77–84.

30. Thal, D. R., Attems, J., and Ewers, M. (2014). Spreading of amyloid, tau, and microvascular pathology in Alzheimer's disease: findings from neuropathological and neuroimaging studies. *J Alzheimers Dis 42 Suppl 4*, S421–429.

31. Whitwell, J. L., Przybelski, S. A., Weigand, S. D., Knopman, D. S., Boeve, B. F., Petersen, R. C., and Jack, C. R., Jr. (2007). 3D maps from multiple MRI illustrate changing atrophy patterns as subjects progress from mild cognitive impairment to Alzheimer's disease. *Brain 130*, 1777–1786.

32. Buckner, R. L., Snyder, A. Z., Shannon, B. J., LaRossa, G., Sachs, R., Fotenos, A. F., Sheline, Y. I., Klunk, W. E., Mathis, C. A., Morris, J. C., et al. (2005). Molecular, structural, and functional characterization of Alzheimer's disease: evidence for a relationship between default activity, amyloid, and memory. *J Neurosci 25*, 7709–7717.

33. Greicius, M. D., Srivastava, G., Reiss, A. L., and Menon, V. (2004). Default-mode network activity distinguishes Alzheimer's disease from healthy aging: evidence from functional MRI. *Proc Natl Acad Sci U S A 101*, 4637–4642.

34. Raj, A., Kuceyeski, A., and Weiner, M. (2012). A network diffusion model of disease progression in dementia. *Neuron 73*, 1204–1215.

35. Seeley, W. W., Crawford, R. K., Zhou, J., Miller, B. L., and Greicius, M. D. (2009). Neurodegenerative diseases target large-scale human brain networks. *Neuron 62*, 42–52.

36. Zhou, J., Gennatas, E. D., Kramer, J. H., Miller, B. L., and Seeley, W. W. (2012). Predicting regional neurodegeneration from the healthy brain functional connectome. *Neuron 73*, 1216–1227.

37. Biswal, B. B., Mennes, M., Zuo, X. N., Gohel, S., Kelly, C., Smith, S. M., Beckmann, C. F., Adelstein, J. S., Buckner, R. L., Colcombe, S., et al. (2010). Toward discovery science of human brain function. *Proc Natl Acad Sci U S A 107*, 4734–4739.

38. Damoiseaux, J. S., Rombouts, S. A. R. B., Barkhof, F., Scheltens, P., Stam, C. J., Smith, S. M., and Beckmann, C. F. (2006). Consistent resting-state networks across healthy subjects. *Proc Natl Acad Sci U S A 103*, 13848–13853.

39. Fox, M. D., and Raichle, M. E. (2007). Spontaneous fluctuations in brain activity observed with functional magnetic resonance imaging. *Nat Rev Neurosci 8*, 700–711.

40. Greicius, M. D., Krasnow, B., Reiss, A. L., and Menon, V. (2003). Functional connectivity in the resting brain: a network analysis of the default mode hypothesis. *Proc Natl Acad Sci U S A 100*, 253–258.

41. Zhou, J., Greicius, M. D., Gennatas, E. D., Growdon, M. E., Jang, J. Y., Rabinovici, G. D., Kramer, J. H., Weiner, M., Miller, B. L., and Seeley, W. W. (2010). Divergent network connectivity changes in behavioural variant frontotemporal dementia and Alzheimer's disease. *Brain 133*, 1352–1367.

42. Biswal, B., Yetkin, F. Z., Haughton, V. M., and Hyde, J. S. (1995). Functional connectivity in the motor cortex of resting human brain using echo-planar MRI. *Magn Reson Med 34*, 537–541.

43. Fox, M. D., Snyder, A. Z., Vincent, J. L., Corbetta, M., Van Essen, D. C., and Raichle, M. E. (2005). The human brain is intrinsically organized into dynamic, anticorrelated functional networks. *Proc Natl Acad Sci U S A 102*, 9673–9678.

44. Raichle, M. E., MacLeod, A. M., Snyder, A. Z., Powers, W. J., Gusnard, D. A., and Shulman, G.

L. (2001). A default mode of brain function. *Proc Natl Acad Sci U S A 98*, 676–682.

45. Vincent, J. L., Patel, G. H., Fox, M. D., Snyder, A. Z., Baker, J. T., Van Essen, D. C., Zempel, J. M., Snyder, L. H., Corbetta, M., and Raichle, M. E. (2007). Intrinsic functional architecture in the anaesthetized monkey brain. *Nature 447*, 83–86.

46. Doria, V., Beckmann, C. F., Arichi, T., Merchant, N., Groppo, M., Turkheimer, F. E., Counsell, S. J., Murgasova, M., Aljabar, P., Nunes, R. G., et al. (2010). Emergence of resting state networks in the preterm human brain. *Proc Natl Acad Sci U S A 107*, 20015–20020.

47. Smith, S. M., Fox, P. T., Miller, K. L., Glahn, D. C., Fox, P. M., Mackay, C. E., Filippini, N., Watkins, K. E., Toro, R., Laird, A. R., et al. (2009). Correspondence of the brain's functional architecture during activation and rest. *Proc Natl Acad Sci U S A 106*, 13040–13045.

48. Beckmann, C. F., DeLuca, M., Devlin, J. T., and Smith, S. M. (2005). Investigations into resting-state connectivity using independent component analysis. *Philos Trans R Soc Lond B Biol Sci 360*, 1001–1013.

49. Yeo, B. T., Krienen, F. M., Sepulcre, J., Sabuncu, M. R., Lashkari, D., Hollinshead, M., Roffman, J. L., Smoller, J. W., Zollei, L., Polimeni, J. R., et al. (2011). The organization of the human cerebral cortex estimated by intrinsic functional connectivity. *J Neurophysiol 106*, 1125–1165.

50. Krajcovicova, L., Marecek, R., Mikl, M., and Rektorova, I. (2014). Disruption of resting functional connectivity in Alzheimer's patients and at-risk subjects. *Curr Neurol Neurosci Rep 14 (10): 491*.

51. Dennis, E. L., and Thompson, P. M. (2014). Functional brain connectivity using fMRI in aging and Alzheimer's sisease. *Neuropsychol Rev 24*, 49–62.

52. He, Y., Chen, Z., and Evans, A. (2008). Structural insights into aberrant topological patterns of large-scale cortical networks in Alzheimer's disease. *J Neurosci 28*, 4756–4766.

53. Horin, P., Sabakova, K., Futas, J., Vychodilova, L., and Necesankova, M. (2010). Immunity-related gene single nucleotide polymorphisms associated with Rhodococcus equi infection in foals. *Int J Immunogenet 37*, 67–71.

54. Lerch, J. P., Worsley, K., Shaw, W. P., Greenstein, D. K., Lenroot, R. K., Giedd, J., and Evans, A. C. (2006). Mapping anatomical correlations across cerebral cortex (MACACC) using cortical thickness from MRI. *Neuroimage 31*, 993–1003.

55. Le Bihan, D., Turner, R., Douek, P., and Patronas, N. (1992). Diffusion MR imaging: clinical applications. *Am J Roentgenol 159*, 591–599.

56. Le Bihan, D., Mangin, J. F., Poupon, C., Clark, C.A., Pappata, S., Molko, N., and Chabriat, H. (2001). Diffusion tensor imaging: concepts and applications. *JMRI 13*, 534–546.

57. Mori, S., Crain, B. J., Chacko, V. P., and Van Zijl, P. C. M. (1999). Three-dimensional tracking of axonal projections in the brain by magnetic resonance imaging. *Ann Neurol 45*, 265–269.

58. Mori, S., and Zhang, J. (2006). Principles of diffusion tensor imaging and its applications to basic neuroscience research. *Neuron 51*, 527–539.

59. Sporns, O., Tononi, G., and Kotter, R. (2005). The human connectome: a structural description of the human brain. *PLoS Comput Biol 1*, e42.

60. Buckner, R. L., Sepulcre, J., Talukdar, T., Krienen, F. M., Liu, H., Hedden, T., Andrews-Hanna, J. R., Sperling, R. A., and Johnson, K. A. (2009a). Cortical hubs revealed by intrinsic functional connectivity: mapping, assessment of stability, and relation to Alzheimer's disease. *J Neurosci 29*, 1860–1873.

61. Crossley, N. A., Mechelli, A., Vertes, P. E., Winton-Brown, T. T., Patel, A. X., Ginestet, C. E., McGuire, P., and Bullmore, E. T. (2013). Cognitive relevance of the community structure of the human brain functional coactivation network. *Proc Natl Acad Sci 110*, 11583–11588.

62. Sporns, O., Honey, C. J., and Kotter, R. (2007). Identification and classification of hubs in brain networks. *PLoS One 2*, e1049.

63. van den Heuvel, M. P., and Sporns, O. (2011). Rich-club organization of the human connectome. *J Neurosci 31*, 15775–15786.

64. Zuo, X. N., Ehmke, R., Mennes, M., Imperati, D., Castellanos, F. X., Sporns, O., and Milham, M. P. (2012). Network centrality in the human functional connectome. *Cereb Cortex 22*, 1862–1875.

65. Braak, H., and Del Tredici, K. (2011). Alzheimer's pathogenesis: is there neuron-to-neuron propagation? *Acta Neuropathol 121*, 589–595.

66. Grinberg, L. T., Rub, U., Ferretti, R. E., Nitrini, R., Farfel, J. M., Polichiso, L., Gierga, K., Jacob-Filho, W., Heinsen, H., and Brazilian Brain Bank Study. (2009). The dorsal raphe nucleus shows phospho-tau neurofibrillary changes before the transentorhinal region in Alzheimer's disease: a precocious onset? *Neuropathol Appl Neurobiol 35*, 406–416.

67. Lomen-Hoerth, C., Anderson, T., and Miller, B. (2002). The overlap of amyotrophic lateral sclerosis and frontotemporal dementia. *Neurology 59*, 1077–1079.

68. Chang, J. L., Lomen-Hoerth, C., Murphy, J., Henry, R. G., Kramer, J. H., Miller, B. L., and

Gorno-Tempini, M. L. (2005). A voxel-based morphometry study of patterns of brain atrophy in ALS and ALS/FTLD. *Neurology 65*, 75–80.

69. Simon, N. G., Turner, M. R., Vucic, S., Al-Chalabi, A., Shefner, J., Lomen-Hoerth, C., and Kiernan, M. C. (2014). Quantifying disease progression in amyotrophic lateral sclerosis. *Ann Neurol 76*, 643–657.

70. Trojsi, F., Monsurro, M. R., Esposito, F., and Tedeschi, G. (2012). Widespread structural and functional connectivity changes in amyotrophic lateral sclerosis: insights from advanced neuroimaging research. *Neural Plast 2012*, 473538.

71. Braak, H., Braak, E., and Bohl, J. (1993). Staging of Alzheimer-related cortical destruction. *Eur Neurol 33*, 403–408.

72. Braak, H., Ghebremedhin, E., Rub, U., Bratzke, H., and Del Tredici, K. (2004). Stages in the development of Parkinson's disease-related pathology. *Cell Tissue Res 318*, 121–134.

73. Jack, C. R., Jr., Shiung, M. M., Gunter, J. L., O'Brien, P. C., Weigand, S. D., Knopman, D. S., Boeve, B. F., Ivnik, R. J., Smith, G. E., Cha, R. H., et al. (2004). Comparison of different MRI brain atrophy rate measures with clinical disease progression in AD. *Neurology 62*, 591–600.

74. Killiany, R. J., Hyman, B. T., Gomez-Isla, T., Moss, M. B., Kikinis, R., Jolesz, F., Tanzi, R., Jones, K., and Albert, M. S. (2002). MRI measures of entorhinal cortex vs hippocampus in preclinical AD. *Neurology 58*, 1188–1196.

75. Varon, D., Loewenstein, D. A., Potter, E., Greig, M. T., Agron, J., Shen, Q., Zhao, W., Celeste Ramirez, M., Santos, I., Barker, W., et al. (2011). Minimal atrophy of the entorhinal cortex and hippocampus: progression of cognitive impairment. *Dement Geriatr Cogn Disord 31*, 276–283.

76. Bondareff, W., Mountjoy, C. Q., and Roth, M. (1981). Selective loss of neurones of origin of adrenergic projection to cerebral cortex (nucleus locus coeruleus) in senile dementia. *Lancet 1*, 783–784.

77. Braak, H., and Del Tredici, K. (2012). Where, when, and in what form does sporadic Alzheimer's disease begin? *Curr Opin Neurol 25*, 708–714.

78. Braak, H., Del Tredici, K., Rub, U., de Vos, R. A., Jansen Steur, E. N., and Braak, E. (2003). Staging of brain pathology related to sporadic Parkinson's disease. *Neurobiol Aging 24*, 197–211.

79. Brettschneider, J., Del Tredici, K., Irwin, D. J., Grossman, M., Robinson, J. L., Toledo, J. B., Lee, E. B., Fang, L., Van Deerlin, V. M., Ludolph, A. C., et al. (2014). Sequential distribution of pTDP-43 pathology in behavioral variant frontotemporal dementia (bvFTD). *Acta Neuropathol 127*, 423–439.

80. Irwin, D. J., McMillan, C. T., Brettschneider, J., Libon, D. J., Powers, J., Rascovsky, K., Toledo, J. B., Boller, A., Bekisz, J., Chandrasekaran, K., et al. (2013). Cognitive decline and reduced survival in C9orf72 expansion frontotemporal degeneration and amyotrophic lateral sclerosis. *J Neurol Neurosurg Psychiatry 84*, 163–169.

81. Seeley, W. W., Menon, V., Schatzberg, A. F., Keller, J., Glover, G. H., Kenna, H., Reiss, A. L., and Greicius, M. D. (2007). Dissociable intrinsic connectivity networks for salience processing and executive control. *J Neurosci 27*, 2349–2356.

82. Kim, E. J., Sidhu, M., Gaus, S. E., Huang, E. J., Hof, P. R., Miller, B. L., Dearmond, S. J., and Seeley, W. W. (2012). Selective frontoinsular von economo neuron and fork cell loss in early behavioral variant frontotemporal dementia. *Cereb Cortex 22*, 251–259.

83. Hedden, T., Van Dijk, K. R., Becker, J. A., Mehta, A., Sperling, R. A., Johnson, K. A., and Buckner, R. L. (2009). Disruption of functional connectivity in clinically normal older adults harboring amyloid burden. *J Neurosci 29*, 12686–12694.

84. Sperling, R. A., Laviolette, P. S., O'Keefe, K., O'Brien, J., Rentz, D. M., Pihlajamaki, M., Marshall, G., Hyman, B. T., Selkoe, D. J., Hedden, T., et al. (2009). Amyloid deposition is associated with impaired default network function in older persons without dementia. *Neuron 63*, 178–188.

85. Damoiseaux, J. S., Seeley, W. W., Zhou, J., Shirer, W. R., Coppola, G., Karydas, A., Rosen, H. J., Miller, B. L., Kramer, J. H., and Greicius, M. D. (2012b). Gender modulates the APOE ε4 effect in healthy older adults: Convergent evidence from functional brain connectivity and spinal fluid Tau levels. *J Neurosci 32*, 8254–8262.

86. Machulda, M. M., Jones, D. T., Vemuri, P., McDade, E., Avula, R., Przybelski, S., Boeve, B. F., Knopman, D. S., Petersen, R. C., and Jack, C. R., Jr. (2011). Effect of APOE epsilon4 status on intrinsic network connectivity in cognitively normal elderly subjects. *Arch Neurology 68*, 1131–1136.

87. Persson, J., Lind, J., Larsson, A., Ingvar, M., Sleegers, K., Van Broeckhoven, C., Adolfsson, R., Nilsson, L. G., and Nyberg, L. (2008). Altered deactivation in individuals with genetic risk for Alzheimer's disease. *Neuropsychologia 46*, 1679–1687.

88. Drzezga, A., Becker, J. A., Van Dijk, K. R., Sreenivasan, A., Talukdar, T., Sullivan, C., Schultz, A. P., Sepulcre, J., Putcha, D., Greve, D., et al. (2011). Neuronal dysfunction and

disconnection of cortical hubs in non-demented subjects with elevated amyloid burden. *Brain* 134, 1635–1646.

89. Bendlin, B. B., Carlsson, C. M., Johnson, S. C., Zetterberg, H., Blennow, K., Willette, A. A., Okonkwo, O. C., Sodhi, A., Ries, M. L., Birdsill, A. C., et al. (2012). CSF T-Tau/Abeta42 predicts white matter microstructure in healthy adults at risk for Alzheimer's disease. *PLoS One 7*, e37720.

90. Chao, L. L., Decarli, C., Kriger, S., Truran, D., Zhang, Y., Laxamana, J., Villeneuve, S., Jagust, W. J., Sanossian, N., Mack, W. J., et al. (2013). Associations between white matter hyperintensities and beta amyloid on integrity of projection, association, and limbic fiber tracts measured with diffusion tensor MRI. *PLoS One 8*, e65175.

91. Gold, B. T., Zhu, Z., Brown, C. A., Andersen, A. H., LaDu, M. J., Tai, L., Jicha, G. A., Kryscio, R. J., Estus, S., Nelson, P. T., et al. (2014). White matter integrity is associated with cerebrospinal fluid markers of Alzheimer's disease in normal adults. *Neurobiol Aging 35*, 2263–2271.

92. Kantarci, K., Schwarz, C. G., Reid, R. I., Przybelski, S. A., Lesnick, T. G., Zuk, S. M., Senjem, M. L., Gunter, J. L., Lowe, V., Machulda, M. M., et al. (2014). White matter integrity determined with diffusion tensor imaging in older adults without dementia: influence of amyloid load and neurodegeneration. *JAMA Neurol 71*, 1547–1554.

93. Molinuevo, J. L., Ripolles, P., Simo, M., Llado, A., Olives, J., Balasa, M., Antonell, A., Rodriguez-Fornells, A., and Rami, L. (2014). White matter changes in preclinical Alzheimer's disease: a magnetic resonance imaging-diffusion tensor imaging study on cognitively normal older people with positive amyloid beta protein 42 levels. *Neurobiol Aging 35*, 2671–2680.

94. Racine, A. M., Adluru, N., Alexander, A. L., Christian, B. T., Okonkwo, O. C., Oh, J., Cleary, C. A., Birdsill, A., Hillmer, A. T., Murali, D., et al. (2014). Associations between white matter microstructure and amyloid burden in preclinical Alzheimer's disease: a multimodal imaging investigation. *Neuroimage Clin 4*, 604–614.

95. Stenset, V., Bjornerud, A., Fjell, A. M., Walhovd, K. B., Hofoss, D., Due-Tonnessen, P., Gjerstad, L., and Fladby, T. (2011). Cingulum fiber diffusivity and CSF T-tau in patients with subjective and mild cognitive impairment. *Neurobiol Aging 32*, 581–589.

96. Filippini, N., MacIntosh, B. J., Hough, M. G., Goodwin, G. M., Frisoni, G. B., Smith, S. M., Matthews, P. M., Beckmann, C. F., and Mackay, C. E. (2009). Distinct patterns of brain activity in young carriers of the APOE-epsilon4 allele. *Proc Natl Acad Sci U S A 106*, 7209–7214.

97. Bai, F., Watson, D. R., Shi, Y., Wang, Y., Yue, C., YuhuanTeng, Wu, D., Yuan, Y., and Zhang, Z. (2011). Specifically progressive deficits of brain functional marker in amnestic type mild cognitive impairment. *PLoS One 6*, e24271.

98. Gili, T., Cercignani, M., Serra, L., Perri, R., Giove, F., Maraviglia, B., Caltagirone, C., and Bozzali, M. (2011). Regional brain atrophy and functional disconnection across Alzheimer's disease evolution. *J Neurol Neurosurg Psychiatry 82*, 58–66.

99. Bendlin, B. B., Ries, M. L., Canu, E., Sodhi, A., Lazar, M., Alexander, A. L., Carlsson, C. M., Sager, M. A., Asthana, S., and Johnson, S. C. (2010). White matter is altered with parental family history of Alzheimer's disease. *Alzheimers Dement 6*, 394–403.

100. Kljajevic, V., Meyer, P., Holzmann, C., Dyrba, M., Kasper, E., Bokde, A. L., Fellgiebel, A., Meindl, T., Hampel, H., Teipel, S., et al. (2014). The epsilon4 genotype of apolipoprotein E and white matter integrity in Alzheimer's disease. *Alzheimers Dement 10*, 401–404.

101. Lyall, D. M., Harris, S. E., Bastin, M. E., Munoz Maniega, S., Murray, C., Lutz, M. W., Saunders, A. M., Roses, A. D., Valdes Hernandez Mdel, C., Royle, N. A., et al. (2014). Alzheimer's disease susceptibility genes APOE and TOMM40, and brain white matter integrity in the Lothian Birth Cohort 1936. *Neurobiol Aging 35*, 1513 e1525–1533.

102. Ringman, J. M., O'Neill, J., Geschwind, D., Medina, L., Apostolova, L. G., Rodriguez, Y., Schaffer, B., Varpetian, A., Tseng, B., Ortiz, F., et al. (2007). Diffusion tensor imaging in preclinical and presymptomatic carriers of familial Alzheimer's disease mutations. *Brain 130*, 1767–1776.

103. Westlye, L. T., Reinvang, I., Rootwelt, H., and Espeseth, T. (2012). Effects of APOE on brain white matter microstructure in healthy adults. *Neurology 79*, 1961–1969.

104. Xiong, C., Roe, C. M., Buckles, V., Fagan, A., Holtzman, D., Balota, D., Duchek, J., Storandt, M., Mintun, M., Grant, E., et al. (2011). Role of family history for Alzheimer biomarker abnormalities in the adult children study. *Arch Neurol 68*, 1313–1319.

105. Fletcher, E., Raman, M., Huebner, P., Liu, A., Mungas, D., Carmichael, O., and DeCarli, C. (2013). Loss of fornix white matter volume as a predictor of cognitive impairment in cognitively normal elderly individuals. *JAMA Neurol 70*, 1389–1395.

106. Zhuang, L., Sachdev, P. S., Trollor, J. N., Kochan, N. A., Reppermund, S., Brodaty, H., and Wen, W. (2012). Microstructural white matter changes in cognitively normal individuals at risk of amnestic MCI. *Neurology 79*, 748–754.

107. Matura, S., Prvulovic, D., Jurcoane, A., Hartmann, D., Miller, J., Scheibe, M., O'Dwyer, L., Oertel-Knochel, V., Knochel, C., Reinke, B., et al. (2014). Differential effects of the ApoE4 genotype on brain structure and function. *Neuroimage 89*, 81–91.

108. Patel, K. T., Stevens, M. C., Pearlson, G. D., Winkler, A. M., Hawkins, K. A., Skudlarski, P., and Bauer, L. O. (2013). Default mode network activity and white matter integrity in healthy middle-aged ApoE4 carriers. *Brain Imaging Behav 7*, 60–67.

109. Heise, V., Filippini, N., Trachtenberg, A. J., Suri, S., Ebmeier, K. P., and Mackay, C.E. (2014). Apolipoprotein E genotype, gender and age modulate connectivity of the hippocampus in healthy adults. *Neuroimage 98*, 23–30.

110. Chen, Y., Chen, K., Zhang, J., Li, X., Shu, N., Wang, J., Zhang, Z., and Reiman, E.M. (2014). Disrupted functional and structural networks in cognitively normal elderly subjects with the APOE varepsilon4 Allele. *Neuropsychopharmacology 40(5), 1181–91*.

111. Dopper, E. G., Rombouts, S. A., Jiskoot, L. C., Heijer, T., de Graaf, J. R., Koning, I., Hammerschlag, A. R., Seelaar, H., Seeley, W. W., Veer, I. M., et al. (2013). Structural and functional brain connectivity in presymptomatic familial frontotemporal dementia. *Neurology 80*, 814–823.

112. Rohrer, J. D., Nicholas, J. M., Cash, D. M., van Swieten, J., Dopper, E., Jiskoot, L., van Minkelen, R., Rombouts, S. A., Cardoso, M. J., Clegg, S., et al. (2015). Presymptomatic cognitive and neuroanatomical changes in genetic frontotemporal dementia in the Genetic Frontotemporal dementia Initiative (GENFI) study: a cross-sectional analysis. *Lancet Neurol 14*, 253–262.

113. Frisoni, G. B., Pievani, M., Testa, C., Sabattoli, F., Bresciani, L., Bonetti, M., Beltramello, A., Hayashi, K. M., Toga, A. W., and Thompson, P. M. (2007). The topography of grey matter involvement in early and late onset Alzheimer's disease. *Brain 130*, 720–730.

114. Koedam, E. L., Lauffer, V., van der Vlies, A. E., van der Flier, W. M., Scheltens, P., and Pijnenburg, Y. A. (2010). Early-versus late-onset Alzheimer's disease: more than age alone. *J Alzheimers Dis 19*, 1401–1408.

115. Crutch, S. J., Lehmann, M., Schott, J. M., Rabinovici, G. D., Rossor, M. N., and Fox, N. C. (2012). Posterior cortical atrophy. *Lancet Neurol 11*, 170–178.

116. Gorno-Tempini, M. L., Brambati, S. M., Ginex, V., Ogar, J., Dronkers, N. F., Marcone, A., Perani, D., Garibotto, V., Cappa, S. F., and Miller, B. L. (2008). The logopenic/phonological variant of primary progressive aphasia. *Neurology 71*, 1227–1234.

117. Snowden, J. S., Stopford, C. L., Julien, C. L., Thompson, J. C., Davidson, Y., Gibbons, L., Pritchard, A., Lendon, C. L., Richardson, A. M., Varma, A., et al. (2007). Cognitive phenotypes in Alzheimer's disease and genetic risk. *Cortex 43*, 835–845.

118. Rogalski, E., Weintraub, S., and Mesulam, M. M. (2013). Are there susceptibility factors for primary progressive aphasia? *Brain Lang 127*, 135–138.

119. Buckner, R. L., Sepulcre, J., Talukdar, T., Krienen, F. M., Liu, H., Hedden, T., Andrews-Hanna, J. R., Sperling, R. A., and Johnson, K. A. (2009b). Cortical hubs revealed by intrinsic functional connectivity: mapping, assessment of stability, and relation to Alzheimer's disease. *J Neurosci 29*, 1860–1873.

120. Saxena, S., and Caroni, P. (2011). Selective neuronal vulnerability in neurodegenerative diseases: from stressor thresholds to degeneration. *Neuron 71*, 35–48.

121. Baker, H. F., Ridley, R. M., Duchen, L. W., Crow, T. J., and Bruton, C. J. (1994). Induction of beta (A4)-amyloid in primates by injection of Alzheimer's disease brain homogenate: comparison with transmission of spongiform encephalopathy. *Mol Neurobiol 8*, 25–39.

122. Frost, B., Ollesch, J., Wille, H., and Diamond, M.I. (2009). Conformational diversity of wild-type Tau fibrils specified by templated conformation change. *J Biol Chem 284*, 3546–3551.

123. Jucker, M., and Walker, L. C. (2011). Pathogenic protein seeding in Alzheimer disease and other neurodegenerative disorders. *Ann Neurol 70*, 532–540.

124. Lee, J. K., Jin, H. K., Endo, S., Schuchman, E. H., Carter, J. E., and Bae, J. S. (2010). Intracerebral transplantation of bone marrow-derived mesenchymal stem cells reduces amyloid-beta deposition and rescues memory deficits in Alzheimer's disease mice by modulation of immune responses. *Stem Cells 28*, 329–343.

125. Prusiner, S. B. (1984). Some speculations about prions, amyloid, and Alzheimer's disease. *N Engl J Med 310*, 661–663.

126. Ridley, R. M., Baker, H. F., Windle, C. P., and Cummings, R. M. (2006). Very long term studies of the seeding of beta-amyloidosis in primates. *J Neural Transm 113*, 1243–1251.

127. Walker, L. C., Levine, H., 3rd, Mattson, M. P., and Jucker, M. (2006). Inducible proteopathies. *Trends Neurosci 29*, 438–443.

128. Appel, S. H. (1981). A unifying hypothesis for the cause of amyotrophic lateral sclerosis,

parkinsonism, and Alzheimer disease. *Ann Neurol 10*, 499–505.

129. Salehi, A., Delcroix, J. D., Belichenko, P. V., Zhan, K., Wu, C., Valletta, J. S., Takimoto-Kimura, R., Kleschevnikov, A. M., Sambamurti, K., Chung, P. P., et al. (2006). Increased App expression in a mouse model of Down's syndrome disrupts NGF transport and causes cholinergic neuron degeneration. *Neuron 51*, 29–42.

130. Richiardi, J., Altmann, A., Milazzo, A. C., Chang, C., Chakravarty, M. M., Banaschewski, T., Barker, G. J., Bokde, A. L., Bromberg, U., Buchel, C., et al. (2015). Brain networks: correlated gene expression supports synchronous activity in brain networks. *Science 348*, 1241–1244.

131. Myers, N., Pasquini, L., Gottler, J., Grimmer, T., Koch, K., Ortner, M., Neitzel, J., Muhlau, M., Forster, S., Kurz, A., et al. (2014). Within-patient correspondence of amyloid-beta and intrinsic network connectivity in Alzheimer's disease. *Brain 137*, 2052–2064.

132. Iturria-Medina, Y., Sotero, R. C., Toussaint, P. J., and Evans, A. C. (2014). Epidemic spreading model to characterize misfolded proteins propagation in aging and associated neurodegenerative disorders. *PLoS Comput Biol 10*, e1003956.

133. Cirrito, J. R., Yamada, K. A., Finn, M. B., Sloviter, R. S., Bales, K. R., May, P. C., Schoepp, D. D., Paul, S. M., Mennerick, S., and Holtzman, D. M. (2005). Synaptic activity regulates interstitial fluid amyloid-beta levels in vivo. *Neuron 48*, 913–922.

134. Spires-Jones, T. L., and Hyman, B. T. (2014). The intersection of amyloid beta and tau at synapses in Alzheimer's disease. *Neuron 82*, 756–771.

135. Ahmed, Z., Cooper, J., Murray, T. K., Garn, K., McNaughton, E., Clarke, H., Parhizkar, S., Ward, M. A., Cavallini, A., Jackson, S., et al. (2014). A novel in vivo model of tau propagation with rapid and progressive neurofibrillary tangle pathology: the pattern of spread is determined by connectivity, not proximity. *Acta Neuropathol 127*, 667–683.

136. Nath, S., Agholme, L., Kurudenkandy, F. R., Granseth, B., Marcusson, J., and Hallbeck, M. (2012). Spreading of neurodegenerative pathology via neuron-to-neuron transmission of beta-amyloid. *J Neurosci 32*, 8767–8777.

137. Lee, S. E., Khazenzon, A. M., Trujillo, A. J., Guo, C. C., Yokoyama, J. S., Sha, S. J., Takada, L. T., Karydas, A. M., Block, N. R., Coppola, G., et al. (2014). Altered network connectivity in frontotemporal dementia with C9orf72 hexanucleotide repeat expansion. *Brain 137*, 3047–3060.

138. Lehmann, M., Madison, C. M., Ghosh, P. M., Seeley, W. W., Mormino, E., Greicius, M. D., Gorno-Tempini, M. L., Kramer, J. H., Miller, B. L., Jagust, W. J., et al. (2013). Intrinsic connectivity networks in healthy subjects explain clinical variability in Alzheimer's disease. *Proc Natl Acad Sci U S A 110*, 11606–11611.

139. Greicius, M. D., and Kimmel, D. L. (2012). Neuroimaging insights into network-based neurodegeneration. *Curr Opin Neurol 25*, 727–734.

140. Zhang, H. Y., Wang, S. J., Liu, B., Ma, Z. L., Yang, M., Zhang, Z. J., and Teng, G. J. (2010). Resting brain connectivity: changes during the progress of Alzheimer disease. *Radiology 256*, 598–606.

141. Damoiseaux, J. S., Prater, K. E., Miller, B. L., and Greicius, M. D. (2012a). Functional connectivity tracks clinical deterioration in Alzheimer's disease. *Neurobiol Aging 33*, 828, e819–830.

142. Migliaccio, R., Agosta, F., Possin, K. L., Canu, E., Filippi, M., Rabinovici, G. D., Rosen, H. J., Miller, B. L., and Gorno-Tempini, M. L. (2015). Mapping the Progression of atrophy in early- and late-onset Alzheimer's disease. *J Alzheimers Dis 46*, 351–364.

143. Binnewijzend, M. A., Schoonheim, M. M., Sanz-Arigita, E., Wink, A. M., van der Flier, W. M., Tolboom, N., Adriaanse, S. M., Damoiseaux, J. S., Scheltens, P., van Berckel, B. N., et al. (2012). Resting-state fMRI changes in Alzheimer's disease and mild cognitive impairment. *Neurobiol Aging 33*, 2018–2028.

144. Petrella, J. R., Sheldon, F. C., Prince, S. E., Calhoun, V. D., and Doraiswamy, P. M. (2011). Default mode network connectivity in stable vs progressive mild cognitive impairment. *Neurology 76*, 511–517.

145. Klupp, E., Grimmer, T., Tahmasian, M., Sorg, C., Yakushev, I., Yousefi, B. H., Drzezga, A., and Forster, S. (2015). Prefrontal hypometabolism in Alzheimer disease is related to longitudinal amyloid accumulation in remote brain regions. *J Nucl Med 56*, 399–404.

146. Odish, O. F., van den Berg-Huysmans, A. A., van den Bogaard, S. J., Dumas, E. M., Hart, E. P., Rombouts, S. A., van der Grond, J., Roos, R. A., and Group, T.-H. I. (2015). Longitudinal resting state fMRI analysis in healthy controls and premanifest Huntington's disease gene carriers: a three-year follow-up study. *Hum Brain Mapp 36*, 110–119.

147. Douaud, G., Menke, R. A., Gass, A., Monsch, A. U., Rao, A., Whitcher, B., Zamboni, G., Matthews, P. M., Sollberger, M., and Smith, S. (2013). Brain microstructure reveals early abnormalities more than two years prior to clinical progression from mild cognitive impairment to Alzheimer's disease. *J Neurosci 33*, 2147–2155.

148. Mielke, M. M., Okonkwo, O. C., Oishi, K., Mori, S., Tighe, S., Miller, M. I., Ceritoglu, C., Brown,

T., Albert, M., and Lyketsos, C. G. (2012). Fornix integrity and hippocampal volume predict memory decline and progression to Alzheimer's disease. *Alzheimers Dement 8*, 105–113.

149. Scola, E., Bozzali, M., Agosta, F., Magnani, G., Franceschi, M., Sormani, M. P., Cercignani, M., Pagani, E., Falautano, M., Filippi, M., et al. (2010). A diffusion tensor MRI study of patients with MCI and AD with a 2-year clinical follow-up. *J Neurol Neurosurg Psychiatry 81*, 798–805.

150. Selnes, P., Aarsland, D., Bjornerud, A., Gjerstad, L., Wallin, A., Hessen, E., Reinvang, I., Grambaite, R., Auning, E., Kjaervik, V. K., et al. (2013). Diffusion tensor imaging surpasses cerebrospinal fluid as predictor of cognitive decline and medial temporal lobe atrophy in subjective cognitive impairment and mild cognitive impairment. *J Alzheimers Dis 33*, 723–736.

151. Fellgiebel, A., Dellani, P. R., Greverus, D., Scheurich, A., Stoeter, P., and Muller, M. J. (2006). Predicting conversion to dementia in mild cognitive impairment by volumetric and diffusivity measurements of the hippocampus. *Psychiatry Res 146*, 283–287.

152. Yacoub, E., Harel, N., and Ugurbil, K. (2008). High-field fMRI unveils orientation columns in humans. *Proc Natl Acad Sci U S A 105*, 10607–10612.

153. Zeineh, M. M., Holdsworth, S., Skare, S., Atlas, S. W., and Bammer, R. (2012). Ultra-high resolution diffusion tensor imaging of the microscopic pathways of the medial temporal lobe. *Neuroimage 62*, 2065–2082.

154. Van der Saag, M., McDonell, D., and Slapeta, J. (2011). Cat genotype Tritrichomonas foetus survives passage through the alimentary tract of two common slug species. *Vet Parasitol 177*, 262–266.

8

Fluid Biomarkers Indicative of Neurodegenerative Diseases

HENRIK ZETTERBERG AND JONATHAN M. SCHOTT

INTRODUCTION

Neurodegeneration is the umbrella term for the progressive loss of function and structure of neurons. Many neurodegenerative diseases, including Alzheimer's disease (AD), Parkinson's disease (PD), frontotemporal dementia (FTD), and amyotrophic lateral sclerosis (ALS), occur as a result of neurodegenerative processes. In addition to neuronal loss, neurodegenerative diseases share several features at the sub-cellular level, most notably misfolding, aggregation, and cell-cell transmission of characteristic disease-related proteins, leading to the sequential dissemination of pathological protein aggregates in specific brain regions, which is often, if not always, accompanied by microglial activation and/or inflammation [1]. Discovering these similarities offers hope for therapeutic advances that could potentially have an impact on many of these diseases. In this chapter, we review established and novel fluid biomarkers for (1) neurodegeneration, (2) protein accumulation and (3) inflammation and microglial activation, in neurodegenerative diseases. We emphasize both overlapping and specific features of each biomarker and highlight areas in need of further research.

BIOMARKER MATRICES

Cerebrospinal Fluid

Cerebrospinal fluid (CSF) is a clear fluid that surrounds and supports the brain. It also carries nutrients and signaling molecules to neurons and helps dispose of metabolites that are further cleared into the blood via arachnoid villi in the intracranial dural sinuses and at the cranial and spinal nerve root sheaths. The total CSF volume is around 150 mL, and the production and clearance rates are around 20 mL per hour. CSF is easily sampled through a lumbar puncture. Standard operating procedures for CSF sampling and handling have been established, and the procedure can be done in outpatients [2]. Lumbar puncture is safe, with post-lumbar puncture headache being the only significant side effect (it affect 2%–20% of patients and can be treated with bed rest, mild analgesics, and, in severe cases, a blood patch) [3, 4]. The main advantage of CSF as a matrix in which to measure markers of CNS injury is that it communicates freely with the brain interstitial fluid that bathes the neurons. Biochemical changes in the brain are thus reflected in the CSF, which may be regarded as an accessible, although not perfect, sample of the brain interstitial fluid. Further, CSF has low protease activity and most molecules do not change upon sampling, provided the sample is not contaminated by blood. The main disadvantage is that lumbar puncture is somewhat more invasive than, say, blood sampling. Further, although CSF allows sampling from the brain side of the blood–brain barrier, it should be remembered that only 20%–30% of the CSF volume is derived directly from the brain; 70%–80% is a choroid plexus-derived filtrate of plasma. Finally, the lack of anatomical information on the biomarker changes is an obvious limitation, and lumbar CSF and ventricular CSF show differences in their composition.

Blood

The other major biofluid for the measurement of biomarkers for neurodegenerative diseases is blood (serum or plasma). Blood is more accessible than CSF, but most CNS-specific markers are present at very low concentrations that necessitate the employment of ultra-sensitive techniques that can measure in the femtomolar range, noting that most standard immunochemical techniques cannot reach this analytical sensitivity. The blood–brain barrier also poses a challenge in the analysis of markers of neurodegeneration in blood. Further, most intra-cellular proteins released into the bloodstream undergo degradation and/or modification by proteases and other enzymes. The dilution of CNS proteins into ~4 L blood instead of ~150 mL CSF may also contribute to the low concentrations of CNS-derived molecules in the blood.

Saliva, Urine, and Tears

It is possible that some CNS-derived proteins are eventually excreted into body fluids other than CSF and blood. The presence of the CNS-specific protein tau in saliva has been demonstrated using mass spectrometry [5]. The same research group has also detected Parkinson-related α-synuclein and DJ-1 in this body fluid [6]. However, the relationship between salivary concentrations of these proteins to processes within the CNS is far from clear, and no conclusive data on disease association have been reported so far. At present, it is hard to imagine how a test based on sampling of saliva, urine, or tears could produce results with a clear link to changes in the brain, given the many barriers and compartments the marker would have to cross on its way to the sampling site. Since these measures are unlikely to yield useful results, there will not be any further consideration of them in this chapter.

MEASUREMENT TECHNIQUES

Most fluid markers of neurodegenerative diseases are proteins or protein fragments. Such proteins may be visualized on Western blots in which proteins in the sample are separated on a gel, transferred to a membrane, and visualized using labeled antibodies to the protein of interest. This technique is often sensitive but not really quantitative and is not suitable for use in clinical laboratory practice. One exception is the neuronal protein 14-3-3, for which a Western blot method is used in the investigation of Creutzfeldt-Jakob disease (CJD) [7].

Enzyme-linked immunosorbent assay (ELISA) and variants thereof have become established as the method of choice for the measurement of specific proteins in biofluids. The general principle is that a capture antibody directed against one epitope on the target analyte is immobilized on a surface. Sample and labeled detector antibody (directed against another epitope on the same analyte) are added sequentially between washing steps to remove unspecific signal. Capture and detector antibodies are in molar excess, so most of the target analyte is captured in a sandwich between the antibody pair. Many ELISAs and ELISA-like techniques can reach lower limits of quantification of 10–100 pg/mL, but reducing this further, as is needed for most brain-specific proteins in the blood, is a challenge.

To that end, two new techniques have entered the market: Erenna and Simoa. The magnetic bead-based Erenna system can detect molecules at femtogram/mL concentrations using Single Molecule Counting technology in which labeled detector antibodies are released from the captured immunocomplexes and are counted one by one. This technique has been successfully used to quantify Alzheimer-associated amyloid β (Aβ) oligomers in CSF [8]. Simoa is based on the isolation of individual immunocomplexes on magnetic beads using standard ELISA reagents and has been used to quantify plasma levels of the neuroaxonal marker total-tau (T-tau) in AD [9]. The main difference between Simoa and conventional immunoassays lies in the ability to trap single beads in femtoliter volume wells, allowing for a digital readout of each individual bead to determine if it is bound to the target analyte or not, thus allowing measurement at the single molecule level.

Mass spectrometry (MS)–based explorative proteomics has been applied to discover novel biomarkers in complex samples such as CSF and plasma for many years [10]. More recently, however, antibody-independent selected reaction monitoring (SRM)–based MS techniques have been developed for the quantitative measurement of proteins and protein fragments in a manner that is stable enough to allow for use on large sample series and in clinical laboratory practice. SRM-based MS is a method that can be expected to grow into a complementary or alternative technique to immunochemical assays in the analysis of protein markers in the near future [11].

CEREBROSPINAL FLUID BIOMARKERS OF NEURODEGENERATION

Neuroaxonal Degeneration

CSF biomarkers of neuroaxonal degeneration include total tau (T-tau, measured using assays that detect all tau isoforms irrespective of phosphorylation state), neurofilament light (NFL), and visinin-like protein 1 (VILIP-1). Whereas tau is a microtubule-stabilizing protein expressed mainly in thin unmyelinated axons of the cerebral cortex [12], NFL is a structural protein of large-caliber myelinated axons that extend subcortically connecting brain regions [2]. Both proteins are CNS-specific [2]. VILIP-1, an intracellular calcium sensor, is also highly expressed in neurons [13], although some expression has also been reported in extracerebral tissues such as heart and pancreas [14, 15]. CSF levels of VILIP-1 correlate closely with T-tau levels [16]. Both CSF T-tau and VILIP-1 levels are robustly elevated in AD but are not specific to the disease process as such [16, 17]. CSF NFL is elevated in FTD, ALS, and other disorders with predominant long tract involvement such as vascular dementia, but is also significantly increased in AD, especially in late-onset disease [18–21]. All three markers correlate positively with measures of disease intensity and predict both clinical disease progression and survival, not only in the dementia stage of AD but also in mild cognitive impairment (MCI), as well as in several other disorders, including FTD and ALS [18, 21–25].

Biomarkers for Synaptic Degeneration

Synaptic degeneration and loss in neurodegenerative diseases may be detected and monitored using CSF levels of the dendritic protein neurogranin [26, 27] and the presynaptic SNARE complex component synaptosomal-associated protein 25 (SNAP-25) [28]. CSF neurogranin levels are elevated in predementia stages of AD and correlate with cognitive decline over time [27]. So far, there is a lack of studies on other neurodegenerative diseases, which is an area in need of further research.

BIOMARKERS FOR PROTEIN ACCUMULATION

Senile Plaque Pathology

Initially, just after the identification of aggregation-prone Aβ proteins ending at amino acids 40 and 42 in senile plaques [29–31], the protein was thought to be an abnormal byproduct of amyloid precursor protein (APP) metabolism invariably associated with AD. The natural secretion of Aβ from untransfected primary cells therefore came as a surprise [32]. Since then, it has been established that APP can enter at least three proteolytic clearance pathways: (1) amyloidogenic processing that primarily leads to production of Aβ42 and Aβ40 (but also some shorter, less aggregation-prone fragments) by successive β- and γ-secretase cleavages; (2) non-amyloidogenic processing that leads to production of sAPPα and possibly also a C-terminal fragment called p3 (this fragment should consist of Aβ17-40/42, but has been difficult to verify using modern techniques; it is possible that it is quickly degraded into shorter

fragments); and (3) another non-amyloidogenic processing pathway involving concerted cleavages of APP by β- and α- secretase, resulting in production of Aβ1-14/15/16 fragments at the expense of longer Aβ fragments [33].

The first (ELISA) assay for CSF Aβ42 was published in 1995 [34]. Using this technique, AD patients were shown to have reduced levels of CSF Aβ42, a finding that has since been replicated and verified in hundreds of papers [35]. This reduction is thought to reflect Aβ42 sequestration in senile plaques in the brain, as evidenced by autopsy, biopsy, and *in vivo* imaging studies [36–39]. Numerous studies have verified that low CSF Aβ42 levels are highly predictive of future AD, both in MCI [40–44] and cognitively normal cohorts [45–47]. Causal mutations aside, CSF Aβ42 remains the earliest biomarker currently available in AD, and as a result CSF Aβ42 is now incorporated into new criteria for the diagnosis of AD, also in predementia stages [48].

Low CSF Aβ42 is also seen in dementia with Lewy bodies (DLB), a disease characterized histologically by intra-neuronal inclusions of α-synuclein, often in conjunction with Alzheimer-like extracellular senile plaques, the latter of which explain the CSF Aβ42 finding [49]. Recent data also suggest that PD patients with CSF Aβ42 levels in the lower range are at increased risk of PD dementia within 5 years, also in the absence of tau changes [50].

Low CSF Aβ42 concentrations in the absence of senile plaque pathology have been reported in neuroinflammatory conditions, for example, bacterial meningitis [51], multiple sclerosis [52], human immunodeficiency virus (HIV)–associated dementia [53], and Lyme neuroborreliosis [54], and are often accompanied by biomarker evidence of a general reduction in APP metabolites, for example, secreted forms of APP, which is not typical of AD [35].

Besides Aβ42, several other Aβ isoforms are present in CSF. The most abundant variant in CSF is Aβ40, which is relatively unchanged in AD. The ratio of CSF Aβ42 to Aβ40 may provide a measurement of cerebral β-amyloidosis that is neutral to general changes in APP expression and processing, which would affect Aβ40 and Aβ42 in parallel. Accordingly, the Aβ40-normalized Aβ42 concentration has been reported to have better diagnostic accuracy for AD compared to CSF Aβ42 alone [55–57]. There are also several other C- or N-terminally truncated Aβ isoforms in CSF, which may be altered in AD [58], also in the earliest clinical stages [59].

Tangle Pathology

Neurofibrillary tangle pathology is one of the core features of AD but is also seen in several other so-called tauopathies, including progressive supranuclear palsy (PSP), some forms of FTD, corticobasal degeneration (CBD), and argyrophilic grain disease [60]. Nevertheless, elevated CSF P-tau levels have been regarded as a rather AD-specific phenomenon [61], which indicates tau phosphorylation in a manner that may be downstream of Aβ pathology [17, 44]. CSF P-tau levels correlate with the presence of tangle pathology in AD [39, 62], and elevated CSF P-tau levels support a diagnosis of AD [61].

A major unresolved question is why the other tauopathies do not show CSF P-tau elevation, at least not as systematically as seen in AD. It is possible that these disorders show disease-specific tau phosphorylation, or that tau is processed or truncated in a way that is not recognized by available assays. However, determining the relative specificity of P-tau elevation and AD has considerable advantages in differentiating different neurodegenerative diseases. For example, the ratio of T-tau to P-tau is a quite specific test for CJD [22, 63]. There are at present only three conditions in addition to AD in which consistently elevated CSF P-tau levels have been reported: (1) term and preterm newborns, possibly reflecting physiological tau phosphorylation in brain development [64]; (2) herpes encephalitis [65]; and (3) superficial CNS siderosis [66, 67]. For obvious reasons, these conditions are not often considered as differential diagnoses for AD. Nevertheless, they may shed light on mechanisms behind CSF P-tau increase by pointing to physiological and pathological conditions in which tau phosphorylation occurs, potentially as a consequence of reduced neuronal activity.

α-Synuclein Pathology

Predominantly expressed in the presynapse, 140-amino-acid-long α-synuclein has been found to be the major constituent of the intracellular aggregates in Lewy bodies, the pathological hallmark of PD and DLB, and in the glial cytoplasmic inclusions of multiple system atrophy (MSA) [68, 69]. These diseases have accordingly been grouped as synucleinopathies. Intracellular α-synuclein has been shown to be released into the extracellular space [70] and may be transmitted between neurons [71]. The exact role of α-synuclein in neurotoxicity remains unclear, but genetic data, including duplications and triplications of the α-synuclein-encoding *SNCA* gene in PD, clearly suggest a primary involvement of the protein in neurodegeneration [72–74].

Full-length α-synuclein has been detected in biological fluids, including CSF, plasma, conditioned cell media, and most recently saliva [6, 70, 75]. Extracerebral expression, particularly in red blood cells [76], is a major problem for this biomarker but can be controlled for in different manners, for example by normalizing its levels to hemoglobin concentration. The quantification of α-synuclein in CSF has been proposed as a potential biomarker for α-synuclein-related diseases [77]. There are, however, discrepant findings by a number of investigators using several different platforms and standard operating procedures, as well as a tremendous overlap of values across studies. Nevertheless, as more and more data accumulate, a trend toward reduced CSF α-synuclein levels in PD and other synucleinopathies has been verified in recent meta-analyses [78, 79]. An outstanding research question is if this reduction correlates with Lewy body counts in the brain and if it can be fine-tuned to better reflect pathology, for example, by developing specific assays against N-terminally acetylated and C-terminally truncated α-synuclein forms that are found in brain tissue [80], or disease-associated multimeric forms of the protein [81, 82]. The hope is that with appropriate quantification, CSF α-synuclein will develop into a biomarker that correlates with pathology in a manner similar to the inverse correlation seen between Aβ42 and senile plaque pathology.

Prions

In recent years, a number of novel molecular techniques for the detection and/or amplification of disease-associated prion protein (PrP) species have been developed. These techniques have the potential to be specific for the basic pathogenic process in prion diseases. Approaches based on the Protein Misfolding Cyclic Amplification (PMCA) technique, whereby the templated misfolding of PrP is seeded by a test sample containing misfolded PrP and the accumulated misfolded protein is then detected, have shown promise [83]. Quaking-Induced Conversion (QuIC), a modified form of PMCA, combined with an immunoprecipitation step, has been shown to detect extremely small amounts of brain-derived, disease-associated PrP when CJD brain homogenate is diluted into human plasma, according to work published by Orrú et al. [84]. Up to 1014-fold dilutions (that would be estimated to contain only a few attograms of abnormal PrP per mL) could be differentiated from dilutions of non-prion disease brain homogenate [84], and the assay can be used to detect CJD-causing misfolded PrP in CSF samples with high analytical sensitivity and specificity and good diagnostic accuracy [85]. However, these techniques are difficult to standardize and are currently being performed only in a few specialized laboratories around the globe. In an attempt to develop a screening test for vCJD, a solid-state binding matrix to capture and concentrate disease-associated prion proteins coupled to direct immunodetection of surface-bound PrP was developed into a blood-based test [86]. This test does not work for sporadic CJD, due to the low amount of misfolded PrP in blood and other peripheral tissues in this disorder, and has unknown performance in CSF. In a recent study, Dorey et al. reported on selective lowering of CSF PrP levels in CJD [87]. This may reflect sequestration of the protein in PrP aggregates in the brain, with lower amounts being able to diffuse via the brain interstitial fluid to reach the lumbar CSF, where it can be sampled and measured. At present, this is only a hypothesis, but if verified, the phenomenon would be very similar to the AD-associated change in the CSF levels of Aβ42.

TDP-43

Transactive response DNA-binding protein of 43 kDa (TDP-43), encoded by the *TARDBP* gene on chromosome 1, is a major component of tau-negative and ubiquitin-positive inclusions that characterize ALS, and a number of forms of FTD linked to TDP-43 pathology (FTD-TDP) [88]. TDP-43 can be measured in CSF [89], but, its levels seem to correlate more with blood levels than CNS pathology [90]. Truncated or modified forms of TDP-43 that better correlate with the presence of inclusions are now being actively sought. A reliable biomarker for TDP-43 would be an important tool for differential diagnosis in neurodegenerative diseases within the FTD spectrum, where there are several causative pathologies, and perhaps as outcome measures for clinical trials in FTD-TDP and ALS.

C9orf72

C9orf72 hexanucleotide repeat expansions are the most common cause of familial FTD and ALS worldwide [91]. Pathogenic repeat lengths are usually in the hundreds or thousands, but the minimum length that increases risk of disease and how or whether the repeat size affects phenotype are unclear. The repeat expansion encodes several dipeptide repeat proteins (poly-[glycine-arginine] and poly-[proline-arginine]) formed by unconventional repeat-associated non-ATG translation. Possible mechanisms of neurodegeneration include loss of C9orf72 protein and function, RNA toxicity, and toxicity from the dipeptide repeat proteins; which of these is the major pathogenic mechanism is not yet certain. At present there are no fluid markers of these types of aberrant proteins, but this is an area of considerable ongoing research, as such markers would be valuable to increase our understanding of the specific role these proteins may have in neurodegeneration.

BIOMARKERS FOR INFLAMMATION AND MICROGLIAL ACTIVATION

Inflammation, oxidative stress, and microglial activation in AD may be downstream phenomena of neurodegeneration, although recent genetic data suggest that they may well contribute to pathogenesis in susceptible individuals [92, 93]. Possible triggers are the accumulation of abnormal proteins (aggregated Aβ in the case of AD) and/or mediators released from dying cells. Such triggers may lead to overshoot inflammation in some individuals, for example, carriers of a recently described loss of function mutation in the microglia-controlling triggering receptor expressed on myeloid cells-2 (*TREM2*) gene [92, 93], perhaps making them more likely to develop clinical AD in response to Aβ.

Many studies have examined potential biomarkers linked to inflammatory processes. Cytokines, such as interleukin 6, transforming growth factor (TGF)-β, tumor necrosis factor α (TNF-α), and interleukin 1β (IL-1β) have been measured in CSF of AD patients, but in one meta-analysis the only consistent finding was of increased CSF levels of TGF-β in AD compared with control groups [94].

Isoprostanes, in particular a subclass called F2-isoprostanes, are the most examined CSF biomarkers for oxidative stress. They are prostaglandin-like compounds produced by free radical–dependent peroxidation of arachidonic acid [95]. Studies report elevated F2-isoprostane levels in AD CSF [96–100] in a manner that appears to be downstream of Aβ pathology [101]. CSF isoprostanes correlate to clinical disease progression in the MCI and dementia stages of AD, especially in *APOE* ε4–carrying patients [102], and may serve as damage response markers. Pilot studies suggest that the levels of oxidative DNA damage repair products are elevated in CSF from mixed vascular and Alzheimer's dementia patients [103], and that reduced levels of mitochondrial DNA in CSF suggest depletion of mitochondria [104], which may reflect oxidative stress, but these studies await replication.

Neuroinflammation is tightly linked to activation of the inflammatory M1 phenotype of microglia, the macrophages of the brain. Chitotriosidase is an enzyme that is secreted by activated macrophages [105], and its plasma levels are increased in patients with the lysosomal storage disorder Gaucher's disease [106]. Increased CSF chitotriosidase activity has been found in AD patients compared with non-demented controls [107]. A glycoprotein that has great homology with chitotriosidase but lacks its enzymatic activity is YKL-40 [108]. YKL-40 is expressed in both microglia and astrocytes, and elevated levels have been reported in both prodromal AD and cerebrovascular disease [109, 110].

Another microglial marker, the C-C chemokine receptor 2, is expressed on monocytes and one of its ligands, C-C chemokine ligand 2 (CCL2), that can be produced by microglia is important for the recruitment of monocytes in the CNS [111]. Higher CSF CCL2 levels have been associated with a faster cognitive decline in MCI patients who developed AD [112]. CCL2 levels in CSF were increased in AD patients compared with healthy controls [113, 114], as well as in the MCI stage of the disease [115]. However, one study failed to report any significant differences between AD patients and controls [116]. Another study found elevated CSF CCL2 levels in AD patients compared with controls, but there was an age-dependent increase in the biomarker level that may have affected the result [117]. Moreover, one study reported elevated levels of a soluble form of CD14 in the CSF from AD (and Parkinson's disease) patients compared with healthy controls [118]. CD14 is a surface protein, mainly expressed by macrophages. As a cofactor for toll-like receptors, CD14 is essential for the recognition of pathogens by the innate immune system of the brain.

Taken together, biomarker studies support involvement of low-grade neuroinflammation, oxidative stress, and microglial activation in the AD process, but to date no single biomarker has emerged as being sufficiently robust to have clinical utility. Future longitudinal studies of healthy individuals will most likely help to determine in what order these markers change in relation to plaque and tangle pathology and neurodegeneration in AD. A recent study found that CSF levels of several proteins possibly associated with microglia

activity predicted longitudinal reduction of CSF Aβ42 in cognitively healthy subjects, suggesting involvement of inflammatory pathways early in the AD disease process [119].

BLOOD BIOMARKERS FOR NEURODEGENERATIVE DISEASES

At present, there are no validate blood biomarkers for neurodegenerative diseases. Several candidate biomarkers exist, the most promising of which is serum NFL level [120]. Plasma levels of tau are quantifiable, but their association with AD is weak and there is no correlation to CSF levels [9]. Aβ42 can be measured in plasma, but there is no correlation to CSF levels, and again the correlation to cerebral β-amyloidosis as measured using amyloid PET is weak [121, 122]. Blood tests for neurodegenerative diseases is an area of intense ongoing research, and one important prerequisite for the generation of reliable results is the standardization of pre-analytical factors, as reviewed elsewhere in detail [123].

CONCLUSIONS

Biomarkers for neurodegenerative diseases are particularly important since the brain is not easily sampled *in vivo*. As well as increasing diagnostic sensitivity and specificity, biomarkers that can reliably allow for quantification of key neuropathological findings are likely to provide vital insights into the etiology of the different neurodegenerative disorders, and how different pathological processes interact to produce different clinical phenotypes. They would also be useful in the evaluation of novel candidate drugs directed against specific pathologies, as the field moves toward personalized treatment. "Generic" biomarkers for neurodegeneration may also be useful in evaluating treatment effects, for example, disease-modifying drugs in AD would be expected to normalize, or lower, CSF tau markers. However, the extent of the reduction will depend on several factors, including the proposed mode of action of the drug and the strength of the disease-modifying effect, These in turn will influence the length of any proposed trial: thus while 6–12-month treatment periods are currently considered, this interval is at present hypothetical and is extrapolated from studies on acute conditions such as stroke and traumatic brain injury [124, 125]. Another important use would be in molecular epidemiology studies, in which potential risk factors could be associated with not only clinical phenotypes but also the prevalence, incidence, and interaction between pathologies. Blood tests would make such studies easier, but cross-sectional and particularly longitudinal CSF and neuromaging studies are already being combined with genetic and detailed clinical data to provide important results in sporadic and familial neurodegenerative diseases and in aging cohorts. Today, we have reasonably good biomarkers for cerebral β-amyloidosis and neurodegeneration, and standardization work is in progress [126]. An important focus in biomarker research is now to develop biomarkers for key pathologies in the non-AD diseases.

ACKNOWLEDGMENTS

We gratefully acknowledge the support of the Leonard Wolfson Experimental Neurology Centre. Work in the authors' laboratories is supported by the Swedish Research Council, the Knut and Alice Wallenberg Foundation, Alzheimer's Association, Swedish State Support for Clinical Research, Alzheimer's Research UK, the MRC, the NIHR Queen Square BRU in dementia and UCL/H BRC. We wish to thank colleagues and patients and their families for generating the extensive literature that was reviewed here.

REFERENCES

1. Brettschneider J, Del Tredici K, Lee VM, Trojanowski JQ: Spreading of pathology in neurodegenerative diseases: a focus on human studies. *Nat Rev Neurosci* 16(2), 109–120 (2015).

2. Blennow K, Hampel H, Weiner M, Zetterberg H: Cerebrospinal fluid and plasma biomarkers in Alzheimer disease. *Nat Rev Neurol* 6(3), 131–144 (2010).

3. Zetterberg H, Tullhog K, Hansson O, Minthon L, Londos E, Blennow K: Low incidence of post-lumbar puncture headache in 1,089 consecutive memory clinic patients. *Eur Neurol* 63(6), 326–330 (2010).

4. Monserrate AE, Ryman DC, Ma S, et al.: Factors associated with the onset and persistence of post-lumbar puncture headache. *JAMA Neurol*, 72(3), 325–332 (2015).

5. Shi M, Sui YT, Peskind ER, et al.: Salivary tau species are potential biomarkers of Alzheimer's disease. *J Alzheimers Dis* 27(2), 299–305 (2011).

6. Devic I, Hwang H, Edgar JS, et al.: Salivary alpha-synuclein and DJ-1: potential biomarkers for Parkinson's disease. *Brain* 134(Pt 7), e178 (2011).

7. Van Everbroeck B, Boons J, Cras P: Cerebrospinal fluid biomarkers in Creutzfeldt-Jakob disease. *Clin Neurol Neurosurg* 107(5), 355–360 (2005).

8. Savage MJ, Kalinina J, Wolfe A, et al.: A sensitive abeta oligomer assay discriminates Alzheimer's and aged control cerebrospinal fluid. *J Neurosci* 34(8), 2884–2897 (2014).

9. Zetterberg H, Wilson D, Andreasson U, et al.: Plasma tau levels in Alzheimer's disease. *Alzheimers Res Ther* 5(2), 9 (2013).

10. Brinkmalm A, Portelius E, Ohrfelt A, et al.: Explorative and targeted neuroproteomics in Alzheimer's disease. *Biochim Biophys Acta* 1854(7), 769–778 (2015).

11. Lemoine J, Fortin T, Salvador A, Jaffuel A, Charrier JP, Choquet-Kastylevsky G: The current status of clinical proteomics and the use of MRM and MRM(3) for biomarker validation. *Expert Rev Mol Diagn* 12(4), 333–342 (2012).

12. Trojanowski JQ, Schuck T, Schmidt ML, Lee VM: Distribution of tau proteins in the normal human central and peripheral nervous system. *J Histochem Cytochem* 37(2), 209–215 (1989).

13. Laterza OF, Modur VR, Crimmins DL, et al.: Identification of novel brain biomarkers. *Clin Chem* 52(9), 1713–1721 (2006).

14. Dai FF, Zhang Y, Kang Y et al.: The neuronal Ca2+ sensor protein visinin-like protein-1 is expressed in pancreatic islets and regulates insulin secretion. *J Biol Chem* 281(31), 21942–21953 (2006).

15. Buttgereit J, Qadri F, Monti J, et al.: Visinin-like protein 1 regulates natriuretic peptide receptor B in the heart. *Regul Pept* 161(1–3), 51–57 (2010).

16. Lee JM, Blennow K, Andreasen N, et al.: The brain injury biomarker VLP-1 is increased in the cerebrospinal fluid of Alzheimer disease patients. *Clin Chem* 54(10), 1617–1623 (2008).

17. Hampel H, Blennow K, Shaw LM, Hoessler YC, Zetterberg H, Trojanowski JQ: Total and phosphorylated tau protein as biological markers of Alzheimer's disease. *Exp Gerontol* 45(1), 30–40 (2010).

18. Skillback T, Farahmand B, Bartlett JW, et al.: CSF neurofilament light differs in neurodegenerative diseases and predicts severity and survival. *Neurology* 83(21), 1945–1953 (2014).

19. Sjogren M, Blomberg M, Jonsson M, et al.: Neurofilament protein in cerebrospinal fluid: a marker of white matter changes. *J Neurosci Res* 66(3), 510–516 (2001).

20. Sjogren M, Rosengren L, Minthon L, Davidsson P, Blennow K, Wallin A: Cytoskeleton proteins in CSF distinguish frontotemporal dementia from AD. *Neurology* 54(10), 1960–1964 (2000).

21. Zetterberg H, Jacobsson J, Rosengren L, Blennow K, Andersen PM: Cerebrospinal fluid neurofilament light levels in amyotrophic lateral sclerosis: impact of SOD1 genotype. *Eur J Neurol* 14(12), 1329–1333 (2007).

22. Skillback T, Rosen C, Asztely F, Mattsson N, Blennow K, Zetterberg H: Diagnostic performance of cerebrospinal fluid total tau and phosphorylated tau in Creutzfeldt-Jakob disease: results from the Swedish Mortality Registry. *JAMA Neurol* 71(4), 476–483 (2014).

23. Wallin AK, Blennow K, Zetterberg H, Londos E, Minthon L, Hansson O: CSF biomarkers predict a more malignant outcome in Alzheimer disease. *Neurology* 74(19), 1531–1537 (2010).

24. Samgard K, Zetterberg H, Blennow K, Hansson O, Minthon L, Londos E: Cerebrospinal fluid total tau as a marker of Alzheimer's disease intensity. *Int J Geriatr Psychiatry* 25(4), 403–410 (2010).

25. Fagan AM, Xiong C, Jasielec MS, et al.: Longitudinal change in CSF biomarkers in autosomal-dominant Alzheimer's disease. *Sci Transl Med* 6(226), 226ra230 (2014).

26. Thorsell A, Bjerke M, Gobom J, et al.: Neurogranin in cerebrospinal fluid as a marker of synaptic degeneration in Alzheimer's disease. *Brain Res* 1362, 13–22 (2010).

27. Kvartsberg H, Duits FH, Ingelsson M, et al.: Cerebrospinal fluid levels of the synaptic protein neurogranin correlates with cognitive decline in prodromal Alzheimer's disease. *Alzheimers Dement* 11(10), 1180–1190 (2014).

28. Brinkmalm A, Brinkmalm G, Honer WG, et al.: SNAP-25 is a promising novel cerebrospinal fluid biomarker for synapse degeneration in Alzheimer's disease. *Mol Neurodegener* 9, 53 (2014).

29. Glenner GG, Wong CW: Alzheimer's disease and Down's syndrome: sharing of a unique cerebrovascular amyloid fibril protein. *Biochem Biophys Res Commun* 122(3), 1131–1135 (1984).

30. Glenner GG, Wong CW: Alzheimer's disease: initial report of the purification and characterization of a novel cerebrovascular amyloid protein. *Biochem Biophys Res Commun* 120(3), 885–890 (1984).

31. Masters CL, Simms G, Weinman NA, Multhaup G, Mcdonald BL, Beyreuther K: Amyloid plaque core protein in Alzheimer disease and Down syndrome. *Proc Natl Acad Sci U S A* 82(12), 4245–4249 (1985).

32. Haass C, Schlossmacher MG, Hung AY, et al.: Amyloid beta-peptide is produced by cultured cells during normal metabolism. *Nature* 359(6393), 322–325 (1992).

33. Portelius E, Price E, Brinkmalm G, et al.: A novel pathway for amyloid precursor protein processing. *Neurobiol Aging* 32(6), 1090–1098 (2011).

34. Motter R, Vigo-Pelfrey C, Kholodenko D, et al.: Reduction of beta-amyloid peptide42 in the cerebrospinal fluid of patients with Alzheimer's disease. *Ann Neurol* 38(4), 643–648 (1995).

35. Rosen C, Hansson O, Blennow K, Zetterberg H: Fluid biomarkers in Alzheimer's disease: current concepts. *Mol Neurodegener* 8, 20 (2013).

36. Strozyk D, Blennow K, White LR, Launer LJ: CSF Abeta 42 levels correlate with amyloid-neuropathology in a population-based autopsy study. *Neurology* 60(4), 652–656 (2003).

37. Fagan AM, Mintun MA, Mach RH et al.: Inverse relation between in vivo amyloid imaging load and cerebrospinal fluid Abeta42 in humans. *Ann Neurol* 59(3), 512–519 (2006).

38. Forsberg A, Engler H, Almkvist O et al.: PET imaging of amyloid deposition in patients with mild cognitive impairment. *Neurobiol Aging* 29(10), 1456–1465 (2008).

39. Seppala TT, Nerg O, Koivisto AM, et al.: CSF biomarkers for Alzheimer disease correlate with cortical brain biopsy findings. *Neurology* 78(20), 1568–1575 (2012).

40. Andreasen N, Minthon L, Vanmechelen E, et al.: Cerebrospinal fluid tau and Abeta42 as predictors of development of Alzheimer's disease in patients with mild cognitive impairment. *Neurosci Lett* 273(1), 5–8 (1999).

41. Hansson O, Zetterberg H, Buchhave P, Londos E, Blennow K, Minthon L: Association between CSF biomarkers and incipient Alzheimer's disease in patients with mild cognitive impairment: a follow-up study. *Lancet Neurol* 5(3), 228–234 (2006).

42. Shaw LM, Vanderstichele H, Knapik-Czajka M, et al.: Cerebrospinal fluid biomarker signature in Alzheimer's disease neuroimaging initiative subjects. *Ann Neurol* 65(4), 403–413 (2009).

43. Visser PJ, Verhey F, Knol DL, et al.: Prevalence and prognostic value of CSF markers of Alzheimer's disease pathology in patients with subjective cognitive impairment or mild cognitive impairment in the DESCRIPA study: a prospective cohort study. *Lancet Neurol* 8(7), 619–627 (2009).

44. Buchhave P, Minthon L, Zetterberg H, Wallin AK, Blennow K, Hansson O: Cerebrospinal fluid levels of beta-amyloid 1–42, but not of tau, are fully changed already 5 to 10 years before the onset of Alzheimer dementia. *Arch Gen Psychiatry* 69(1), 98–106 (2012).

45. Skoog I, Davidsson P, Aevarsson O, Vanderstichele H, Vanmechelen E, Blennow K: Cerebrospinal fluid beta-amyloid 42 is reduced before the onset of sporadic dementia: a population-based study in 85-year-olds. *Dement Geriatr Cogn Disord* 15(3), 169–176 (2003).

46. Fagan AM, Head D, Shah AR, et al.: Decreased cerebrospinal fluid Abeta(42) correlates with brain atrophy in cognitively normal elderly. *Ann Neurol* 65(2), 176–183 (2009).

47. Gustafson DR, Skoog I, Rosengren L, Zetterberg H, Blennow K: Cerebrospinal fluid beta-amyloid 1–42 concentration may predict cognitive decline in older women. *J Neurol Neurosurg Psychiatry* 78(5), 461–464 (2007).

48. Dubois B, Feldman HH, Jacova C, et al.: Advancing research diagnostic criteria for Alzheimer's disease: the IWG-2 criteria. *Lancet Neurol* 13(6), 614–629 (2014).

49. Hall S, Ohrfelt A, Constantinescu R, et al.: Accuracy of a panel of 5 cerebrospinal fluid biomarkers in the differential diagnosis of patients with dementia and/or parkinsonian disorders. *Arch Neurol* 69(11), 1445–1452 (2012).

50. Alves G, Lange J, Blennow K, et al.: CSF Abeta42 predicts early-onset dementia in Parkinson disease. *Neurology* 82(20), 1784–1790 (2014).

51. Sjogren M, Gisslen M, Vanmechelen E, Blennow K: Low cerebrospinal fluid beta-amyloid 42 in patients with acute bacterial meningitis and normalization after treatment. *Neurosci Lett* 314(1–2), 33–36 (2001).

52. Mattsson N, Axelsson M, Haghighi S, et al.: Reduced cerebrospinal fluid BACE1 activity in multiple sclerosis. *Mult Scler* 15(4), 448–454 (2009).

53. Gisslen M, Krut J, Andreasson U, et al.: Amyloid and tau cerebrospinal fluid biomarkers in HIV infection. *BMC Neurol* 9, 63 (2009).

54. Mattsson N, Bremell D, Anckarsater R, et al.: Neuroinflammation in Lyme neuroborreliosis affects amyloid metabolism. *BMC Neurol* 10, 51 (2010).

55. Schoonenboom NS, Mulder C, Van Kamp GJ, et al.: Amyloid beta 38, 40, and 42 species in cerebrospinal fluid: more of the same? *Ann Neurol* 58(1), 139–142 (2005).

56. Hansson O, Zetterberg H, Buchhave P, et al.: Prediction of Alzheimer's disease using the CSF Abeta42/Abeta40 ratio in patients with mild cognitive impairment. *Dement Geriatr Cogn Disord* 23(5), 316–320 (2007).

57. Wiltfang J, Esselmann H, Bibl M, et al.: Amyloid beta peptide ratio 42/40 but not A beta 42 correlates with phospho-Tau in patients with low- and high-CSF A beta 40 load. *J Neurochem* 101(4), 1053–1059 (2007).

58. Portelius E, Zetterberg H, Andreasson U, et al.: An Alzheimer's disease-specific beta-amyloid fragment signature in cerebrospinal fluid. *Neurosci Lett* 409(3), 215–219 (2006).

59. Mattsson N, Portelius E, Rolstad S, et al.: Longitudinal cerebrospinal fluid biomarkers over four years in mild cognitive impairment. *J Alzheimers Dis* 30(4), 767–778 (2012).

60. Kovacs GG: Invited review: Neuropathology of tauopathies: principles and practice. *Neuropathol Appl Neurobiol* 41(1), 3–23 (2015).

61. Hampel H, Buerger K, Zinkowski R, et al.: Measurement of phosphorylated tau epitopes in the differential diagnosis of Alzheimer disease: a comparative cerebrospinal fluid study. *Arch Gen Psychiatry* 61(1), 95–102 (2004).

62. Buerger K, Ewers M, Pirttila T, et al.: CSF phosphorylated tau protein correlates with neocortical neurofibrillary pathology in Alzheimer's disease. *Brain* 129(Pt 11), 3035–3041 (2006).

63. Riemenschneider M, Wagenpfeil S, Vanderstichele H, et al.: Phospho-tau/total tau ratio in cerebrospinal fluid discriminates Creutzfeldt-Jakob disease from other dementias. *Mol Psychiatry* 8(3), 343–347 (2003).

64. Mattsson N, Savman K, Osterlundh G, Blennow K, Zetterberg H: Converging molecular pathways in human neural development and degeneration. *Neurosci Res* 66(3), 330–332 (2010).

65. Grahn A, Hagberg L, Nilsson S, Blennow K, Zetterberg H, Studahl M: Cerebrospinal fluid biomarkers in patients with varicella-zoster virus CNS infections. *J Neurol* 260(7), 1813–1821 (2013).

66. Kondziella D, Zetterberg H: Hyperphosphorylation of tau protein in superficial CNS siderosis. *J Neurol Sci* 273(1–2), 130–132 (2008).

67. Ikeda T, Noto D, Noguchi-Shinohara M, et al.: CSF tau protein is a useful marker for effective treatment of superficial siderosis of the central nervous system: two case reports. *Clin Neurol Neurosurg* 112(1), 62–64 (2010).

68. Spillantini MG, Schmidt ML, Lee VM, Trojanowski JQ, Jakes R, Goedert M: Alpha-synuclein in Lewy bodies. *Nature* 388(6645), 839–840 (1997).

69. Gai WP, Power JH, Blumbergs PC, Blessing WW: Multiple-system atrophy: a new alpha-synuclein disease? *Lancet* 352(9127), 547–548 (1998).

70. El-Agnaf OM, Salem SA, Paleologou KE, et al.: Alpha-synuclein implicated in Parkinson's disease is present in extracellular biological fluids, including human plasma. *Faseb J* 17(13), 1945–1947 (2003).

71. Desplats P, Lee HJ, Bae EJ, et al.: Inclusion formation and neuronal cell death through neuron-to-neuron transmission of alpha-synuclein. *Proc Natl Acad Sci U S A* 106(31), 13010–13015 (2009).

72. Singleton AB, Farrer M, Johnson J, et al.: Alpha-synuclein locus triplication causes Parkinson's disease. *Science* 302(5646), 841 (2003).

73. Simon-Sanchez J, Schulte C, Bras JM, et al.: Genome-wide association study reveals genetic risk underlying Parkinson's disease. *Nat Genet* 41(12), 1308–1312 (2009).

74. Fuchs J, Nilsson C, Kachergus J, et al.: Phenotypic variation in a large Swedish pedigree due to SNCA duplication and triplication. *Neurology* 68(12), 916–922 (2007).

75. Lee HJ, Patel S, Lee SJ: Intravesicular localization and exocytosis of alpha-synuclein and its aggregates. *J Neurosci* 25(25), 6016–6024 (2005).

76. Barbour R, Kling K, Anderson JP, et al.: Red blood cells are the major source of alpha-synuclein in blood. *Neurodegener Dis* 5(2), 55–59 (2008).

77. Mollenhauer B, El-Agnaf OM, Marcus K, Trenkwalder C, Schlossmacher MG: Quantification of alpha-synuclein in cerebrospinal fluid as a biomarker candidate: review of the literature and considerations for future studies. *Biomark Med* 4(5), 683–699 (2010).

78. Zetterberg H, Petzold M, Magdalinou N: Cerebrospinal fluid alpha-synuclein levels in Parkinson's disease: changed or unchanged? *Eur J Neurol* 21(3), 365–367 (2014).

79. Sako W, Murakami N, Izumi Y, Kaji R: Reduced alpha-synuclein in cerebrospinal fluid in synucleinopathies: evidence from a meta-analysis. *Mov Disord* 29(13), 1599–1605 (2014).

80. Ohrfelt A, Zetterberg H, Andersson K, et al.: Identification of novel alpha-synuclein isoforms in human brain tissue by using an online nanoLC-ESI-FTICR-MS method. *Neurochem Res* 36(11), 2029–2042 (2011).

81. Bartels T, Choi JG, Selkoe DJ: Alpha-synuclein occurs physiologically as a helically folded tetramer that resists aggregation. *Nature* 477(7362), 107–110 (2011).

82. Hansson O, Hall S, Ohrfelt A, et al.: Levels of cerebrospinal fluid alpha-synuclein oligomers are increased in Parkinson's disease with dementia and dementia with Lewy bodies compared to Alzheimer's disease. *Alzheimers Res Ther* 6(3), 25 (2014).

83. Gonzalez-Montalban N, Makarava N, Ostapchenko VG, et al.: Highly efficient protein misfolding cyclic amplification. *PLoS Pathog* 7(2), e1001277 (2011).

84. Orru CD, Wilham JM, Raymond LD, et al.: Prion disease blood test using immunoprecipitation and improved quaking-induced conversion. *MBio* 2(3), e00078–00011 (2011).

85. Mcguire LI, Peden AH, Orru CD, et al.: Real time quaking-induced conversion analysis of cerebrospinal fluid in sporadic Creutzfeldt-Jakob disease. *Ann Neurol* 72(2), 278–285 (2012).

86. Edgeworth JA, Farmer M, Sicilia A, et al.: Detection of prion infection in variant Creutzfeldt-Jakob disease: a blood-based assay. *Lancet* 377(9764), 487–493 (2011).

87. Dorey A, Tholance Y, Vighetto A, et al.: Cerebrospinal fluid prion protein levels discriminate Alzheimer's disease from Creutzfeldt-Jakob's disease. *JAMA Neurol* 72(3), 267–275 (2015).

88. Neumann M, Sampathu DM, Kwong LK, et al.: Ubiquitinated TDP-43 in frontotemporal lobar degeneration and amyotrophic lateral sclerosis. *Science* 314(5796), 130–133 (2006).

89. Steinacker P, Hendrich C, Sperfeld AD, et al.: TDP-43 in cerebrospinal fluid of patients with frontotemporal lobar degeneration and amyotrophic lateral sclerosis. *Arch Neurol* 65(11), 1481–1487 (2008).

90. Feneberg E, Steinacker P, Lehnert S, et al.: Limited role of free TDP-43 as a diagnostic tool in neurodegenerative diseases. *Amyotroph Lateral Scler Frontotemporal Degener* 15(5–6), 351–356 (2014).

91. Rohrer JD, Isaacs AM, Mizlienska S, et al.: C9orf72 expansions in frontotemporal dementia and amyotrophic lateral sclerosis. *Lancet Neurol* 14(3), 291–301 (2015).

92. Guerreiro R, Wojtas A, Bras J, et al.: TREM2 variants in Alzheimer's disease. *N Engl J Med* 368(2), 117–127 (2013).

93. Jonsson T, Stefansson H, Steinberg S, et al.: Variant of TREM2 associated with the risk of Alzheimer's disease. *N Engl J Med* 368(2), 107–116 (2013).

94. Swardfager W, Lanctot K, Rothenburg L, Wong A, Cappell J, Herrmann N: A meta-analysis of cytokines in Alzheimer's disease. *Biol Psychiatry* 68(10), 930–941 (2010).

95. Morrow JD, Roberts LJ: The isoprostanes: unique bioactive products of lipid peroxidation. *Prog Lipid Res* 36(1), 1–21 (1997).

96. Brys M, Pirraglia E, Rich K, et al.: Prediction and longitudinal study of CSF biomarkers in mild cognitive impairment. *Neurobiol Aging* 30(5), 682–690 (2009).

97. De Leon MJ, Desanti S, Zinkowski R, et al.: Longitudinal CSF and MRI biomarkers improve the diagnosis of mild cognitive impairment. *Neurobiol Aging* 27(3), 394–401 (2006).

98. Grossman M, Farmer J, Leight S, et al.: Cerebrospinal fluid profile in frontotemporal dementia and Alzheimer's disease. *Ann Neurol* 57(5), 721–729 (2005).

99. Montine TJ, Beal MF, Cudkowicz ME, et al.: Increased CSF F2-isoprostane concentration in probable AD. *Neurology* 52(3), 562–565 (1999).

100. Montine TJ, Markesbery WR, Morrow JD, Roberts LJ, 2nd: Cerebrospinal fluid F2-isoprostane levels are increased in Alzheimer's disease. *Ann Neurol* 44(3), 410–413 (1998).

101. Ringman JM, Younkin SG, Pratico D, et al.: Biochemical markers in persons with preclinical familial Alzheimer disease. *Neurology* 71(2), 85–92 (2008).

102. Duits FH, Kester MI, Scheffer PG, et al.: Increase in cerebrospinal fluid F2-isoprostanes is related to cognitive decline in APOE epsilon4 carriers. *J Alzheimers Dis* 36(3), 563–570 (2013).

103. Gackowski D, Rozalski R, Siomek A, et al.: Oxidative stress and oxidative DNA damage is characteristic for mixed Alzheimer disease/vascular dementia. *J Neurol Sci* 266(1–2), 57–62 (2008).

104. Podlesniy P, Figueiro-Silva J, Llado A, et al.: Low cerebrospinal fluid concentration of mitochondrial DNA in preclinical Alzheimer disease. *Ann Neurol* 74(5), 655–668 (2013).

105. Renkema GH, Boot RG, Au FL, et al.: Chitotriosidase, a chitinase, and the 39-kDa human cartilage glycoprotein, a chitin-binding lectin, are homologues of family 18 glycosyl hydrolases secreted by human macrophages. *Eur J Biochem* 251(1–2), 504–509 (1998).

106. Hollak CE, Van Weely S, Van Oers MH, Aerts JM: Marked elevation of plasma chitotriosidase activity: a novel hallmark of Gaucher disease. *J Clin Invest* 93(3), 1288–1292 (1994).

107. Watabe-Rudolph M, Song Z, Lausser L, et al.: Chitinase enzyme activity in CSF is a powerful biomarker of Alzheimer disease. *Neurology* 78(8), 569–577 (2012).

108. Hakala BE, White C, Recklies AD: Human cartilage gp-39, a major secretory product of articular chondrocytes and synovial cells, is a mammalian member of a chitinase protein family. *J Biol Chem* 268(34), 25803–25810 (1993).

109. Craig-Schapiro R, Perrin RJ, Roe CM, et al.: YKL-40: a novel prognostic fluid biomarker for preclinical Alzheimer's disease. *Biol Psychiatry* 68(10), 903–912 (2010).

110. Olsson B, Hertze J, Lautner R, et al.: Microglial markers are elevated in the prodromal phase of Alzheimer's disease and vascular dementia. *J Alzheimers Dis* 33(1), 45–53 (2013).

111. Sokolova A, Hill MD, Rahimi F, Warden LA, Halliday GM, Shepherd CE: Monocyte chemoattractant protein-1 plays a dominant role in the chronic inflammation observed in Alzheimer's disease. *Brain Pathol* 19(3), 392–398 (2009).

112. Westin K, Buchhave P, Nielsen H, Minthon L, Janciauskiene S, Hansson O: CCL2 is associated with a faster rate of cognitive decline during early stages of Alzheimer's disease. *PLoS ONE* 7(1), e30525 (2012).

113. Correa JD, Starling D, Teixeira AL, Caramelli P, Silva TA: Chemokines in CSF of Alzheimer's disease patients. *Arq Neuropsiquiatr* 69(3), 455–459 (2011).

114. Galimberti D, Schoonenboom N, Scheltens P, et al.: Intrathecal chemokine levels in Alzheimer disease and frontotemporal lobar degeneration. *Neurology* 66(1), 146–147 (2006).

115. Galimberti D, Schoonenboom N, Scheltens P, et al.: Intrathecal chemokine synthesis in mild cognitive impairment and Alzheimer disease. *Arch Neurol* 63(4), 538–543 (2006).

116. Mattsson N, Tabatabaei S, Johansson P, et al.: Cerebrospinal fluid microglial markers in Alzheimer's disease: elevated chitotriosidase activity but lack of diagnostic utility. *Neuromolecular Med* 13(2), 151–159 (2011).

117. Blasko I, Lederer W, Oberbauer H, et al.: Measurement of thirteen biological markers in CSF of patients with Alzheimer's disease and other dementias. *Dement Geriatr Cogn Disord* 21(1), 9–15 (2006).

118. Yin GN, Jeon H, Lee S, Lee HW, Cho JY, Suk K: Role of soluble CD14 in cerebrospinal fluid as a regulator of glial functions. *J Neurosci Res* 87(11), 2578–2590 (2009).

119. Mattsson N, Insel P, Nosheny R, et al.: CSF protein biomarkers predicting longitudinal reduction of CSF beta-amyloid42 in cognitively healthy elders. *Transl Psychiatry* 3, e293 (2013).

120. Gaiottino J, Norgren N, Dobson R, et al.: Increased neurofilament light chain blood levels in neurodegenerative neurological diseases. *PLoS ONE* 8(9), e75091 (2013).

121. Hansson O, Zetterberg H, Vanmechelen E, et al.: Evaluation of plasma Abeta(40) and Abeta(42) as predictors of conversion to Alzheimer's disease in patients with mild cognitive impairment. *Neurobiol Aging* 31(3), 357–367 (2010).

122. Rembach A, Watt AD, Wilson WJ, et al.: Plasma amyloid-beta levels are significantly associated with a transition toward Alzheimer's disease as measured by cognitive decline and change in neocortical amyloid burden. *J Alzheimers Dis* 40(1), 95–104 (2014).

123. O'bryant SE, Gupta V, Henriksen K, et al.: Guidelines for the standardization of preanalytic variables for blood-based biomarker studies in Alzheimer's disease research. *Alzheimers Dement* 11(5), 549–560 (2014).

124. Hesse C, Rosengren L, Andreasen N, et al.: Transient increase in total tau but not phospho-tau in human cerebrospinal fluid after acute stroke. *Neurosci Lett* 297(3), 187–190 (2001).

125. Neselius S, Brisby H, Granholm F, Zetterberg H, Blennow K: Monitoring concussion in a knocked-out boxer by CSF biomarker analysis. *Knee Surg Sports Traumatol Arthrosc* 23(9), 2536–2539 (2014).

126. Carrillo MC, Blennow K, Soares H, et al.: Global standardization measurement of cerebral spinal fluid for Alzheimer's disease: an update from the Alzheimer's Association Global Biomarkers Consortium. *Alzheimers Dement* 9(2), 137–140 (2013).

9

Predementia Disorders

Neurodegenerative Disorder Predecessor States as Unifying Clinical Features

JAGAN A. PILLAI

INTRODUCTION

Neurodegenerative disorders (NDDs) are proteinopathies, and they share this theme in their underlying pathophysiology. The kaleidoscope of clinical syndromes results from the predilection of the abnormal protein deposits for specific regions of the central nervous system (CNS), resulting in neuronal dysfunction and loss. Identifying the drivers of abnormal protein deposition has been a focus of intense recent research efforts. This focus has also made us acutely aware of the time course of pathophysiological changes in NDDs. Molecular changes related to NDDs can now be identified years, sometimes decades, before the diagnosis of dementia. In the predementia state, early in the course of these diseases, irrevocable significant damage to the CNS has yet to occur. Identifying predementia states and developing therapeutic interventions targeting this time period are therefore of interest to forestall future clinical decline and dementia in NDDs.

CLINICAL IMPERATIVES ON TACKLING PREDEMENTIA STATES: A HISTORICAL PERSPECTIVE

Currently there is an emphasis on identifying predementia states using biomarkers of the underlying proteinopathy, but the interest in predementia states itself is not recent. Investigators have been focusing their attention for many decades on characterizing the cognitive and biological changes between "normal aging" and Alzheimer's disease (AD) dementia, where individuals often share similar amyloid plaque and neurofibrillary tangle pathology at autopsy. The focus during this earlier era was on delineating cognitive profiles among the elderly that were less likely to proceed to dementia. The focus on this clinical state was driven by practical imperatives when no medical therapies were available to dementia patients and it was as important to identify and reassure patients and families who will not develop cognitive decline over time toward dementia [1].

The term "benign senescent forgetfulness" was proposed by Kral in the 1960s [2]. It denoted memory changes of normal aging not evolving to dementia. "Age associated memory impairment" (AAMI) was proposed by a workgroup of the National Institute of Health. AAMI had a more defined criterion, with memory scores that are one standard deviation (SD) below the mean of young people [3]. A more general term, "age associated cognitive decline" (AACD) (not just memory being affected), was proposed by a workgroup of the International Psychogeriatric Association [4], and the similar term "cognitive impairment no dementia" (CIND) was coined by the Canadian Study of Health and Aging [5]. These criteria, as they were not based on underlying pathophysiology, were broadly inclusive; individuals with a host of medical, psychiatric, or neurological diseases were included [1]. The common feature was that they were all elderly individuals who were not demented but did not have normal cognition.

The clinical and research focus shifted with the definition of mild cognitive impairment (MCI), where the imperative was to identify individuals at risk of developing AD dementia in the future. MCI individuals have a memory impairment beyond that expected for age and education, yet are not demented. With the start of multiple therapeutic trails for AD, the hope was that MCI patients could potentially be targeted before the development of significant AD pathology and neuronal loss that correlates with the severity of dementia [6]. MCI as a clinical category was best articulated by Petersen and colleagues, although several other groups have articulated a similar construct [7, 8]. A diagnosis of MCI, according to the Petersen criteria, is established by (1) evidence of memory impairment, (2) preservation of general cognitive and functional abilities, and (3) absence of diagnosed dementia. Memory deficit in MCI is quantitated by scores greater than 1.0, 1.5, or 2.0 SDs below that of age-appropriate norms on measures of episodic memory [6, 9, 10]. Although advantageous in many clinical circumstances, the challenges of a purely clinical construct like MCI have been well recognized. Progression of patients with MCI to *diagnosable AD dementia* is often confounded by the subjective threshold for a dementia diagnosis, variability on cognitive test performance and informant measures, and the heterogeneity of pathology underlying MCI [1, 10]. These challenges have led to further revisions in the MCI criteria, with increasing use of biological markers of disease progression in AD.

ROLE OF BIOMARKERS IN CHARACTERIZING PREDEMENTIA STATES

Clinical measures alone have been poorly sensitive to early changes in NDD. Insights gained from individuals certain to develop NDD symptoms, who could be identified through genetic testing before clinical signs of the disease begin, have revolutionized our understanding of NDDs. Studies on individuals from families with a known mutation causing an NDD (e.g., Dominantly Inherited Alzheimer Network [DIAN] for AD, PREDICT-HD for Huntington's disease [HD]), along with data from large longitudinal cohorts (e.g., Alzheimer's Disease Neuroimaging Initiative [ADNI], ENROLL -HD), have led to validation of novel biological markers (neuroimaging, cerebrospinal fluid assays, and other biomarkers) that can track disease progression and conversion to dementia. In AD, convergent biomarker findings from autosomal dominant mutation cohorts, non-deterministic genetic-at-risk populations, and age-at-risk cohorts provide a window into pathophysiological processes before dementia onset [11, 12, 13]. New diagnostic criteria proposed for clinical constructs like MCI now have a biological marker of AD pathology, along with the clinical measures traditionally collected [14]. The combination of detailed clinical history, cognitive evaluation, and biomarker signatures are currently used mainly in research settings, but the advantages and clinical confidence they generate in some circumstances (e.g.,. early onset AD) have seen their use increase in a clinical setting.

With early treatment trials targeting mild to moderate AD dementia having failed to demonstrate clinical benefit, there is a growing consensus that NDDs could be more optimally treated prior to significant cognitive impairment during the predementia state. With the availability of disease-related biomarkers, predementia states in sporadic NDD individuals are being diagnosed and treatment trials designed based on a combination of clinical measures and biomarker status [15]. Secondary prevention studies, to treat "cognitively normal" individuals with only biomarker evidence of AD pathology, in order to delay the onset of clinical symptoms, have been initiated.

PREDEMENTIA ACROSS NDDS

Though the existence of a continuum of pathology burden (from completely asymptomatic individuals at risk of developing an NDD to those at the final stage of dementia) and the need to distinguish an intermediate state (those with biomarker evidence of neuropathological changes but not at the stage of dementia) have been recognized, the specific terminology of the predementia state varies across NDDs.

Terms including MCI and prodromal AD usually denote predementia states with some early clinical signs and symptoms, whereas *presymptomatic, premanifest, asymptomatic, at risk, latent*, or *preclinical* (and *prodromal* in HD) are terms often used interchangeably for subjects with biomarker or genetic mutation for an NDD but who are as yet clinically asymptomatic. These terms have been used to capture predementia states across NDDs, but there are differences on what these terms convey and how they apply to a specific NDD, including AD, HD, or frontotemporal lobar degeneration (FTLD).

Among some NDDs, including HD or AD, the early expression of the disease is better understood and the specific categories of preclinical AD and MCI or premanifest HD have proposed clinical criteria to help consistency in diagnosis [14, 16]. For other NDDs, including behavioral variant FTLD or dementia with Lewy bodies (DLB), where even though a model of disease progression over time and a pattern of regional spread of disease are being revealed by recent researches, the implications of these new findings in defining a predementia state are more challenging. The common challenges regarding predementia states in NDDs often relate to poorly understood factors including (1) variability in initial symptoms, which could often be overlooked or misattributed to other psychiatric or neurological conditions; (2) the length of the predementia state before onset of dementia may be different due to variability in the underlying biology with the same clinical syndrome (FTLD from tau [τ], and TDP-43 pathologies) and differences in rate and regions of spread of specific pathology (α-synuclein versus β-amyloid); (3) the role of initial clinical symptoms (motor symptoms or frontal lobe deficits or visuospatial deficits) in disease subtyping and future rate of progression; (4) modifying factors in the predementia states impacting disease manifestation and rate of progression (cognitive reserve, vascular disease, and non-determinant risk genes like apolipoprotein (APOɛ 4 gene) are incompletely characterized in the initial stages of the disease. The predementia state, even as it is shared across NDDs, is currently difficult to operationalize in specific NDDs and has unique features in many NDDs (Figure 9.1).

PREDEMENTIA IN AD

Research in AD has helped define the paradigm in characterizing and developing therapeutic interventions for predementia states. The term *Alzheimer's disease* has often been used to refer to the clinical syndrome of progressive cognitive and behavioral impairment, typically at the stage of dementia while others use it in reference to the neuropathological criteria for AD diagnosis [17] or for the prodromal and dementia symptomatic

phases of AD where an amyloid biomarker is present. Clinical evidence supporting the postulate that AD is characterized by a sequence of neuropathological changes that begins far in advance of clinical dementia and the development of surrogate biomarkers of these changes has seen a shift in the use of the term *AD* to stages prior to dementia if the presence of biomarkers supportive of AD pathology can be demonstrated [17, 18].

Currently, five AD biomarkers are commonly used in the diagnostic criteria for AD. They include two CSF measures, Aβ and tau (τ), (reduced Aβ, increased total τ, and phospho- τ; more specifically, abnormal ratio of Aβ to τ) and three neuroimaging markers, positive amyloid positron emission tomography (PET) (with Pittsburgh compound B or other radioligands (18F-AV-45, florbetaben) measuring fibrillar Aβ deposition), medial temporal lobe and hippocampal atrophy and reduced glucose metabolism in temporoparietal regions on fluorodeoxyglucose PET [19, 20, 21]. The last two neuroimaging markers relate to downstream changes after neurodegeneration and generally follow the Braak stages of neurofibrillary tangle accumulation [21].

The biomarker signature model of AD progression by Jack et al. [22, 23], attaches temporal ordering of different biomarkers to the cumulative burden of multiple pathological changes in the brain relating to different stages of AD progression before dementia. Biomarkers of Aβ deposition are

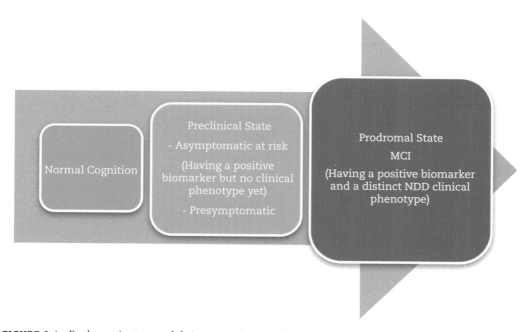

FIGURE 9.1. Predementia states and their progression over time.

hypothesized to become abnormal initially, before neurodegeneration and clinical symptoms occur. Cognitive symptoms are not expected to parallel initial biomarkers of Aβ deposition. Biomarkers of neuronal injury, dysfunction, and neurodegeneration become abnormal later in the disease and correlate with clinical symptom severity. Rates of change in each biomarker change over time are thought to follow a nonlinear time course with a late plateau [22, 23] so that biomarkers changing initially (Aβ) do not change significantly later in the disease course. MRI measures of atrophy that are noted later in the temporal progression of changes than other biomarkers continue to change and correlate with cognitive performance later into the disease [22]. A schema of biomarker changes versus cognitive decline over time is shown in Figure 9.2.

Two groups, the International Working Group (IWG) and the National Institute on Aging together with the Alzheimer's Association (NIA/ AA), have developed clinical criteria for operationalizing stages of AD using a combination of biomarkers and clinical tests but use different terminologies [24, 25, 26]. The predementia states of AD include both the preclinical at risk and prodromal (or MCI) phases before the disease reaches the dementia state. In the preclinical phase (per NIA/AA), the subjects are all cognitively normal (or only on detailed neurocognitive testing may have subtle cognitive changes), but some have AD pathological changes (abnormal Aβ and/or τ) and others have a genetic predisposition to developing AD. The prodromal phase of AD (MCI due

to AD) is characterized by the onset of the earliest cognitive symptoms (commonly deficits in episodic memory) that do not meet the criteria for dementia in addition to AD pathological changes. The severity of cognitive impairment in the prodromal stage of AD varies from early episodic memory changes to more widespread cognitive dysfunction in other domains [25]. It is important to note that AD is not currently excluded in these two diagnostic criteria by a negative amyloid signature on PET imaging, while a positive amyloid signature is not limited to patients with AD and can occur in DLB type or amyloid angiopathy as well as in cognitively normal persons [27]. Points of lack in consistency among the guidelines at the present time indicate areas of evolving consensus and ongoing research on the specific relationship between neurodegeneration and amyloid deposition. Deepening insights into the initial stages of AD pathophysiology could help define future diagnostic criteria that are pathophysiologically consistent and clinically relevant.

IWG criteria (1 & 2) emphasize a single clinico-biological approach that includes all symptomatic phases of AD and uses the same diagnostic framework across the spectrum of symptomatic disease [24, 25]. Biomarkers are an integrated and required part of the IWG criteria, but if no symptoms are present then it is not considered a disease state. The IWG-1 criteria require episodic memory impairment and at least one abnormal AD biomarker (medial temporal lobe atrophy on MRI or parietotemporal hypoperfusion or increased CSF amyloid-$\beta_{1\text{-}42}$, increased

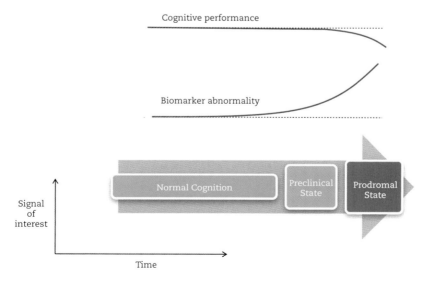

FIGURE 9.2. Schema of biomarker signal abnormality that increases over time versus cognitive decline over time.

CSF τ, or increased amyloid PET uptake). The presence of the biomarker alone represents a risk factor for progressing to AD in the future, for which the time frame is not defined [24]. The updated IWG-2 criteria require cognitive impairment in any cognitive domain and either the AD CSF signature (decreased CSF amyloid-β_{1-42} and increased τ) or increased amyloid PET uptake and specify typical and atypical prodromal AD with/without initial episodic memory loss [25]. The NIA/AA criteria apply slightly different diagnostic approaches to the AD stages. Biomarkers are optional in the NIA/AA approach in diagnosing MCI or AD dementia [26, 28]. A notable aspect of the NIA/AA criteria for the preclinical asymptomatic phase of AD is the description of a sequential appearance of abnormalities from stage 1 with abnormalities of amyloid only, to stage 2 with biomarkers of both amyloid abnormalities and neurodegeneration, to stage 3 with both types of biomarkers and minimal clinical decline not meeting criteria for MCI [17]. Preliminary reports with over 1 year and 5-year longitudinal follow-up support this trajectory of the preclinical stages; subjects with β-amyloidosis (stages 1–3) were at greater risk for progression to MCI or dementia than those subjects with normal biomarkers and normal cognition [29, 30], and compared with individuals classed as normal, subjects with preclinical AD had an increased risk of death after adjusting for covariates [30].

Even as the clinical implications of predementia states are increasingly recognized, current diagnosis of these states is dependent also on an underlying hypothesis of initial Aβ accumulation. The evidence for the key hypothesis supporting Aβ accumulation as necessary and sufficient for the development of AD cognitive decline is still unclear [18, 22]. Whether individuals having preclinical AD will eventually go on to develop AD dementia is also debatable, as some of these individuals will die without ever expressing clinical symptoms [18, 22]. Even as new biomarkers have been crucial in defining predementia states in AD, a few questions remain: (1) What role do biomarkers and the characterizing of predementia states play in our understanding of the future progression and the eventual emergence of clinical symptoms of AD in the lifetime of an individual? (2) Do the temporal relationships between Aβ, τ, atrophy, and cognitive changes in the current biomarker model of AD progression hold true in all individuals with AD? (3) How do biomarker changes characterized in predementia stages of AD with cross-sectional studies relate to the longitudinal time course of changes in sporadic AD? Answers to these questions are important in order to extrapolate with confidence the findings of the predementia stage in AD as defined in special research cohorts to specific individual histories evaluated in the clinical setting. Clarifying predementia states under a single pathophysiological model represents a conceptual advance, but the field still wrestles with issues of significant heterogeneity within the disease, the role of amyloid as a sufficient marker for AD, the threshold of pathology needed for diagnosis and intervention, and factors mediating the rate of progression.

PRECLINICAL DISEASE IN HD

Huntington's disease (HD) is an autosomal dominant NDD caused by an expanded number of CAG repeats in the Huntingtin gene on chromosome 4. Cognitive deficits, psychiatric manifestations, and abnormal motor function, including chorea, are noted with disease progression. Patients are often diagnosed with HD once the motor signs are judged as clinically significant. As the clinical diagnosis of the HD precedes the stage of dementia that occurs many years later, the predementia state in HD is broad and includes a significant proportion of the clinical early stage HD population.

The availability of genetic testing has made it possible to study the natural history of HD prior to the traditional clinical diagnosis, termed *preclinical HD* (other terms used include *premanifest, pre-HD,* and *prodromal*). New criteria for premanifest HD require that these individuals do not exhibit symptoms and have no changes in function. Thus, no relevant changes are seen in the total motor score of the Unified Huntington's Disease Rating Scale (UHDRS) [16]. Approximately 15 years before clinical diagnosis, subtle cognitive and motor difficulties and related changes in brain structure can be observed in some affected individuals [31, 32, 33, 34]. Psychiatric changes (depression, irritability, anxiety, paranoid ideation, and psychoticism) and changes in cognitive functioning are also noted in the preclinical state [34, 35]. Nearly 40% of preclinical HD individuals meet criteria for MCI, and those closer to HD diagnosis have higher rates of MCI, with nonamnestic MCI being the more common presentation [36].

The overarching focus in studying the preclinical HD population has been on developing replicable biomarkers that track neuronal integrity for eventual use in clinical trials. Structural imaging techniques have revealed significant regional cerebral cortical atrophy and basal ganglia volume loss years before clinical onset in a preclinical HD cohort [32, 34, 37, 38]. Low glucose metabolism in the basal ganglia has been reported in preclinical individuals [39, 40]. Preclinical HD individuals also show reduced levels of striatal dopamine receptors as well as abnormal metabolic network signatures [41, 42]. Blood markers, such as interleukin (IL)–6 levels, have been reported to be increased as many as 16 years before clinical diagnosis [43], and correlate with disease progression [44].

Although preclinical HD populations have been intensively researched, there are still significant limitations in our current understanding. Clinical heterogeneity in HD is well recognized, and neuropathological changes of HD do not appear to be uniform across all cases, specifically with age (comparing later disease onset disease with earlier onset) [45]. Heterogeneity in a well-defined genetic disease like HD is also starting to be understood, even at the cellular level where differences in region-specific degeneration of cortical interneurons are now thought to be an important factor [46]. Given this heterogeneity, with potential modifying factors (comorbidities, cognitive reserve, etc.) coming into play, predicting the future rate of clinical decline and defining a robust biomarker signature that relates to burden of neuropathology, clinical severity, and rate of progression are challenging. Insights that may be important in defining the preclinical stage at the group level have still to be carefully parsed when attempting to counsel a specific individual.

PRECLINICAL STATES IN PD AND DLB

Parkinson's disease (PD), the second most common NDD, is characterized by both motor and non-motor features. Clinical diagnosis of PD has classically focused on the motor signs: rest tremor, bradykinesia, rigidity, and loss of postural reflexes. By the time the clinical diagnosis is made, about 70%–80% of striatal dopamine (DA) [47] and at least one-third of substantia nigra (SN) neurons and striatal dopaminergic fibers are lost [48, 49]. The pathological process leading to PD is hypothesized to be ongoing decades before onset of the typical motor symptoms. Based on clinicopathological studies, preclinical PD is thought to precede the classic motor signs by approximately 4 to 7 years [see 50, for a review]. At this preclinical stage, several premotor symptoms are present and include olfactory dysfunction, sleep disturbances, essential tremor, dysautonomia (constipation and

other features), and behavioral changes (depression, anxiety, apathy) [50]. Subclinical abnormalities may also exist that can be detected only by specialized neuroimaging or by biological or physiological tests [50, 51]. The goals of identifying a preclinical PD population have been well articulated: (1) detection of at-risk individuals at a phase in which neuroprotective therapies are expected to have their greatest impact; (2) discriminate PD from other causes of parkinsonism; and (3) accelerate research into pathogenesis-targeted therapeutics of PD [50]. In addition to preclinical PD, the predementia state in PD also includes the clinical diagnostic category of PD-MCI.

Identifying preclinical PD currently faces significant challenges. The clear delineation of a preclinical state in PD rests on a model of progression of the disease that has been best articulated by the Braak hypothesis [52]. This hypothesis proposes that α-synuclein pathological changes in PD start in the lower brainstem and progress following a predictable caudal-rostral pattern, reaching the SN in the mesencephalon only after extensive involvement of the brainstem has occurred. This model lends support to the concept that non-motor features reflecting this prenigral involvement can antedate the classic motor features of PD [50, 52]. Although supported by early non-motor features in PD, the staging proposal probably needs modifications to account for a wider array of observations and alternate sequences [50, 53].

Additional hypotheses to model the preclinical stage that currently are being debated include α-synuclein possibly spreading from the periphery like a prion protein [54] and the role of incidental LBs (iLBs) (10% of clinically normal people older than 60 year have iLBs) as representing a preclinical PD state [55, 56]. The field is yet to come to a conclusion regarding the pathophysiology and development of the preclinical stage in PD. Furthermore, current biomarkers of PD, such as neuroimaging abnormalities detected by dopamine transporter SPECT, meta-iodobenzyl guanidine I 123 (MIBG-scintigraphy), fluorodexoyglucose or dopamine transporter PET, or MRI, have been tested in patients with moderate or advanced PD, but are not specific to PD, and have not been validated in early preclinical stages of PD [50]. Due to current limitations in our understanding of the pathophysiological mechanisms driving PD progression, there is a lack of reliable predictive risk markers for PD, and preclinical therapeutic targets in PD are still at an early stage along with disease-modifying therapies.

As with HD, cognitive deficits often occur years after the initial diagnosis of the PD, with up to 80% of cases fulfilling criteria for dementia by 15 years of disease [57]. But up to 20% of PD patients at initial diagnosis exhibit evidence of some cognitive impairment [58], although not at the stage of dementia. The predementia state in PD therefore includes PD-MCI and the preclinical stage of PD. PD-MCI is defined as cognitive decline in PD that is not normal for age but with essentially normal functional activities [59]. In 2012, a Movement Disorder Society group clarified criteria for the diagnosis of PD-MCI [60]. MCI criteria utilize a two-level operational schema, depending on the comprehensiveness of neuropsychological testing. Among subjects on whom comprehensive neuropsychology testing was performed, it recognizes MCI subtypes for research purposes [60]. Supporting rationales have been put forward to distinguish PD-MCI as a separate population with a distinct clinical focus, requiring interventions to delay functional impairment and improve quality of life [59]. Currently, cognitive features in PD-MCI that predict progression to dementia are unclear. This limits PD-MCI as a useful clinical entity in PD predementia clinical trials and is an area of active research.

In common with other NDDs, the predementia state in PD has significant heterogeneity in presentation and in the time line of clinical progression regarding its motor and non-motor symptoms. Furthermore, there is overlap between PD dementia and the closely related DLB, making clinical differentiation of these two closely aligned disorders difficult. The DLB consortium proposed the "1-year rule" to separate DLB and PD dementia (PDD) clinically [61]. The MCI predementia stage has been studied in DLB, and investigations have documented the development of DLB among MCI subtypes based on neuropsychology (deficits in visuospatial domains, executive function, and attention are commonly noted) [62]. Biomarkers at the MCI-stage of DLB are yet to be well characterized. The cognitive changes in the PDD/DLB spectrum and lack of biomarkers mirroring initial changes add to the difficulty of easily delineating a predementia stage in PD.

PRECLINICAL DISEASE IN FTLD

FTLD is an NDD with a spectrum of clinical syndromes. They include behavioral variant FTD (bvFTD), the primary progressive aphasia (PPA) variants, corticobasal syndrome (CBS), progressive supranuclear palsy (PSP), FTD with Parkinsonism (FTD-P), and the FTD motor neuron variant (FTD-MND). These varying clinical syndromes share similar abnormal protein deposition signatures. About 30%–40% of FTD patients are tauopathies, usually displaying a three amino acid repeat (3R) form of τ in bvFTD and PPA; or a four amino acid repeat (4R) in PSP, CBS, and FTD-P. In approximately 50% of FTD patients, the proteinopathy is a mutant transactive response DNA-binding protein 43 (TDP-43). TDP-43 proteinopathy also occurs in sporadic FTD and in chromosome 9 open reading frame 72 gene (C9ORF72) mutation-identified FTD-MND [see 63, 64 for reviews].

Common FTD autosomal dominant mutations are progranulin (GRN), the microtubule associated protein τ (MAPT), and the C9ORF72. Genetic mutations in four other genes (valosin containing protein [VCP[, fused in sarcoma [FUS], chromatin modifying protein 2B [CHMP2B], and transactive repeat DNA binding protein [TARDBP]) have been documented, but are rare, occurring in only a few families. Insights from families with autosomal dominant FTD mutations have in general supported the model of progressive neuropathological changes with subclinical changes occurring well before onset of characteristic clinical syndromes [63, 64].

There are far fewer data on the clinical, neuropsychological, and radiological features among preclinical carriers of FTLD mutations compared to AD or HD. Cross-sectional analysis of a large Danish family with autosomal dominant FTLD and a mutation in the CHMP2B gene (19 mutation carriers and 32 non-carriers) followed for more than two decades showed that clinically asymptomatic mutation carriers as a group scored lower on several neuropsychological tests of psychomotor speed, working memory, executive functions, and verbal memory compared to a control group consisting of family members without the CHMP2B mutation and spouses [65]. A gradual decline was noted among the predementia mutation carriers over 8 years in psychomotor speed, working memory capacity, and global executive measures compared to non-carriers. The study also noted significant individual variation in the phenotypic presentations in patients with CHMP2B mutations, some showing a typical FTLD dysexecutive syndrome, others developing dementia with a more general cognitive decline; a few patients manifested severe anomia [65].

Case reports of longitudinal follow-up among family members with FTLD who go on to develop dementia later have been reported [66, 67].

A longitudinal case report of two probands with FTLD with S305N τ mutations on chromosome 17 noted many similarities in the behavioral symptoms at onset and cognitive decline over time among the probands, along with a similar topographic pattern of progressive atrophy on MRI [67]. There were also significant differences between the probands, in the rates of change in whole-brain volume and ventricular volume and in their neuropsychology profile, including differences in episodic memory loss [67]. This case report sheds light on the critical issue of members of the same kindred with the same mutation exhibiting different features and rates of change for the disease. It highlights the challenges inherent in a predementia diagnosis and designing therapeutic interventions for these subjects. Neuroimaging studies on preclinical carriers of CHMP2B l mutations have noted significantly lower cerebral blood flow in multiple brain regions (temporal, hippocampus, parietal, and occipital) compared with first-degree relatives without the mutation [68]. Structural changes, measured both as decreased whole-brain volume [66, 67] and as reduced fractional anisotropy in white matter [67], have also been reported in case reports of preclinical mutation carriers.

Formulating a predementia diagnosis is even more challenging in the FTLD spectrum due to the FTD phenocopy syndrome or slowly progressive bvFTD (bvFTD-SP) [68, 69]. They tend to have a slow progressive course and plateau at mild symptom severity [69]. Although many of them have been reported to be devoid of FTLD pathology at autopsy, a recent report noted two individuals who were bvFTD-SP and subsequently were found to carry the C9ORF72 expansion [71]. A combination of heterogeneity in clinical presentations and underlying proteinopathy, along with varying rates of clinical progression, makes defining a predementia stage in FTLD unusually challenging. Novel ways to identify and therapeutically intervene in patients with FTLD pathology at the preclinical state are being debated [63, 67].

PRECLINICAL DISEASE IN OTHER NEURODEGENERATIVE DISEASES

The spinocerebellar ataxias (SCAs) are a group of autosomal dominant inherited NDDs with progressive ataxia as a prominent symptom. They are caused by CAG repeat expansions that code for elongated polyglutamine tracts within the proteins associated with each subtype. Currently, at least 43 SCA subtypes are described, and the causative molecular defects in 27 of them are identified and useful in making a clear clinical diagnosis and provide molecular testing for at risk. [72]. The most common are SCA1, SCA2, SCA3, and SCA6, which together affect more than half of all SCA families [73]. Cognitive decline has been reported for SCA types 1, 2, 3, 6, and 17, with a distinct profile of executive dysfunction with variable affects among subtypes on other cognitive domains [74]. The cognitive dysfunction does not appear to relate to CAG length in most subtypes. Dementia as part of the clinical picture is common in SCA 2 and 17, but could be seen in other subtypes on disease progression [74]. On investigating the mechanism of cognitive dysfunction in SCA, correlations have been found between the scores on neuropsychological tests and perfusion in the prefrontal cortices in patients of the SCA6 type. These results suggest that cognitive impairments in SCA result from prefrontal dysfunction [75]. However, disruption of the cerebrocerebellar circuitry or cortico-striatal-thalamocortical circuitry may also cause prefrontal dysfunction, so the mechanism of such dysfunction remains unresolved [74]. The CAG repeat mutations that cause SCA types 1, 2, 3, and 6 are fully penetrant, and preclinical stage before ataxia can therefore be distinguished [76]. Mild coordination deficits gradually increase before the onset of clinically manifest ataxia. Onset of gait ataxia is typically the first symptom described [77, 78].

As in other NDDs discussed, preclinical stage studies in SCAs are made difficult by the heterogeneity of this disease group. SCA2 mutation carriers with no signs of ataxia were shown to have slowing of saccades [79], disordered rapid eye movement sleep [80], impaired motor performance in a prism adaptation task [81], reduced heart rate variability [82], and nerve conduction abnormalities [83]. Early manifestation of non-ataxia signs described include spontaneous cramps in carriers of SCA1 and SCA2 mutations [76]. MRI also notes the development of cerebellar atrophy in SCA1 and SCA2 and brainstem atrophy in SCA2 before the clinical onset of ataxia and loss of brainstem volume in SCA3 [76]. Characteristics of preclinical stage among SCA subtypes described have to be taken as preliminary due to the small number of subjects described within each subtype.

Preclinical stages of SCA subtypes are especially of interest as the expanded proteins are ubiquitously expressed in neurons, but strikingly distinct regional susceptibility differences among the SCA subtypes are noted on structural MRI in the preclinical stages. Even as SCAs are genetically determined (unlike sporadic AD, for example), they provoke questions on the relationship between variations in genetic predisposition and distinct early regional CNS changes that determine the clinical phenotype.

Preclinical stages, although expected to be found in other NDDs, including dentatorubral-pallidoluysian atrophy (DRPLA; cognitive changes similar to subcortical dementia with executive dysfunction) [74] and Friedreich's ataxia (FA; cognitive changes with lower baseline IQ, speed of processing, and executive dysfunction) [84], have yet to be carefully characterized.

CLINICAL TRIALS IN PREDEMENTIA STATES

The goal of identifying predementia populations in NDD has been to help target these diseases at a stage before significant neuronal damage, when neuroprotective therapies are expected to have their greatest impact. Therapeutic interventions, when planned early in the disease process among asymptomatic individuals, before clinical symptoms and biologic markers are observed, is termed *primary prevention*; in *secondary prevention*, the focus is on asymptomatic individuals with biologic evidence of underlying disease; *tertiary prevention* aims at slowing or deferring the progression of mild symptoms of symptomatic individuals (or it can be said to target the prodromal/MCI stage of NDD) [15].

Autosomal dominant AD has provided a model to study disease progression and test primary or secondary prevention interventions in as-yet asymptomatic persons. A large study involving familial AD is the Alzheimer Prevention Initiative (API). Cognitively normal *PS1 E280A* mutation carriers, at least 35 years of age (i.e., within 10 years of the carriers' estimated median age at clinical onset), from the world's largest known early-onset AD kindred, located in Antioquia, Colombia, are to be randomized to active treatment or placebo with the non-carriers assigned only to placebo. Changes in amyloid PET, FDG-PET, volumetric MRI, CSF, and cognitive scores serve as endpoints. Crenezumab, a monoclonal antibody, will be the interventional agent [85]. A larger undertaking is the Dominantly Inherited Alzheimer Network (DIAN), a worldwide network of centers studying autosomal-dominant AD. DIAN has determined the timing and order of changes in autosomal-dominant AD in a large cohort with the disease [11]. The DIAN therapeutic trials unit has recently started a 2-year study of the effects of anti-amyloid treatment in the preclinical population.

Predementia trials among non-autosomal dominant AD subjects are also being undertaken. A trial in asymptomatic subjects is the Anti-Amyloid Treatment in Asymptomatic Alzheimer's Disease (A4) trial by the Alzheimer's Disease Cooperative Study (ADCS). The A4 trial aims to study the impact of anti-amyloid treatment on downstream markers of neurodegeneration (τ and pτ proteins in the CSF, alterations in functional brain imaging, and brain atrophy and cortical thinning) and to explore whether there is a critical window for anti-amyloid therapy within the preclinical stages of AD [86]. The A4 trial will enroll cognitively normal older individuals (ages 65–85) with positive amyloid imaging into a phase 3 double-blind trial of solanezumab versus placebo. The primary outcome of the A4 Study is rate of change on a composite cognitive outcome measure, but it also includes novel participant-reported outcomes and computerized testing on an iPad [18]. A novel preclinical AD subject enrichment algorithm is being tested by a Takeda/Zinfandel clinical trial consortium for a therapeutic trail of the PPARγ (Peroxisome proliferator-activated receptor gamma) agonist, pioglitazone. Asymptomatic gene-positive individuals who carry the *TOMM40* gene (long alleles of this locus were nearly always linked to APOE ε4 and associated with greater disease risk) [87] are being targeted to track pioglitazone's impact on the rate of future cognitive decline [15].

Successful interventions in secondary AD prevention are expected to decrease the burden of neuropathology or to delay its accrual and influence biomarkers, with a corresponding impact on progression of clinical symptoms. Secondary prevention trials can be focused on specific biomarkers and neuropsychological measures. Similarities in trials across NDD are described in the Chapter 18 on clinical trials and drug development.

HD PREDEMENTIA CLINICAL TRIALS

Interest in designing trials for preclinical HD has had significant increase in the last decade, but preventive clinical trials are hampered by the lack of sensitive markers early in the disease course. Therapeutic trials using clinical scores, such as the Total Functional Capacity (TFC) and UHDRS, typically require studying large cohorts over long periods of time [88]. The two longitudinal studies tracking preclinical HD (PREDICT-HD and

TRACK-HD) are providing important biomarker data in this population [32, 34]. PREQUEL (study in <u>PRE</u>-manifest Huntington's disease of coenzyme Q10 [<u>U</u>biquinon<u>E</u>] <u>L</u>eading to preventive trials), a Phase II trial, was the first multicenter interventional trial among preclinical HD, with 90 participants. CoQ10 is critically involved in the electron transport chain and is a scavenger of free radicals. The trial attempted to demonstrate the biological activity of CoQ10 through changes in plasma 8-hydroxy-2′-deoxyguanosine (8-OHdG). No reductions in 8-OHdG were observed in this trial, but the effect showed that such trials can be designed and carried out successfully in the preclinical HD population [89]. A second phase III clinical trial examining the efficacy of CoQ10 (2CARE) is being carried out among early HD patients (many not yet at the stage of dementia). This trial is to have 608 participants followed for 5 years, with the primary outcome of change in TFC [90]. Dietary creatine supplementation (1%–3%) was shown to delay disease progression in HD mice, but a low dose trial (5–10 mg/day) in HD patients was not promising [90]. In a higher dose (40 mg/day) phase II prevention and biomarker trial (PRECREST) of creatine among preclincial HD, neuroimaging demonstrated treatment-related slowing of cortical and striatal atrophy at 6 and 18 months. This study suggested a role for intervention in the preclinical course, although its clinical benefit is still unproven [91]. Another approach being investigated in HD is the increasing PGC-1α, by activation of peroxisome proliferator-activated receptor (PPAR) gamma coactivator 1 alpha (PGC-1α) nuclear receptors to improve energy metabolism [89]. This mechanism is also being tested in a trial of preclinical AD subjects by the Takeda/Zinfandel clinical trial consortium. Shared druggable targets in the preclinical stages across some NDDs may be feasible given shared pathogenic mechanisms.

FUTURE CHALLENGES IN NDD PRECLINICAL STATES

Although biomarkers have revolutionized the study of NDD, these markers are proxies for the underlying pathology and may not fully reflect the biological progression in the living brain. Temporal sequence of biomarker changes and rate of change of the biomarkers are incompletely understood and make prognostication for an individual patient in the predementia stage fraught with pitfalls, even as the group-level findings have often been robust. Relatively few biomarkers have been developed to track disease progression.

Additionally, there is significant heterogeneity in the clinical presentation and progression of NDDs. Characterization of a predementia state does not always allow for a linear extrapolation into future rate of clinical decline into dementia. Finally, it is important to acknowledge that the relationship between biomarkers, neuropathology, and cognition may vary significantly across age and genetic cohorts. For example, older onset in some NDDs (AD and HD) have been described as more likely to have mixed pathology and less severe clinical course than in young onset subjects. Discerning a predementia state necessarily would have to reflect these nuances.

Lessons learned in clinical trials of MCI populations will have significant bearing on future predementia trials. In the MCI trials of AD, tests used to operationalize MCI criteria were not uniform, and the trial populations were not homogeneous; there was substantial heterogeneity in MCI populations across trials [92]. The primary endpoint of prevention trials was not always defined as the development of dementia, and a variety of surrogate measures have been used to track decline across multiple trials, making conclusions less generalizable [93]. Most of the measures had not been developed specifically for the MCI stage and therefore are without validation, raising additional questions [93]. There is epidemiological evidence that the diagnosis of MCI is sometimes unstable, and some persons labeled as having MCI may revert over time to normal cognition [94, 95]; similar studies on the stability of biomarker-supported predementia populations are lacking. Targeting a predementia population in clinical trials has to answer important questions to overcome pitfalls in earlier MCI trials.

1. Definition of predementia state is to be made effective in the clinic. This requires replicability (across multiple sites and over a specified time period) and validity (tests that characterize predementia stage effectively). Prevalence and prognosis of predementia states are being clarified based on the new biomarker based research criteria in this regard [96].
2. The time line of a predementia state is to be clarified to provide a quantitative estimate of the risk and/or rate of progression from a predementia state to dementia.
3. Are biomarker thresholds and/or clinical thresholds that are targeted to measure rate of decline clinically meaningful? The

progression of non-amnestic MCI and suspected non-Alzheimer pathology to AD dementia is challenging prior assumptions [94, 96].

4. Modifying factors in the predementia state (e.g., age, risk genes, vascular disease, cognitive reserve, inflammation) are to be made part of the staging and prognostication of future decline.

CONCLUSION

Predementia has been generally recognized across NDDs as a promising stage where efforts aimed at preventing the increase in neuropathology can have the greatest and most meaningful long-term clinical impact. The initial successes have stemmed from identifying promising biomarkers in some NDDs (notably AD, HD) to better characterize this stage, while other NDDs await similar characterization (FTLD, DLB). The future challenges involve understanding the initial pathophysiology of these diseases at the preclinical stage. This will help develop prognostic elements in the preclinical stages of NDDs, render disease heterogeneity comprehensible, identify subjects at varying degrees of risk of decline while cognitively normal, and help develop new therapeutic targets and agents.

REFERENCES

1. Gainotti G. Origins, controversies and recent developments of the MCI construct. *Curr Alzheimer Res.* 2010;7(3):271–279.
2. Kral VA. Senescent forgetfulness: benign and malignant. *Can Med Assoc J.* 1962;86:257–260.
3. Crook T, Bahar H, Sudilovsky A. Age-associated memory impairment: diagnostic criteria and treatment strategies. *Int J Neurol.* 1987;21–22:73–82.i
4. Levy R. Aging-associated cognitive decline. Working Party of the International Psychogeriatric Association in collaboration with the World Health Organization. *Int Psychogeriatr.* 1994;6(1):63–68.
5. Graham JE, Rockwood K, Beattie BL, Eastwood R, Gauthier S, Tuokko H, et al. Prevalence and severity of cognitive impairment with and without dementia in an elderly population. Lancet. 1997;349(9068):1793–1796.
6. Petersen RC, Smith GE, Waring SC, Ivnik RJ, Tangalos EG, Kokmen E. Mild cognitive impairment: clinical characterization and outcome. *Arch Neurol.* 1999;56(3):303–308.
7. Flicker C, Ferris SH, Reisberg B. Mild cognitive impairment in the elderly: predictors of dementia. *Neurology.* 1991;41(7):1006–1009.
8. Morris JC, Storandt M, Miller JP, McKeel DW, Price JL, Rubin EH, et al. Mild cognitive impairment represents early-stage Alzheimer disease. *Arch Neurol.* 2001;58(3):397–405.
9. Petersen RC, Stevens JC, Ganguli M, Tangalos EG, Cummings JL, DeKosky ST. Practice parameter: early detection of dementia: mild cognitive impairment (an evidence-based review). Report of the Quality Standards Subcommittee of the American Academy of Neurology. *Neurology.* 2001;56(9):1133–1142.
10. Winblad B, Palmer K, Kivipelto M, Jelic V, Fratiglioni L, Wahlund LO, et al. Mild cognitive impairment—beyond controversies, towards a consensus: report of the International Working Group on Mild Cognitive Impairment. *J Intern Med.* 2004;256(3):240–246.
11. Bateman RJ, Xiong C, Benzinger TL, Fagan AM, Goate A, Fox NC, et al. Clinical and biomarker changes in dominantly inherited Alzheimer's disease. *N Engl J Med.* 2012;367(9):795–804.
12. Reiman EM, Quiroz YT, Fleisher AS, Chen K, Velez-Pardo C, Jimenez-Del-Rio M, et al. Brain imaging and fluid biomarker analysis in young adults at genetic risk for autosomal dominant Alzheimer's disease in the presenilin 1 E280A kindred: a case-control study. *Lancet Neurol.* 2012;11(12):1048–1056.
13. Villemagne VL, Burnham S, Bourgeat P, Brown B, Ellis KA, Salvado O, et al. Amyloid beta deposition, neurodegeneration, and cognitive decline in sporadic Alzheimer's disease: a prospective cohort study. *Lancet Neurol.* 2013;12(4):357–367.
14. Albert MS, DeKosky ST, Dickson D, Dubois B, Feldman HH, Fox NC, et al. The diagnosis of mild cognitive impairment due to Alzheimer's disease: recommendations from the National Institute on Aging-Alzheimer's Association workgroups on diagnostic guidelines for Alzheimer's disease. *Alzheimers Dement.* 2011;7(3):270–279.
15. Pillai JA, Cummings JL. Clinical trials in predementia stages of Alzheimer disease. *Med Clin North Am.* 2013;97(3):439–457.
16. Reilmann R, Leavitt BR, Ross CA. Diagnostic criteria for Huntington's disease based on natural history. *Mov Disord.* 2014;29(11):1335–1341.
17. Sperling RA, Aisen PS, Beckett LA, Bennett DA, Craft S, Fagan AM, et al. Toward defining the preclinical stages of Alzheimer's disease: recommendations from the National Institute on Aging-Alzheimer's Association workgroups on diagnostic guidelines for Alzheimer's disease. *Alzheimers Dement.* 2011;7(3):280–292.
18. Sperling R, Mormino E, Johnson K. The evolution of preclinical Alzheimer's disease: implications for prevention trials. *Neuron.* 2014;84(3):608–622.

19. Blennow K, Zetterberg H, Fagan AM. Fluid biomarkers in Alzheimer disease. *Cold Spring Harb Perspect Med.* 2012;2(9):a006221.

20. Humpel C. Identifying and validating biomarkers for Alzheimer's disease. *Trends Biotechnol.* 2011;29(1):26–32.

21. Frisoni GB, Fox NC, Jack CR, Jr., Scheltens P, Thompson PM. The clinical use of structural MRI in Alzheimer disease. *Nat Rev Neurol.* 2010;6(2):67–77.

22. Jack CR, Jr., Knopman DS, Jagust WJ, Shaw LM, Aisen PS, Weiner MW, et al. Hypothetical model of dynamic biomarkers of the Alzheimer's pathological cascade. *Lancet Neurol.* 2010;9(1):119–128.

23. Jack CR, Jr., Knopman DS, Jagust WJ, Petersen RC, Weiner MW, Aisen PS, et al. Tracking pathophysiological processes in Alzheimer's disease: an updated hypothetical model of dynamic biomarkers. *Lancet Neurol.* 2013;12(2):207–216.

24. Dubois B, Feldman HH, Jacova C, Dekosky ST, Barberger-Gateau P, Cummings J, et al. Research criteria for the diagnosis of Alzheimer's disease: revising the NINCDS-ADRDA criteria. *Lancet Neurol.* 2007;6(8):734–746.

25. Dubois B, Feldman HH, Jacova C, Hampel H, Molinuevo JL, Blennow K, et al. Advancing research diagnostic criteria for Alzheimer's disease: the IWG-2 criteria. *Lancet Neurol.* 2014; 13(6):614–629.

26. Jack CR, Jr., Albert MS, Knopman DS, McKhann GM, Sperling RA, Carrillo MC, et al. Introduction to the recommendations from the National Institute on Aging-Alzheimer's Association workgroups on diagnostic guidelines for Alzheimer's disease. *Alzheimers Dement.* 2011;7(3):257–262.

27. Cummings J. Alzheimer's disease diagnostic criteria: practical applications. *Alzheimers Res Ther.* 2012;4(5):35.

28. Albert MS, DeKosky ST, Dickson D, Dubois B, Feldman HH, Fox NC, et al. The diagnosis of mild cognitive impairment due to Alzheimer's disease: recommendations from the National Institute on Aging-Alzheimer's Association workgroups on diagnostic guidelines for Alzheimer's disease. *Alzheimers Dement.* 2011;7(3):270–279.

29. Knopman DS, Jack CR, Jr., Wiste HJ, Weigand SD, Vemuri P, Lowe V, et al. Short-term clinical outcomes for stages of NIA-AA preclinical Alzheimer disease. *Neurology.* 2012;78(20):1576–1582.

30. Vos SJ, Xiong C, Visser PJ, Jasielec MS, Hassenstab J, Grant EA, et al. Preclinical Alzheimer's disease and its outcome: a longitudinal cohort study. *Lancet Neurol.* 2013;12(10):957–965.

31. Tabrizi SJ, Scahill RI, Durr A, Roos RA, Leavitt BR, Jones R, et al. Biological and clinical changes in premanifest and early stage Huntington's disease in the TRACK-HD study: the 12-month longitudinal analysis. *Lancet Neurol.* 2011;10(1):31–42.

32. Tabrizi SJ, Scahill RI, Owen G, Durr A, Leavitt BR, Roos RA, et al. Predictors of phenotypic progression and disease onset in premanifest and early-stage Huntington's disease in the TRACK-HD study: analysis of 36-month observational data. *Lancet Neurol.* 2013;12(7):637–649.

33. Biglan KM, Zhang Y, Long JD, Geschwind M, Kang GA, Killoran A, et al. Refining the diagnosis of Huntington disease: the PREDICT-HD study. *Front Aging Neurosci.* 2013;5:12.

34. Paulsen JS, Smith MM, Long JD, investigators PH, Coordinators of the Huntington Study G. Cognitive decline in prodromal Huntington Disease: implications for clinical trials. *J Neurol Neurosurg Psychiatry.* 2013;84(11):1233–1239.

35. Marshall J, White K, Weaver M, Flury Wetherill L, Hui S, Stout JC, et al. Specific psychiatric manifestations among preclinical Huntington disease mutation carriers. *Arch Neurol.* 2007;64(1):116–121.

36. Duff K, Paulsen J, Mills J, Beglinger LJ, Moser DJ, Smith MM, et al. Mild cognitive impairment in prediagnosed Huntington disease. *Neurology.* 2010;75(6):500–507.

37. Aylward EH, Nopoulos PC, Ross CA, Langbehn DR, Pierson RK, Mills JA, et al. Longitudinal change in regional brain volumes in prodromal Huntington disease. *J Neurol Neurosurg Psychiatry.* 2011;82(4):405–410.

38. Majid DS, Aron AR, Thompson W, Sheldon S, Hamza S, Stoffers D, et al. Basal ganglia atrophy in prodromal Huntington's disease is detectable over one year using automated segmentation. *Mov Disord.* 2011;26(14):2544–2551.

39. Hayden MR, Martin WR, Stoessl AJ, Clark C, Hollenberg S, Adam MJ, et al. Positron emission tomography in the early diagnosis of Huntington's disease. *Neurology.* 1986;36(7):888–894.

40. Ciarmiello A, Giovacchini G, Orobello S, Bruselli L, Elifani F, Squitieri F. 18F-FDG PET uptake in the pre-Huntington disease caudate affects the time-to-onset independently of CAG expansion size. *Eur J Nucl Med Mol Imaging.* 2012;39(6):1030–1036.

41. Antonini A, Leenders KL, Spiegel R, Meier D, Vontobel P, Weigell-Weber M, et al. Striatal glucose metabolism and dopamine D2 receptor binding in asymptomatic gene carriers and patients with Huntington's disease. *Brain.* 1996;119 (Pt 6):2085–2095.

42. Tang CC, Feigin A, Ma Y, Habeck C, Paulsen JS, Leenders KL, et al. Metabolic network as a progression biomarker of premanifest Huntington's disease. *J Clin Invest.* 2013;123(9):4076–4088.

43. Bjorkqvist M, Wild EJ, Thiele J, Silvestroni A, Andre R, Lahiri N, et al. A novel pathogenic pathway of immune activation detectable before clinical onset in Huntington's disease. *J Exp Med.* 2008;205(8):1869–1877.

44. Dalrymple A, Wild EJ, Joubert R, Sathasivam K, Bjorkqvist M, Petersen A, et al. Proteomic profiling of plasma in Huntington's disease reveals neuroinflammatory activation and biomarker candidates. *J Proteome Res.* 2007;6(7):2833–2840.

45. Pillai JA, Hansen LA, Masliah E, Goldstein JL, Edland SD, Corey-Bloom J. Clinical severity of Huntington's disease does not always correlate with neuropathologic stage. *Mov Disord.* 2012;27(9):1099–1103.

46. Nana AL, Kim EH, Thu DC, Oorschot DE, Tippett LJ, Hogg VM, et al. Widespread heterogeneous neuronal loss across the cerebral cortex in Huntington's disease. *J Huntingtons Dis.* 2014;3(1):45–64.

47. Bohnen NI, Albin RL, Koeppe RA, Wernette KA, Kilbourn MR, Minoshima S, et al. Positron emission tomography of monoaminergic vesicular binding in aging and Parkinson disease. *J Cereb Blood Flow Metab.* 2006;26(9):1198–1212

48. Hilker R, Schweitzer K, Coburger S, Ghaemi M, Weisenbach S, Jacobs AH, et al. Nonlinear progression of Parkinson disease as determined by serial positron emission tomographic imaging of striatal fluorodopa F 18 activity. *Arch Neurol.* 2005;62(3):378–382.

49. Marek K, Jennings D. Can we image premotor Parkinson disease? *Neurology.* 2009;72(7 Suppl):S21–26.

50. Wu Y, Le W, Jankovic J. Preclinical biomarkers of Parkinson disease. *Arch Neurol.* 2011;68(1):22–30

51. Siderowf A, Stern MB. Preclinical diagnosis of Parkinson's disease: are we there yet? *Curr Neurol Neurosci Rep.* 2006;6(4):295–301.

52. Braak H, Del Tredici K, Rub U, de Vos RA, Jansen Steur EN, Braak E. Staging of brain pathology related to sporadic Parkinson's disease. *Neurobiol Aging.* 2003;24(2):197–211.

53. Halliday GM, Del Tredici K, Braak H. Critical appraisal of brain pathology staging related to presymptomatic and symptomatic cases of sporadic Parkinson's disease. *J Neural Transm Suppl.* 2006(70):99–103.

54. Olanow CW, Prusiner SB. Is Parkinson's disease a prion disorder? *Proc Natl Acad Sci U S A.* 2009;106(31):12571–12572.

55. DelleDonne A, Klos KJ, Fujishiro H, Ahmed Z, Parisi JE, Josephs KA, et al. Incidental Lewy body disease and preclinical Parkinson disease. *Arch Neurol.* 2008;65(8):1074–1080.

56. Dickson DW, Fujishiro H, DelleDonne A, Menke J, Ahmed Z, Klos KJ, et al. Evidence that incidental Lewy body disease is pre-symptomatic Parkinson's disease. *Acta Neuropathol.* 2008;115(4):437–444.

57. Aarsland D, Litvan I, Salmon D, Galasko D, Wentzel-Larsen T, Larsen JP. Performance on the dementia rating scale in Parkinson's disease with dementia and dementia with Lewy bodies: comparison with progressive supranuclear palsy and Alzheimer's disease. *J Neurol Neurosurg Psychiatry.* 2003;74(9):1215–1220.

58. Aarsland D, Bronnick K, Larsen JP, Tysnes OB, Alves G, Norwegian ParkWest Study G. Cognitive impairment in incident, untreated Parkinson disease: the Norwegian ParkWest study. *Neurology.* 2009;72(13):1121–1126.

59. Litvan I, Aarsland D, Adler CH, Goldman JG, Kulisevsky J, Mollenhauer B, et al. MDS Task Force on mild cognitive impairment in Parkinson's disease: critical review of PD-MCI. *Mov Disord.* 2011;26(10):1814–1824.

60. Litvan I, Goldman JG, Troster AI, Schmand BA, Weintraub D, Petersen RC, et al. Diagnostic criteria for mild cognitive impairment in Parkinson's disease: Movement Disorder Society Task Force guidelines. *Mov Disord.* 2012;27(3):349–356.

61. McKeith IG, Dickson DW, Lowe J, Emre M, O'Brien JT, Feldman H, et al. Diagnosis and management of dementia with Lewy bodies: third report of the DLB Consortium. *Neurology.* 2005;65(12):1863–1872.

62. Ferman TJ, Smith GE, Kantarci K, Boeve BF, Pankratz VS, Dickson DW, et al. Nonamnestic mild cognitive impairment progresses to dementia with Lewy bodies. *Neurology.* 2013;81(23):2032–2038.

63. Rabinovici GD, Miller BL. Frontotemporal lobar degeneration: epidemiology, pathophysiology, diagnosis and management. *CNS Drugs.* 2010;24(5):375–398.

64. Rohrer JD, Warren JD. Phenotypic signatures of genetic frontotemporal dementia. *Curr Opin Neurol.* 2011;24(6):542–549.

65. Stokholm J, Teasdale TW, Johannsen P, Nielsen JE, Nielsen TT, Isaacs A, et al. Cognitive impairment in the preclinical stage of dementia in FTD-3 CHMP2B mutation carriers: a longitudinal prospective study. *J Neurol Neurosurg Psychiatry.* 2013;84(2):170–176.

66. Janssen JC, Schott JM, Cipolotti L, Fox NC, Scahill RI, Josephs KA, et al. Mapping the onset and progression of atrophy in familial frontotemporal lobar degeneration. *J Neurol Neurosurg Psychiatry.* 2005;76(2):162–168.

67. Boeve BF, Tremont-Lukats IW, Waclawik AJ, Murrell JR, Hermann B, Jack CR, Jr., et al. Longitudinal characterization of two siblings with frontotemporal dementia and parkinsonism linked to chromosome 17 associated with

the S305N tau mutation. *Brain*. 2005;128(Pt 4): 752–772.

68. Lunau L, Mouridsen K, Rodell A, Ostergaard L, Nielsen JE, Isaacs A, et al. Presymptomatic cerebral blood flow changes in CHMP2B mutation carriers of familial frontotemporal dementia (FTD-3), measured with MRI. *BMJ Open*. 2012;2(2):e000368

69. Hornberger M, Shelley BP, Kipps CM, Piguet O, Hodges JR. Can progressive and non-progressive behavioural variant frontotemporal dementia be distinguished at presentation? *J Neurol Neurosurg Psychiatry*. 2009;80(6):591–593.

70. Kipps CM, Hodges JR, Hornberger M. Nonprogressive behavioural frontotemporal dementia: recent developments and clinical implications of the 'bvFTD phenocopy syndrome.' *Curr Opin Neurol*. 2010;23(6):628–632.

71. Khan BK, Yokoyama JS, Takada LT, Sha SJ, Rutherford NJ, Fong JC, et al. Atypical, slowly progressive behavioural variant frontotemporal dementia associated with C9ORF72 hexanucleotide expansion. *J Neurol Neurosurg Psychiatry*. 2012;83(4):358–364.

72. Matilla-Duenas A. The ever expanding spinocerebellar ataxias. Editorial. *Cerebellum*. 2012;11(4): 821–827.

73. Schols L, Bauer P, Schmidt T, Schulte T, Riess O. Autosomal dominant cerebellar ataxias: clinical features, genetics, and pathogenesis. *Lancet Neurol*. 2004;3(5):291–304.

74. Kawai Y, Suenaga M, Watanabe H, Sobue G. Cognitive impairment in spinocerebellar degeneration. *Eur Neurol*. 2009;61(5):257–268.

75. Kawai Y, Suenaga M, Watanabe H, Ito M, Kato K, Kato T, et al. Prefrontal hypoperfusion and cognitive dysfunction correlates in spinocerebellar ataxia type 6. *J Neurol Sci*. 2008;271(1–2):68–74.

76. Jacobi H, Reetz K, du Montcel ST, Bauer P, Mariotti C, Nanetti L, et al. Biological and clinical characteristics of individuals at risk for spinocerebellar ataxia types 1, 2, 3, and 6 in the longitudinal RISCA study: analysis of baseline data. *Lancet Neurol*. 2013;12(7):650–658.

77. Jacobi H, Hauser TK, Giunti P, Globas C, Bauer P, Schmitz-Hubsch T, et al. Spinocerebellar ataxia types 1, 2, 3 and 6: the clinical spectrum of ataxia and morphometric brainstem and cerebellar findings. *Cerebellum*. 2012;11(1):155–166.

78. Storey E. Presymptomatic features of spinocerebellar ataxias. *Lancet Neurol*. 2013;12(7):625–626.

79. Velazquez-Perez L, Seifried C, Abele M, Wirjatijasa F, Rodriguez-Labrada R, Santos-Falcon N, et al. Saccade velocity is reduced in presymptomatic spinocerebellar ataxia type 2. *Clin Neurophysiol*. 2009;120(3):632–635.

80. Rodriguez-Labrada R, Velazquez-Perez L, Ochoa NC, Polo LG, Valencia RH, Cruz GS, et al. Subtle rapid eye movement sleep abnormalities in presymptomatic spinocerebellar ataxia type 2 gene carriers. *Mov Disord*. 2011;26(2):347–350.

81. Velazquez-Perez L, Diaz R, Perez-Gonzalez R, Canales N, Rodriguez-Labrada R, Medrano J, et al. Motor decline in clinically presymptomatic spinocerebellar ataxia type 2 gene carriers. *PLoS One*. 2009;4(4):e5398.

82. Montes-Brown J, Machado A, Estevez M, Carricarte C, Velazquez-Perez L. Autonomic dysfunction in presymptomatic spinocerebellar ataxia type-2. *Acta Neurol Scand*. 2012;125(1):24–29.

83. Velazquez Perez L, Sanchez Cruz G, Canales Ochoa N, Rodriguez Labrada R, Rodriguez Diaz J, Almaguer Mederos L, et al. Electrophysiological features in patients and presymptomatic relatives with spinocerebellar ataxia type 2. *J Neurol Sci*. 2007;263(1–2):158–164.

84. Mantovan MC, Martinuzzi A, Squarzanti F, Bolla A, Silvestri I, Liessi G, Macchi C, Ruzza G, Trevisan CP, Angelini C. Exploring mental status in Friedreich's ataxia: a combined neuropsychological, behavioral and neuroimaging study. *Eur J Neurol*. 2006;13:827–835.

85. Reiman EM, Langbaum JB, Fleisher AS, Caselli RJ, Chen K, Ayutyanont N, et al. Alzheimer's Prevention Initiative: a plan to accelerate the evaluation of presymptomatic treatments. *J Alzheimers Dis*. 2011;26 Suppl 3:321–329.

86. Sperling RA, Jack CR, Jr., Aisen PS. Testing the right target and right drug at the right stage. *Sci Transl Med*. 2011;30;3(111):111cm33. doi:10.1126/scitranslmed.3002609.

87. Roses AD, Lutz MW, Amrine-Madsen H, Saunders AM, Crenshaw DG, Sundseth SS, et al. A TOMM40 variable-length polymorphism predicts the age of late-onset Alzheimer's disease. *Pharmacogenomics J*. 2010;10(5):375–384.

88. Henry PG, Mochel F. The search for sensitive biomarkers in presymptomatic Huntington disease. *J Cereb Blood Flow Metab*. 2012;32(5):769–770.

89. Chandra A, Johri A, Beal MF. Prospects for neuroprotective therapies in prodromal Huntington's disease. *Mov Disord*. 2014;29(3): 285–293.

90. Duan W, Jiang M, Jin J. Metabolism in HD: still a relevant mechanism? *Mov Disord*. 2014;29(11): 1366–1374.

91. Rosas HD, Doros G, Gevorkian S, Malarick K, Reuter M, Coutu JP, et al. PRECREST: a phase II prevention and biomarker trial of creatine in at-risk Huntington disease. *Neurology*. 2014;82(10): 850–857.

92. Raschetti R, Albanese E, Vanacore N, Maggini M. Cholinesterase inhibitors in mild cognitive

impairment: a systematic review of randomised trials. *PLoS Med.* 2007;4(11):e338.

93. Jelic V, Kivipelto M, Winblad B. Clinical trials in mild cognitive impairment: lessons for the future. *J Neurol Neurosurg Psychiatry.* 2006; 77(4):429–438.

94. Busse A, Hensel A, Guhne U, Angermeyer MC, Riedel-Heller SG. Mild cognitive impairment: long-term course of four clinical subtypes. *Neurology.* 2006;67(12):2176–2185.

95. Han JW, Kim TH, Lee SB, Park JH, Lee JJ, Huh Y, et al. Predictive validity and diagnostic stability of mild cognitive impairment subtypes. *Alzheimers Dement.* 2012;8(6):553–559.

96. Vos SJ, Verhey F, Frolich L, Kornhuber J, Wiltfang J, Maier W, et al. Prevalence and prognosis of Alzheimer's disease at the mild cognitive impairment stage. *Brain.* 2015;138(Pt 5): 1327–1338.

10

Genetics of Neurodegenerative Diseases

Sporadic and Autosomal Dominant Forms

LYNN M. BEKRIS AND JAMES B. LEVERENZ

INTRODUCTION

A great deal has been discovered about aging-associated cognitive disorders. This includes genetic variants associated with both sporadic and autosomal dominant disease. While much is still to be learned, these findings will play an important role in the future of neurodegenerative prediction, diagnosis, and treatment. This chapter will summarize the current genetic knowledge related to both the sporadic and autosomal dominant forms of neurodegenerative disease.

ALZHEIMER'S DISEASE

Alzheimer's disease (AD) is the most common irreversible and progressive brain disease of aging adults. It is characterized by a gradual loss of memory and cognitive skills. AD accounts for over 50% of all dementia cases, and presently affects more than 24 million people worldwide, with over 5 million new cases each year, a figure that is likely to increase as a greater proportion of the population ages.[1]

Age is the largest known risk factor, with AD prevalence increasing significantly with age. AD incidence increases from 2.8 per 1,000 person years at age 65–69 years to 56.1 per 1,000 person years for those older than 90 years.[2] The disease can be divided into two subtypes based on the age of onset: early-onset AD (EOAD) and late-onset AD (LOAD). EOAD accounts for approximately 1%–6% of all cases and ranges roughly from the age of 30 years to 60 or 65 years. On the other hand, the most common form of AD, LOAD, is defined as an age at onset later than 60 or 65 years. Both EOAD and LOAD may have a positive family history of AD. With the exception of a few autosomal dominant families that have single gene disorders, most AD appears to be a complex disorder that is likely to involve multiple susceptibility genes

and environmental factors.[3–7] Approximately 60% of EOAD is familial, with multiple cases of AD within a family, of which 13% are inherited in an autosomal-dominant manner with at least three generations affected.[8,9] Early-onset cases can also occur in families with late-onset disease.[3]

At autopsy, AD is characterized by the extra-neuronal deposition of the amyloid β protein in the form of plaques and the intraneuronal aggregation of the microtubule-associated protein tau in the form of neurofibrillary tangles.[1]

To date, autosomal dominant early onset familial AD (EOFAD) is associated with three genes: the amyloid precursor protein gene (*APP*), the presenilin 1 gene (*PSEN1*) and the presenilin 2 gene (*PSEN2*).[10] However, it is likely that other genes will be identified as a cause of EOFAD because there are still kindreds with autosomal-dominant EOFAD without known mutations in these three genes.[3,11,12] Despite evidence from family studies that genetic mutations cause EOFAD, more than 90% of AD cases are LOAD and appear to be sporadic (without a family history).[13] Twin studies support the existence of a strong genetic component in LOAD.[14] However, the only gene consistently found to be associated with sporadic LOAD, across multiple studies, is the apolipoprotein E gene (*APOE*) *ε4* risk allele.[15–19] However, many carriers of the *APOE* risk allele (*ε4*) survive into their 10th decade without dementia, suggesting the existence of other LOAD genetic and/or environmental risk factors that are yet to be identified. Recently, a rare genetic variant in the triggering receptor expressed on myeloid cells 2 gene (*TREM2*) has been described as a LOAD risk gene.[20–23] In addition, an amyloid precursor protein (*APP*) variant has been described as protective against LOAD (Table 10.1).[24] Several other genetic variants have also been reported and suggest that there may be five to seven major LOAD

TABLE 10.1 GENES ASSOCIATED WITH SPORADIC AND AUTOSOMAL DOMINANT
NEURODEGENERATIVE DISEASE

Gene	Gene Name	Chromosome Location	Neurodegenerative Disease
Familial Alzheimer Disease			
APP	Amyloid Precursor Protein	21q21.3	Early Onset Familial Alzheimer's disease, Cerebral Amyloid Angiopathy
PSEN1	Presenilin 1	14q24.2	Early Onset Familial Alzheimer's disease, Pick's disease, Frontotemporal Dementia, Cardiomyopathy
PSEN2	Presenilin 2	1q42.13	Early Onset Familial Alzheimer's disease, Cardiomyopathy
Sporadic Alzheimer Disease			
APOE	Apolipoprotein E	19q13.32	Late Onset Alzheimer's disease Susceptibility, Hyperlipoproteinemia, Dysbetalipoproteinemia, Hypercholesterolemia, Hypertriglyceridemia, Coronary Artery Disease
TREM2	Triggering receptor expressed on myeloid cells 2	6p21.1	Late Onset Alzheimer's disease Susceptibility, Polycystic Lipomembrainous Osteodysplasia with Sclerosing Leukoencephalopathy
APP	Amyloid Precursor Protein	21q21.3	One mutation confers protection against Late Onset Alzheimer's disease
Familial Parkinson Disease and Dementia with Lewy Body			
SNCA	α-Synuclein	4q22.1	Autosomal Dominant Parkinson's disease, Dementia with Lewy Body, Multiple System Atrophy
LRRK2	Dardarin	12q12	Autosomal Dominant PD, Corticobasal Degeneration, Primary Progressive Aphasia, Late Onset PD Susceptibility
PRKN/PARK2	Parkin	6q26	Autosomal Recessive Juvenile PD
DJ1/PARK7	Parkinson disease protein 7	1p36.23	Early Onset Autosomal Recessive PD
ATP13A2	Probable cation-transporting ATPase 13A2	1p36.13	Kufor-Rakeb (Autosomal Recessive Parkinsonism with Dementia, juvenile onset) Neuronal Ceroid Lipofuscinosis (1 family)
Sporadic Parkinson Disease and Dementia with Lewy Body			
SNCA	α-Synuclein	4q22.1	Some genetic variants associated with PD susceptibility
LRRK2	Dardarin	12q12	Some genetic variants associated with PD susceptibility
GBA	Glucosidase beta acid	1q22	Gauche Disease, Dementia with Lewy Body Susceptibility, Late Onset PD Susceptibility
PINK1	Phosphatase and Tensin (PTEN) Induced Kinase 1	1p36.12	Late Onset AD Susceptibility, Autosomal Recessive Early Onset PD

(continued)

TABLE 10.1 CONTINUED

Gene	Gene Name	Chromosome Location	Neurodegenerative Disease
SCARB2	Scavenger receptor class B member 2	4q21.1	Autosomal Recessive Progressive MyoclonicEpilepsy-4 with or without Renal Failure, Dementia with Lewy Body Susceptibility
Omi/HtrA2	High temperature requirement protein A2	2p13.1	Autosomal Dominant PD and PD Susceptibility (Not replicated)
UCHL1	Ubiquitin Carboxy-terminal Esterase L1	4p14	Autosomal Dominant PD (1 family not replicated), Childhood Onset Neurodegeneration Optical Atrophy (1 family)

Familial and Sporadic Frontal Temporal Lobar Dementia and Amyotrophic Lateral Sclerosis

SOD1	Superoxide dismutase 1	21q22.11	Autosomal Dominant and Autosomal Recessive Amyotrophic Lateral Sclerosis
C9orf72	Chromosome 9 open reading frame 72	9p21.2	Autosomal Dominant Frontotemporal Dementia, Amyotrophic Lateral Sclerosis, Progressive Supranuclear Palsy, Corticobasal Degeneration
GRN	Granulin	17q21.31	Frontotemporal Lobar Degeneration with Ubiquitin-Postive Inclusions, Primary Progressive Aphasia
MAPT	Microtubule associated protein tau	17q21.31	Progressive Supranuclear Palsy, Frontotemporal Dementia, Pick's disease
TARDBP	TAR DNA binding protein 43 (TDP-43)	1p36.22	Amyotrophic Lateral Sclerosis with and without Frontotemporal Dementia with TDP43 Inclusions, Frontotemporal Dementia with TDP43 Inclusions
FUS	FUS RNA binding protein	16p11.2	Amyotrophic Lateral Sclerosis with and without Frontotemporal Dementia, Auosomal Rescessive Amyotrophic Lateral Sclerosis, Hereditary Essential Tremor
CHMP2B	Charged multivesicular body protein 2B	3p11.2	Frontotemporal Dementia, Amyotrophic Lateral Sclerosis
DCNT1	Dynactin subunit 1	2p13.1	Distal Hereditary Motor Neuronopathy (type VIIB), Amyotrophic Lateral Sclerosis Susceptibility, Perry Syndrome
SMPD1	Sphingomyelin Phosphodiesterase 1	11p15.4	Niemann-Pick Disease (Type A and Type B)
VCP	Valosin containing protein	9p13.3	Amyotrophic Lateral Sclerosis with or without Frontotemporal Dementia, Inclusion Body Myopathy with Early-onset Paget Disease and Frontotemporal Dementia
TMEM106B	Transmembrane protein 106B	7p21.3	Frontotemporal Dementia with TDP43 Inclusions
TBK1	TANK-binding Kinase 1	12q14.1	Frontotemporal Dementia with TDP43 Inclusions
OPTN	Optineurin	10p13	Frontotemporal Dementia with TDP43 Inclusions

susceptibility genes. However, many are without replication among studies.[3,25,26]

AUTOSOMAL DOMINANT ALZHEIMER'S DISEASE

Amyloid Precursor Protein Gene: APP
Inheritance and Clinical Features

The purification of both plaque and vascular amyloid deposits and the isolation of their 40-residue constituent peptide (Aβ) led to the cloning of the APP type I integral membrane glycoprotein from which Aβ is proteolytically derived.[27] The APP gene was mapped to chromosome 21q, which accounts for the observation that Down syndrome patients (trisomy 21) can develop amyloid deposits and the neuropathological features of AD at a very early age, and universally by their forties.[28–32] Subsequent searches for autosomal dominant EOAD families with genetic linkage to chromosome 21 resulted in the identification of six different missense mutations in APP, five associated with familial AD[33–37] and one with the neuropathologically related syndrome of hereditary cerebral hemorrhage with amyloidosis of the Dutch type.[38]

Subsequently, over 20 different APP missense mutations have been identified in 60 families, most with onset in the mid-forties and fifties.[39] Interestingly, most of these mutations are located at exons 16 and 17, where the secretase cleavage sites or the APP transmembrane domain are located, suggesting altered processing of APP is pathobiologically linked to AD.[40,41] Information regarding APP mutations are available in the Alzheimer Disease Mutation Database (www.molgen.ua.ac.be/ADMutations).[12] Mutations within APP account for 10%–15% of EOFAD,[3,11,42,43] appear to be family specific, and do not occur within the vast majority of sporadic AD cases.

Structure, Function, and Expression

Sequences encoding APP were first cloned by screening cDNA libraries.[27] The APP gene is alternatively spliced into several products, named according to their length in amino acids (i.e., APP695, APP714, APP751, APP770, and APP563) and expressed differentially by tissue type. Three isoforms, most relevant to AD, are restricted to the central nervous system (APP695) or are expressed in both the peripheral and CNS tissues (APP751 and APP770).[27,44–50]

APP is a type I integral membrane protein[27] that resembles a signal-transduction receptor. It is expressed in many tissues and is concentrated in the synapses of neurons. Its primary function is not known, though it has been implicated in neural plasticity[51] and as a regulator of synapse formation.[52]

Proteolysis of APP by α-secretase or β-secretase leads to the secretion of sAPPα or sAPPβ. These fragments can be cut by γ-secretase to release the Aβ peptide extracellularly[53] and a cytoplasmic fragment identified as AICD intracellularly.[54] The majority of early-onset AD mutations alter processing of APP in such a way that the relative level of Aβ42 is increased, either by increasing Aβ42 or decreasing Aβ40 peptide levels, or both.[55,56] The first described, and best characterized APP mutation (V717I), was identified in a London family and is located within the transmembrane domain near the γ-secretase cleavage site.[33] Subsequently other substitutions at this site have been identified and many other groups have reported the V717I mutation in other families. Many other mutations have been identified, most of which are located near the gamma-secreatase cleavage site and have been associated with modulation of Aβ levels.

Transgenic mouse models of APP mutations have been developed, including PDAPP, Tg2576, APP23, TgCRND8, and J20.[57] Each of these transgenic mouse models have different mutations and different promoters that lead to different expression levels and different levels of neuroanatomical abnormalities.[57,58] For example, the Tg2576 mouse model that carries the "Swedish" mutation has high APP levels, high Aβ, and cognitive disturbances[59] that are progressive and start as early as 6 months of age.[60]

Presenilin 1: PSEN1
Inheritance and Clinical Features

Linkage studies established the presence of a locus on chromosome 14 linked to AD,[61] and positional cloning led to the identification of mutations in the presenilin-1 (PSEN1) gene.[62] Mutations in PSEN1 are the most common cause of EOFAD. PSEN1 missense mutations account for 18%–50% of the autosomal dominant EOFAD.[63] PSEN1 mutations' influence on γ-secretase function is still unclear but appears to impact levels of Aβ production in cell and mouse models.[64] In preclinical cases with PSEN1 mutations, deposition of Aβ42 may be an early event.[65]

Mutations in PSEN1 cause the most severe forms of autosomal dominant AD, with complete penetrance and an onset occurring as early as 30 years of age.[10,66] There is considerable phenotypic variability in EOFAD, including some patients with spastic paraparesis and other atypical AD symptoms, such as parkinsonism. Some of these variable clinical phenotypes have been linked to specific mutations. Neuropathogical studies usually confirm the presence of AD pathology, including both severe amyloid plaque and neurofibrillary tangle pathology. Other pathologies have also been described in *PSEN1* mutation–associated AD, including Lewy bodies, corticospinal tract degeneration, and atypical plaques.[67–70]

Structure, Function, and Expression

PSEN1 consists of 12 exons that encode a 467–amino acid protein that is predicted to traverse the membrane 6–10 times; the ammino and carboxyl termini are both oriented toward the cytoplasm.[71]

PSEN1 is a polytopic membrane protein that forms the catalytic core of the gamma-secretase complex.[72,73] As previously mentioned, the gamma-secretase complex is an integral membrane protein important in the processing of APP. *PSEN1*, nicastrin (Nct), anterior pharynx defective 1 (Aph-1), and presenilin enhancer 2 (PSENEN) are required for the stability and activity of the γ-secretase complex.[74–78] *PSEN1* knock-out mice are not viable,[79] but a conditional *PSEN1* knock-out mouse model, where the loss of the gene is limited to the postnatal forebrain, shows mild cognitive impairments in long-term spatial reference memory and retention.[80] Knock-in mouse models with missense mutations of the endogenous murine *PSEN1* express high levels of Aβ42 levels and perform poorly on the object recognition test.[81,82] Double *PSEN1/APP* transgenics have been developed and suggest that *PSEN1*, *APP*, and mutations within these genes play a role in the production of Aβ and the development of the senile plaques characteristic of AD neuropathology.[58,83]

Genetic Variants

To date, there have been 123 *PSEN1* mutations reported. A comprehensive list of *PSEN1* mutations is available through the National Center for Biotechnology Information (NCBI) database (http://www.molgen.ua.ac.be/ADmutations). The majority of these mutations are missense mutations. These missense mutations cause amino acid substitutions throughout the *PSEN1* protein and appear to result in a relative increase in the ratio of the Aβ42 to Aβ40 peptides via either increased Aβ42 or decreased Aβ40 generation, or a combination of both.[55]

Presenilin 2: *PSEN2*
Inheritance and Clinical Features

A candidate gene on chromosome 1 was identified in 1995 in a Volga-German AD kindred with a high homology to *PSEN1* and was later named presenilin 2 (*PSEN2*).[42,84,85] In contrast to mutations in the *PSEN1* gene, missense mutations in the *PSEN2* gene are a rare cause of EOFAD, at least in Caucasian populations. Clinical features of *PSEN2*-affected families appear to differ from those of *PSEN1*; in general, the age of onset is older (45–88 years) than that observed for most *PSEN1* mutations (25–65 years), and is more highly variable among affected members within the same family.[8,42,62,84,86]

Structure, Function, and Expression

The *PSEN2* gene was identified by sequence homology and cloned.[84,85] *PSEN2* has 12 exons and is organized into 10 translated exons that encode a 448–amino acid peptide. The *PSEN2* protein is predicted to consist of nine transmembrane domains and a large loop structure between the sixth and seventh domains. *PSEN2* also displays tissue-specific alternative splicing.[84,85,87–90] *PSEN2* is expressed in a variety of tissues, including the brain, where it is expressed primarily in neurons.[91]

Like *PSEN1*, *PSEN2* has been described as a component of the atypical aspartyl protease called γ-secretase that is responsible for the cleavage of Aβ.[72,92] *PSEN2*-associated mutations have been reported to increase the ratio of Aβ42 to Aβ40 (Aβ42/Aβ40) in mice and humans,[55,64] indicating that presenilins might modify the way in which γ-secretase cuts *APP*. *APP* processing at the gamma-secretase site has been reported to be affected in variable ways by the presenilin mutations. For example, *PSEN1*-L166P mutations cause a reduction in Aβ production, whereas *PSEN1*-G384A mutant significantly increased Aβ42. In contrast, *PSEN2* appears to be a less efficient producer of Aβ than *PSEN1*.[93]

Genetic Variation

Mutations in *PSEN2* are a much rarer cause of FAD than are *PSEN1* mutations, having been described in only six families, including the Volga-German kindred where a founder effect has been demonstrated.[12,42,84,85] One of the first mutations to be identified was a point mutation resulting in the substitution of an isoleucine for an asparagine at residues 141 (N141l) located within the second transmembrane domain.[85] More recently, a V393M mutation located within the seventh transmembrane domain has been described.[94]

A comprehensive list of *PSEN2* mutations is available through the NCBI database (http://www.molgen.ua.ac.be/ADmutations).

SPORADIC LATE-ONSET ALZHEIMER'S DISEASE

Apolipoprotein E: APOE

Inheritance and Clinical Features

The *APOE* gene has been associated with both familial late-onset and sporadic late-onset AD, and in numerous studies of multiple ethnic groups. There are three major protein isoforms of human apoE (apoE2, apoE3, and apoE4), which are the products of three alleles (ε2, ε3, and ε4). The frequency of the *APOE* ε4 allele varies between ethnic groups, but the *APOE* ε4 carriers are the most frequent in AD patients across all ethnic groups.[15-17,95-104]

The *APOE* ε4 genotype is associated with higher risk of AD,[105] earlier age of dementia onset for both AD[106] and Down syndrome,[107] and also with a worse outcome after head trauma[108] and stroke.[109] In addition, individuals carrying apoE4 have higher amyloid and tangle pathology,[110] and have an increase in mitochondrial damage[111] compared to those carrying other forms.

Structure, Function, and Expression

The *APOE* gene consists of four exons that encode a 299–amino acid protein. The three *APOE* ε4 alleles (ε2, ε3, and ε4) are defined by two single nucleotide polymorphisms; rs429358 and rs7412 encode the three protein isoforms (E2, E3, and E4). The most frequent isoform is apoE3, which contains cysteine and arginine at amino acid positions 112 and 158. Both positions contain cysteine residues in apoE2 and arginine residues in apoE4. This substitution affects the three-dimensional structure and the lipid-binding properties between isoforms.[112] In humans the greatest expression of apoE is found in the liver, followed by the brain. Animal and *in vitro* models show that in the brain, astrocytes and microglia are the main producers of secreted apoE,[113,114] while neurons appear to produce apoE under stress conditions.[115,116]

The mechanisms that govern apoE4 toxicity in the brain are not fully understood. Some proposed mechanisms include isoform specific toxicity, apoE4–mediated amyloid aggregation, and apoE4-mediated tau hyperphosphorylation.[117] In the brain, lipidated apoE binds aggregated Aβ in a isoform-specific manner, apoE4 being much more effective than the other forms,

and has been proposed to enhance deposition of the Aβ peptide.[118]

Brain cells from *APOE* knock-out mice (*APOE*−/−) are more sensitive to excitotoxic and age-related synaptic loss,[119] while Aβ-induced synaptosomal dysfunction is also enhanced compared to control animals.[120] When human apoE isoforms are expressed in *APOE*−/− mice, the expression of apoE3, but not apoE4, is protective against age-related neurodegeneration[119] and Aβ toxicity.[120] In addition, astrocytes, from *APOE*−/− mice that express human apoE3, release more cholesterol than those expressing apoE4, suggesting that apoE isoforms may modulate the amount of lipid available for neurons. Other studies report apoE-specific effects on Aβ removal from the extracellular space whereby the apoE3 isoform has a higher Aβ binding capacity than apoE4 when associated with lipids.[121,122]

Genetic Variation

The gene dose of *APOE* ε4 is a major risk factor for AD, with many studies reporting an association between gene dose, age at onset,[123] and cognitive decline.[124] However, a 44% risk of AD by age 93 among family members of *APOE* 4/4 carriers indicates that as many as 50% of people having at least one ε4 allele do not develop AD. Furthermore, if an *APOE* ε4 carrier lives past 85 without developing AD, then his or her risk is drastically diminished. In addition, 40%–60% of AD cases are not *APOE* ε4 carriers.[96-104]

Triggering Receptor Expressed on Myeloid Cells 2: TREM2
Inheritance and Clinical Features

Inheritance of two *TREM2* mutations (homozygous) is a cause of a rare autosomal recessive disorder, polycystic lipomembranous osteodysplasia with sclerosing leukoencephalopathy (PLOSL: also called Nasu-Hakola disease).[21] In 2013, inheritance of a single *TREM2* mutation was linked to an increased risk of AD by two groups of investigators.[22,125] Patients with the *TREM2* variant pathologically have the typical plaques and neurofibrillary tangles of AD, some with additional Lewy body and transactive response DNA-binding protein 43 (TDP-43) pathology and amyloid angiopathy.[126]

Structure, Function, and Expression

TREM2 encodes a membrane protein that forms a receptor signaling complex with the TYRO protein tyrosine kinase-binding protein. The encoded protein functions in immune response and may be involved in chronic inflammation by triggering the production of constitutive inflammatory cytokines. *TREM2* expression differed compared to control mice in the mouse model of AD.[21] Some debate exists as to how the presence of a *TREM2* mutation increases risk for AD; however, given its normal role, it implicates the inflammatory system in the pathobiology of AD.

Genetic Variation

In patients with PLOSL, four different homozygous mutations in the *TREM2* gene have been identified (W78X, K186N, D134G, W44X, V126G, Q33X).[127,128] In a large GWAS in an Icelandic cohort, there was an association between AD risk and the T allele of *TREM2* R47H (rs75932628).[22]

Sporadic Late-Onset AD Genome-Wide Association Study Genes

Genome-wide association studies (GWAS) have investigated the genetics of sporadic AD and have identified over 20 candidate loci. Ten novel AD candidate loci within or near genes *CLU*, *CR1*, *BIN1*, *PICALM*, *MS4A4/MS4A6E*, *CD2AP*, *CD33*, *EPHA1*, and *ABCA7* were identified and replicated, including the *APOE* locus[129-134] (see alzgene.org for a comprehensive list). In addition, a GWAS meta-analysis of 74,046 individuals further validated these 10 loci, as well as the *TREM2* locus.[23] Furthermore, this large analysis identified new candidate susceptibility loci: *SORL1*, *CASS4*, *FERMT2*, *HLA-DRB5–DRB1*, *INPP5D*, *PTK2B*, *MEF2C*, *CELF1*, *NME8*.[23] The odds ratios for AD risk are small and can range between 0.80 and 1.20 depending on the variant, suggesting that each locus individually has a small impact on AD. In addition, although there is intense research effort to understand the functional impact of these loci on pathophysiology of AD, it remains unclear.

For a catalog of candidate gene association studies, refer to the AlzGene online database (http://www.alzforum.org/res/com/gen/alzgene/default.asp).

Summary

AD is characterized by an irreversible, progressive loss of memory and cognitive skills that can occur in rare familial cases as early as the third decade. Currently there is no cure for AD, and treatments only slow AD progression slightly in some patients.[135,136] The early onset familial forms of AD have an autosomal dominant inheritance linked to three genes: *APP*, *PSEN1*, and *PSEN2*. The most common sporadic form of AD occurs after the age of 60 and has thus far been consistently, across numerous studies, associated with only one gene, the *APOE* gene. The mechanistic contribution of these genes in AD pathogenesis has been studied extensively and suggests that the processing of APP and the inflammatory response are important in AD pathogenesis. However, given the range of genes linked to AD, the pathobiology of AD likely involves a complex interplay of genes and environment.

PARKINSON'S DISEASE

Parkinson disease (PD) is the second most common neurodegenerative disorder. The incidence is similar worldwide, with the prevalence increasing in proportion to regional increases in population longevity, with more than 1% affected over the age of 65 years and more than 4% of the population affected by the age of 85 years.[137] While PD has generally been considered a largely sporadic disease, increasing evidence suggests that there is a genetic influence either through an autosomal dominant/recessive pathway or through inheritance of risk genes.[138,139]

There is an overlap of the clinical, pathological, and clinical characteristics of Parkinson's disease (PD)/PD with dementia (PDD) and dementia with Lewy bodies (DLB). PD/PDD and DLB both share similar features of parkinsonism, behavioral disturbances, and sleep and autonomic dysfunction. PDD and DLB also are characterized by dementia, generally differentiated based on whether the motor parkinsonism preceded the dementia by one or more years (the "one year rule"). A key pathologic hallmark in these disorders is the presence of Lewy body pathology. The Lewy body is an intraneuronal cytoplasmic inclusion in which α-synuclein is the key aggregated protein and is also associated with aggregated α-synuclein in neuronal processes ("Lewy neurites").[140]

Historically, PD was considered to be largely sporadic in nature, without genetic origin. However, in the past decade, genetic studies of PD families from different geographical regions worldwide have strengthened the hypothesis that PD has a substantial genetic component. One of the first autosomal dominant inherited forms of PD was identified in an Italian family, the gene initially designated as *PARK1*.[141] Since then 13 loci, *PARK 1–13*, have been linked to rare forms of PD, autosomal dominant and autosomal recessive PD.[142,143] Of these 13 loci, eight genes have been described as causing PD: four autosomal dominant (*SNCA*, *LRRK2*, *UCHL1*, *HTRA2*) and four autosomal recessive (*PRKN*, *DJ1*, *PINK1*,

ATP13A2). Mutations in *SNCA, LRRK2, PRKN*, and *PINK1* genes are the most well characterized as causing PD, whereas mutations in the other genes listed do not have as much supporting evidence as causes of PD. Recently, a clinical association has been reported between type 1 Gaucher's disease and PD, which is caused by a glucocerebrosidase deficiency owing to mutations in the glucocerebrosidase gene (*GBA*), and several studies have found an association between *GBA* mutations and increased risk for PD.[144–157] The *GBA* gene has not yet been named as a PD gene but will be described briefly here. Some PD genes, where mutations have been linked to familial forms of PD, are also candidate genes for sporadic forms of PD, as those genes (*SNCA, LRRK2*) may also carry other mutations that merely increase risk (Table 10.1).[144–157]

AUTOSOMAL DOMINANT PARKINSON'S DISEASE

α-synuclein: SNCA
Inheritance and Clinical Features
PARK1- and PARK4-linked PD are both of autosomal dominant inheritance and are linked to the α-synuclein gene (*SNCA*). However, PARK1 is caused by missense SNCA mutations, while PARK4 by multiplications of *SNCA*. Affected family members are mostly of juvenile-onset with atypical clinical features, including myoclonus and hypoventilation, with rapid progression of symptoms. PARK1 missense mutations and PARK4 multiplications are both extremely rare causes of familial parkinsonism.[158–163]

Structure, Function, and Expression
SNCA has six exons and encodes a 140–amino acid protein. The N-terminus consists of an amphipathic α-helical domain that associates with membrane microdomains, known as lipid rafts.[164] The central region contains a fibrillization region and the C-terminus contains an aggregation inhibition region.[165] *SNCA* is expressed throughout the mammalian brain and is enriched in presynaptic nerve terminals.[166] The protein can adopt partially folded structures, but in its native form is unfolded and can assume both monomeric and oligomeric alpha-helix and beta-sheet conformations, as well as morphologically diverse aggregates, ranging from those that are amorphous to amyloid-like fibrils.[167] These fibrillar moieties are a component of LBs in both familial and idiopathic PD,[168] but it is unclear whether the fibrils themselves, or the oligomeric fibrilization

intermediates (protofibrils), are toxic to the cell. Interestingly, *SNCA* genomic multiplications in familial PD are associated with an increase in protein expression,[163] and brain samples of triplication mutant carriers show that protofibril formation is enhanced with an increase in *SNCA* expression.[169] *In vitro*, A30P, A53T, and E46K mutant proteins show an increased propensity for self-aggregation and oligomerization into protofibrils, compared with wild-type protein,[170,171] that may be related to the membrane permeabilization activity of these protofibrils, which form pore-like and tubular structures.[172] It appears that only A53T and E46K promote formation of the fibrils,[173,174] whereas A30P has been reported to disrupt the interaction between α-synuclein and the lipid raft and possibly redistributing the protein away from the synapse.[164]

A mouse spontaneous deletion strain is viable, fertile, and phenotypically normal,[175] whereas overexpression of wild-type *SNCA* in a mouse model has many features of PD, such as loss of dopaminergic terminals in the striatum, mislocalization and accumulation of insoluble α-synuclein, and motor abnormalities.[176–178] Both A30P and A53T mutant mouse models display neuronal cell loss and motor changes.[179]

Increased tendency for oligomer and aggregate formation in *SNCA* mutants has been suggested to be a cause of PARK1-linked PD, and PARK4-linked PD multiplications with an increased amount of normal α-synuclein may predispose neurons to oligomer and aggregate formations.[180,181]

Genetic Variation
Multiple *SNCA* mutations and multiplications have been described. Genetic variation in *SNCA* appears to contribute to PD phenotype. For example, PARK4 American and European families with *SNCA* triplication show different clinical features from families with the *SNCA* duplication where the phenotype closely resembles idiopathic PD.[158,159] *SNCA* duplications are rarely associated with dementia.[160,161] Both the E46K mutation and the triplication are associated with Parkinsonism and dementia, and the age of onset is younger than the other mutations with diffuse Lewy body disease. A30P mutation is usually not associated with dementia. The A53T mutation has been associated with dementia and the presence of cortical Lewy bodies.[182,183]

In addition, *SNCA* promoter polymorphisms have been associated with idiopathic PD disease risk,[184–186] and recently *SNCA* polymorphic mutations associated with increased α-synuclein expression have been reported to be significant risk factors for sporadic PD.[187,188]

Leucine Repeat Rich Kinase 2: LRRK2
Inheritance and Clinical Features

Autosomal dominant PARK8-linked PD was first identified in a Japanese family known as the Samagihara kindred.[189] Clinical features were first described in 1978 in a large Japanese family[190] with similar symptoms as sporadic PD with a slightly earlier onset of age, and this linkage has been replicated in Caucasian families.[191] Although affected individuals have clinically typical PD, pathologically the disease appears to be heterogeneous with reports of Lewy body pathology and tau pathology, andneuronal loss without intracellular inclusions,[192,193] as well as motor neuron disease.[191] Cognitive impairment and dementia appear to be less common in these cases.[194]

Structure, Function, and Expression

The gene for PARK8 was identified as Leucine Repeat Rich Kinase 2 (*LRRK2*) (also called *dardarin*, from the Basque word for tremor), in families from the Basque region of Spain, Britain, western Nebraska, and in an American kindred of German descent.[191,195] It is a large gene encompassing 144 kb in the genome, consisting of 51 exons (7449 bp cDNA), and encodes a protein consisting of 2,517 amino acids. The function of *LRRK2* is not well known, although it has been identified as a tyrosine kinase-like protein.[196] The ROC domain is able to bind GTP and is essential for the MAPKKK domain to exert kinase activity, but does not have GTPase activity.[197] Some of the *LRRK2* mutations appear to exert increased kinase activity.[198,199] Other functional domains are believed to be important in protein-protein interactions.[191] *LRRK2* also interacts with other proteins linked to familial PD. For example, *LRRK2* appears to interact with parkin through the ROC domain.[200] *LRRK2* expression has been described in the central nervous system (cerebral cortex, medulla, cerebellum, spinal cord, putamen, and substantia nigra), heart, kidney, lung, liver, and peripheral leukocytes.[191,195] *LRRK2* protein is found in the cytosol and mitochondrial outer membrane,[199] plasma membrane, lysosomes, endosomes, transport vesicles, Golgi apparatus, a cytoskeleton protein microtubule, synaptic vesicles, and lipid rafts.[201,202] Interestingly, α-synuclein is also expressed in the presynaptic membranes and lipid rafts.[164]

There is currently limited postmortem data on pathogenic *LRRK2* mutations, but it appears that typical LB pathology is seen in most, but not all, *LRRK2*-related patients.[203] The mechanism that links *LRRK2* protein to *SNCA* protein accumulation remains unknown, but evidence suggests that there may be a direct interaction between *LRRK2* and the *SNCA* protein.[200,204]

Genetic Variation

Over 20 missense or nonsense mutations are concentrated in these functional domains.[189,191,195,196] Several coding mutations have been identified in the *LRRK2* gene, including Y1699C, R1441C, I1122V, I2020T, and R1369G, and a splice-site mutation, 3342A. The most frequent mutation is G2019S, which accounts for as many as 40% of patients of Arabic descent and about 20% of Ashkenazi Jewish patients, and is the most frequent *LRRK2* mutation in a large British kindred.[205–208] *LRRK2* mutations have also been reported in some apparently sporadic PD patients.[209] Reduced penetrance is common for some of the LRRK2 mutations.[210] In addition, the mean age at onset (64 years) in a British kindred and the occurrence of mutations in apparently sporadic PD patients suggests that mutations in this gene may be more widely distributed in the late-onset PD population than the alpha-synuclein gene.[193]

AUTOSOMAL RECESSIVE PARKINSON'S DISEASE

Parkin: PRKN
Inheritance and Clinical Features

Clinical features of the autosomal recessive young onset PARK2-linked PD include an age of onset between 20 and 40 years, but the age of onset can be earlier than 10 years and above 60 years.[211] When the age of onset is young, dystonia is a characteristic symptom and patients are L-dopa responsive, although with frequent dyskinesias. Pathologically, the substantia nigra undergoes severe neuronal loss and gliosis and usually no Lewy bodies are seen, although Lewy body positive cases have been reported.[212]

Structure, Function, and Expression

Linkage analysis of several PD families mapped the PARK2 disease locus to chromosome 6q26, near the sod2 locus.[213–215] By screening a BAC library using the D6S305 marker at this region, a cDNA was cloned consisting of the open reading frame of the novel gene *PRKN*.[216] PRKN protein belongs to the RING-IBR-RING family, which is a subgroup of RING finger-type E3 ubiquitin ligase. The PRKN protein is 465 amino acids, with 12 exons and a 1,395 bp open reading frame. It contains two RING finger domains at the carboxyl (C) terminus. RING stands for "rare interesting gene," and RING-like structures have been found in proteins with ubiquitin ligase activity.[217] Similar to other RING finger proteins, the PRKN protein has been found to function as an E3 ubiquitin ligase.[218]

PRKN appears to be a cytosolic protein normally, but it may also co-localize to synaptic vesicles, the Golgi complex, endoplasmic reticulum, and the mitochondrial outer membrane.[218–221] Many of the single amino acid substitutions appear to alter wild-type PRKN cellular localization, solubility, and propensity to aggregate.[222–224] Many ubiquitination substrates have been proposed, including the aminoacyl-tRNA synthetase cofactor, p38, and a rare, 22-kD glycosylated form of α-synuclein.[225–227] Some mutations appear to result in *PRKN* loss of function, although *PRKN* knock-out mice have only subtle behavior and glutaminergic transmission alterations and do not suffer nigral neuronal degeneration or clinical manifestations of parkinsonism;[228,229] reduced numbers of noradrenergic neurons in the locus ceruleus were reported in one strain.[230] Accumulation of p38 leading to catecholaminergic cell death has been shown in one strain, as well as in PARK2-linked PD and idiopathic PD brain.[231]

PRKN knock-out mice also have reduced numbers of mitochondrial oxidative phosphorylation proteins, decrease in mitochondrial respiratory capacity, and age-dependent increases in oxidative damage.[232] Mitochondrial defects have also been reported in parkin knock-out *Drosophila*, suggesting that PRKN ubiquination dysfunction may be secondary in the course of pathogenic events.[233,234]

Genetic Variation

Reported mutations in parkin now exceed 100, including missense and nonsense mutations as well as exonic deletions, rearrangements, and duplications.[235–240] Exonic deletions in the Parkin gene were first identified in Japanese families with autosomal recessive juvenile parkinsonism.[216] Parkin mutations have been found to account for about 50% of familial cases and about 70% of sporadic cases, with very early onset at age 20 years, depending on the ethnicity of the population sample.[241–243] Parkin mutational frequency in late-onset PD is lower than early-onset cases, accounting for between 0% to 11%, depending largely on whether the sample is familial or sporadic.[243–245]

Many *PRKN* mutations, including deletion mutations and point mutations, have been detected in the *PRKN* gene of PARK2-linked patients. The site of these mutations spans almost all regions including the N-terminal UBL domain and the RING-IBR-RING domain. *PRKN*-linked PD has been initially characterized as a recessively inherited disease with a deleterious alteration on both alleles with the presumption that heterozygous carriers are unaffected. More recently, it has been suggested that carriers of a single mutation could have an increased risk for PD, although not all evidence supports this hypothesis.[246,247]

In summary, over 100 different mutations have been identified in the parkin gene including, but not limited to, 40 exon rearrangements (26 deletions and 14 multiplications), 43 single base pair substitutions, and 12 small deletions or insertions of one or several base pairs. The most common mutations appear to be (1) deletions of exon 4 ($n = 28$); (2) deletions of exon 3 ($n = 27$); (3) deletions of exons 3 to 4 ($n = 23$); (4) a point mutation in exon 7 (924C>T; $n = 38$); and (5) a single base pair deletion in exon 2 (255/256delA; $n = 17$). These five common alterations account for 35% of all parkin mutations. Hot spots for common parkin mutations appear to be concentrated in exons 2 and 7, whereas hot spots for exon rearrangements are more likely to occur in introns 2 through 4.[248]

Parkinson Protein 7: PARK7 (DJ1) Inheritance and Clinical Features

DJ1 recessively inherited missense and exonic deletion mutations were first identified in two European families with an age of onset of 20–40 years.[249] PARK7-linked PD appears to be very rare.[249–251] Very few *DJ1* patients have been reported in the literature; thus clinical features and correlations with *DJ1* mutations are still difficult to determine. Some clinical features, such as psychiatric symptoms,[252] short stature, and brachydactyly,[253] have been reported. *DJ1* mutations rarely associate with PD, but some missense, splice-site, and exonic deletion mutations have been identified, accounting for less than 1% of early-onset PD.[251,254–256]

Structure, Function, and Expression

DJ1 has a transcript length of 949 bps with seven exons.[257] It encodes a protein consisting of 189 amino acids. Expression of *DJ1* is ubiquitous and abundant in most mammalian tissues, including in the brain, where it is found in both neuronal and glial cells.[258] *DJ1* is a homodimer that belongs to the peptidase C56 family of proteins.[259] It is a cytoplasmic protein, but can also translocate into the mitochondria[260] and appears to act as an antioxidant.[257,261–263] *DJ1* may act as either a redox sensor protein that can prevent the aggregation of α-synuclein or an antioxidant.[262,264–268] *DJ1* may also act as a reactive oxygen species scavenger through auto-oxidation.[269] *DJ1* null mice are sensitive to oxidative stress and MPTP.[270] *DJ1* knock-out strains show normal numbers of dopaminergic neurons but sensitivity to the PD-associated environmental toxins, paraquat and rotenone.[271,272] Thus, it has been proposed that since substantia nigra neurons are exposed to high oxidative stress, *DJ1* may be acting as a strong antioxidative protein.[263] Mutant *DJ1* also appears to interact with parkin, whereby parkin acts as an E3 ligase to remove mutated *DJ1*.[263]

DJ1 does not appear to be an essential component of Lewy bodies in sporadic cases.[258] *DJ1* mutations are rare in sporadic PD, but recent studies suggest that *DJ1* may play an important role in common forms of the disease. Sporadic PD brain has oxidative damage to *DJ1* and a significant increase in total protein levels, compared with normal controls,[273] as well as significantly higher cerebrospinal fluid *DJ1* levels in sporadic PD, especially in the early stages of disease.[274]

Genetic Variation

In general, *DJ1* mutations are found in the homozygous or compound heterozygous state, putatively resulting in a loss of protein function. The L166P mutation causes destabilization through unfolding of the C-terminus, inhibiting dimerization and enhancing degradation by the proteasome.[259,275,276] In addition, probably consequential to instability, L166P reduces the neuroprotective function of *DJ1*.[269] Reduced nuclear localization, in favor of the mitochondria, is also seen for L166P, as well as for the M26I and D149A mutations.[249,277] In addition, there appear to be structural perturbations associated with *DJ1* mutations L166P, E64D, M26I, A104T, and D149A, which can lead to global destabilization, unfolding of the protein structure, heterodimer formation, or reduced antioxidant activity, implicating these mutations in pathogenicity associated with *DJ1*.[278–280]

Phosphotase and Tensin (PTEN) Induced Kinase 1: PINK1
Inheritance and Clinical Features

Mutations in the phosphatase and Tensin (PTEN) Induced Kinase 1 gene (*PINK1*) were first identified in patients with recessive young onset autosomal recessive PD, designated as PARK6. The age of onset is from 32 to 48 years.[281] *PINK1* mutations account for approximately 1%–7% of autosomal recessive PD in Caucasians,[281–283] about 9% in Japanese autosomal recessive PD families,[284] and 2%–3% in sporadic and familial PD of Chinese origin.[285,286] Clinical features of PARK6 are similar to late onset PD, with rare features such as dystonia at onset, sleep benefit, and psychiatric disturbances.[281,286,287] Clinical characteristics of *PINK1* are similar to *PRKN*, with dystonia at onset and increased reflexes, which were originally thought to be related only to parkin.[288]

Structure, Function, and Expression

PINK1 has eight exons and cDNA that spans 1.8 kb. It encodes a protein with 581 amino acids. It has a serine/threonine protein kinase domain. It is a mitochondrial protein located in the matrix and the intermembrane space that is ubiquitously expressed in the brain and systemic organs and that contains a mitochondrial-targeting motif and a conserved serine/threonine kinase domain.[289] Functional studies have shown that *PINK1* can be localized to mitochondria both *in vitro* and *in vivo*.[290] Wild-type *PINK1* appears to be important in neuroprotection against mitochondrial dysfunction and proteasome-induced apoptosis, whereas the G309D mutation impairs this protective effect, possibly by interfering with adenosine diphosphate (ADP) binding and thus inhibiting kinase activity.[281,291] E240K and L489P mutants disrupt *PINK1*'s protectivity by either enhancing the instability of the protein or disrupting the kinase activity of the protein.[292] *In vitro* studies indicate that cells transfected with *PINK1* mutants have disrupted mitochondrial membrane potential under stressful conditions.[293] Knock-out models of the *Drosophila PINK1* ortholog have defects in mitochondrial morphology and increased sensitivity to oxidative stress and appear to be rescued by human parkin.[294]

PINK1 haploinsufficiency may be sufficient to cause disease because *PINK1* is detected in some LBs in sporadic PD, as well as in samples carrying only one mutant *PINK1* allele, which are clinically and pathologically indistinguishable from sporadic cases.[290]

Genetic Variation

The first mutations discovered were the G309D missense and a W437X truncating mutation found in families of Italian and Spanish descent.[281,291] Several point mutations, frameshifts, and truncating mutants have been identified.[286,288,295] Interestingly, in contrast to *PRKN*, most of the *PINK1* mutations reported are either missense or nonsense mutations.[283,284,287,291,296]

Japanese and Israeli *PINK1*-linked families and a sporadic PD patient of Chinese ethnicity have an R246X mutation.[286] Most of the reported mutations are located in a highly conserved amino acid position in the protein kinase domain and are absent in healthy controls, thus suggesting that these mutations are pathogenic,[293] and homozygous mutation carriers appear to be clinically affected, whereas heterozygous carriers are not.[297]

Probable Cation–Transporting ATPase 13A2: ATP13A2
Inheritance and Clinical Features

Homozygous and compound heterozygous mutations in the P-type ATPase gene (*ATP13A2*) have been demonstrated in a Jordanian family[298,299] and a Chilean family[300] with Kufor-Rakeb syndrome, a form of recessively inherited atypical parkinsonism which is clinically characterized by very early age of onset (11–16 years), levodopa-responsive parkinsonism, pyramidal signs, dementia, a supranuclear gaze palsy.[298,301] MRI shows significant atrophy of the globus pallidus and the pyramids, and generalized brain atrophy in later stages. Some develop facial–faucial–finger minimyoclonus, visual hallucinations, and oculogyric dystonic spasm.[301]

Structure, Function, and Expression

The disease locus designated as PARK9 was mapped to 1p36.13 with a maximum LOD score of 3.6, a hot spot for autosomal recessive familial PD.[300] The disease gene was subsequently identified as *ATP13A2*. The transcript has 29 exons and is 3,854 bps in length. The ATP13A2 protein contains 1,180 amino acids and has 10 transmembrane domains. ATP13A2 is a lysosomal membrane protein with an ATPase domain.[300] It is a member of the P5 subfamily of ATPases, which transports inorganic cations and other substrates. The exact function of the ATP13A2 protein is still unknown. *ATP13A2* is predominantly expressed in brain tissues, and

ATP13A2 mRNA levels are about 10-fold higher in the substantia nigra dopaminergic neurons of sporadic patients than control subject brains.[300]

Genetic Variation

All known *ATP13A2* mutations appear to directly or indirectly impact transmembrane domains.[300] In vitro evidence indicates that wild-type *ATP13A2* is localized to the lysosome membrane of transiently transfected cells, whereas unstable truncated mutants are retained in the endoplasmic reticulum and are degraded by the proteasome.[300]

SPORADIC PARKINSON'S DISEASE

Glucocerebrosidase: GBA
Inheritance and Clinical Features

An association between mutations within the glucocerebrosidase gene (*GBA*) and PD has been reported in multiple studies, initially suspecting a link due to parkinsonism in Gaucher's disease patients (a metabolic autosomal recessive disease due to *GBA* mutations).[144] The frequency for *GBA* mutations appears to be less than 1% in the general population and 6%–7% in Ashkenazi Jews, varies according to ethnicity, and is associated with PD as well as PD age at onset.[144–157,302]

A family history of parkinsonism is often reported in patients with Gaucher's disease (GD), which is an autosomal recessive disorder caused by mutations in *GBA*.[303] GD is a lysosomal storage disease characterized by an accumulation of glucocerebrosides.[304] Recent studies show that the neuropathological features associated with *GBA* mutations include a variety of LB synucleinopathies, suggesting that the clinical phenotype of PD with *GBA* mutations may be diverse.[304,305] Of note, GBA mutations have also been linked to an increased risk of pathologically confirmed DLB.[305,306]

Structure, Function, and Expression

GBA is located on chromosome 1 (1q21). The *GBA* cDNA is approximately 2 kb in length.[307,308] A *GBA* pseudogene has a 96% homology to *GBA* and is located approximately 12 kb downstream. There are two in-frame translational start sites in exon 1 and exon 2. Initiation at each exon leads to a different leader sequence, but both are processed into a mature functional enzyme of the same length. The protein is cleaved to produce a mature polypeptide of 497 amino acids with a molecular weight of 55.5 kDa. The *GBA* gene encodes the lysosomal membrane protein, glucocerebrosidase, which cleaves the beta-glucosidic linkage of glycosylceramide, an intermediate in glycolipid metabolism.[309] *GBA* mRNA levels vary among cell lines, with high, moderate, low, and negligible levels reported in epithelial, fibroblast, macrophage, and B-cell lines, respectively.[310–312] There appears to be a poor correlation between the levels of mRNA and the amount of identified enzymatic activity,[311,313] implicating a complex regulatory system for the expression of glucocerebrosidase at the level of transcription, translation, and post-translational modification.[314]

Genetic Variation

Over 250 mutations have been reported in *GBA*: 203 missense mutations, 18 nonsense mutations, 36 small insertions or deletions that lead to either frameshifts or in-frame alterations, 14 splice junction mutations, and 13 complex alleles carrying two or more mutations in cis.[315] Recombination events with a highly homologous pseudogene downstream of the *GBA* locus also have been identified, resulting from gene conversion, fusion, or duplication. Some of the alleles for disease mutations are also found in the pseudogene, making analysis complicated. The *GBA* mutations that influence GD or PD are not necessarily disease specific. For example, N370S and L444P are the most common mutations associated with both GD and PD whereas, while R120W is found mainly in PD but not GD, and R463C is found in mainly in GD but not PD.[144–157,315]

Sporadic PD Genome Wide Association Study Genes

The discovery of mutations in a small number of genes associated with autosomal dominant and autosomal recessive forms of PD (e.g., *SNCA, LRRK2, PRKN, PINK1, DJ-1*) account for a small minority of PD cases.[316–318] Analyses of sporadic PD has demonstrated that variants in multiple genes influence risk rather than cause disease in an autosomal dominant or recessive manner. GWAS and GWAS meta-analyses have identified more than 20 loci that confer relatively small association with PD.[316–318] Interestingly, many of these loci are near genes that cause autosomal forms of PD (e.g., *SNCA, LRRK2*). However, many may represent rare PD genes and some are yet to be replicated across multiple studies (e.g., *SCARB2, Omi/HtrA2, UCHL1*; see PDgene.org for a comprehensive list).[316–318]

There has been substantial progress in the discovery of PD risk loci over the past decade.

However, the risk attributable to identified genetic variants still does not account for all the genetic heritability observed in PD. This gap indicates that multiple genetic variants not yet described likely play a role in PD pathophysiology. This missing heritability in PD is estimated to represent approximately 27% of PD, while 3%–5% is attributable to the top PD GWAS SNPs identified to date.[318] This finding suggests that many more yet to be discovered genetic variants may influence PD risk.

Summary

Multiple loci have been linked to PD, of which eight genes have been described: two autosomal dominant (*SNCA, LRRK2*), and four autosomal recessive, (*PRKN, DJ1, PINK1, ATP13A2*). In addition, another gene has recently been described as a robust risk factor for sporadic PD (*GBA*), and several loci have been identified in GWAS. The characterization of these PD genes suggests that PD pathology involves a strong genetic component and provides numerous clues to the etiology of the disease. The function of these genes and their contribution to PD pathogenesis remain unclear. However, many of these genes play a role in ubiquitination, oxidative stress, and apoptosis, suggesting that PD may be a genetically complex and heterogenous disease. In addition to the link between these genes and familial forms of PD, many are also candidate genes for sporadic forms of the disease, suggesting that some of these genes carry other mutations that simply increase risk.

AMYOTROPHIC LATERAL SCLEROSIS, FRONTOTEMPORAL DEMENTIA

Amyotrophic lateral sclerosis (ALS), also known as Lou Gehrig's disease, is a neurodegenerative disease of the motor system. Disease onset typically ranges between 40 and 70 years of age. The gradual loss of motor neurons in the cerebral cortex, the brainstem, and the spinal cord leads to devastatingly rapid progressive loss of motor function. Familial ALS accounts for 5%–10% of all cases, while the remainder appear to be sporadic.

Frontotemporal dementia (FTD) is an early onset dementia characterized by progressive degeneration of the frontal and temporal lobes of the brain. FTD is a group of disorders that are identified according to multiple distinct subtypes of clinical signs and symptoms. The subtypes of FTD are diagnosed according to the most prominent symptoms that appear first. These clinical subtypes include behavioral variant FTD (bvFTD), primary progressive aphasia (PPA), FTD with motor neuron disease, progressive supranuclear palsy (PSP), and corticobasal degeneration (CBD).[319–321] Upon autopsy, the FTDs are subsumed under the umbrella term of frontotemporal lobar degeneration (FTLD). Further neuropathologic subcategorization depends on the type of aggregated protein observed, including tau (FTLD-tau), TDP-43 (FTLD-TDP), ubiquitin only (FTLD-U), or FUS (FTLD-FUS), and by the distribution of the pathology (e.g., cortical versus subcortical tau pathology in CBD and PSP, respectively).

ALS and FTD have traditionally been considered as two different neurological disorders with discordant clinical features. However, motor dysfunctions have been described in approximately 15% of FTD patients[322,323] and FTD is present in 15%–18% of patients with ALS.[324]

These disorders can share pathological and genetic features. TDP-43 inclusions are considered a common hallmark of both ALS and some forms of FTLD.[325] However, mutations within the TDP-43 gene are rare in familial or sporadic FTD with TDP-43 inclusions and present more often in familial or sporadic ALS.326 A notable example of genetic overlap between FTD and ALS is *C9orf72* (chromosome 9 open reading frame 72), described in both ALS and FTD.[327,328] Other genes that show overlap between ALS and FTD include *FUS*, *TARDBP*, and *CHMP2* (Table 10.1). There is an ongoing attempt to categorize ALS/FTD according to clinical phenotype, pathological features, and genetics. These efforts may have contributed to the emergence of evidence suggesting that ALS and FTLD represent a spectrum of disorders.[319–321,329]

A strong family history of FTD and/or ALS accounts for about 10%–15% of FTD. The majority, but not all, have a mutation in a currently known FTD gene. Some family history of a neurodegenerative disease accounts for about 20%–25% of FTD, of which less than half have a mutation in a currently known FTD gene. Sporadic, or patients with an unknown family history, account for about 60%–70% of FTD, of which less than 10% have a mutation in a currently known FTD gene.[319–321,329,330]

Autosomal Dominant and Recessive ALS/FTD
Superoxide Dismutase 1: SOD1
Inheritance and Clinical Features
Autosomal and recessive inherited mutations in superoxide dismutase 1 (*SOD1*) were first identified in the 1990s in multiple families with ALS and account for 15%–20% of cases of familial ALS.[331–335] Compared to those with ALS caused by mutations in other genes, those with *SOD1* mutations tend to

have predominantly lower limb onset. The clinical features of the disease can vary somewhat according to mutation. One-third of ALS patients with a *SOD1* mutation survive for more than 7 years, and they tend to have an earlier disease onset compared to those with a more rapid course. ALS patients with *SOD1* mutations typically are without signs of cognitive impairment.[335,336] At autopsy, neuropathological assessment generally finds inclusions that can be positive for SOD1, ubiquitin, and phosphorylated neurofilaments, but notably are usually TDP-43 negative.[337,338]

Structure, Function, and Expression
The *SOD1* gene encodes a cytoplasmic antioxidant enzyme that contains copper and zinc and metabolizes superoxide radicals to molecular oxygen and hydrogen peroxide, providing a major cellular defense against oxygen toxicity.[339,340] The 153-residue protein has a molecular mass of approximately 18.5 kD.[340–342] RT-PCR analysis has identified five splice variants of SOD1. The mRNA variants are expressed in a tissue-specific manner, including expression in the brain, and are found in both ALS patients and controls.[343]

Genetic Variation
The *SOD1* A4V substitution in exon 1 is the most common, occurring in approximately 50% of *SOD1* families. Other *SOD1* missense mutations have been identified in family studies and are located throughout the gene within different exons, including L38V, D90A, and G93C.[336] *SOD1* A4V is thought to be the most clinically severe and is associated with reduced survival time after onset: 1.2 years as compared to 2.5 years for other familial ALS patients.[344]

Transactive Response DNA-Binding Protein TDP-43: TARDBP
Inheritance and Clinical Features
Transactive response (TAR) DNA-binding protein is 43 kD in size and is therefore called TDP-43, and is encoded by the gene *TARDBP*. The TDP-43 protein was first identified as the major pathologic protein of ubiquitin-positive, tau-negative inclusions in FTLD-ubiquitin positive disease (FTLD-U), as well as FTD with motor neuron disease (MND) and ALS with MND. These disorders are now thought to represent different clinical manifestations of the same underlying TDP-43 proteinopathy that differ by the selective vulnerability of different segments of the neuroaxis to neurodegeneration. It has been estimated that *TARDBP* mutations occur in about 3% of patients

with familial ALS, and in 1.5% of patients with sporadic disease.[326,337,345]

Structure, Function, and Expression

The *TARDBP* gene encodes the 43-kD TAR DNA-binding protein (TDP-43). It was originally identified as a transcriptional repressor that binds to TAR DNA of human immunodeficiency virus type 1.[346] TDP-43 is a nuclear protein that binds both DNA and RNA and is widely expressed throughout multiple tissues. It shuttles between the nucleus and cytoplasm and is involved in many aspects of RNA and microRNA processing, such as splicing, trafficking, and stabilization.[347–351] In neurodegenerative diseases, it is thought that neuronal and glial TDP-43 becomes mislocalized to the cytoplasm, where it aggregates into stress granules and insoluble inclusion bodies.[352,353] This aggregation appears to be reflected in ALS biofluids, such as cerebrospinal fluid and serum, where there is a detectable, mutation-dependent, dysregulation of TDP-43 binding to microRNAs.[354]

Genetic Variation

Three mutations in the *TARDBP* gene were identified in a family segregating as autosomal dominant ALS and in two sporadic cases.[355] These three mutations, M337V, Q331K, and G294A, occurred in a conserved region of the C terminus of TDP-43 involved in protein-protein interactions. Multiple other *TARDBP* heterozygous mutations have been identified in patients with both familial and sporadic ALS; for example, Q343R[356] and A315T,[357] and many others, including G290A, G298S, A382T, K263E, G295S, and a 2076G-A transition in the 3-prime untranslated region.[326,337,349,358–360]

Interestingly, with each new discovery of *TARDBP* mutation carriers diagnosed with ALS/FTD, it has become increasingly clear that a larger clinical phenotypic spectrum is associated with the *TARDBP* gene. For example, a patient presenting with semantic dementia at age 50 years later developed ritual behaviors, apathy, social avoidance, aggressiveness, and bulimia, consistent with bvFTD. She also had bulbar symptoms of ALS and upper and lower motor neuron disease in all four limbs. Her sister had dysarthria and dysphagia at age 57, later developed upper and lower limb motor neuron disease, and died at age 60. Both patients carried the same heterozygous mutation in the *TARDBP* gene (G295S).[349] Other families with *TARDBP* mutations have also been described with substantial clinical heterogeneity.[337,359,360] Despite the clinical heterogeneity, pathologically these cases are similar to sporadic ALS, where the predominant inclusions are cytoplasmic and TDP-43 immunopositive.

Microtubule Associated Protein Tau: MAPT
Inheritance and Clinical Features

FTLD-tau is caused by mutations in the gene encoding microtubule-associated protein tau (*MAPT*) on chromosome 17q21. Most FTLD-tau cases are caused by heterozygous mutations, although rare homozygous mutations have been reported. There are considerable differences in clinical and pathologic presentation of patients with *MAPT* mutations.[361]

In several families with FTD linked to chromosome 17 (FTDP-17), multiple exonic and intronic mutations in the *MAPT* gene have been identified, including mutations in the 5-prime splice site of exon 10.[362,363] All of the splice site mutations destabilize a stem-loop structure involved in regulating the alternative splicing of exon 10,[364,365] leading to an increase in tau transcripts that included exon 10 and the number of transcripts with four microtubule-binding repeats (4R), consistent with the neuropathology described in these families. Further evaluation of *MAPT* mutations suggests that they reduce the ability of tau to bind microtubules and promote microtubule assembly and result in hyperphosphorylation of tau protein, assembly into filaments, and subsequent cell death.[363,366] In addition, the H1 *MAPT* haplotype has been identified as a risk factor for two of the sporadic 4R tauopathies, PSP and CBD.[367]

Tau pathology can vary considerably in both its quantity and characteristics and appears to be not necessarily associated with any given mutation.[363–366] Depending on the specific mutation in *MAPT*, familial FTLD-tau can have 3R, 4R, or a combination of 3R and 4R tau. As mentioned, sporadic PSP and CBD are associated with the H1 *MAPT* haplotype.[368–371] It is thought that this haplotype association can be described largely by its influence on *MAPT* gene expression, where variants in the H1 haplotypes confer risk and the H2 haplotype protects against disease by altering expression at the locus, with the risky H1 haplotype expressing higher levels of MAPT.[372–374] PSP and CBD are characterized by a predominant 4R tau deposition. Pick's disease is another usually sporadic FTLD characterized by cytoplasmic inclusions, "Pick bodies," that are predominantly composed of 3R tau with a stereotypic appearance and neuroanatomical distribution.[375]

Structure, Function, and Expression

There are six tau isoforms produced in the adult human brain by alternative mRNA splicing. The tau isoforms that predominate in the human brain are encoded by 11 exons. The tau proteins are composed of 352 to 441 amino acids. The isoforms differ from each other by the presence or absence of 29-amino acid or 58-amino acid inserts located in the N terminus and a 31-amino repeat located in the C terminus. Inclusion of the latter, which is encoded by exon 10 of the tau gene, gives rise to the three repeat (3R) and four repeat (4R) isoforms. The normal cerebral cortex contains similar levels of 3-repeat and 4-repeat tau isoforms. The repeats and some adjoining sequences constitute the microtubule-binding domains of tau. The tau isoforms that predominate in the human brain are encoded by 11 exons.[362,376–378]

Genetic Variation

In one study of 37 patients with FTD, a mutation in the MAPT gene was found in 17.8% of the group of patients with FTD and in 43% of patients with FTD who also had a positive family history of the disorder. Three distinct missense mutations, G272V, P301L, and R406W, accounted for 15.6% of the mutations.[366] In another report, 22 patients with FTLD due to a MAPT mutation presented with different patterns of gray matter atrophy using MRI voxel-based morphometry. All patients showed gray matter loss in the anterior temporal lobes, with varying degrees of involvement of the frontal and parietal lobes. Carriers of the IVS10+16, IVS10+3, N279K, or S305N mutations (all predicted to increase 4R tau isoforms levels) showed gray matter loss particularly affecting the medial temporal lobes, including the hippocampus and amygdala. In contrast, patients with the P301L or V337M mutations showed gray matter loss particularly affecting the inferior and lateral temporal lobes, but not the medial temporal lobe, and gray matter loss in the basal ganglia.[379]

Chromosome 9 Open Reading Frame 72: C9orf72
Inheritance and Clinical Features

A GGGGCC hexanucleotide repeat within the non-coding region of the C9orf72 gene accounts for 30%–50% of familial ALS, depending on the population. Nearly 50% of familial ALS cases in Finland and more than a third of familial cases in other European populations carry the mutation. A research team at the Mayo Clinic found that in healthy individuals the C9orf72 repeat is normally repeated only 2 to 23 times, but in ALS or FTD patients it is repeated 700–1,600 times. These changes were found in almost 12% of familial FTD and more than 23% of familial ALS samples studied at the Mayo Clinic.[327,328] The C9orf72 repeat expansion is more than twice as common as the SOD1 gene in familial ALS, and four times as common as TARDBP, FUS, VCP combined. The identification of this repeat and the rapid, reliable method of screening individuals for repeat expansion may have immediate utility identification of ALS patients at risk of cognitive impairment and FTLD cases at risk of progressive motor neuron disease.[327,328]

Structure, Function, and Expression

Three C9orf72 transcripts have been described.[327] Transcripts 1 and 3 contain different non-coding first exons (exons 1b and 1a) fused to coding exons 2 through 11. Both encode the same 481-amino acid protein.[327,328] C9orf72 transcript 2 contains exon 1a fused to coding exons 2 through 5 and encodes a deduced 222-amino acid protein. Exon 1a in transcript 2 uses a different 3-prime donor site than that used by exon 1a in transcript 3. Transcript-specific primers detect expression of transcripts 1 and 3 in all tissues examined, whereas transcript 2 is highly expressed in testis, fetal brain, cerebellum, and frontal cortex, with lower expression in kidney, lung, and hippocampus, and no expression in liver and lymphoblasts. Expression array analyses find C9orf72 expression in all brain regions examined and spinal cord, with highest expression in the cerebellum.[328] Immunohistochemical analyses show nuclear expression of C9orf72 in a normal human fibroblast cell line and a mouse motor neuron cell line.[328] Western blot analysis reveals 55 and 25 kD C9orf72 proteins in human lymphoblasts. Immunohistochemical analysis of brain suggests that C9orf72 is largely a neuronal cytoplasmic protein, but also can localize to large presynaptic terminals.[327] Tissue from affected individuals shows reduced or absent mRNA levels of C9orf72 transcripts 1 and 3, consistent with a loss-of-function mechanism in repeat expansion carriers. However, protein levels of these variants were similar to controls, and analysis of patient frontal cortex and spinal cord tissue shows that the transcribed expanded GGGGCC repeat formed nuclear RNA foci, suggesting a gain-of-function mechanism.[327]

Genetic Variation

The polymorphic C9orf72 hexanucleotide repeat (GGGGCC) is located between the non-coding exons 1a and 1b of the *C9orf72* gene within the promoter region of transcript variant 1 and in intron 1 of transcript variants 2 and 3. Normally the maximum size of the repeat in healthy controls is 23, whereas it is expanded in patients with frontotemporal dementia and/or amyotrophic lateral sclerosis mapping to chromosome 9p21.[327,380] Affected individuals have expanded repeats ranging from 700 to 1,600. The expanded hexanucleotide repeat was reported present in 16 (61.5%) of a series of 26 families with the disorder, as well as in 11.7% of familial FTD and 23.5% of familial ALS from three other patient series. Sporadic cases with the expansion were also identified. Overall, 75 (10.4%) of 722 unrelated patients with FTD, ALS, or both were found to carry an expanded GGGGCC repeat, making it is the most common genetic abnormality in FTD/ALS.[327] The SNP rs3849942 A allele is associated with the longer repeats, possibly tagging the disease haplotype.

In a meta-analysis of 2,668 FTD patients (not ALS) from 15 European countries, there was a frequency of *C9orf72* expansions in Western Europe of 9.98% in FTD, with 18.52% in familial and 6.26% in sporadic FTD patients.[381] Finland, Sweden, and Spain had an overall frequency of 29.33%, 20.73%, and 25.49%, respectively. Interestingly, the prevalence in Germany was low, at 4.82%.[381] The disease phenotype was predominately bvFTD (95.7%). Postmortem examination of a small number of cases showed TDP-43 deposits in the brain.[381] Intermediate repeats (7 to 24 repeat units) were found to be strongly correlated with a risk haplotype tagged by a T allele of SNP rs2814707.[381]

In another report, in five European populations where known ALS genes were excluded, the *C9orf72* expanded hexanucleotide repeat was identified in 226 (17%) of 1,347 patients with ALS with or without FTD.[382] The expansion was observed in 3 (0.3%) of 856 controls, suggesting incomplete penetrance.[382]

Expanded *C9orf72* repeats were identified in 9 (8.2%) of 109 individuals in a Spanish cohort with FTD.[383] Four individuals had 30 repeats, four had 20 repeats, and one had 22 repeats. None of the other 100 cases had greater than 13 repeats, and none of 216 controls had more than 14 repeats. In addition, in four families, 20–22 repeats segregated consistently in all affected sibs, with unaffected sibs having 2–9 repeats. There was no phenotypic difference between those with longer or shorter expansions. Most of the expansion carriers had extended periods with psychiatric symptoms and subjective cognitive complaints before

neurologic deterioration was evident. These findings suggested that short C9orf72 hexanucleotide expansions in the 20- to 22-repeat range can be related to FTD.[383]

Taken together, these reports show that the *C9orf72* expanded repeat is the most common genetic cause of ALS, with or without FTD, across Europe.[382,383]

Granulin: *GRN*
Inheritance and Clinical Features
Mutations in the granulin (*GRN*) gene were originally described as a cause of autosomal dominant FTD with ubiquitin-positive (FTLD-U), and later included patients with TDP-43 positive inclusions.[384,385] Subsequently, a number of studies described *GRN* mutations in a variety of FTD phenotypes. Nine novel null mutations in the *GRN* gene were identified in 10 (4.8%) of 210 unrelated patients with FTD with a frequency of 12.8% in familial and 3.2% in sporadic cases. These patients exhibited a heterogeneous phenotype. The age at onset was 45–74 years, with frequent occurrence of early apraxia (50%), visual hallucinations (30%), and parkinsonism (30%). No *GRN* mutations were found in 43 patients with dementia and motor neuron disease.[386] In another report, a *GRN* mutation was found in one of 78 unrelated families with FTD, with an incidence of 1.3% lower than previous reports.[387] A quantitative analysis of *GRN* in 103 Belgian patients with frontotemporal dementia identified one (1%) patient with a heterozygous 54- to 69-kb genomic deletion encompassing the *GRN* gene as well as two centromeric neighboring genes: *RUNDC3A* and *SLC25A39*. This patient developed classic bvFTD at age 71 years without additional symptoms, and died 3 years later. This finding suggests that *GRN* haploinsufficiency results in the disease phenotype.[388] Pathologically, *GRN* mutations are associated with cytoplasmic TDP-43 inclusions.[389]

The majority of *GRN* mutations are nonsense mutations, resulting in nonsense-mediated mRNA decay and reduced protein levels or secretion consistent with haploinsufficiency. More than 63 heterozygous loss-of-function mutations had been identified in 163 families worldwide, representing about 5%–10% of FTLD.[388]

Other reports have identified additional pathogenic *GRN* mutations, several novel mutations,[390] and a 3'UTR SNP.[390,391] In a large collaborative study, a *GRN* mutation frequency was described as 21.4% (9 of 42) in those with a pathologically confirmed diagnosis of FTLD-U; 16.0% (28 of 175) of FTD-spectrum cases with a family history; and 56.2% (9 of 16) of FTLD-U with a family history.[390]

Structure, Function, and Expression

The *GRN* gene is located on 17q21.32. The protein-coding region of the *GRN* gene comprises 12 exons covering about 3,700 bp.[385,392] Granulins are a family of secreted, glycosylated peptides that are cleaved from a single precursor protein with 7.5 repeats of a highly conserved 12-cysteine granulin/epithelin motif. The precursor protein, progranulin, is 88 kDa. Cleavage of the signal peptide produces mature granulin. Mature granulin can be further cleaved into a variety of active, 6 kDa peptides. These cleavage products are named granulin A, granulin B, and granulin C.[393] The peptides and intact granulin regulate cell growth, acting as inhibitors, stimulators, or even with dual actions on cell growth. Granulin family members play important roles in normal development, wound healing, and tumorigenesis in multiple tissues, including the brain.[394–402]

Genetic Variation

Genetic studies of families with FTLD-U autosomal dominant inheritance have identified multiple GRN mutations, including a G-to-C transversion at the +5 position of the intron following the first non-coding exon of the *GRN* gene (IVS0+5G-C);[384,385,403,404] a C-to-T transition at nucleotide 373 resulting in a substitution of a termination codon for glutamine-125 (Q125X);[384,385,405] a T-to-C transition of the second nucleotide in exon 1 that alters the initiating methionine codon (2T-C);[384,385] a G-to-A transition in exon 1 that destroys the native Kozak sequence surrounding the met1 translation initiation codon (3G-A); a 4-bp insertion of CTGC between coding nucleotides 90 and 91 (90insCTGC) resulting in a frameshift and premature termination in progranulin (Cys31LeufsTer34); and a splice site mutation at the +1 position of intron 8 of the *GRN* gene (IVS8+1G-A) resulting in a frameshift (Val279GlyfsTer4).[378] The mean age at onset ranged from 57 to 65 years old.[384,406,407] Most also had features suggestive of parietal lobe involvement, including dyscalculia, visuoperceptual/visuospatial dysfunction, and limb apraxia.[384,406,407]

GRN A9D results in transcription of the protein with a defect in trafficking resulting in functional haploinsufficiency.[408–410] It has been reported that patients with the A9D mutation have earlier disease onset and more parkinsonian features compared to patients with other *GRN* mutations.[411] To date, the most frequently found mutation is a heterozygous mutation resulting in an arg493-to-ter (R493X) substitution. Many other *GRN* mutations have been described, most resulting in functional haploinsufficiency.[380, 387,401,409,411–414,415–424]

In summary, the majority of *GRN* pathogenic mutations in FTD are nonsense, frameshift, and splice-site mutations that cause premature termination of the coding sequence and degradation of the mutant RNA by nonsense-mediated decay. Thus, evidence suggests that all *GRN* mutations exert this pathogenic effect through reduced progranulin protein levels, loss of transcript (nonsense or frameshift mutations), reduced transcription (promoter mutations), loss of translation (mutation of initiating methionine), or loss of protein function (missense mutations)

Charged Multivesicular Body Protein 2B: CHMP2B
Inheritance and Clinical Features

A large Danish family with an FTD-like disorder without typical neuropathological features was mapped to chromosome 3. Heterozygous mutation in the *CHMP2B* gene on chromosome 3 was identified in 11 affected members from this Danish family.[425–428] The average age at onset in the Danish family was 57 years, with an insidious change in personality and behavior, including memory loss, cognitive decline, apathy, aggressiveness, stereotyped behavior, and disinhibition. Most patients developed a motor syndrome with abnormal gait, rigidity, hyperreflexia, and pyramidal signs. PET scan of two affected individuals showed global reduction in cerebral blood flow, and neuropathologic examination of several individuals showed generalized cerebral atrophy, most prominent in the frontal and parietal lobes, cortical neuronal loss, astrocytosis, and white matter changes due to loss of myelin, without plaques, fibrillary tangles, or inclusions.[425,426,429] Once linkage to chromosome 3 markers were described in some of these patients,[426] later a truncating mutation in the *CHMP2B* gene on chromosome 3 was identified in autosomal-dominant FTLD families.[430]

However, a later study of a cohort of 141 FTD patients from the United States and the United Kingdom failed to identify any pathogenic *CHMP2B* mutations and the splice site mutation reported was not found in 450 control individuals.[431] In another screen, *CHMP2B* pathogenic mutations were not identified in 128 probands with FTD without *MAPT* mutations.[432] These findings suggest that *CHMP2B* mutations are an uncommon cause of FTD.

Structure, Function, and Expression

Chmp2b is part of the chromatin-modifying protein/charged multivesicular body protein (CHMP) family. This family consists of components of ESCRT-III (endosomal sorting complex required for transport III), a complex involved in the degradation of surface receptor proteins and the formation of endocytic multivesicular bodies (MVBs).

The *CHMP2B* gene contains six exons and is located at 3p11.2.[428] Chmp2b is expressed in all neuronal populations, especially in the hippocampus, frontal and temporal lobes, and cerebellum. Vps2, the yeast ortholog of *CHMP2B,* was first identified in a mutagenesis screen seeking unusual vacuolar protein sorting (vps) phenotypes in S. cerevisiae.[433] It was characterized as part of the ESCRTIII complex (endosomal secretory complex required for transport), which participates in endosomal trafficking.[433] It was later described to participate in endosomal pathology in *CHMP2B* mutation-positive patient brains and to influence abnormal endosomes in patient fibroblasts.[434] Functional studies further demonstrated a specific disruption of endosome-lysosome fusion but not protein sorting by the multivesicular body (MVB), suggesting a mechanism for impaired endosome-lysosome fusion whereby mutant *CHMP2B* constitutively binds to MVBs and prevents recruitment of proteins, such as Rab7, that are necessary for fusion to occur.[434]

Genetic Variation and Clinical Features

Skibinski et al. (2005) identified a heterozygous G-to-C transversion in the acceptor splice site of exon 6 (IVS5AS, G-C) of the *CHMP2B* gene.[428] The mutation results in either inclusion of the 201-bp intronic sequence spanning exons 5 and 6 or a short deletion resulting from the use of a cryptic splice site mapping 10 bp from the 5-prime end of exon 6.[428] Functional studies in rat PC12 cells suggest that the mutant proteins accumulated on the outer membrane of large aberrant cytoplasmic bodies, consistent with the formation of dysmorphic organelles of the late endosomal pathway.[428] Another mutation was also identified, a 442G-T transversion in exon 5 (ASP148TYR), resulting in an asp148-to-tyr (D148Y) substitution in the conserved Snf-7 domain.[428]

A heterozygous 493C-T transition in exon 5, resulting in a gln165-to-ter (Q165X) substitution, was identified in a Belgian woman with onset of FTD at age 58.[430] Expression studies confirmed the presence of a mutant transcript in patient cells. The mutation was not found in 459 Belgian control individuals. Overexpression of the Q165X mutant in human neuroblastoma cells resulted in the accumulation of truncated protein in enlarged vesicular structures. Normally, the C terminal of CHMP2B functions as an autoinhibitor, allowing the protein to shuttle between the inactive and active states. This mutation results in a truncation that eliminates this inhibitory effect, resulting in constitutive activation and involvement in the endosomal complex and accumulation on the endosomal membrane.[430]

Two mutations in the *CHMP2B* gene were identified (Q206H; I29V) in two ALS patients without SOD1 mutations.[435] Neuropathology of the Q206H case showed lower motor neuron predominant disease with ubiquitinated inclusions in motor neurons.[435] The mutation was not identified in 640 control samples. The Q206H carrier died of respiratory failure 15 months after symptom onset. There was no evidence of dementia or other non-motor neurologic involvement.[435]

A heterozygous 161A-G transition, resulting in an ile29-to-val (I29V) substitution located between two conserved regions of the protein, was identified in a man with onset of progressive FTLD in his late sixties, followed by ALS.[435] The mutation was not found in 640 controls or in 400 FTLD samples. The patient had brisk tendon reflexes and extensor plantar responses. Interestingly, the I29V variant was found in one of 141 patients with FTLD and at a frequency of 0.5% among 200 control chromosomes, suggesting that it may be a benign variant.[431] However, Cox et al. (2010) also identified a heterozygous I29V substitution, resulting in an 85A-G transition, in two unrelated patients with onset of ALS at ages 64 and 49 years, respectively. In addition, in a 54-year-old man with ALS, a *CHMP2B* heterozygous 311C-A transversion in exon 3 was identified, resulting in a thr104-to-asn (T104N) substitution in a highly conserved residue.[436] The mutations were not found in 1,000 control chromosomes. Patients had involvement of the upper and lower limbs, as well as bulbar symptoms, but no signs of upper motor neuron involvement. Functional studies showed that cells expressing the mutant protein had large cytoplasmic vacuoles with an accumulation of mutant CHMP2B on the outer membrane, termed *halos*, and an overall defect in the autophagic pathway.[436] The authors concluded that in this population drawn from North of England, pathogenic *CHMP2B* mutations account for approximately 1% of cases of ALS and 10% of those with lower motor neuron predominant ALS.[436]

Fused in Sarcoma RNA Binding Protein: FUS
Inheritance and Clinical Features
In eight families with ALS, mutations in the *FUS* gene were identified. The 20 affected individuals showed an even gender distribution, lack of cognitive deficits, an average age at onset of 44.5 years, and an average survival of 33 months. The site of onset varied among these 20 individuals and included cervical, lumbar or bulbar. Neuropathologic examination of three patients showed severe lower motor neuron loss in the spinal cord, and to a lesser degree in the brainstem, while the dorsal horn neurons appeared unaffected. FUS immunostaining indicated large globular and elongated cytoplasmic inclusions in spinal cord motor neurons and dystrophic neurites in all affected individuals.[437] In another report, a 69-year-old man who presented with predominantly lower motor neuron ALS involving both the lower and upper limbs[438] also showed neuronal and glial cytoplasmic inclusions that stained for *FUS*.[438] In a cohort of 101 patients from 25 unrelated families with ALS, who carry heterozygous mutations in the *FUS* gene, the average age at symptom onset was 43.6 years, which was earlier than that observed in patients with *SOD1* or *TARDBP* mutations.[439] Some patients with *FUS* mutations have onset in adolescence. The average duration of symptoms for those with *FUS* mutations was 3.4 years, with almost 90% with a duration of less than 4 years, indicating a more rapid disease progression compared to those with *SOD1* or *TARDBP* mutations. Approximately 33.3% of those with *FUS* mutations presented with bulbar onset, and some affected members of three families also developed FTD. It appears that the *FUS* gene mutations are not an uncommon cause of familial ALS, and have a prevalence of 5.6% in non-*SOD1* and non-*TARDBP* familial ALS, and approximately 4.79% in all familial ALS. The pathogenicity of some of these novel mutations awaits further studies. In summary, patients with *FUS* mutations manifest earlier symptom onset, a higher rate of bulbar onset, and shorter duration of symptoms.[439]

Structure, Function, and Expression
The *FUS* gene consists of 15 exons located within 12 kb of genomic DNA. *FUS* exon 1 contains a 72-bp untranslated region and the translation initiation codon. The gene has multiple glycine repeats and an RNP region encoded by exons 9, 10, and 11. The gene is likely to share a common ancestral gene with *RBP56* and *EWSR1*.[440,441]

The *FUS* gene has been mapped to chromosome 16p11.2.[442–444] *FUS* might function as a regulator of growth factor independence and prevent differentiation via modulation of cytokine receptor expression,[445] and it may act as a key transcriptional regulatory sensor of DNA damage signals.[446,447] For example, the recruitment of *FUS* to the *CCND1* promoter causes gene-specific repression that is directed by single-stranded, low copy-number non-coding RNA transcripts tethered to the five prime regulatory regions of *CCND1* that are induced in response to DNA damage signals.[446,447] *FUS* is a nucleoprotein that functions in DNA and RNA metabolism, including DNA repair, and the regulation of transcription, RNA splicing, and export to the cytoplasm. Translocation of the FUS transcriptional activation domain results in fusion proteins and has been implicated in tumorigenesis.[443,446–448] The full-length 526–amino acid FUS protein contains an N-terminal serine-, tyrosine-, glycine-, and glutamine-rich domain, followed by a glycine-rich region, an RNA recognition motif, and a zinc finger domain. Interspersed between these domains are 3 RGG repeat regions.[449] Vance et al. determined that *FUS* also has a C-terminal proline-tyrosine nuclear localization signal by showing that an epitope-tagged *FUS* localized predominantly to the nucleus of transfected human neuroblastoma cells.[449]

Genetic Variation
A *FUS* homozygous 1551C-G transversion in exon 15 (H517Q) has been identified in ALS families.[450] In addition, a heterozygous 1561C-G transversion in exon 15 of the *FUS* gene was identified (R521G) where the inheritance is autosomal dominant with incomplete penetrance, and the mean age at onset was 39.6 years. Other mutations include a 1562G-A transition in exon 15 (R521H) and a 1553G-A transition in exon 15 (R518K). Inheritance was autosomal dominant, and the mean age at onset was 40.3 years. None of these mutations was detected in 1,446 control DNA samples from North America.[450,451]

A heterozygous R521C mutation in families with ALS has been described,[336,437,452,453] as well as a heterozygous R521H substitution in some affected members.[437] Onset occurs between age 34 and 54 years.[453] Other familial mutations include G507D, R216C, R524W, and R495X.[438,454]

ALS/FTD Genome Wide Association Study Genes

The ALS/FTD spectrum is a genetically heterogeneous disorder that shows the typical dichotomy of familial inherited forms and sporadic disease. While the former is caused by rare, highly penetrant, and pathogenic mutations, the risk for sporadic ALS/FTD is thought to be the result of combined effects of common genetic polymorphisms with minor to moderate effect sizes. The search for common genetic polymorphisms in GWAS studies has yielded a few novel gene candidates, but mostly has revealed the same genes identified in family studies.[455,456] ALS/FTD GWAS genes include *UNC13A, RAB38, HLA-DRB5, SUN3,* and *LAMA3,* as well as genes identified in familial forms of the disease, such as *C9orf72, MAPT,* and *GRN*.[457,458] A comprehensive up-to-date list of mutations and polymorphisms associated with ALS/FTLD can be found at ALSoD http://alsod.iop.kcl.ac.uk/ and ALSGene (http://www.alsgene.org).

Summary

Most ALS and FTD cases are sporadic. However, multiple gene loci have been linked to familial ALS/FTD with autosomal or recessive inheritance, most commonly due to *C9orf72, MAPT,* or *GRN* mutations. Other genes not described here include *DCNT1, VCP, TMEM106B,* and more recently reported, *TBK1* and *OPTN*.[459–464] The association between specific genes and distinct ALS/FTD pathology suggests that this disease or disease spectrum involves a strong genetic component and provides numerous clues to the etiology of the disease. Sporadic ALS and FTD studies have identified the same genes identified in familial forms of the disease, and have provided additional gene candidates. The functional contribution of these genes to ALS and FTD pathogenesis remains to be fully characterized.

REFERENCES

1. Ferri, C. P., et al. Global prevalence of dementia: a Delphi consensus study. *Lancet* **366**, 2112–2117 (2005).
2. Kukull, W. A., et al. Dementia and Alzheimer disease incidence: a prospective cohort study. *Arch Neurol* **59**, 1737–1746 (2002).
3. Bird, T. D. Genetic aspects of Alzheimer disease. *Genet Med* **10**, 231–239 (2008).
4. Roses, A. D. On the discovery of the genetic association of Apolipoprotein E genotypes and common late-onset Alzheimer disease. *J Alzheimers Dis* **9**, 361–366 (2006).
5. Kamboh, M. I. Molecular genetics of late-onset Alzheimer's disease. *Ann Hum Genet* **68**, 381–404 (2004).
6. Bertram, L., & Tanzi, R. E. The current status of Alzheimer's disease genetics: what do we tell the patients? *Pharmacol Res* **50**, 385–396 (2004).
7. Serretti, A., Artioli, P., Quartesan, R., & De Ronchi, D. Genes involved in Alzheimer's disease, a survey of possible candidates. *J Alzheimers Dis* **7**, 331–353 (2005).
8. Campion, D., et al. Early-onset autosomal dominant Alzheimer disease: prevalence, genetic heterogeneity, and mutation spectrum. *Am J Hum Genet* **65**, 664–670 (1999).
9. Brickell, K. L., et al. Early-onset Alzheimer disease in families with late-onset Alzheimer disease: a potential important subtype of familial Alzheimer disease. *Arch Neurol* **63**, 1307–1311 (2006).
10. Goedert, M., & Spillantini, M. G. A century of Alzheimer's disease. *Science* **314**, 777–781 (2006).
11. Raux, G., et al. Molecular diagnosis of autosomal dominant early onset Alzheimer's disease: an update. *J Med Genet* **42**, 793–795 (2005).
12. Cruts, M., & Van Broeckhoven, C. Molecular genetics of Alzheimer's disease. *Ann Med* **30**, 560–565 (1998).
13. Bertram, L., & Tanzi, R. E. Alzheimer's disease: one disorder, too many genes? *Hum Mol Genet* **13** Spec No 1, R135–R141 (2004).
14. Gatz, M., et al. Role of genes and environments for explaining Alzheimer disease. *Arch Gen Psychiatry* **63**, 168–174 (2006).
15. Roses, A. D., et al. Apolipoprotein E E4 allele and risk of dementia. *JAMA* **273**, 374–375; author reply 375–376 (1995).
16. Schellenberg, G. D. Genetic dissection of Alzheimer disease, a heterogeneous disorder. *Proc Natl Acad Sci U S A* **92**, 8552–8559 (1995).
17. Selkoe, D. J. Alzheimer's disease: genes, proteins, and therapy. *Physiol Rev* **81**, 741–766 (2001).
18. Couzin, J. Genetics: once shunned, test for Alzheimer's risk headed to market. *Science* **319**, 1022–1023 (2008).
19. Coon, K. D., et al. A high-density whole-genome association study reveals that APOE is the major susceptibility gene for sporadic late-onset Alzheimer's disease. *J Clin Psychiatry* **68**, 613–618 (2007).
20. Benitez, B. A., et al. TREM2 is associated with the risk of Alzheimer's disease in Spanish population. *Neurobiol Aging* **34**, 1711, e15–e17 (2013).

21. Guerreiro, R. J., et al. Using exome sequencing to reveal mutations in TREM2 presenting as a frontotemporal dementia-like syndrome without bone involvement. *JAMA Neurol* **70**, 78–84 (2013).

22. Jonsson, T., et al. Variant of TREM2 associated with the risk of Alzheimer's disease. *N Engl J Med* **368**, 107–116 (2013).

23. Lambert, J. C., et al. Meta-analysis of 74,046 individuals identifies 11 new susceptibility loci for Alzheimer's disease. *Nat Genet* **45**, 1452–1458 (2013).

24. Jonsson, T., et al. A mutation in APP protects against Alzheimer's disease and age-related cognitive decline. *Nature* **488**, 96–99 (2012).

25. Chai, C. K. The genetics of Alzheimer's disease. *Am J Alzheimers Dis Other Demen* **22**, 37–41 (2007).

26. Daw, E. W., et al. The number of trait loci in late-onset Alzheimer disease. *Am J Hum Genet* **66**, 196–204 (2000).

27. Kang, J., et al. The precursor of Alzheimer's disease amyloid A4 protein resembles a cell-surface receptor. *Nature* **325**, 733–736 (1987).

28. Giaccone, G., et al. Down patients: extracellular preamyloid deposits precede neuritic degeneration and senile plaques. *Neurosci Lett* **97**, 232–238 (1989).

29. Mann, D. M., et al. Immunocytochemical profile of neurofibrillary tangles in Down's syndrome patients of different ages. *J Neurol Sci* **92**, 247–260 (1989).

30. Iwatsubo, T., et al. Visualization of A beta 42(43) and A beta 40 in senile plaques with end-specific A beta monoclonals: evidence that an initially deposited species is A beta 42(43). *Neuron.* **13**, 45–53 (1994).

31. Lemere, C. A., et al. Sequence of deposition of heterogeneous amyloid beta-peptides and APO E in Down syndrome: implications for initial events in amyloid plaque formation. *Neurobiol Dis* **3**, 16–32 (1996).

32. Leverenz, J. B., & Raskind, M. A. Early amyloid deposition in the medial temporal lobe of young Down syndrome patients: a regional quantitative analysis. *Exp Neurol* **150**, 296–304 (1998).

33. Goate, A., et al. Segregation of a missense mutation in the amyloid precursor protein gene with familial Alzheimer's disease. *Nature* **349**, 704–706 (1991).

34. Chartier-Harlin, M. C., et al. Early-onset Alzheimer's disease caused by mutations at codon 717 of the beta-amyloid precursor protein gene. *Nature* **353**, 844–846 (1991).

35. Chartier-Harlin, M. C., et al. Screening for the beta-amyloid precursor protein mutation (APP717: Val—Ile) in extended pedigrees with early onset Alzheimer's disease. *Neurosci Lett* **129**, 134–135 (1991).

36. Murrell, J., Farlow, M., Ghetti, B., & Benson, M. D. A mutation in the amyloid precursor protein associated with hereditary Alzheimer's disease. *Science* **254**, 97–99 (1991).

37. Mullan, M. Familial Alzheimer's disease: second gene locus located. *BMJ* **305**, 1108–1109 (1992).

38. Levy, E., et al. Mutation of the Alzheimer's disease amyloid gene in hereditary cerebral hemorrhage, Dutch type. *Science* **248**, 1124–1126 (1990).

39. Hardy, J. The genetic causes of neurodegenerative diseases. *J Alzheimers Dis* **3**, 109–116 (2001).

40. Suzuki, N., et al. An increased percentage of long amyloid beta protein secreted by familial amyloid beta protein precursor (beta APP717) mutants. *Science.* **264**, 1336–1340 (1994).

41. Esler, W. P., & Wolfe, M. S. A portrait of Alzheimer secretases: new features and familiar faces. *Science* **293**, 1449–1454 (2001).

42. Sherrington, R., et al. Alzheimer's disease associated with mutations in presenilin 2 is rare and variably penetrant. *Hum Mol Genet* **5**, 985–988 (1996).

43. Janssen, J. C., et al. Early onset familial Alzheimer's disease: mutation frequency in 31 families. *Neurology* **60**, 235–239 (2003).

44. Goldgaber, D., Lerman, M. I., McBride, O. W., Saffiotti, U., & Gajdusek, D. C. Characterization and chromosomal localization of a cDNA encoding brain amyloid of Alzheimer's disease. *Science* **235**, 877–880 (1987).

45. Tanzi, R. E., et al. Protease inhibitor domain encoded by an amyloid protein precursor mRNA associated with Alzheimer's disease. *Nature* **331**, 528–530 (1988).

46. Ponte, P., et al. A new A4 amyloid mRNA contains a domain homologous to serine proteinase inhibitors. *Nature* **331**, 525–527 (1988).

47. Kitaguchi, N., Takahashi, Y., Tokushima, Y., Shiojiri, S., & Ito, H. Novel precursor of Alzheimer's disease amyloid protein shows protease inhibitory activity. *Nature* **331**, 530–532 (1988).

48. Golde, T. E., Estus, S., Usiak, M., Younkin, L. H., & Younkin, S. G. Expression of beta amyloid protein precursor mRNAs: recognition of a novel alternatively spliced form and quantitation in Alzheimer's disease using PCR. *Neuron* **4**, 253–267 (1990).

49. de Sauvage, F., & Octave, J. N. A novel mRNA of the A4 amyloid precursor gene coding for a possibly secreted protein. *Science* **245**, 651–653 (1989).

50. Yoshikai, S., Sasaki, H., Doh-ura, K., Furuya, H., & Sakaki, Y. Genomic organization of the

human amyloid beta-protein precursor gene. *Gene* **87**, 257–263 (1990).

51. Turner, P. R., O'Connor, K., Tate, W. P., & Abraham, W. C. Roles of amyloid precursor protein and its fragments in regulating neural activity, plasticity and memory. *Prog Neurobiol* **70**, 1–32 (2003).

52. Priller, C., et al. Synapse formation and function is modulated by the amyloid precursor protein. *J Neurosci* **26**, 7212–7221 (2006).

53. Walter, J., Kaether, C., Steiner, H., & Haass, C. The cell biology of Alzheimer's disease: uncovering the secrets of secretases. *Curr Opin Neurobiol* **11**, 585–590 (2001).

54. Sastre, M., et al. Presenilin-dependent gamma-secretase processing of beta-amyloid precursor protein at a site corresponding to the S3 cleavage of Notch. *EMBO Rep* **2**, 835–841 (2001).

55. Scheuner, D., et al. Secreted amyloid beta-protein similar to that in the senile plaques of Alzheimer's disease is increased in vivo by the presenilin 1 and 2 and APP mutations linked to familial Alzheimer's disease. *Nat Med* **2**, 864–870 (1996).

56. Walker, L. C., et al. Emerging prospects for the disease-modifying treatment of Alzheimer's disease. *Biochem Pharmacol* **69**, 1001–1008 (2005).

57. Higgins, G. A., & Jacobsen, H. Transgenic mouse models of Alzheimer's disease: phenotype and application. *Behav Pharmacol* **14**, 419–438 (2003).

58. Mineur, Y. S., McLoughlin, D., Crusio, W. E., Sluyter, F., & Huynh, L. X. Genetic mouse models of Alzheimer's disease social behavior deficits in the Fmr1 mutant mouse Genetic dissection of learning and memory in mice. *Neural Plast* **12**, 299–310 (2005).

59. Irizarry, M. C., McNamara, M., Fedorchak, K., Hsiao, K., & Hyman, B. T. APPSw transgenic mice develop age-related A beta deposits and neuropil abnormalities, but no neuronal loss in CA1. *J Neuropathol Exp Neurol* **56**, 965–973 (1997).

60. Westerman, M. A., et al. The relationship between Abeta and memory in the Tg2576 mouse model of Alzheimer's disease. *J Neurosci* **22**, 1858–1867 (2002).

61. Schellenberg, G. D., et al. Genetic linkage evidence for a familial Alzheimer's disease locus on chromosome 14. *Science* **258**, 668–671 (1992).

62. Sherrington, R., et al. Cloning of a gene bearing missense mutations in early-onset familial Alzheimer's disease. *Nature* **375**, 754–760 (1995).

63. Theuns, J., et al. Genetic variability in the regulatory region of presenilin 1 associated with risk for Alzheimer's disease and variable expression. *Hum Mol Genet* **9**, 325–331 (2000).

64. Citron, M., et al. Mutant presenilins of Alzheimer's disease increase production of 42-residue amyloid beta-protein in both transfected cells and transgenic mice. *Nat Med* **3**, 67–72 (1997).

65. Lippa, C. F., Nee, L. E., Mori, H., & St George-Hyslop, P. Abeta-42 deposition precedes other changes in PS-1 Alzheimer's disease. *Lancet* **352**, 1117–1118 (1998).

66. Wolfe, M. S. When loss is gain: reduced presenilin proteolytic function leads to increased Abeta42/Abeta40. Talking point on the role of presenilin mutations in Alzheimer disease. *EMBO Rep* **8**, 136–140 (2007).

67. Moehlmann, T., et al. Presenilin-1 mutations of leucine 166 equally affect the generation of the Notch and APP intracellular domains independent of their effect on Abeta 42 production. *Proc Natl Acad Sci U S A* **99**, 8025–8030 (2002).

68. Rudzinski, L. A., et al. Early onset familial Alzheimer disease with spastic paraparesis, dysarthria, and seizures and N135S mutation in PSEN1. *Alzheimer Dis Assoc Disord* **22**, 299–307 (2008).

69. Leverenz, J. B., et al. Lewy body pathology in familial Alzheimer disease: evidence for disease- and mutation-specific pathologic phenotype. *Arch Neurol* **63**, 370–376 (2006).

70. Crook, R., et al. A variant of Alzheimer's disease with spastic paraparesis and unusual plaques due to deletion of exon 9 of presenilin 1. *Nat Med* **4**, 452–455 (1998).

71. Hutton, M., & Hardy, J. The presenilins and Alzheimer's disease. *Hum Mol Genet* **6**, 1639–1646 (1997).

72. De Strooper, B., et al. Deficiency of presenilin-1 inhibits the normal cleavage of amyloid precursor protein. *Nature* **391**, 387–390 (1998).

73. Wolfe, M. S., De Los Angeles, J., Miller, D. D., Xia, W., & Selkoe, D. J. Are presenilins intramembrane-cleaving proteases? Implications for the molecular mechanism of Alzheimer's disease. *Biochemistry* **38**, 11223–11230 (1999).

74. Francis, R., et al. aph-1 and pen-2 are required for Notch pathway signaling, gamma-secretase cleavage of betaAPP, and presenilin protein accumulation. *Dev Cell* **3**, 85–97 (2002).

75. Goutte, C., Tsunozaki, M., Hale, V. A., & Priess, J. R. APH-1 is a multipass membrane protein essential for the Notch signaling pathway in Caenorhabditis elegans embryos. *Proc Natl Acad Sci U S A* **99**, 775–779 (2002).

76. Edbauer, D., et al. Reconstitution of gamma-secretase activity. *Nat Cell Biol* **5**, 486–488 (2003).

77. Kimberly, W. T., et al. Gamma-secretase is a membrane protein complex comprised of presenilin, nicastrin, Aph-1, and Pen-2. *Proc Natl Acad Sci U S A* **100**, 6382–6387 (2003).

78. Takasugi, N., et al. The role of presenilin cofactors in the gamma-secretase complex. *Nature* **422**, 438–441 (2003).

79. Shen, J., et al. Skeletal and CNS defects in Presenilin-1-deficient mice. *Cell* **89**, 629–639 (1997).

80. Yu, H., et al. APP processing and synaptic plasticity in presenilin-1 conditional knockout mice. *Neuron* **31**, 713–726 (2001).

81. Huang, X. G., Yee, B. K., Nag, S., Chan, S. T., & Tang, F. Behavioral and neurochemical characterization of transgenic mice carrying the human presenilin-1 gene with or without the leucine-to-proline mutation at codon 235. *Exp Neurol* **183**, 673–681 (2003).

82. Janus, C., et al. Spatial learning in transgenic mice expressing human presenilin 1 (PS1) transgenes. *Neurobiol Aging* **21**, 541–549 (2000).

83. Holcomb, L., et al. Accelerated Alzheimer-type phenotype in transgenic mice carrying both mutant amyloid precursor protein and presenilin 1 transgenes. *Nat Med* **4**, 97–100 (1998).

84. Rogaev, E. I., et al. Familial Alzheimer's disease in kindreds with missense mutations in a gene on chromosome 1 related to the Alzheimer's disease type 3 gene. *Nature* **376**, 775–778 (1995).

85. Levy-Lahad, E., et al. A familial Alzheimer's disease locus on chromosome 1. *Science* **269**, 970–973 (1995).

86. Tandon, A., & Fraser, P. The presenilins. *Genome Biol* **3**, reviews 3014 (2002).

87. Alzheimer's Disease Collaborative Group. The structure of the presenilin 1 (S182) gene and identification of six novel mutations in early onset AD families. *Nat Genet* **11**, 219–222 (1995).

88. Hutton, M., et al. Complete analysis of the presenilin 1 gene in early onset Alzheimer's disease. *Neuroreport* **7**, 801–805 (1996).

89. Prihar, G., et al. Structure and alternative splicing of the presenilin-2 gene. *Neuroreport* **7**, 1680–1684 (1996).

90. Anwar, R., et al. Molecular analysis of the presenilin 1 (S182) gene in "sporadic" cases of Alzheimer's disease: identification and characterisation of unusual splice variants. *J Neurochem* **66**, 1774–1777 (1996).

91. Kovacs, D. M., et al. Alzheimer-associated presenilins 1 and 2: neuronal expression in brain and localization to intracellular membranes in mammalian cells. *Nat Med* **2**, 224–229 (1996).

92. Wolfe, M. S., et al. Two transmembrane aspartates in presenilin-1 required for presenilin endoproteolysis and gamma-secretase activity. *Nature* **398**, 513–517 (1999).

93. Bentahir, M., et al. Presenilin clinical mutations can affect gamma-secretase activity by different mechanisms. *J Neurochem* **96**, 732–742 (2006).

94. Lindquist, S. G., et al. A novel presenilin 2 mutation (V393M) in early-onset dementia with profound language impairment. *Eur J Neurol* **15**, 1135–1139 (2008).

95. Chauhan, N. B. Membrane dynamics, cholesterol homeostasis, and Alzheimer's disease. *J Lipid Res* **44**, 2019–2029 (2003).

96. Poirier, J., et al. Apolipoprotein E polymorphism and Alzheimer's disease. *Lancet* **342**, 697–699 (1993).

97. Tsai, M. S., et al. Apolipoprotein E: risk factor for Alzheimer disease. *Am J Hum Genet* **54**, 643–649 (1994).

98. Lucotte, G., Turpin, J. C., & Landais, P. Apolipoprotein E-epsilon 4 allele doses in late-onset Alzheimer's disease. *Ann Neurol* **36**, 681–682 (1994).

99. Mayeux, R., et al. The apolipoprotein epsilon 4 allele in patients with Alzheimer's disease. *Ann Neurol* **34**, 752–754 (1993).

100. Liddell, M., Williams, J., Bayer, A., Kaiser, F., & Owen, M. Confirmation of association between the e4 allele of apolipoprotein E and Alzheimer's disease. *J Med Genet* **31**, 197–200 (1994).

101. Brousseau, T., et al. Confirmation of the epsilon 4 allele of the apolipoprotein E gene as a risk factor for late-onset Alzheimer's disease. *Neurology* **44**, 342–344 (1994).

102. Hendrie, H. C., et al. Apolipoprotein E genotypes and Alzheimer's disease in a community study of elderly African Americans. *Ann Neurol* **37**, 118–120 (1995).

103. Farrer, L. A., et al. Apolipoprotein E genotype in patients with Alzheimer's disease: implications for the risk of dementia among relatives. *Ann Neurol* **38**, 797–808 (1995).

104. Farrer, L. A., et al. Effects of age, sex, and ethnicity on the association between apolipoprotein E genotype and Alzheimer disease: a meta-analysis. APOE and Alzheimer Disease Meta Analysis Consortium. *JAMA.* **278**, 1349–1356 (1997).

105. Corder, E. H., et al. Gene dose of apolipoprotein E type 4 allele and the risk of Alzheimer's disease in late onset families. *Science* **261**, 921–923 (1993).

106. Tang, M. X., et al. Relative risk of Alzheimer disease and age-at-onset distributions, based on APOE genotypes among elderly African Americans, Caucasians, and Hispanics in New York City. *Am J Hum Genet* **58**, 574–584 (1996).

107. Schupf, N., & Sergievsky, G. H. Genetic and host factors for dementia in Down's syndrome. *Br J Psychiatry* **180**, 405–410 (2002).

108. Nicoll, J. A., Roberts, G. W., & Graham, D. I. Apolipoprotein E epsilon 4 allele is associated with deposition of amyloid beta-protein following head injury. *Nat Med* **1**, 135–137 (1995).

109. Liu, Y., et al. Apolipoprotein E polymorphism and acute ischemic stroke: a diffusion- and perfusion-weighted magnetic resonance imaging study. *J Cereb Blood Flow Metab* **22**, 1336–1342 (2002).

110. Nagy, Z., et al. Influence of the apolipoprotein E genotype on amyloid deposition and neurofibrillary tangle formation in Alzheimer's disease. *Neuroscience* **69**, 757–761 (1995).

111. Gibson, G. E., et al. Mitochondrial damage in Alzheimer's disease varies with apolipoprotein E genotype. *Ann Neurol* **48**, 297–303 (2000).

112. Mahley, R. W., Weisgraber, K. H., & Huang, Y. Apolipoprotein E4: a causative factor and therapeutic target in neuropathology, including Alzheimer's disease. *Proc Natl Acad Sci U S A.* **103**, 5644–5651 (2006).

113. Pitas, R. E., Boyles, J. K., Lee, S. H., Foss, D., & Mahley, R. W. Astrocytes synthesize apolipoprotein E and metabolize apolipoprotein E-containing lipoproteins. *Biochim Biophys Acta.* **917**, 148–161 (1987).

114. Uchihara, T., et al. ApoE immunoreactivity and microglial cells in Alzheimer's disease brain. *Neurosci Lett* **195**, 5–8 (1995).

115. Aoki, K., et al. Expression of apolipoprotein E in ballooned neurons-comparative immunohistochemical study on neurodegenerative disorders and infarction. *Acta Neuropathol* **106**, 436–440 (2003).

116. Xu, P. T., et al. Specific regional transcription of apolipoprotein E in human brain neurons. *Am J Pathol.* **154**, 601–611 (1999).

117. Huang, Y. Molecular and cellular mechanisms of apolipoprotein E4 neurotoxicity and potential therapeutic strategies. *Curr Opin Drug Discov Devel* **9**, 627–641 (2006).

118. Stratman, N. C., et al. Isoform-specific interactions of human apolipoprotein E to an intermediate conformation of human Alzheimer amyloid-beta peptide. *Chem Phys Lipids* **137**, 52–61 (2005).

119. Buttini, M., et al. Expression of human apolipoprotein E3 or E4 in the brains of Apoe-/- mice: isoform-specific effects on neurodegeneration. *J Neurosci* **19**, 4867–4880 (1999).

120. Keller, J. N., et al. Amyloid beta-peptide effects on synaptosomes from apolipoprotein E-deficient mice. *J Neurochem* **74**, 1579–1586 (2000).

121. LaDu, M. J., et al. Purification of apolipoprotein E attenuates isoform-specific binding to beta-amyloid. *J Biol Chem* **270**, 9039–9042 (1995).

122. Canevari, L., & Clark, J. B. Alzheimer's disease and cholesterol: the fat connection. *Neurochem Res* **32**, 739–750 (2007).

123. Blacker, D., et al. ApoE-4 and age at onset of Alzheimer's disease: the NIMH genetics initiative. *Neurology* **48**, 139–147 (1997).

124. Martins, C. A., Oulhaj, A., de Jager, C. A., & Williams, J. H. APOE alleles predict the rate of cognitive decline in Alzheimer disease: a nonlinear model. *Neurology* **65**, 1888–1893 (2005).

125. Guerreiro, R., et al. TREM2 variants in Alzheimer's disease. *N Engl J Med* **368**, 117–127 (2013).

126. Korvatska, O., et al. R47H variant of TREM2 associated with Alzheimer disease in a large late-onset family: clinical, genetic, and neuropathological study. *JAMA Neurol* **72**, 920–927 (2015).

127. Klunemann, H. H., et al. The genetic causes of basal ganglia calcification, dementia, and bone cysts: DAP12 and TREM2. *Neurology* **64**, 1502–1507 (2005).

128. Paloneva, J., et al. Mutations in two genes encoding different subunits of a receptor signaling complex result in an identical disease phenotype. *Am J Hum Genet* **71**, 656–662 (2002).

129. Bertram, L., McQueen, M. B., Mullin, K., Blacker, D., & Tanzi, R. E. Systematic meta-analyses of Alzheimer disease genetic association studies: the AlzGene database. *Nat Genet* **39**, 17–23 (2007).

130. Harold, D., et al. Genome-wide association study identifies variants at CLU and PICALM associated with Alzheimer's disease. *Nat Genet* **41**, 1088–1093 (2009).

131. Hollingworth, P., et al. Common variants at ABCA7, MS4A6A/MS4A4E, EPHA1, CD33, and CD2AP are associated with Alzheimer's disease. *Nat Genet* **43**, 429–435 (2011).

132. Lambert, J. C., et al. Genome-wide association study identifies variants at CLU and CR1 associated with Alzheimer's disease. *Nat Genet* **41**, 1094–1099 (2009).

133. Naj, A. C., et al. Common variants at MS4A4/MS4A6E, CD2AP, CD33 and EPHA1 are associated with late-onset Alzheimer's disease. *Nat Genet* **43**, 436–441 (2011).

134. Seshadri, S., et al. Genome-wide analysis of genetic loci associated with Alzheimer disease. *JAMA* **303**, 1832–1840 (2010).

135. Raschetti, R., Albanese, E., Vanacore, N., & Maggini, M. Cholinesterase inhibitors in mild cognitive impairment: a systematic review of randomised trials. *PLoS Med* **4**, e338 (2007).

136. Raina, P., et al. Effectiveness of cholinesterase inhibitors and memantine for treating dementia: evidence review for a clinical practice guideline. *Ann Intern Med* **148**, 379–397 (2008).

137. de Rijk, M. C., et al. Prevalence of Parkinson's disease in Europe: a collaborative study of population-based cohorts. Neurologic Diseases in the Elderly Research Group. *Neurology* **54**, S21–S23 (2000).

138. Volta, M., Milnerwood, A. J., & Farrer, M. J. Insights from late-onset familial parkinsonism on the pathogenesis of idiopathic Parkinson's disease. *Lancet Neurol* **14**, 1054–1064 (2015).

139. Verstraeten, A., Theuns, J., & Van Broeckhoven, C. Progress in unraveling the genetic etiology of Parkinson disease in a genomic era. *Trends Genet* **31**, 140–149 (2015).

140. McKeith, I. Dementia with Lewy bodies and Parkinson's disease with dementia: where two worlds collide. *Pract Neurol* **7**, 374–382 (2007).

141. Polymeropoulos, M. H., et al. Mapping of a gene for Parkinson's disease to chromosome 4q21-q23. *Science* **274**, 1197–1199 (1996).

142. Farrer, M. J. Genetics of Parkinson disease: paradigm shifts and future prospects. *Nat Rev Genet* **7**, 306–318 (2006).

143. Belin, A. C., & Westerlund, M. Parkinson's disease: a genetic perspective. *FEBS J* **275**, 1377–1383 (2008).

144. Lwin, A., Orvisky, E., Goker-Alpan, O., LaMarca, M. E., & Sidransky, E. Glucocerebrosidase mutations in subjects with parkinsonism. *Mol Genet Metab* **81**, 70–73 (2004).

145. Aharon-Peretz, J., Rosenbaum, H., & Gershoni-Baruch, R. Mutations in the glucocerebrosidase gene and Parkinson's disease in Ashkenazi Jews. *N Engl J Med* **351**, 1972–1977 (2004).

146. Clark, L. N., et al. Pilot association study of the beta-glucocerebrosidase N370S allele and Parkinson's disease in subjects of Jewish ethnicity. *Mov Disord* **20**, 100–103 (2005).

147. Sato, C., et al. Analysis of the glucocerebrosidase gene in Parkinson's disease. *Mov Disord* **20**, 367–370 (2005).

148. Eblan, M. J., et al. Glucocerebrosidase mutations are also found in subjects with early-onset parkinsonism from Venezuela. *Mov Disord* **21**, 282–283 (2006).

149. Toft, M., Pielsticker, L., Ross, O. A., Aasly, J. O., & Farrer, M. J. Glucocerebrosidase gene mutations and Parkinson disease in the Norwegian population. *Neurology* **66**, 415–417 (2006).

150. Bras, J., et al. Complete screening for glucocerebrosidase mutations in Parkinson disease patients from Portugal. *Neurobiol Aging* **30**, 1515–1517 (2007).

151. Clark, L. N., et al. Mutations in the glucocerebrosidase gene are associated with early-onset Parkinson disease. *Neurology* **69**, 1270–1277 (2007).

152. De Marco, E. V., et al. Glucocerebrosidase gene mutations are associated with Parkinson's disease in southern Italy. *Mov Disord* **23**, 460–463 (2008).

153. Spitz, M., Rozenberg, R., Pereira Lda, V., & Reis Barbosa, E. Association between Parkinson's disease and glucocerebrosidase mutations in Brazil. *Parkinsonism Relat Disord* **14**, 58–62 (2008).

154. Wu, Y. R., et al. Glucocerebrosidase gene mutation is a risk factor for early onset of Parkinson disease among Taiwanese. *J Neurol Neurosurg Psychiatry* **78**, 977–979 (2007).

155. Ziegler, S. G., et al. Glucocerebrosidase mutations in Chinese subjects from Taiwan with sporadic Parkinson disease. *Mol Genet Metab* **91**, 195–200 (2007).

156. Tan, E. K., et al. Glucocerebrosidase mutations and risk of Parkinson disease in Chinese patients. *Arch Neurol* **64**, 1056–1058 (2007).

157. Gan-Or, Z., et al. Genotype-phenotype correlations between GBA mutations and Parkinson disease risk and onset. *Neurology* **70**, 2277–2283 (2008).

158. Chartier-Harlin, M. C., et al. Alpha-synuclein locus duplication as a cause of familial Parkinson's disease. *Lancet* **364**, 1167–1169 (2004).

159. Ibanez, P., et al. Causal relation between alpha-synuclein gene duplication and familial Parkinson's disease. *Lancet* **364**, 1169–1171 (2004).

160. Nishioka, K., et al. Clinical heterogeneity of alpha-synuclein gene duplication in Parkinson's disease. *Ann Neurol* **59**, 298–309 (2006).

161. Fuchs, J., et al. Phenotypic variation in a large Swedish pedigree due to SNCA duplication and triplication. *Neurology* **68**, 916–922 (2007).

162. Singleton, A. B., et al. alpha-Synuclein locus triplication causes Parkinson's disease. *Science* **302**, 841 (2003).

163. Farrer, M., et al. Comparison of kindreds with parkinsonism and alpha-synuclein genomic multiplications. *Ann Neurol* **55**, 174–179 (2004).

164. Fortin, D. L., et al. Lipid rafts mediate the synaptic localization of alpha-synuclein. *J Neurosci* **24**, 6715–6723 (2004).

165. Bisaglia, M., Mammi, S., & Bubacco, L. Structural insights on physiological functions and pathological effects of {alpha}-synuclein. *FASEB J* (2008).

166. George, J. M. The synucleins. *Genome Biol* **3**, reviews 3002 (2002).

167. Uversky, V. N. A protein-chameleon: conformational plasticity of alpha-synuclein, a disordered protein involved in neurodegenerative disorders. *J Biomol Struct Dyn* **21**, 211–234 (2003).

168. Spillantini, M. G., et al. Alpha-synuclein in Lewy bodies. *Nature* **388**, 839–840 (1997).

169. Miller, D. W., et al. Alpha-synuclein in blood and brain from familial Parkinson disease with SNCA locus triplication. *Neurology* **62**, 1835–1838 (2004).

170. Conway, K. A., Harper, J. D., & Lansbury, P. T. Accelerated in vitro fibril formation by a mutant alpha-synuclein linked to early-onset Parkinson disease. *Nat Med* **4**, 1318–1320 (1998).

171. Pandey, N., Schmidt, R. E., & Galvin, J. E. The alpha-synuclein mutation E46K promotes aggregation in cultured cells. *Exp Neurol* **197**, 515–520 (2006).

172. Lashuel, H. A., et al. Alpha-synuclein, especially the Parkinson's disease-associated mutants, forms pore-like annular and tubular protofibrils. *J Mol Biol* **322**, 1089–1102 (2002).

173. Conway, K. A., Harper, J. D., & Lansbury, P. T., Jr. Fibrils formed in vitro from alpha-synuclein and two mutant forms linked to Parkinson's disease are typical amyloid. *Biochemistry* **39**, 2552–2563 (2000).

174. Greenbaum, E. A., et al. The E46K mutation in alpha-synuclein increases amyloid fibril formation. *J Biol Chem* **280**, 7800–7807 (2005).

175. Specht, C. G., & Schoepfer, R. Deletion of the alpha-synuclein locus in a subpopulation of C57BL/6J inbred mice. *BMC Neurosci* **2**, 11 (2001).

176. Rockenstein, E., et al. Differential neuropathological alterations in transgenic mice expressing alpha-synuclein from the platelet-derived growth factor and Thy-1 promoters. *J Neurosci Res* **68**, 568–578 (2002).

177. Masliah, E., et al. Dopaminergic loss and inclusion body formation in alpha-synuclein mice: implications for neurodegenerative disorders. *Science* **287**, 1265–1269 (2000).

178. Fleming, S. M., et al. Early and progressive sensorimotor anomalies in mice overexpressing wild-type human alpha-synuclein. *J Neurosci* **24**, 9434–9440 (2004).

179. Melrose, H. L., Lincoln, S. J., Tyndall, G. M., & Farrer, M. J. Parkinson's disease: a rethink of rodent models. *Exp Brain Res* **173**, 196–204 (2006).

180. El-Agnaf, O. M., et al. Aggregates from mutant and wild-type alpha-synuclein proteins and NAC peptide induce apoptotic cell death in human neuroblastoma cells by formation of beta-sheet and amyloid-like filaments. *FEBS Lett* **440**, 71–75 (1998).

181. Fredenburg, R. A., et al. The impact of the E46K mutation on the properties of alpha-synuclein in its monomeric and oligomeric states. *Biochemistry* **46**, 7107–7118 (2007).

182. Golbe, L. I., Di Iorio, G., Bonavita, V., Miller, D. C., & Duvoisin, R. C. A large kindred with autosomal dominant Parkinson's disease. *Ann Neurol* **27**, 276–282 (1990).

183. Golbe, L. I. The genetics of Parkinson's disease: a reconsideration. *Neurology* **40**, suppl 7–14; discussion 14–16 (1990).

184. Pals, P., et al. alpha-Synuclein promoter confers susceptibility to Parkinson's disease. *Ann Neurol* **56**, 591–595 (2004).

185. Maraganore, D. M., et al. Collaborative analysis of alpha-synuclein gene promoter variability and Parkinson disease. *JAMA* **296**, 661–670 (2006).

186. Tan, E. K., et al. Alpha-synuclein haplotypes implicated in risk of Parkinson's disease. *Neurology* **62**, 128–131 (2004).

187. Mueller, J. C., et al. Multiple regions of alpha-synuclein are associated with Parkinson's disease. *Ann Neurol* **57**, 535–541 (2005).

188. Mizuta, I., et al. Multiple candidate gene analysis identifies alpha-synuclein as a susceptibility gene for sporadic Parkinson's disease. *Hum Mol Genet* **15**, 1151–1158 (2006).

189. Funayama, M., et al. A new locus for Parkinson's disease (PARK8) maps to chromosome 12p11.2-q13.1. *Ann Neurol* **51**, 296–301 (2002).

190. Nukada, H., Kowa, H., Saitoh, T., Tazaki, Y., & Miura, S. [A big family of paralysis agitans (author's transl)]. *Rinsho Shinkeigaku* **18**, 627–634 (1978).

191. Zimprich, A., et al. The PARK8 locus in autosomal dominant parkinsonism: confirmation of linkage and further delineation of the disease-containing interval. *Am J Hum Genet* **74**, 11–19 (2004).

192. Wszolek, Z. K., et al. Autosomal dominant parkinsonism associated with variable synuclein and tau pathology. *Neurology* **62**, 1619–1622 (2004).

193. Nicholl, D. J., et al. Two large British kindreds with familial Parkinson's disease: a clinicopathological and genetic study. *Brain* **125**, 44–57 (2002).

194. Srivatsal, S., et al. Cognitive profile of LRRK2-related Parkinson's disease. *Mov Disord* **30**, 728–733 (2015).

195. Paisan-Ruiz, C., et al. Cloning of the gene containing mutations that cause PARK8-linked Parkinson's disease. *Neuron* **44**, 595–600 (2004).

196. Mata, I. F., et al. LRRK2 mutations are a common cause of Parkinson's disease in Spain. *Eur J Neurol* **13**, 391–394 (2006).

197. Ito, G., et al. GTP binding is essential to the protein kinase activity of LRRK2, a causative gene product for familial Parkinson's disease. *Biochemistry* **46**, 1380–1388 (2007).

198. Gloeckner, C. J., et al. The Parkinson disease causing LRRK2 mutation I2020T is associated

with increased kinase activity. *Hum Mol Genet* **15**, 223–232 (2006).

199. West, A. B., et al. Parkinson's disease-associated mutations in leucine-rich repeat kinase 2 augment kinase activity. *Proc Natl Acad Sci U S A* **102**, 16842–16847 (2005).

200. Smith, W. W., et al. Leucine-rich repeat kinase 2 (LRRK2) interacts with parkin, and mutant LRRK2 induces neuronal degeneration. *Proc Natl Acad Sci U S A* **102**, 18676–18681 (2005).

201. Biskup, S., et al. Localization of LRRK2 to membranous and vesicular structures in mammalian brain. *Ann Neurol* **60**, 557–569 (2006).

202. Hatano, T., et al. Leucine-rich repeat kinase 2 associates with lipid rafts. *Hum Mol Genet* **16**, 678–690 (2007).

203. Wider, C., Dickson, D. W., & Wszolek, Z. K. Leucine-rich repeat kinase 2 gene-associated disease: redefining genotype-phenotype correlation. *Neurodegener Dis* **7**, 175–179 (2010).

204. Silveira-Moriyama, L., et al. Hyposmia in G2019S LRRK2-related parkinsonism: clinical and pathologic data. *Neurology* **71**, 1021–1026 (2008).

205. Zabetian, C. P., et al. LRRK2 G2019S in families with Parkinson disease who originated from Europe and the Middle East: evidence of two distinct founding events beginning two millennia ago. *Am J Hum Genet* **79**, 752–758 (2006).

206. Lesage, S., et al. LRRK2 G2019S as a cause of Parkinson's disease in North African Arabs. *N Engl J Med* **354**, 422–423 (2006).

207. Lesage, S., et al. G2019S LRRK2 mutation in French and North African families with Parkinson's disease. *Ann Neurol* **58**, 784–787 (2005).

208. Khan, N. L., et al. Mutations in the gene LRRK2 encoding dardarin (PARK8) cause familial Parkinson's disease: clinical, pathological, olfactory and functional imaging and genetic data. *Brain* **128**, 2786–2796 (2005).

209. Gilks, W. P., et al. A common LRRK2 mutation in idiopathic Parkinson's disease. *Lancet* **365**, 415–416 (2005).

210. Dachsel, J. C., & Farrer, M. J. LRRK2 and Parkinson disease. *Arch Neurol* **67**, 542–547 (2010).

211. Yamamura, Y., Sobue, I., Ando, K., Iida, M., & Yanagi, T. Paralysis agitans of early onset with marked diurnal fluctuation of symptoms. *Neurology* **23**, 239–244 (1973).

212. Doherty, K. M., et al. Parkin disease: a clinicopathologic entity? *JAMA Neurol* **70**, 571–579 (2013).

213. Matsumine, H., et al. Localization of a gene for an autosomal recessive form of juvenile Parkinsonism to chromosome 6q25.2–27. *Am J Hum Genet* **60**, 588–596 (1997).

214. Jones, A. C., et al. Autosomal recessive juvenile parkinsonism maps to 6q25.2-q27 in four ethnic groups: detailed genetic mapping of the linked region. *Am J Hum Genet* **63**, 80–87 (1998).

215. Tassin, J., et al. Chromosome 6-linked autosomal recessive early-onset Parkinsonism: linkage in European and Algerian families, extension of the clinical spectrum, and evidence of a small homozygous deletion in one family. The French Parkinson's Disease Genetics Study Group, and the European Consortium on Genetic Susceptibility in Parkinson's Disease. *Am J Hum Genet* **63**, 88–94 (1998).

216. Kitada, T., et al. Mutations in the parkin gene cause autosomal recessive juvenile parkinsonism. *Nature* **392**, 605–608 (1998).

217. Lorick, K. L., et al. RING fingers mediate ubiquitin-conjugating enzyme (E2)-dependent ubiquitination. *Proc Natl Acad Sci U S A* **96**, 11364–11369 (1999).

218. Shimura, H., et al. Familial Parkinson disease gene product, parkin, is a ubiquitin-protein ligase. *Nat Genet* **25**, 302–305 (2000).

219. Kubo, S. I., et al. Parkin is associated with cellular vesicles. *J Neurochem* **78**, 42–54 (2001).

220. Mouatt-Prigent, A., et al. Ultrastructural localization of parkin in the rat brainstem, thalamus and basal ganglia. *J Neural Transm* **111**, 1209–1218 (2004).

221. Darios, F., et al. Parkin prevents mitochondrial swelling and cytochrome c release in mitochondria-dependent cell death. *Hum Mol Genet* **12**, 517–526 (2003).

222. Cookson, M. R., et al. RING finger 1 mutations in Parkin produce altered localization of the protein. *Hum Mol Genet* **12**, 2957–2965 (2003).

223. Gu, W. J., et al. The C289G and C418R missense mutations cause rapid sequestration of human parkin into insoluble aggregates. *Neurobiol Dis* **14**, 357–364 (2003).

224. Wang, C., et al. Alterations in the solubility and intracellular localization of parkin by several familial Parkinson's disease-linked point mutations. *J Neurochem* **93**, 422–431 (2005).

225. Shimura, H., et al. Ubiquitination of a new form of alpha-synuclein by parkin from human brain: implications for Parkinson's disease. *Science* **293**, 263–269 (2001).

226. Corti, O., et al. The p38 subunit of the aminoacyl-tRNA synthetase complex is a parkin substrate: linking protein biosynthesis and neurodegeneration. *Hum Mol Genet* **12**, 1427–1437 (2003).

227. von Coelln, R., Dawson, V. L., & Dawson, T. M. Parkin-associated Parkinson's disease. *Cell Tissue Res* **318**, 175–184 (2004).

228. Goldberg, M. S., et al. Parkin-deficient mice exhibit nigrostriatal deficits but not loss of

dopaminergic neurons. *J Biol Chem* **278**, 43628–43635 (2003).

229. Itier, J. M., et al. Parkin gene inactivation alters behaviour and dopamine neurotransmission in the mouse. *Hum Mol Genet* **12**, 2277–2291 (2003).

230. Von Coelln, R., et al. Loss of locus coeruleus neurons and reduced startle in parkin null mice. *Proc Natl Acad Sci U S A* **101**, 10744–10749 (2004).

231. Ko, H. S., et al. Accumulation of the authentic parkin substrate aminoacyl-tRNA synthetase cofactor, p38/JTV-1, leads to catecholaminergic cell death. *J Neurosci* **25**, 7968–7978 (2005).

232. Palacino, J. J., et al. Mitochondrial dysfunction and oxidative damage in parkin-deficient mice. *J Biol Chem* **279**, 18614–18622 (2004).

233. Greene, J. C., et al. Mitochondrial pathology and apoptotic muscle degeneration in Drosophila parkin mutants. *Proc Natl Acad Sci U S A* **100**, 4078–4083 (2003).

234. Pesah, Y., et al. Drosophila parkin mutants have decreased mass and cell size and increased sensitivity to oxygen radical stress. *Development* **131**, 2183–2194 (2004).

235. Hattori, N., et al. Point mutations (Thr240Arg and Gln311Stop) [correction of Thr240Arg and Ala311Stop] in the Parkin gene. *Biochem Biophys Res Commun* **249**, 754–758 (1998).

236. Abbas, N., et al. A wide variety of mutations in the parkin gene are responsible for autosomal recessive parkinsonism in Europe. French Parkinson's Disease Genetics Study Group and the European Consortium on Genetic Susceptibility in Parkinson's Disease. *Hum Mol Genet* **8**, 567–574 (1999).

237. Klein, C., et al. Parkin deletions in a family with adult-onset, tremor-dominant parkinsonism: expanding the phenotype. *Ann Neurol* **48**, 65–71 (2000).

238. Kann, M., et al. Role of parkin mutations in 111 community-based patients with early-onset parkinsonism. *Ann Neurol* **51**, 621–625 (2002).

239. Klein, C., et al. Frequency of parkin mutations in late-onset Parkinson's disease. *Ann Neurol* **54**, 415–416; author reply 416–417 (2003).

240. Hedrich, K., et al. Evaluation of 50 probands with early-onset Parkinson's disease for Parkin mutations. *Neurology* **58**, 1239–1246 (2002).

241. Lucking, C. B., et al. Association between early-onset Parkinson's disease and mutations in the parkin gene. *N Engl J Med* **342**, 1560–1567 (2000).

242. Periquet, M., et al. Parkin mutations are frequent in patients with isolated early-onset parkinsonism. *Brain* **126**, 1271–1278 (2003).

243. Mata, I. F., Lockhart, P. J., & Farrer, M. J. Parkin genetics: one model for Parkinson's disease. *Hum Mol Genet* **13** Spec No 1, R127–133 (2004).

244. Foroud, T., et al. Heterozygosity for a mutation in the parkin gene leads to later onset Parkinson disease. *Neurology* **60**, 796–801 (2003).

245. Oliveri, R. L., et al. The parkin gene is not a major susceptibility locus for typical late-onset Parkinson's disease. *Neurol Sci* **22**, 73–74 (2001).

246. West, A., et al. Complex relationship between Parkin mutations and Parkinson disease. *Am J Med Genet* **114**, 584–591 (2002).

247. Kay, D. M., et al. Heterozygous parkin point mutations are as common in control subjects as in Parkinson's patients. *Ann Neurol* **61**, 47–54 (2007).

248. Hedrich, K., et al. Distribution, type, and origin of Parkin mutations: review and case studies. *Mov Disord* **19**, 1146–1157 (2004).

249. Bonifati, V., et al. DJ-1(PARK7), a novel gene for autosomal recessive, early onset parkinsonism. *Neurol Sci* **24**, 159–160 (2003).

250. Hague, S., et al. Early-onset Parkinson's disease caused by a compound heterozygous DJ-1 mutation. *Ann Neurol* **54**, 271–274 (2003).

251. Hering, R., et al. Novel homozygous p.E64D mutation in DJ1 in early onset Parkinson disease (PARK7). *Hum Mutat* **24**, 321–329 (2004).

252. Dekker, M. C., et al. A clinical-genetic study of Parkinson's disease in a genetically isolated community. *J Neurol* **250**, 1056–1062 (2003).

253. Dekker, M. C., et al. Brachydactyly and short stature in a kindred with early-onset parkinsonism. *Am J Med Genet A* **130A**, 102–104 (2004).

254. Lockhart, P. J., et al. DJ-1 mutations are a rare cause of recessively inherited early onset parkinsonism mediated by loss of protein function. *J Med Genet* **41**, e22 (2004).

255. Clark, L. N., et al. Analysis of an early-onset Parkinson's disease cohort for DJ-1 mutations. *Mov Disord* **19**, 796–800 (2004).

256. Tan, E. K., et al. Genetic analysis of DJ-1 in a cohort Parkinson's disease patients of different ethnicity. *Neurosci Lett* **367**, 109–112 (2004).

257. Nagakubo, D., et al. DJ-1, a novel oncogene which transforms mouse NIH3T3 cells in cooperation with ras. *Biochem Biophys Res Commun* **231**, 509–513 (1997).

258. Bandopadhyay, R., et al. The expression of DJ-1 (PARK7) in normal human CNS and idiopathic Parkinson's disease. *Brain* **127**, 420–430 (2004).

259. Moore, D. J., Zhang, L., Dawson, T. M., & Dawson, V. L. A missense mutation (L166P) in DJ-1, linked to familial Parkinson's disease, confers reduced protein stability and impairs homo-oligomerization. *J Neurochem* **87**, 1558–1567 (2003).

260. Zhang, L., et al. Mitochondrial localization of the Parkinson's disease related protein DJ-1: implications for pathogenesis. *Hum Mol Genet* **14**, 2063–2073 (2005).

261. Abou-Sleiman, P. M., Healy, D. G., Quinn, N., Lees, A. J., & Wood, N. W. The role of pathogenic DJ-1 mutations in Parkinson's disease. *Ann Neurol* **54**, 283–286 (2003).

262. Canet-Aviles, R. M., et al. The Parkinson's disease protein DJ-1 is neuroprotective due to cysteine-sulfinic acid-driven mitochondrial localization. *Proc Natl Acad Sci U S A* **101**, 9103–9108 (2004).

263. Moore, D. J., et al. Association of DJ-1 and parkin mediated by pathogenic DJ-1 mutations and oxidative stress. *Hum Mol Genet* **14**, 71–84 (2005).

264. Mitsumoto, A., et al. Oxidized forms of peroxiredoxins and DJ-1 on two-dimensional gels increased in response to sublethal levels of paraquat. *Free Radic Res* **35**, 301–310 (2001).

265. Mitsumoto, A., & Nakagawa, Y. DJ-1 is an indicator for endogenous reactive oxygen species elicited by endotoxin. *Free Radic Res* **35**, 885–893 (2001).

266. Zhou, W., Zhu, M., Wilson, M. A., Petsko, G. A., & Fink, A. L. The oxidation state of DJ-1 regulates its chaperone activity toward alpha-synuclein. *J Mol Biol* **356**, 1036–1048 (2006).

267. Zhou, W., & Freed, C.R. DJ-1 up-regulates glutathione synthesis during oxidative stress and inhibits A53T alpha-synuclein toxicity. *J Biol Chem* **280**, 43150–43158 (2005).

268. Batelli, S., et al. DJ-1 modulates alpha-synuclein aggregation state in a cellular model of oxidative stress: relevance for Parkinson's disease and involvement of HSP70. *PLoS ONE* **3**, e1884 (2008).

269. Taira, T., et al. DJ-1 has a role in antioxidative stress to prevent cell death. *EMBO Rep* **5**, 213–218 (2004).

270. Kim, R. H., et al. Hypersensitivity of DJ-1-deficient mice to 1-methyl-4-phenyl-1,2,3,6-tetrahydropyrindine (MPTP) and oxidative stress. *Proc Natl Acad Sci U S A* **102**, 5215–5220 (2005).

271. Meulener, M. C., et al. DJ-1 is present in a large molecular complex in human brain tissue and interacts with alpha-synuclein. *J Neurochem* **93**, 1524–1532 (2005).

272. Goldberg, M. S., et al. Nigrostriatal dopaminergic deficits and hypokinesia caused by inactivation of the familial Parkinsonism-linked gene DJ-1. *Neuron* **45**, 489–496 (2005).

273. Choi, J., et al. Oxidative damage of DJ-1 is linked to sporadic Parkinson and Alzheimer diseases. *J Biol Chem* **281**, 10816–10824 (2006).

274. Waragai, M., et al. Increased level of DJ-1 in the cerebrospinal fluids of sporadic Parkinson's disease. *Biochem Biophys Res Commun* **345**, 967–972 (2006).

275. Miller, D. W., et al. L166P mutant DJ-1, causative for recessive Parkinson's disease, is degraded through the ubiquitin-proteasome system. *J Biol Chem* **278**, 36588–36595 (2003).

276. Olzmann, J. A., et al. Familial Parkinson's disease-associated L166P mutation disrupts DJ-1 protein folding and function. *J Biol Chem* **279**, 8506–8515 (2004).

277. Xu, J., et al. The Parkinson's disease-associated DJ-1 protein is a transcriptional co-activator that protects against neuronal apoptosis. *Hum Mol Genet* **14**, 1231–1241 (2005).

278. Takahashi-Niki, K., Niki, T., Taira, T., Iguchi-Ariga, S. M., & Ariga, H. Reduced anti-oxidative stress activities of DJ-1 mutants found in Parkinson's disease patients. *Biochem Biophys Res Commun* **320**, 389–397 (2004).

279. Malgieri, G., & Eliezer, D. Structural effects of Parkinson's disease linked DJ-1 mutations. *Protein Sci* **17**, 855–868 (2008).

280. Anderson, P. C., & Daggett, V. Molecular basis for the structural instability of human DJ-1 induced by the L166P mutation associated with Parkinson's disease. *Biochemistry* **47**, 9380–9393 (2008).

281. Valente, E. M., et al. Localization of a novel locus for autosomal recessive early-onset parkinsonism, PARK6, on human chromosome 1p35-p36. *Am J Hum Genet* **68**, 895–900 (2001).

282. Healy, D. G., et al. PINK1 (PARK6) associated Parkinson disease in Ireland. *Neurology* **63**, 1486–1488 (2004).

283. Rohe, C. F., et al. Homozygous PINK1 C-terminus mutation causing early-onset parkinsonism. *Ann Neurol* **56**, 427–431 (2004).

284. Li, Y., et al. Clinicogenetic study of PINK1 mutations in autosomal recessive early-onset parkinsonism. *Neurology* **64**, 1955–1957 (2005).

285. Tan, E. K., et al. Analysis of PINK1 in Asian patients with familial parkinsonism. *Clin Genet* **68**, 468–470 (2005).

286. Tan, E. K., et al. PINK1 mutations in sporadic early-onset Parkinson's disease. *Mov Disord* **21**, 789–793 (2006).

287. Hatano, Y., et al. PARK6-linked autosomal recessive early-onset parkinsonism in Asian populations. *Neurology* **63**, 1482–1485 (2004).

288. Ibanez, P., et al. Mutational analysis of the PINK1 gene in early-onset parkinsonism in Europe and North Africa. *Brain* **129**, 686–694 (2006).

289. Silvestri, L., et al. Mitochondrial import and enzymatic activity of PINK1 mutants associated

to recessive parkinsonism. *Hum Mol Genet* **14**, 3477–3492 (2005).

290. Gandhi, S., et al. PINK1 protein in normal human brain and Parkinson's disease. *Brain* **129**, 1720–1731 (2006).

291. Valente, E. M., et al. Hereditary early-onset Parkinson's disease caused by mutations in PINK1. *Science* **304**, 1158–1160 (2004).

292. Petit, A., et al. Wild-type PINK1 prevents basal and induced neuronal apoptosis, a protective effect abrogated by Parkinson disease-related mutations. *J Biol Chem* **280**, 34025–34032 (2005).

293. Abou-Sleiman, P. M., et al. A heterozygous effect for PINK1 mutations in Parkinson's disease? *Ann Neurol* **60**, 414–419 (2006).

294. Clark, I. E., et al. Drosophila pink1 is required for mitochondrial function and interacts genetically with parkin. *Nature* **441**, 1162–1166 (2006).

295. Bonifati, V., et al. Early-onset parkinsonism associated with PINK1 mutations: frequency, genotypes, and phenotypes. *Neurology* **65**, 87–95 (2005).

296. Hatano, Y., et al. Novel PINK1 mutations in early-onset parkinsonism. *Ann Neurol* **56**, 424–427 (2004).

297. Hiller, A., et al. Phenotypic spectrum of PINK1-associated parkinsonism in 15 mutation carriers from 1 family. *Mov Disord* **22**, 145–147 (2007).

298. Najim al-Din, A. S., Wriekat, A., Mubaidin, A., Dasouki, M., & Hiari, M. Pallido-pyramidal degeneration, supranuclear upgaze paresis and dementia: Kufor-Rakeb syndrome. *Acta Neurol Scand* **89**, 347–352 (1994).

299. Myhre, R., et al. Significance of the parkin and PINK1 gene in Jordanian families with incidences of young-onset and juvenile parkinsonism. *BMC Neurol* **8**, 47 (2008).

300. Ramirez, A., et al. Hereditary parkinsonism with dementia is caused by mutations in ATP13A2, encoding a lysosomal type 5 P-type ATPase. *Nat Genet* **38**, 1184–1191 (2006).

301. Williams, D. R., Hadeed, A., al-Din, A. S., Wreikat, A. L., & Lees, A. J. Kufor Rakeb disease: autosomal recessive, levodopa-responsive parkinsonism with pyramidal degeneration, supranuclear gaze palsy, and dementia. *Mov Disord* **20**, 1264–1271 (2005).

302. Nichols, W. C., et al. Mutations in GBA are associated with familial Parkinson disease susceptibility and age at onset. *Neurology* **72**, 310–316 (2009).

303. Neudorfer, O., et al. Occurrence of Parkinson's syndrome in type I Gaucher disease. *QJM* **89**, 691–694 (1996).

304. Goker-Alpan, O., et al. The spectrum of parkinsonian manifestations associated with

glucocerebrosidase mutations. *Arch Neurol* **65**, 1353–1357 (2008).

305. Mata, I. F., et al. Glucocerebrosidase gene mutations: a risk factor for Lewy body disorders. *Arch Neurol* **65**, 379–382 (2008).

306. Bras, J., et al. Genetic analysis implicates APOE, SNCA and suggests lysosomal dysfunction in the etiology of dementia with Lewy bodies. *Hum Mol Genet* **23**, 6139–6146 (2014).

307. Horowitz, M., et al. The human glucocerebrosidase gene and pseudogene: structure and evolution. *Genomics* **4**, 87–96 (1989).

308. Reiner, O., Wigderson, M., & Horowitz, M. Structural analysis of the human glucocerebrosidase genes. *DNA* **7**, 107–116 (1988).

309. Dinur, T., et al. Human acid beta-glucosidase: isolation and amino acid sequence of a peptide containing the catalytic site. *Proc Natl Acad Sci U S A* **83**, 1660–1664 (1986).

310. Reiner, O., Wilder, S., Givol, D., & Horowitz, M. Efficient in vitro and in vivo expression of human glucocerebrosidase cDNA. *DNA* **6**, 101–108 (1987).

311. Reiner, O., & Horowitz, M. Differential expression of the human glucocerebrosidase-coding gene. *Gene* **73**, 469–478 (1988).

312. Wigderson, M., et al. Characterization of mutations in Gaucher patients by cDNA cloning. *Am J Hum Genet* **44**, 365–377 (1989).

313. Doll, R. F., & Smith, F. I. Regulation of expression of the gene encoding human acid beta-glucosidase in different cell types. *Gene* **127**, 255–260 (1993).

314. Xu, Y. H., Wenstrup, R., & Grabowski, G. A. Effect of cellular type on expression of acid beta-glucosidase: implications for gene therapy in Gaucher disease. *Gene Ther* **2**, 647–654 (1995).

315. Hruska, K. S., LaMarca, M. E., Scott, C. R., & Sidransky, E. Gaucher disease: mutation and polymorphism spectrum in the glucocerebrosidase gene (GBA). *Hum Mutat* **29**, 567–583 (2008).

316. Nalls, M. A., et al. Large-scale meta-analysis of genome-wide association data identifies six new risk loci for Parkinson's disease. *Nat Genet* **46**, 989–993 (2014).

317. Lill, C. M., et al. Comprehensive research synopsis and systematic meta-analyses in Parkinson's disease genetics: The PDGene database. *PLoS Genet* **8**, e1002548 (2012).

318. Keller, M. F., et al. Using genome-wide complex trait analysis to quantify "missing heritability" in Parkinson's disease. *Hum Mol Genet* **21**, 4996–5009 (2012).

319. Lomen-Hoerth, C. Characterization of amyotrophic lateral sclerosis and frontotemporal

dementia. *Dement Geriatr Cogn Disord* **17**, 337–341 (2004).

320. Trojsi, F., et al. Functional overlap and divergence between ALS and bvFTD. *Neurobiol Aging* **36**, 413–423 (2015).

321. Lattante, S., Ciura, S., Rouleau, G. A., & Kabashi, E. Defining the genetic connection linking amyotrophic lateral sclerosis (ALS) with frontotemporal dementia (FTD). *Trends Genet* **31**, 263–273 (2015).

322. Burrell, J. R., Kiernan, M. C., Vucic, S., & Hodges, J. R. Motor neuron dysfunction in frontotemporal dementia. *Brain* **134**, 2582–2594 (2011).

323. Lomen-Hoerth, C., Anderson, T. & Miller, B. The overlap of amyotrophic lateral sclerosis and frontotemporal dementia. *Neurology* **59**, 1077–1079 (2002).

324. Ringholz, G. M., et al. Prevalence and patterns of cognitive impairment in sporadic ALS. *Neurology* **65**, 586–590 (2005).

325. Feiguin, F., et al. Depletion of TDP-43 affects Drosophila motoneurons terminal synapsis and locomotive behavior. *FEBS Lett* **583**, 1586–1592 (2009).

326. Van Deerlin, V. M., et al. TARDBP mutations in amyotrophic lateral sclerosis with TDP-43 neuropathology: a genetic and histopathological analysis. *Lancet Neurol* **7**, 409–416 (2008).

327. DeJesus-Hernandez, M., et al. Expanded GGGGCC hexanucleotide repeat in noncoding region of C9ORF72 causes chromosome 9p-linked FTD and ALS. *Neuron* **72**, 245–256 (2011).

328. Renton, A. E., et al. A hexanucleotide repeat expansion in C9ORF72 is the cause of chromosome 9p21-linked ALS-FTD. *Neuron* **72**, 257–268 (2011).

329. Bennion Callister, J., & Pickering-Brown, S. M. Pathogenesis/genetics of frontotemporal dementia and how it relates to ALS. *Exp Neurol* **262 Pt B**, 84–90 (2014).

330. Guerreiro, R., Bras, J., & Hardy, J. SnapShot: genetics of ALS and FTD. *Cell* **160**, 798, e1 (2015).

331. Rosen, D. R., et al. Mutations in Cu/Zn superoxide dismutase gene are associated with familial amyotrophic lateral sclerosis. *Nature* **362**, 59–62 (1993).

332. Deng, H. X., et al. Amyotrophic lateral sclerosis and structural defects in Cu,Zn superoxide dismutase. *Science* **261**, 1047–1051 (1993).

333. Orrell, R. W., Marklund, S. L., & deBelleroche, J. S. Familial ALS is associated with mutations in all exons of SOD1: a novel mutation in exon 3 (Gly72Ser). *J Neurol Sci* **153**, 46–49 (1997).

334. Cudkowicz, M. E., et al. Epidemiology of mutations in superoxide dismutase in amyotrophic lateral sclerosis. *Ann Neurol* **41**, 210–221 (1997).

335. Al-Chalabi, A., et al. Recessive amyotrophic lateral sclerosis families with the D90A SOD1 mutation share a common founder: evidence for a linked protective factor. *Hum Mol Genet* **7**, 2045–2050 (1998).

336. Millecamps, S., et al. SOD1, ANG, VAPB, TARDBP, and FUS mutations in familial amyotrophic lateral sclerosis: genotype-phenotype correlations. *J Med Genet* **47**, 554–560 (2010).

337. Gitcho, M. A., et al. TARDBP 3'-UTR variant in autopsy-confirmed frontotemporal lobar degeneration with TDP-43 proteinopathy. *Acta Neuropathol* **118**, 633–645 (2009).

338. Saberi, S., Stauffer, J. E., Schulte, D. J., & Ravits, J. Neuropathology of Amyotrophic Lateral Sclerosis and Its Variants. *Neurol Clin* **33**, 855–876 (2015).

339. Niwa, J., et al. Disulfide bond mediates aggregation, toxicity, and ubiquitylation of familial amyotrophic lateral sclerosis-linked mutant SOD1. *J Biol Chem* **282**, 28087–28095 (2007).

340. Sherman, L., Dafni, N., Lieman-Hurwitz, J., & Groner, Y. Nucleotide sequence and expression of human chromosome 21-encoded superoxide dismutase mRNA. *Proc Natl Acad Sci U S A* **80**, 5465–5469 (1983).

341. Barra, D., et al. The complete amino acid sequence of human Cu/Zn superoxide dismutase. *FEBS Lett* **120**, 53–56 (1980).

342. Jabusch, J. R., Farb, D. L., Kerschensteiner, D. A., & Deutsch, H. F. Some sulfhydryl properties and primary structure of human erythrocyte superoxide dismutase. *Biochemistry* **19**, 2310–2316 (1980).

343. Hirano, M., et al. Multiple transcripts of the human Cu, Zn superoxide dismutase gene. *Biochem Biophys Res Commun* **276**, 52–56 (2000).

344. Rosen, D. R., et al. A frequent ala 4 to val superoxide dismutase-1 mutation is associated with a rapidly progressive familial amyotrophic lateral sclerosis. *Hum Mol Genet* **3**, 981–987 (1994).

345. Kuhnlein, P., et al. Two German kindreds with familial amyotrophic lateral sclerosis due to TARDBP mutations. *Arch Neurol* **65**, 1185–1189 (2008).

346. Ou, S. H., Wu, F., Harrich, D., Garcia-Martinez, L. F., & Gaynor, R. B. Cloning and characterization of a novel cellular protein, TDP-43, that binds to human immunodeficiency virus type 1 TAR DNA sequence motifs. *J Virol* **69**, 3584–3596 (1995).

347. Buratti, E., et al. Nuclear factor TDP-43 and SR proteins promote in vitro and in vivo CFTR exon 9 skipping. *EMBO J* **20**, 1774–1784 (2001).

348. Wang, H. Y., Wang, I. F., Bose, J., & Shen, C. K. Structural diversity and functional implications

of the eukaryotic TDP gene family. *Genomics* **83**, 130–139 (2004).

349. Benajiba, L., et al. TARDBP mutations in motoneuron disease with frontotemporal lobar degeneration. *Ann Neurol* **65**, 470–473 (2009).

350. Kawahara, Y., & Mieda-Sato, A. TDP-43 promotes microRNA biogenesis as a component of the Drosha and Dicer complexes. *Proc Natl Acad Sci U S A* **109**, 3347–3352 (2012).

351. Ling, S. C., et al. ALS-associated mutations in TDP-43 increase its stability and promote TDP-43 complexes with FUS/TLS. *Proc Natl Acad Sci U S A* **107**, 13318–13323 (2010).

352. McDonald, K. K., et al. TAR DNA-binding protein 43 (TDP-43) regulates stress granule dynamics via differential regulation of G3BP and TIA-1. *Hum Mol Genet* **20**, 1400–1410 (2011).

353. Di Carlo, V., et al. TDP-43 regulates the microprocessor complex activity during in vitro neuronal differentiation. *Mol Neurobiol* **48**, 952–963 (2013).

354. Freischmidt, A., Muller, K., Ludolph, A. C., & Weishaupt, J. H. Systemic dysregulation of TDP-43 binding microRNAs in amyotrophic lateral sclerosis. *Acta Neuropathol Commun* **1**, 42 (2013).

355. Sreedharan, J., et al. TDP-43 mutations in familial and sporadic amyotrophic lateral sclerosis. *Science* **319**, 1668–1672 (2008).

356. Yokoseki, A., et al. TDP-43 mutation in familial amyotrophic lateral sclerosis. *Ann Neurol* **63**, 538–542 (2008).

357. Gitcho, M. A., et al. TDP-43 A315T mutation in familial motor neuron disease. *Ann Neurol* **63**, 535–538 (2008).

358. Kabashi, E., et al. TARDBP mutations in individuals with sporadic and familial amyotrophic lateral sclerosis. *Nat Genet* **40**, 572–574 (2008).

359. Synofzik, M., et al. Targeted high-throughput sequencing identifies a TARDBP mutation as a cause of early-onset FTD without motor neuron disease. *Neurobiol Aging* **35**, 1212, e1–5 (2014).

360. Kovacs, G. G., et al. TARDBP variation associated with frontotemporal dementia, supranuclear gaze palsy, and chorea. *Mov Disord* **24**, 1843–1847 (2009).

361. Rademakers, R., Cruts, M., & van Broeckhoven, C. The role of tau (MAPT) in frontotemporal dementia and related tauopathies. *Hum Mutat* **24**, 277–295 (2004).

362. Hutton, M., et al. Association of missense and 5'-splice-site mutations in tau with the inherited dementia FTDP-17. *Nature* **393**, 702–705 (1998).

363. Hong, M., et al. Mutation-specific functional impairments in distinct tau isoforms of hereditary FTDP-17. *Science* **282**, 1914–1917 (1998).

364. Goedert, M., Spillantini, M. G., Potier, M. C., Ulrich, J., & Crowther, R. A. Cloning and sequencing of the cDNA encoding an isoform of microtubule-associated protein tau containing four tandem repeats: differential expression of tau protein mRNAs in human brain. *EMBO J* **8**, 393–399 (1989).

365. Varani, L., et al. Structure of tau exon 10 splicing regulatory element RNA and destabilization by mutations of frontotemporal dementia and parkinsonism linked to chromosome 17. *Proc Natl Acad Sci U S A* **96**, 8229–8234 (1999).

366. Rizzu, P., et al. High prevalence of mutations in the microtubule-associated protein tau in a population study of frontotemporal dementia in the Netherlands. *Am J Hum Genet* **64**, 414–421 (1999).

367. Verpillat, P., et al. Association between the extended tau haplotype and frontotemporal dementia. *Arch Neurol* **59**, 935–939 (2002).

368. Conrad, C., et al. Genetic evidence for the involvement of tau in progressive supranuclear palsy. *Ann Neurol* **41**, 277–281 (1997).

369. Baker, M., et al. Association of an extended haplotype in the tau gene with progressive supranuclear palsy. *Hum Mol Genet.* **8**, 711–715 (1999).

370. Litvan, I., Baker, M., & Hutton, M. Tau genotype: no effect on onset, symptom severity, or survival in progressive supranuclear palsy. *Neurology* **57**, 138–140 (2001).

371. Pittman, A. M., et al. The structure of the tau haplotype in controls and in progressive supranuclear palsy. *Hum Mol Genet.* **13**, 1267–1274 (2004).

372. Rademakers, R., et al. High-density SNP haplotyping suggests altered regulation of tau gene expression in progressive supranuclear palsy. *Hum Mol Genet* **14**, 3281–3292 (2005).

373. Pittman, A. M., et al. Linkage disequilibrium fine mapping and haplotype association analysis of the tau gene in progressive supranuclear palsy and corticobasal degeneration. *J Med Genet.* **42**, 837–846 (2005).

374. Kwok, J. B., et al. Glycogen synthase kinase-3beta and tau genes interact in Alzheimer's disease. *Ann Neurol* **64**, 446–454 (2008).

375. Piguet, O., et al. Clinical phenotypes in autopsy-confirmed Pick disease. *Neurology* **76**, 253–259 (2011).

376. Goedert, M., Spillantini, M. G., Jakes, R., Rutherford, D., & Crowther, R. A. Multiple isoforms of human microtubule-associated protein tau: sequences and localization in neurofibrillary tangles of Alzheimer's disease. *Neuron* **3**, 519–526 (1989).

377. Andreadis, A., Brown, W. M., & Kosik, K. S. Structure and novel exons of the human tau gene. *Biochemistry* **31**, 10626–10633 (1992).

378. Conrad, C., Vianna, C., Freeman, M., & Davies, P. A polymorphic gene nested within an intron of the tau gene: implications for Alzheimer's disease. *Proc Natl Acad Sci U S A* **99**, 7751–7756 (2002).

379. Whitwell, J. L., et al. Atrophy patterns in IVS10+16, IVS10+3, N279K, S305N, P301L, and V337M MAPT mutations. *Neurology* **73**, 1058–1065 (2009).

380. Boxer, A. L., et al. Clinical, neuroimaging and neuropathological features of a new chromosome 9p-linked FTD-ALS family. *J Neurol Neurosurg Psychiatry* **82**, 196–203 (2011).

381. van der Zee, J., et al. A pan-European study of the C9orf72 repeat associated with FTLD: geographic prevalence, genomic instability, and intermediate repeats. *Hum Mutat* **34**, 363–373 (2013).

382. Smith, B. N., et al. The C9ORF72 expansion mutation is a common cause of ALS+/-FTD in Europe and has a single founder. *Eur J Hum Genet* **21**, 102–108 (2013).

383. Gomez-Tortosa, E., et al. C9ORF72 hexanucleotide expansions of 20–22 repeats are associated with frontotemporal deterioration. *Neurology* **80**, 366–370 (2013).

384. Baker, M., et al. Mutations in progranulin cause tau-negative frontotemporal dementia linked to chromosome 17. *Nature* **442**, 916–919 (2006).

385. Cruts, M., et al. Null mutations in progranulin cause ubiquitin-positive frontotemporal dementia linked to chromosome 17q21. *Nature* **442**, 920–924 (2006).

386. Le Ber, I., et al. Progranulin null mutations in both sporadic and familial frontotemporal dementia. *Hum Mutat* **28**, 846–855 (2007).

387. Bruni, A. C., et al. Heterogeneity within a large kindred with frontotemporal dementia: a novel progranulin mutation. *Neurology* **69**, 140–147 (2007).

388. Gijselinck, I., et al. Progranulin locus deletion in frontotemporal dementia. *Hum Mutat* **29**, 53–58 (2008).

389. Mackenzie, I. R. The neuropathology and clinical phenotype of FTD with progranulin mutations. *Acta Neuropathol* **114**, 49–54 (2007).

390. Yu, C. E., et al. The spectrum of mutations in progranulin: a collaborative study screening 545 cases of neurodegeneration. *Arch Neurol* **67**, 161–170 (2010).

391. Rademakers, R., et al. Common variation in the miR-659 binding-site of GRN is a major risk factor for TDP43-positive frontotemporal dementia. *Hum Mol Genet* **17**, 3631–3642 (2008).

392. Bhandari, V., & Bateman, A. Structure and chromosomal location of the human granulin gene. *Biochem Biophys Res Commun* **188**, 57–63 (1992).

393. He, Z., & Bateman, A. Progranulin gene expression regulates epithelial cell growth and promotes tumor growth in vivo. *Cancer Res* **59**, 3222–3229 (1999).

394. Liau, L. M., et al. Identification of a human glioma-associated growth factor gene, granulin, using differential immuno-absorption. *Cancer Res* **60**, 1353–1360 (2000).

395. He, Z., Ong, C. H., Halper, J., & Bateman, A. Progranulin is a mediator of the wound response. *Nat Med* **9**, 225–229 (2003).

396. Ashcroft, G. S., et al. Secretory leukocyte protease inhibitor mediates non-redundant functions necessary for normal wound healing. *Nat Med* **6**, 1147–1153 (2000).

397. Zhu, J., et al. Conversion of proepithelin to epithelins: roles of SLPI and elastase in host defense and wound repair. *Cell* **111**, 867–878 (2002).

398. Tangkeangsirisin, W., & Serrero, G. PC cell-derived growth factor (PCDGF/GP88, progranulin) stimulates migration, invasiveness and VEGF expression in breast cancer cells. *Carcinogenesis* **25**, 1587–1592 (2004).

399. Hu, F., et al. Sortilin-mediated endocytosis determines levels of the frontotemporal dementia protein, progranulin. *Neuron* **68**, 654–667 (2010).

400. Tang, W., et al. The growth factor progranulin binds to TNF receptors and is therapeutic against inflammatory arthritis in mice. *Science* **332**, 478–484 (2011).

401. Park, B., et al. Granulin is a soluble cofactor for toll-like receptor 9 signaling. *Immunity* **34**, 505–513 (2011).

402. Huang, K., et al. Progranulin is preferentially expressed in patients with psoriasis vulgaris and protects mice from psoriasis-like skin inflammation. *Immunology* **145**, 279–287 (2015).

403. van der Zee, J., et al. A Belgian ancestral haplotype harbours a highly prevalent mutation for 17q21-linked tau-negative FTLD. *Brain* **129**, 841–852 (2006).

404. Brouwers, N., et al. Alzheimer and Parkinson diagnoses in progranulin null mutation carriers in an extended founder family. *Arch Neurol* **64**, 1436–1446 (2007).

405. Rademakers, R., et al. Tau negative frontal lobe dementia at 17q21: significant finemapping of the candidate region to a 4.8 cM interval. *Mol Psychiatry* **7**, 1064–1074 (2002).

406. Mackenzie, I. R., et al. A family with tau-negative frontotemporal dementia and neuronal intranuclear inclusions linked to chromosome 17. *Brain* **129**, 853–867 (2006).

407. Rohrer, J. D., et al. Parietal lobe deficits in frontotemporal lobar degeneration caused by a

mutation in the progranulin gene. *Arch Neurol* **65**, 506–513 (2008).

408. Mukherjee, O., et al. HDDD2 is a familial frontotemporal lobar degeneration with ubiquitin-positive, tau-negative inclusions caused by a missense mutation in the signal peptide of progranulin. *Ann Neurol* **60**, 314–322 (2006).

409. Mukherjee, O., et al. Molecular characterization of novel progranulin (GRN) mutations in frontotemporal dementia. *Hum Mutat* **29**, 512–521 (2008).

410. Shankaran, S. S., et al. Missense mutations in the progranulin gene linked to frontotemporal lobar degeneration with ubiquitin-immunoreactive inclusions reduce progranulin production and secretion. *J Biol Chem* **283**, 1744–1753 (2008).

411. Chen-Plotkin, A. S., et al. Genetic and clinical features of progranulin-associated frontotemporal lobar degeneration. *Arch Neurol* **68**, 488–497 (2011).

412. Huey, E. D., et al. Characteristics of frontotemporal dementia patients with a Progranulin mutation. *Ann Neurol* **60**, 374–380 (2006).

413. Mesulam, M., et al. Progranulin mutations in primary progressive aphasia: the PPA1 and PPA3 families. *Arch Neurol* **64**, 43–47 (2007).

414. Davion, S., et al. Clinicopathologic correlation in PGRN mutations. *Neurology* **69**, 1113–1121 (2007).

415. Rademakers, R., et al. Phenotypic variability associated with progranulin haploinsufficiency in patients with the common 1477C-->T (Arg493X) mutation: an international initiative. *Lancet Neurol* **6**, 857–868 (2007).

416. Seelaar, H., et al. Distinct genetic forms of frontotemporal dementia. *Neurology* **71**, 1220–1226 (2008).

417. Morris, J. C., Cole, M., Banker, B. Q., & Wright, D. Hereditary dysphasic dementia and the Pick-Alzheimer spectrum. *Ann Neurol* **16**, 455–466 (1984).

418. Froelich, S., et al. Mapping of a disease locus for familial rapidly progressive frontotemporal dementia to chromosome 17q12–21. *Am J Med Genet* **74**, 380–385 (1997).

419. Basun, H., et al. Clinical characteristics of a chromosome 17-linked rapidly progressive familial frontotemporal dementia. *Arch Neurol* **54**, 539–544 (1997).

420. Skoglund, L., et al. Frontotemporal dementia in a large Swedish family is caused by a progranulin null mutation. *Neurogenetics* **10**, 27–34 (2009).

421. Kelley, B. J., et al. Alzheimer disease-like phenotype associated with the c.154delA mutation in progranulin. *Arch Neurol* **67**, 171–177 (2010).

422. Moreno-Luna, R., et al. Two independent apolipoprotein A5 haplotypes modulate postprandial lipoprotein metabolism in a healthy Caucasian population. *J Clin Endocrinol Metab* **92**, 2280–2285 (2007).

423. Borroni, B., et al. Progranulin genetic variations in frontotemporal lobar degeneration: evidence for low mutation frequency in an Italian clinical series. *Neurogenetics* **9**, 197–205 (2008).

424. Krefft, T. A., Graff-Radford, N. R., Dickson, D. W., Baker, M., & Castellani, R. J. Familial primary progressive aphasia. *Alzheimer Dis Assoc Disord* **17**, 106–112 (2003).

425. Gydesen, S., Hagen, S., Klinken, L., Abelskov, J., & Sorensen, S. A. Neuropsychiatric studies in a family with presenile dementia different from Alzheimer and Pick disease. *Acta Psychiatr Scand* **76**, 276–284 (1987).

426. Brown, J., et al. Familial non-specific dementia maps to chromosome 3. *Hum Mol Genet* **4**, 1625–1628 (1995).

427. Gydesen, S., et al. Chromosome 3 linked frontotemporal dementia (FTD-3). *Neurology* **59**, 1585–1594 (2002).

428. Skibinski, G., et al. Mutations in the endosomal ESCRTIII-complex subunit CHMP2B in frontotemporal dementia. *Nat Genet* **37**, 806–808 (2005).

429. Poduslo, S. E., et al. A familial case of Alzheimer's disease without tau pathology may be linked with chromosome 3 markers. *Hum Genet* **105**, 32–37 (1999).

430. van der Zee, J., et al. CHMP2B C-truncating mutations in frontotemporal lobar degeneration are associated with an aberrant endosomal phenotype in vitro. *Hum Mol Genet* **17**, 313–322 (2008).

431. Cannon, A., et al. CHMP2B mutations are not a common cause of frontotemporal lobar degeneration. *Neurosci Lett* **398**, 83–84 (2006).

432. Momeni, P., et al. Genetic variability in CHMP2B and frontotemporal dementia. *Neurodegener Dis* **3**, 129–133 (2006).

433. Babst, M., Katzmann, D. J., Estepa-Sabal, E. J., Meerloo, T., & Emr, S. D. Escrt-III: an endosome-associated heterooligomeric protein complex required for mvb sorting. *Dev Cell* **3**, 271–282 (2002).

434. Urwin, H., et al. Disruption of endocytic trafficking in frontotemporal dementia with CHMP2B mutations. *Hum Mol Genet* **19**, 2228–2238 (2010).

435. Parkinson, N., et al. ALS phenotypes with mutations in CHMP2B (charged multivesicular body protein 2B). *Neurology* **67**, 1074–1077 (2006).

436. Cox, L. E., et al. Mutations in CHMP2B in lower motor neuron predominant amyotrophic lateral sclerosis (ALS). *PLoS One* **5**, e9872 (2010).

437. Vance, C., et al. Mutations in FUS, an RNA processing protein, cause familial amyotrophic

lateral sclerosis type 6. *Science* **323**, 1208–1211 (2009).

438. Hewitt, C., et al. Novel FUS/TLS mutations and pathology in familial and sporadic amyotrophic lateral sclerosis. *Arch Neurol* **67**, 455–461 (2010).

439. Yan, J., et al. Frameshift and novel mutations in FUS in familial amyotrophic lateral sclerosis and ALS/dementia. *Neurology* **75**, 807–814 (2010).

440. Aman, P., et al. Expression patterns of the human sarcoma-associated genes FUS and EWS and the genomic structure of FUS. *Genomics* **37**, 1–8 (1996).

441. Morohoshi, F., et al. Genomic structure of the human RBP56/hTAFII68 and FUS/TLS genes. *Gene* **221**, 191–198 (1998).

442. Eneroth, M., et al. Localization of the chromosomal breakpoints of the t(12;16) in liposarcoma to subbands 12q13.3 and 16p11.2. *Cancer Genet Cytogenet* **48**, 101–107 (1990).

443. Crozat, A., Aman, P., Mandahl, N., & Ron, D. Fusion of CHOP to a novel RNA-binding protein in human myxoid liposarcoma. *Nature* **363**, 640–644 (1993).

444. Mrozek, K., Karakousis, C. P., & Bloomfield, C. D. Chromosome 12 breakpoints are cytogenetically different in benign and malignant lipogenic tumors: localization of breakpoints in lipoma to 12q15 and in myxoid liposarcoma to 12q13.3. *Cancer Res* **53**, 1670–1675 (1993).

445. Perrotti, D., et al. TLS/FUS, a pro-oncogene involved in multiple chromosomal translocations, is a novel regulator of BCR/ABL-mediated leukemogenesis. *EMBO J* **17**, 4442–4455 (1998).

446. Yang, L., Embree, L. J., & Hickstein, D. D. TLS-ERG leukemia fusion protein inhibits RNA splicing mediated by serine-arginine proteins. *Mol Cell Biol* **20**, 3345–3354 (2000).

447. Wang, X., et al. Induced ncRNAs allosterically modify RNA-binding proteins in cis to inhibit transcription. *Nature* **454**, 126–130 (2008).

448. Rabbitts, T. H., Forster, A., Larson, R., & Nathan, P. Fusion of the dominant negative transcription regulator CHOP with a novel gene FUS by translocation t(12;16) in malignant liposarcoma. *Nat Genet* **4**, 175–180 (1993).

449. Vance, C., et al. ALS mutant FUS disrupts nuclear localization and sequesters wild-type FUS within cytoplasmic stress granules. *Hum Mol Genet* **22**, 2676–2688 (2013).

450. Kwiatkowski, T. J., Jr., et al. Mutations in the FUS/TLS gene on chromosome 16 cause familial amyotrophic lateral sclerosis. *Science* **323**, 1205–1208 (2009).

451. Sapp, P. C., et al. Identification of two novel loci for dominantly inherited familial amyotrophic lateral sclerosis. *Am J Hum Genet* **73**, 397–403 (2003).

452. Ruddy, D. M., et al. Two families with familial amyotrophic lateral sclerosis are linked to a novel locus on chromosome 16q. *Am J Hum Genet* **73**, 390–396 (2003).

453. Corrado, L., et al. Mutations of FUS gene in sporadic amyotrophic lateral sclerosis. *J Med Genet* **47**, 190–194 (2010).

454. Waibel, S., Neumann, M., Rabe, M., Meyer, T., & Ludolph, A. C. Novel missense and truncating mutations in FUS/TLS in familial ALS. *Neurology* **75**, 815–817 (2010).

455. Lill, C. M., Abel, O., Bertram, L., & Al-Chalabi, A. Keeping up with genetic discoveries in amyotrophic lateral sclerosis: the ALSoD and ALSGene databases. *Amyotroph Lateral Scler* **12**, 238–249 (2011).

456. Ferrari, R., Hardy, J., & Momeni, P. Frontotemporal dementia: from Mendelian genetics towards genome wide association studies. *J Mol Neurosci* **45**, 500–515 (2011).

457. Ferrari, R., et al. Frontotemporal dementia and its subtypes: a genome-wide association study. *Lancet Neurol* **13**, 686–699 (2014).

458. Diekstra, F. P., et al. C9orf72 and UNC13A are shared risk loci for amyotrophic lateral sclerosis and frontotemporal dementia: a genome-wide meta-analysis. *Ann Neurol* **76**, 120–133 (2014).

459. Maruyama, H., et al. Mutations of optineurin in amyotrophic lateral sclerosis. *Nature* **465**, 223–226 (2010).

460. Freischmidt, A., et al. Haploinsufficiency of TBK1 causes familial ALS and fronto-temporal dementia. *Nat Neurosci* **18**, 631–636 (2015).

461. Pottier, C., et al. Whole-genome sequencing reveals important role for TBK1 and OPTN mutations in frontotemporal lobar degeneration without motor neuron disease. *Acta Neuropathol* **130**, 77–92 (2015).

462. Gijselinck, I., et al. Loss of TBK1 is a frequent cause of frontotemporal dementia in a Belgian cohort. *Neurology* **85**, 2116–2125 (2015).

463. Tsai, P. C., et al. Mutational analysis of TBK1 in Taiwanese patients with amyotrophic lateral sclerosis. *Neurobiol Aging* **40**, 191e11–191e16 (2016).

464. Goldstein, O., et al. OPTN 691_692insAG is a founder mutation causing recessive ALS and increased risk in heterozygotes. *Neurology* **86**, 446–453 (2016).

11

An Epigenetics Perspective on Diseases of the Central Nervous System

DIEGO F. MASTROENI

WHAT IS EPIGENETICS?

All cells in the body contain the same DNA. What then determines whether a cell will become skin, muscle, neuron, or glia? What mechanisms dictate that some cells atrophy, age, and die, whereas immediately adjacent cells with the same DNA remain functional? And what overarching mechanisms can help account for the enormous connectional plasticity required for learning and memory? Epigenetics may help answer some of these questions.

The term *epigenetics* is generally attributed to Waddington's (1942) seminal work in developmental biology, where he referred to this type of study as the "causal mechanisms" by which "the genes of the genotype bring about phenotypic effects." Since then, the term has come to have different meanings to different people. For example, epigenetics has been defined as "the study of mitotically and/or meiotically heritable changes in gene function that cannot be explained by changes in DNA sequence," "the entire series of interactions among cells and cell products which leads to morphogenesis and differentiation," as well as "heritable changes that do not involve changes in DNA sequence" (1). Unfortunately, most of these definitions hinge on the heritability of epigenetic mechanisms, a key concept in the earlier developmental biology research on epigenetics that may be less appropriate today, particularly with respect to neuroepigenetic mechanisms of brain function and dysfunction. The key to a definition of epigenetics may lie essentially in its prefix, *epi-* (over, above, or before). Epigenetics is the set of overarching mechanisms that regulate subsequent genetic mechanisms and, thereby, the myriad biological pathways that follow from selective gene transcription and expression. In this chapter we adopt the simple and broad definition of epigenetics as those mechanisms that affect the structure of chromatin to regulate the availability of selected components of the genome for transcription.

The roles of epigenetics can be viewed from a number of different perspectives, but here we emphasize the role of epigenetics in the modulation of gene expression. The ability of epigenetic mechanisms to broadly modulate gene expression is indicative of the importance of epigenetics in development, in diseases of the brain and the body, in learning and memory, in effects of environmental exposures—in fact, in all the changes of phenotype that take place from fertilization to death. There are two broad categories of mechanisms by which epigenetic changes may modulate gene expression: (1) those that operate at the level of DNA to alter accessibility of DNA for transcription, and (2) those that operate at the level of transcription by modulating translation of messenger RNA to protein.

Epigenetic Mechanisms at the Level of DNA

To comprehend epigenetic mechanisms at the level of DNA, it is best to visualize the structure of the nucleosome, which consists of a segment of DNA wrapped around a core made up of histone protein molecules. Thread wrapped around a spool is a reasonably approximate visualization. However, the entire DNA is not wrapped around one spool, but rather 146–147 base pairs of DNA are wrapped around one histone core two and a half times (2). These strung-together protein/DNA (histone DNA) complexes form what is known as chromatin. When DNA is tightly wrapped around the histone "spool" and the nucleosomes (spool plus DNA) are tightly packed together, the chromatin is "closed" and DNA is not accessible to transcription factors, RNA polymerase, and other modulators (2, 3). In other words, the DNA is not accessible to the mechanisms of transcription. On the other hand, when a segment of chromatin is "open," or permissive, a gene, or genes, within that segment are available to the transcription machinery and can be expressed (3). There are two basic epigenetic mechanisms that regulate the winding/unwinding of DNA around the histone spool and the spacing of the spools (i.e., the structure of chromatin). These are DNA methylation/ hydroxymethylation and histone modifications.

DNA Methylation

In DNA methylation a methyl group (CH3) is placed on the fifth carbon of cytosine, and this modification is generally considered to have a repressive effect on the structure of chromatin. However, it must be emphasized that this repression is frequently not the case for many reasons, including complex interactions among DNA methylation, hydroxymethylation, histone modifications, and other proteins.

DNA methylation typically takes place at the tens of millions of cytosine-guanine dinucleotides (CpG) sequences in the human genome, but methylation at non-CpG sites is also common. Unmethylated CpG sites frequently cluster in "CpG islands," often in the regulatory regions of genes that are to be expressed. DNA methylation by itself may impede the binding of the transcription machinery to DNA.

It is now well established that the cytosine base can be methylated by the actions of the DNA methyltransferases DNMT1, DNMT2, DNMT3a/b, and DNMT4. Current research has implicated DNMT1 as the primary maintenance enzyme that targets hemimethylated DNA after DNA replication, whereas DNMT3a and DNMT3b are particularly important for *de novo* methylation. The generation of the methyl group transferred to cytosine by the DNMTs is derived from folate through its interactions with S-adenosylmethionine (SAM) and, further upstream, the one-carbon metabolic cycle (4). The addition of a methyl group to the cytosine base attracts methyl CpG binding domain proteins (MBDs), which in turn recruit histone-modifying proteins (see later discussion) to alter chromatin structure (Figure 11.1). More recently it has become known that rather than DNA methylation, ten-eleven translocation (TET) enzymes can modulate the formation of a hydroxyl group (OH) at the fifth carbon of cytosine to form a hydroxymethylated site. The possible functions of hydroxymethylation are under intense investigation.

Histone Modifications

Histone modifications play crucial roles in regulating the structure of chromatin and, consequently,

the ability of transcription machinery to access the DNA of specific genes. Structurally, one may consider the histone molecules as the core that contributes to the formation of the "spool," and a tail. The histones that form the core are histones H2A, H2B, H3, and H4, each of which has a tail. The histone modifications that are important to the structure of chromatin take place at specific amino acid sites along the histone tails. Here, histone acetyltransferases (HATs) catalyze the transfer of an acetyl group from acetyl-coenzyme A to lysine residues on the N-termini of histone proteins. Conversely, the histone deacetylases (HDACs) transfer acetyl groups from acetylated histone proteins back to coenzyme A, producing a more condensed chromatin state and decreased or silenced gene transcription. Recent studies have suggested that histone acetylation and deacetylation are dynamic, rapid-turnover processes that can "poise" genes for transcription (5). The types of modifications that take place on histone tails include methylation, acetylation, phosphorylation, ubiquitination, and palmitoylation. In specifying histone modifications, the histone involved is listed first, then the amino acid and its location on the histone tail, and, finally, the nature of the modification. Thus, H3K9ac signifies acetylation of lysine 4 of histone H3.

Selected histone modifications are known to be repressive or permissive for gene expression. For example, H3K4me3 and H3K9ac are associated with active transcription of the genes on which these modifications are found. On the other hand, H3K27me3 or H3K9me2/3 are associated with repression of expression (6). It is important to note that multiple histone modifications, as well as DNA methylations, often interact to produce a final common result—chromatin structure.

MicroRNA

Although the existence of microRNA has been known for about 25 years, it was not until the first decade of the 2000s that their role as epigenetic regulators of gene expression began to be recognized. MicroRNAs are products of gene expression that recognize target messenger RNAs (mRNAs) by complementarity of a short sequence of nucleotides, usually about 19–25 nucleotides in length (reviewed in 7, 8). The binding of microRNA to specific mRNA disrupts translation by a variety of mechanisms. Because the binding can occur with only a relatively short sequence of nucleotides, any given microRNA can bind to and modulate translation of large numbers of mRNAs. This also means that any given mRNA can be affected by multiple

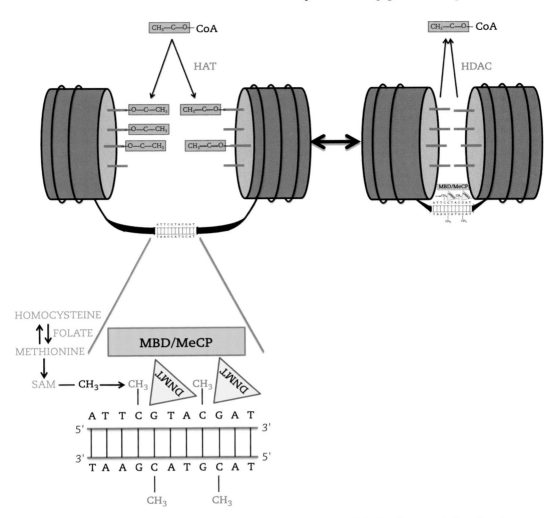

FIGURE 11.1. Simplified schematic of histone acetylation and DNA methylation. In transcriptionally active genes the chromatin, made up of histones (blue cylinders) around which DNA is wrapped, is in a relaxed state, permitting transcriptional access to unwound DNA. This relaxed, euchromatin state is, in part, mediated by acetylation of histone tails (red rods) in which acetyl groups (green blocks) are transferred from acetyl-coenzyme A (acetyl-CoA) to the histone tails by histone acetyltransferases (HATs). (Bottom left) Within the DNA, the cytosines of adjacent C-G dinucleotides (CpGs) may be methylated. The methyl group ultimately derives from folate as part of the methionine/ homocysteine cycle, and is transferred from S-adenosylmethionine (SAM) to the cytosine by DNA methyltransferases (DNMTs). CpG-methyl-binding-domain proteins (MBDs) and methylation complex proteins (MeCPs) (which may contain MBDs) become associated with methylated CpGs, further inhibiting transcriptional access and repression of the gene. (Upper right) DNA methylation and histone modifications are integrally linked, because MBDs and MeCPs attract histone deacetylases (HDACs) that transfer acetyl groups on the histone tail back to CoA. Histone deacetylation, in turn, promotes the condensed, heterochromatin state characteristic of silenced or repressed genes.

Figure reproduced with permission from Mastroeni et al. (2011), *Neurobiology of Aging*.

microRNAs binding at different sequences of the target RNA. Such wide-ranging capacities of microRNAs allow them to play significant roles in events that require coordinated changes in expression of large numbers of genes, such as during development, learning and memory, and many diseases. Thus, multiple binding capacities of microRNAs lead to a role in the coordination of expression of large numbers of genes required to execute complex changes in phenotype.

BRIEF OVERVIEW OF METHODS FOR EPIGENETIC INVESTIGATION

Methods to Quantify DNA Methylation

Although a number of methods for examination of DNA methylation exist, the most common are global methylation, methylation sensitive restriction enzymes, methylated DNA immunoprecipitation (MeDIP), and bisulfite conversion, the most widely used technique.

Global methylation levels are determined using an antibody to 5-methylcytosine for such downstream applications as histochemistry, cytochemistry, enzyme-linked immunosorbent assays (ELISAs), and dot blots. Although these methods are adequate, they are not without ambiguity, as will be seen in the coming sections.

Nucleotide specific methylation is accomplished by sodium bisulfite conversion of the DNA. Sodium bisulfite deaminates cytosine bases to uracil unless the 5' cytosine carbon is already methylated (i.e., 5-methylcytosine or 5-hydroxymethylcytosine). With PCR amplification, the uracils become thymines and the unmodified 5-methylcytosines (or 5-hydroxymethylcytosines) become cytosines (9). Comparison to the original sequence then reveals sites at which the cytosines were initially methylated (or hydroxymethylated). Downstream applications of bisulfite-treated DNA include methylation-specific PCR (10), bisulfite sequencing (9), pyrosequencing (11), BeadChip arrays (12), and next-generation sequencing (13). A weakness of bisulfite conversion is that it does not differentiate 5-methylcytosine from 5-hydroxymethylcytosine. The two less common methods for nucleotide-specific analysis, which are gaining momentum, use either methylation-sensitive restriction enzymes (e.g., HpaII and MspI) (14) or MeDIP, an enrichment technique wherein methyl CpG binding domain proteins (e.g., MBD2) are employed to pull down methylated DNA (15). Both of these methods consistently use PCR for downstream applications, but other methods have been reported (15).

Analysis of other DNA modifications (e.g., hydroxymethylation) are gaining relevance but not with the same vigor as methylated DNA assays. Common methods of analysis for determining 5-hydroxymethylation (5hMeC) include global 5hMeC levels using antibody-based technology; oxidative bisulfite sequencing, which introduces an additional oxidative step to the aforementioned bisulfite method (16); and TET-assisted bisulfite sequencing, which relies on the TET enzyme to discriminate between 5hMeC and 5MeC (17). Likewise, J-binding protein-1 (JB-1) has been used in pull-down assays to bind to glucosylated enriched hydroxymethylated DNA that is then simply separated from its methylated counterpart (18). Downstream applications range from global to sequence- and locus-specific analysis (18).

Methods to Determine Histone Modifications Levels

Analysis of histone proteins (e.g., histone 3) and the post-translational modifications (e.g., lysine 4 tri-methylation) are primarily accomplished using basic immunohistochemical/cytochemical methods, as well as the more refined chromatin immunoprecipitation method (ChIP) (19). Briefly, chromatin extracts are fixed, sheared into smaller fragments, incubated with an antibody to a specific post-translational modification, and analyzed, invariably by gene-specific PCR. However, more recent work has focused on whole-genome chromatin immunoprecipitation sequencing (CHIP-seq) (20). This genome-wide profiling is a step up from its array-based predecessor, ChIP-chip (21), but effective computational analysis is still in question (22).

Methods to Determine the Expression of MicroRNA

Unlike the large chromatin dependent methods, microRNA (miRNA) analysis is focused on significantly smaller stretches of nucleotides, ~22 base pairs long. Isolation of miRNAs is typically accomplished by phenol-chloroform/guanidinium extraction of RNA, size fractionation, column-based cleanup, and the addition of stem-loop structure or poly-A tail. From here, further investigation is conducted using one of several technologies: miRNA qPCR (23), miRNA array (24), or RNA-sequencing (RNAseq) (25). The latter is the most sophisticated of the three, combining high-throughput sequencing on next-generation platforms. Unlike the array-based and standard qPCR methods, RNAseq is not limited to specific sequences selected by the scientist; it is unbiased in that all individual nucleotides in the sequence are quantified without the need of primer design. Although this method has remarkable coverage, it has nowhere near the sensitivity of qPCR methods; in fact, most studies follow up the aforementioned methods with qPCR validation (26).

Ultimately, all of the methods have specific applications that depend on the experimental questions asked, the number of samples available, and cost. Each assay has weaknesses, some more than others.

AN EPIGENETICS PERSPECTIVE ON ALZHEIMER'S DISEASE

Alzheimer's Disease (AD) is a progressive, irreversible neurodegenerative disorder culminating in dementia. Clinically, AD is characterized by a decline in multiple cognitive functions (27). Although the field is evolving to address interindividual variability of the clinical presentations of the disease, the frequency of overlap between neurodegenerative diseases generally presents a major problem.

Pathologically, the classical diagnostic hallmarks of AD, amyloid β peptide plaques and neurofibrillary tangles, still remain much the same as those in Alois Alzheimer's seminal report on AD. However, it has become increasingly recognized that AD is likely to be a multifactorial disorder, with many aberrant biological events that contribute to its pathogenesis and progression—perhaps none of which is absolute. In fact, the most salient risk factor for developing AD is age. This makes the etiology and pathogenesis of AD particularly difficult to dissect because most, if not all, of the best-studied abnormalities in AD also occur with age, including increased inflammation, altered glucose and energy metabolism, protein misfolding, synaptic dysfunction, mitochondrial dysfunction, oxidative stress, and abnormalities in lysosomal/proteasomal pathways, to name a few. Although these parallels between aging and AD provide interpretive problems, they may also provide clues to the importance of epigenetics, since one of the best-known drivers of aging processes is epigenetic mechanisms (28). Perhaps they, too, drive many of the changes in AD (Table 11.1).

From the standpoint of genetics, with the exception of the rare 3% of familial, early-onset AD cases, no one gene seems to predict the outcome for the more common late-onset AD cases (LOAD). Although there are polymorphisms in genes that increase risk, such as the E4 variant of apolipoprotein E (*ApoE*) gene (29, 30), none has complete penetrance. This makes defining the disease based on genetic standards quite as difficult as defining it on clinical and pathological standards.

Global DNA Methylation Analysis

In an attempt to address the genetic and environmental complexities of AD, the field of epigenetics has exploded in the last decade. With respect to DNA methylation, two major methods of analysis

TABLE 11.1. ADDITIONAL EPIGENETIC MODIFICATION IN ALZHEIMER'S DISEASE

	References
DNA Methylation	
(Hypo)methylation in AD brain/blood/model	(32–34, 39, 45, 47, 48, 51, 52, 59, 61, 185, 198–217)
(Hyper)methylation in AD brain/blood/model	(37, 39, 40, 59, 212, 214, 215, 218–222)
No change in methylation in AD brain/blood/model	(46, 50, 223–226)
Histone Alterations	
Histone alterations and related molecules (e.g., HDACs, HATs, methylation, phosphorylation) in AD brain/blood/model	(32, 78, 79, 89, 195, 199, 227–238)
MicroRNA	
Upregulation of microRNAs in AD brain/blood/model	(239–260)
Downregulation of microRNAs in AD brain/blood/model	(75, 76, 246, 251, 261–268)
No change in microRNAs in AD brain/blood/model	(259, 260)

have been performed: nucleotide-specific methylation and global methylation levels. The latter has yielded some very interesting results, but not without ambiguity. As observed in normal aging (31), in 2008 Mastroeni and colleagues reported significant immunohistochemical decrements (hypomethylation) in DNA methylation levels in the entorhinal cortex using the first generation of antibodies to 5-methylcytosine (32). This research was followed by a study, in 2009, wherein temporal cortex samples from monozygotic twins discordant for AD were analyzed using the same methods. Despite having identical DNA, the AD twin showed a significant decrease in levels of DNA methylation compared to his unaffected sibling, consistent with the previous findings (33). These results were confirmed several years later by an independent researcher at another institution using hippocampus CA1 samples, albeit from the same AD Brain Bank as the Mastroeni samples (34). Similarly, studies employing an in vitro cell model (H4-sw) harboring the Swedish mutation found that of the 6,296 differentially methylated genes, 77% were hypomethylated (35). In contrast, Lashley and colleagues, using immunocytochemical and ELISA methods, reported that there was no significant difference in DNA methylation levels between AD and controls (36), and Coppieters and colleagues found a significant increase in DNA methylation levels in the middle frontal gyrus and middle temporal gyrus of AD cases (37).

The reasons for these conflicting results remain unclear. It could be that in the antibody studies the sample sizes were relatively small, the tissues were prepared differently, antibody specificities may have differed, and postmortem intervals and immuohistochemial methods were not equivalent. For example, the study conducted by Lashley and colleagues reported a mean postmortem interval of 59 hours for the brain samples, nearly 56 hours longer than samples used in the Mastroeni and Chorlleius studies. Likewise, Coppieters reported an average postmortem interval of nearly 14 hours. Although further research is needed to confirm or refute the preceding findings, it is the case that they paved the way to a new wave of research on the epigenetics of AD.

More recently, epigenetic-wide association studies (EWAS) have looked at multiple CpG sites per gene across the entire human genome using bisulfite conversion, followed by hybridization on Illumna Infinium 450k chips. The most recent publications by Jager (38, 39) and by Mills (40) both revealed only modest changes in global DNA methylation levels among AD brains compared to control brains. However, both studies were able to identify a similar pattern of hypermethylation in the ankyrin 1 (ANK1) gene across multiple cortical regions, including replication in several additional, independent sample cohorts (39, 40). One of the most interesting findings regarding the list of the most affected genes was that it contained very few of the most commonly studied molecules in AD research. This may be due to the complexity of the regulation of gene expression that extends well beyond DNA methylation, as well as the inability to account for different types of neurons or disease states.

Despite important advances, global methylation analysis at the level of the entire genome is still in its infancy and faces a number of significant technical problems, from analysis to probe design (41, 42). The future of global methylation analysis will involve the more expensive, but necessary genome-wide next-generation sequencing-based approaches in order to analyze every methylated nucleotide in the human genome, but these approaches, too, have their own complexities, particularly with respect to large-scale data analysis methods.

Gene-Specific DNA Methylation Studies on AD-Specific Genes
Amyloid Precursor Protein

Analysis of DNA methylation data using bisulfite sequencing has been primarily focused on the pathogenic pathway of amyloid beta peptide (Aβ). The literature covering the amyloid cascade is extensive and thoroughly reviewed (43, 44). Briefly, Aβ is approximately 39–42 amino acids in length, embedded within a larger molecule, the amyloid precursor protein (APP). Cleavage of APP by the enzyme α-secretase cuts APP near the midpoint of Aβ, so that no intact Aβ can be formed. However, cleavage of APP at the N-terminus of Aβ by the enzyme β-secretase (BACE) and at the C-terminus of Aβ by the γ-secretase complex can release Aβ species of various lengths. The most intensely studied species are Aβ40 and Aβ42, the latter being generally considered the more toxic of the two. Mutations in the APP gene or in the genes coding for two members of the γ-secretase complex, presenilin 1 (PSEN-1) and presenilin 2 (PSEN-2) are known to cause hereditary AD. Wide ranges of neurotoxic effects, from synapse damage to stimulation of inflammation, have been reported for Aβ.

Analyses of the APP Promoter

Preliminary studies using array and single-base technology were quick to analyze the CpG-rich regions within the promoter of the APP gene, the typical sites of gene activation. Reports from human brain (45) to human blood (46) to human cells (47) have shown site-specific hypomethylation in diseased samples. More recent studies, however, have found significant hypermethylation of the APP gene in sporadic AD cases using pyrosequencing methods (48). As described previously, this method allows for deeper sequencing and greater coverage over the length of the gene. Further complicating interpretation of these results, other studies in humans have found no significant differences in APP promoter methylation (49, 50).

Proteolytic Enzymes and Proteolytic Mediators That Cleave APP

The obvious next pathways for the analysis of epigenetic modifications of the amyloid cascade were the enzymes that mediate production of the various lengths of Aβ. Over the past decade, many studies have shown that BACE activity is directly related to its methylation levels, which, in turn, are dependent on folate/B_{12} levels (51). *In vitro* exposure of cultured neurons to folate/B_{12}-deficient medium results in hypomethylation of PS1 and BACE, increased PS1 and BACE expression, and enhanced Aß production (52, 53). Similarly, exposure of APP-overexpressing transgenic mice to a folate/B_{12}/B_6-deficient diet is associated with PS1 and BACE upregulation, increased γ-secretase activity, enhanced Aß deposition, and an accelerated appearance of intraneuronal Aß and cognitive deficits (54). Treatment with s-adenosylmethionine, a substrate for methyl-group transfer, reduces the expression of PS1 and Aß production, making a strong case for an environmental influence on APP regulators. In fact, many studies have shown that the environment inside and outside our bodies can influence the epigenetic signature in a wide range of enzymatic genes (55–57). Finally, neprilysin (NEP), an enzymatic protein that degrades Aß (58), is conversely affected. It has been shown that Aβ peptide induces hypermethylation of the NEP gene (59), downregulating the expression of this very important clearing mechanism (60).

Molecules That Regulate Tau

A second classical neuropathological hallmark of AD is the neurofibrillary tangle, a fibrillar inclusion in neurons that occurs throughout the AD cortex. Like Aβ, neurofibrillary tangles have been intensely studied as an important pathogenic factor in AD, including research on epigenetic markers associated with tau, a phosphoprotein and a major constituent of neurofibrillary tangles that normally interacts with tubulin to stabilize and promote assembly of microtubules. As we have reported in a previous review (61), in normal adults the AP2 binding site of the tau promoter is demethylated, whereas the SP1 (transcriptional activator site) and GCF binding sites (promoter repressor site) are significantly methylated with increasing age, suggesting an overall downregulation of tau gene expression (62). Although an age-related decrease in normal tau protein has been reported, there was no correlation with neurofibrillary tangle pathology in the same subjects (63).

Moreover, tau phosphorylation mechanisms are subject to cytoplasmic alterations, and have been the subject of many reports. Our studies, for example, showed co-localized immunoreactivity for the methyl binding complex component p66α, HDAC1, and DNMT1 with PHF1-positive neurofibrillary tangles (64). Furthermore, PP2A

is an enzyme that can remove phosphate groups from hyperphosphorylated tau, an action that may be potently activated by methylation of the PP2A catalytic subunit at its L309 site. In N2a cultured cells carrying the APP Swedish mutation (APPswe) and in APPswe/PS1 transgenic mice, levels of demethylated PP2A at L309 were significantly upregulated, corresponding with increases in tau phosphorylation at the Tau-1 and PHF-1 sites (65). Zhou and colleagues have shown that treatment with Aß25-35 led to demethylation and enhanced tau phosphorylation (66). Similarly, exposure of rodent primary neuron cultures to methotrexate (folate antagonist) results in demethylation of PP2A, with an increase in tau phosphorylation, APP, and BACE (67). Vena caudalis injection of homocysteine into rats for 2 weeks yielded decreased PP2A (Leu) 309 methylation and PP2A activity; administration of folate and vitamin B_{12} reversed this affect. Hippocampal samples from both rats and AD patients exhibited immunohistochemical co-localization of demethylated, but not methylated PP2A with hyperphosphorylated tau (68).

Moreover, an imbalance between phosphorylation (kinases) and de-phosphorylation (phosphatases) has been suggested to be a causative factor in AD pathogenesis in general and aberrant tau pathology in particular. Thus, studies of the methylation status of the serine/threonine kinase, glycogen synthase kinase 3 beta (GSK3β), and the phosphatase PP2A have been strongly associated with tau hyperphosphorylation levels (69). The authors further suggest that alterations in one-carbon metabolism (e.g., vitamin B deficiency) are responsible for the disequilibrium between kinases and phosphatases observed in AD (70).

MicroRNAs

Epigenetic regulation occurs not only with respect to DNA, but also with respect to RNA in the form of the newest epigenetic mediators, microRNA (miRNA). These small, ~22 nucleotides have promise as the next wave of therapeutic targets to treat AD, particularly because of the association with synapse formation and neurite outgrowth (71, 72), both of which are affected in the earliest stages of AD (73). Over the past few years this promise has motivated investigators to examine the complexity of miRNA, and considerable efforts have been expended toward study of the 1,400 (and counting) miRNAs in the human genome. Studies by Lukiw and colleagues several years ago were some of the first to address differences between miRNAs miR-9, miR-124a, miR-125b, miR-128, miR-132, and miR-219 in development, aging, and AD (74). These early reports, showing that alterations in miRNA exist in select disease states, generated great interest in scaling up efforts to use genome-wide technology toward better understanding the roles of microRNAs in both brain and blood.

In brain, investigators have identified several key miRNAs that reliably turn up as potential therapeutic targets for gene manipulation. For example, miR-29a, -29b-1, and -9 were found to be significantly reduced in AD and to correlate significantly with changes in BACE1 activity *in vitro* (75). These correlations were further tested to determine causation by showing that manipulation of the miR-29a/b-1 cluster resulted in an increase in Aβ production. Likewise, Wang and colleagues determined that another miRNA, miR-107, decreased early in the course of disease, exhibiting an inverse correlation with BACE1 activity (76). Both studies strongly implicate multiple miRNAs in accelerated disease pathogenesis through the regulation of BACE1 activity.

Though research into brain miRNAs is gaining momentum, the most significant push in the field is in peripheral compartments. The reason for this is that blood and all of its components are easily accessible using relatively noninvasive methods. Thus, if blood changes in miRNAs are found to be a reliable surrogate of brain changes, they may have great potential utility as a biomarker. Using next-generation sequencing, Leidinger and colleagues identified 140 unique miRNAs that were significantly altered in peripheral blood of AD patients (77). Of the 140 miRNAs identified, 12 were used to develop what the authors termed a "12-miRNA signature." This signature was able to differentiate AD and controls with a reported accuracy of 93%, which represents improvement over accuracy achieved in primary care offices. Differentiating between AD and other neurodegenerative diseases was lower, however (74%–78%). Although these findings are important in distinguishing disease versus non-disease, the current emphasis is on finding blood changes before the onset of disease. For this reason, Wang and colleagues recruited amnestic mild cognitive impairment (MCI) cases for their studies. Based on miRNA-107 levels in plasma, the investigators were able to discriminate between MCI cases and healthy controls with 91.9% accuracy, 98.3% sensitivity, and 82.7% specificity (76). These data and others (Table 11.1) show that miR-107 expression levels in plasma may be a significant candidate in discriminating between the early stages of disease and healthy control cases. Although these studies suggest promise, it remains to be seen whether they will be successfully replicated in other laboratories and in the clinic.

Seeking Answers in the Histone Code

Although cytosine methylation embodies the bulk of epigenetic studies, histone tail alterations and their modification-specific enzymes could be even more clinically and pathologically relevant. Hundreds of publications have shown histone changes from mislocalization of key histone molecules to post-translational modifications of the histone proteins (Table 11.1). Immunohistochemical studies have shown an increase in histone 3 phosphorylation in AD hippocampal neurons (78), and an upregulation of a non-nuclear form of histone 1 in astrocytes and neurons (79). Protein-protein association studies have shown that linker Histone H1 preferentially binds Aβ-42, as well as Aβ-like structures of numerous proteins (80). In addition, the H1 molecule has been shown to target poly-(ADP-ribosyl)ation in high pathology areas in the AD brain (81).

Moreover, manipulation of histone tails with HDAC inhibitors has been investigated in several animal models of AD. Treatment with the HDAC inhibitor Trichostatin A, for example, increased acetylated H4 levels and contextual freezing performance to wild-type values in APP/PS1 mice (82). Treatment with HDAC inhibitors has also been shown to increase the number of synapses, and to re-establish access to long-term memories (83, 84). Another HDAC inhibitor, valproic acid, has been shown to decrease Aβ production and plaque burden in the brains of AD transgenic mice (85). Similarly, a daily dose of phenylbutyrate in the Tg2576 mouse model of AD normalized levels of phosphorylated tau, but failed to alter Aβ levels (86). In a cellular model, overexpression of APP resulted in a decrease in histone 3 and histone 4 acetylation, as well as a decrease in CREB-binding protein levels (87, 88). The most recent and promising work has focused on the manipulation of HDAC6. Investigators have identified selective HDAC6 inhibitors (e.g., tubastatin A and ACY-1215), both of which have been shown to rescue cognitive deficits in AD mice (89, 90). With these studies in mind, Sung and colleagues have developed HDAC inhibitors (HDACI) with improved pharmacological properties such as stability and blood–brain barrier penetration. They show that two specific HDACIs, mercaptoacetamide (class II HDACI) and hydroxamide-based (class I HDACI), decrease the expression of beta and gamma secretase, and increase the expression of Aβ degradation enzymes, while mercaptoacetamide decreases tau phosphorylation at Thr181(91).

It is evident from the literature that histone modifications are integral components for active learning, memory, and storage consolidation, which are altered in AD, AD-like animal models, and AD-like cellular models (Table 11.1). The biggest conundrum with respect to HDACs is specificity, or the lack thereof. The patterns of changes in HDACs are too complex for one class of current HDAC manipulations to address both histone acetylation increases and decreases at specific loci, not to mention crossing the blood–brain barrier.

AN EPIGENETIC PERSPECTIVE ON PARKINSON'S DISEASE

Parkinson's disease (PD), like Alzheimer's, is a progressive, irreversible neurodegenerative disorder culminating in a host of debilitating motor and non-motor features. Clinically, PD is characterized by the presence of resting tremors, rigidity, loss of postural reflexes, and bradykinesia (92). Pathologically, PD is characterized by the loss of dopamine neurons in the substantia nigra pars compacta, but other neocortical brain regions have also been reported to be affected (92). Neurons residing in these pathogenic regions are often riddled with cytoplasmic inclusions known as Lewy bodies. These inclusions consist of α-synuclein-containing protein aggregates that become fibrillar and neurotoxic in the later stages of disease (93). The α-synuclein gene (*SNCA*) was the first gene identified to harbor a mutation, and is by far the most studied of all PD-related genes. Although a broad understanding of the clinical presentations and pathological features of PD are known, the origin of the disease, particularly in those with sporadic PD, is unknown. Although several disease-causing mutations exist (94), 90% of cases are considered sporadic.

Global DNA Methylation Analysis

The role of DNA methylation in the pathogenesis of PD is several years behind AD methylation studies, but early reports indicate similar phenomena. Desplats and colleagues reported a significant reduction in DNA methylation in the frontal cortex of PD cases (95). The authors also found a strong association with the ectopic localization of DNMT1 and subsequent alterations to the "normal" methylation patterns, similar to findings from our laboratory in AD (32, 96). Using the infinium Human 450K beadchip, Masliah and colleagues analyzed brain and blood samples from PD and normal control cases. The investigators determined that 317 probes in the brain and 476 probes in the blood were hypermethylated, while 2,591 and 3,421 respectfully, were hypomethylated (97). Further work conducted in a larger cohort also identified many of the same hypomethylated/hypermethylated PD-related genes. For example, further genome-wide methylation studies by several investigators found significantly hypomethylated genes in both brain (CYPE1) (Kaut et al. 2012) and blood (PER1, PER2, CRY1, CRY2, Clock, NPAS2 and BMAL1) (Lin et al. 2012). These data indicate that DNA methylation may be a major player in the disease process. Future work addressing the heterogeneity in both brain and blood will be extremely important. Without knowing the exact classes of cells that are affected or the sites of methylation changes, pharmacologic or other therapies would be difficult to conceive.

DNA Methylation Studies on PD-Specific Genes

Much as in AD, Parkinson's investigators have focused on gene-causing mutations such as those occuring in *SNCA, PARK2, UCHL1, DJ1*, and *LRRK2*, although genome-wide methylation studies indicate that other genes may be just as important (Table 11.2). In fact, several investigators have determined that many of the disease-causing mutations in genes such as *PARK2* show no significant difference in methylation levels between PD carriers, PD non-carriers, and normal control subjects (98). Similar results have been found in analyzing the UCHL1 promoter in PD, which revealed no significant differences (49). Perhaps this is because the focus of these studies was to detect changes in flanking specific sites within the promoter region, whereas hundreds of other influential sites are contained in the gene.

α-Synuclein Encoding Gene, SNCA

The disease-causing mutations in the *SNCA* gene, on the other hand, have led to much work both at methylation and expression levels. Genome-wide association studies and gene-specific studies have demonstrated a strong association between *SNCA* variability and susceptibility to developing PD (99, 100). Likewise, many studies, looking at both brain and blood, have made strong cases for association between promoter methylation levels of non-mutated *SNCA* and disease risk. Pihlstrom and colleagues, for example, assessed variant 1 of the *SNCA* gene and found a significant reduction in DNA methylation levels in PD cases compared to normal controls (101). This association

TABLE 11.2. ADDITIONAL EPIGENETIC MODIFICATION IN PARKINSON'S DISEASE

	References
DNA Methylation	
(Hypo)methylation in PD brain/blood/model	(95, 102, 103, 269–277)
(Hyper)methylation in PD brain/blood/model	(270–272)
No change in methylation in PD brain/blood/model	(49, 103, 278–280)
Histone Alterations	
Histone alterations and related molecules (e.g., HDACs, HATs, methylation, phosphorylation) in PD brain/blood/model	(87, 108, 109, 281–288)
MicroRNA	
Upregulation of microRNAs AD brain/blood/model	(289–291)
Downregulation of microRNAs in PD brain/blood/model	(105, 290, 292–302)
No change in microRNAs in PD brain/blood/model	(303–305)

was detected in both brain and blood, although it was stronger in blood. In another complementary study analyzing SNCA methylation in blood, Tan and colleagues analyzed 14 different CpG sites within the SNCA promoter region, one of which flanked intron 1. Among the 14 CpG sites, four were found to be significantly hypomethylated in PD, including the CpG site within variant 1 (102). As one would predict, both studies showed an increase in SNCA mRNA levels when the active sites were hypomethylated. Likewise, Matsumoto and colleagues studied the same CpG island within intron 1 in the brain of PD cases, and they too determined significant decrements in methylation levels, as well as the same association between methylation and the expression of the SNCA gene (103). These data indicate that methylation patterns in brain SNCA genes can parallel those in blood, and that alterations in methylation can contribute to the increase in expression of the SNCA gene observed in disease.

MicroRNAs

As noted, because of the accessibility of blood compared to brain, the most clinically relevant target for biomarkers of disease progression in PD may lie in analysis of circulating miRNAs. Moreover, of all the epigenetic marks, miRNAs are of particular interest because of their ability to specifically reduce the expression of key overexpressing pathogenic genes (e.g., SNCA).

To date, there are 20 or so miRNAs that have been implicated in PD (Table 11.2), but two, miR-7 and miR-153, show the greatest promise (104, 105). Human α-synuclein mRNA has a 3'-UTR, which is the preferential binding site for both miR-7 and miR-153 (105). Upon binding, these miRNAs destabilize α-synuclein mRNA, resulting in a decrease in the rate of translation. In fact, PD models have been used to identify the specificity of miR-7 and miR-153 by blocking their function with specific anti-miRNA inhibitors, which resulted in an increase in α-synuclein production (105, 106). Experiments from the same investigators using overexpression models of the same miRNAs found significantly reduced endogenous α-synuclein, and protection against cytotoxicity and oxidative stress (104, 105). Interestingly, they also reported that miR-7 and miR-153 have a synergistic relationship, in that they work better together. These data indicate that MiR-7 and miR-153 might be used as pharmacological tools to rewrite the α-synuclein signaling pathway in PD, provided that the findings are applicable to sporadic PD and not simply to PD involving mutations to the SNCA gene (the model system on which the previous research was based). It is also the case that, although miRNAs hold great promise to restore "normal" function in the early stages of PD, there is a notable lack of evidence for change in miRNAs in early PD.

Seeking Answers in the Histone Code

As described earlier, both promoter methylation and miRNA binding sites within the promoter region are important determinants of transcriptional state. However, histone modifications are the true regulators of open (euchromatin) or closed (heterochromatin) chromatin structure (reviewed in Figure 11.1). More than a decade has passed since the first reports of histone proteins and their involvement in the pathogenesis of PD (107). Since these initial reports, the majority of the field has moved from living systems to cellular models in an attempt to address the heterogeneity and molecular mechanism(s) that contribute to disease.

It has been known for some time that α-synuclein directly binds to histone H3, and inhibits histone acetylation (107, 108), presumably through inhibition of some unknown selective histone acetyltransferases (HATs) or the activation of histone deacetylases (HDACs). In fact, non-specific HDAC inhibitors (e.g., sodium butyrate) have been used successfully to minimize the effect of α-synuclein on H3 acetylation (108). Another study, using a different PD model and a different non-specific HDAC inhibitor (valproic acid), also found the same neuroprotective effects and similar increases in histone acetylation (109). More recent work, however, has focused on more selective HDAC inhibitors, such as NAD-dependent protein deacetylase sirtuin-2 (SIRT2). Outeiro and colleagues have identified specific SIRT2 inhibitors that rescue α-synuclein-induced toxicity in several dosing models and in genetic knock-down models (110, 111). In addition to its actions on HDAC activity, α-synuclein also appears to inhibit HAT pathways. For example, using α-synuclein transgenic mice, Jin and colleagues found that α-synuclein negatively regulates p300 levels and its HAT activity, reducing protein kinase Cδ expression (112), a key oxidative stress kinase that has been associated with apoptotic processes, particularly in dopaminergic neurons (113, 114).

Collectively these findings and many others (see Table 11.2) suggest the need for studies that determine the proper balance between HATs and HDACs. A whole host of other inhibitors, both specific and non-specific, competitive and non-competitive, have been identified as useful therapeutic targets for PD (Table 11.2), but the future is not in finding more specific inhibitors, but rather (1) determining the balance between HDACs and HATs, and (2) determining how to affect a specific cell or class of cells.

AN EPIGENETIC PERSPECTIVE ON AMYOTROPHIC LATERAL SCLEROSIS

Amyotrophic lateral sclerosis (ALS) is the third most common neurodegenerative disorder. It primarily affects motor neurons in the cerebral cortex, brainstem, and spinal cord, which develop cytoplasmic inclusions containing ubiquitin, transactive response (TAR) DNA-binding protein (TDP-43), and other elements (reviewed in 115). Clinical presentation typically includes weakness in the hands, feet, legs, and ankles, often leading to walking difficulties and clumsiness. Muscle cramps/twitching, slurring of speech, and trouble swallowing are also classical hallmarks of the disease (115). Like AD and PD, several

disease-causing mutations (e.g., *SOD1*) have been identified in ALS, but most cases are sporadic, and the sporadic and familial forms are clinically and neuropathologically indistinguishable (115). Also like AD and PD, there is an emerging consensus that the pathogenesis of ALS may be multifactorial, including much recent work on epigenetic mechanisms (Table 11.3).

Global DNA Methylation Analysis

Global immunohistochemical studies of DNA methylation levels have shown an accumulation of the 5meC mark in diseased motor neurons in spine and in brain, suggesting hypermethylation. Displacement of the 5hmeC mark was also observed in astrocytes (116). Global methylation levels in sporadic ALS have also been analyzed in a handful of candidate genes (*SOD1*, *VEGF*, and *EAAT2*). Although none thus far has revealed significant alterations (117, 118), genome-wide analysis of human brain using chromatin immunoprecipitation technology, followed by microarray hybridization, has identified new candidate genes for sporadic ALS, many of which have previously received little attention.

TABLE 11.3. ADDITIONAL EPIGENETIC MODIFICATION IN ALS

	References
DNA Methylation	
(Hypo)methylation in ALS brain/blood/model	(118–120, 306)
(Hyper)methylation in ALS brain/blood/model	(116, 119, 120, 307–309)
No change in methylation in ALS brain/blood/model	(117, 310–312)
Histone Alterations	
Histone alterations and related molecules (e.g., HDACs, HATs, methylation, phosphorylation) in ALS brain/blood/model	(127, 128, 313–327)
MicroRNA	
Upregulation of microRNAs in ALS brain/blood/model	(121, 328–340)
Downregulation of microRNAs in ALS brain/blood/model	(330, 340, 341)
No change in microRNAs in ALS brain/blood/model	(330)

Genes encoding calcium channels (*CACNA1B* and *CACNA1C*) were found to be significantly hypermethylated, while genes encoding neurexin-1 (*NRXN1*), glial cell-derived neurotrophic factor receptors (*GFRA1* and *GFRA2*), and phospholipid metabolism (*PLA2G4C*) were significantly hypomethylated (119).

Further studies on postmortem ALS and control spinal cord using more sophisticated bead-chip arrays have yielded interesting findings primarily targeted to inflammation and innate immunity (120). In addition to gene-specific alterations, the investigators analyzed global changes in methylation and hydroxymethylation levels by ELISA and determined that both were upregulated in ALS, a phenomenon they attribute to the overactivation of the key methylating enzyme DNMT1 (120). Collectively, it will be important to extend these studies on DNA methylation in ALS to specific cell classes (e.g., astrocytes, microglia, vascular cells, neurons) to identify specific targets for cell-based therapy.

MicroRNAs

As previously discussed, miRNAs may represent a reliable and specific epigenetic modification that could prove useful in terms of identifying and targeting disease-causing genes. This would be particularly valuable in ALS, where only a handful of disease-causing genes have been reported. To date, one of the most promising leads follows from research on a skeletal muscle microRNA, miR-206. Because the effects of ALS are muscular in nature, Williams and colleagues investigated involvement of miR-206 in the bidirectional signaling between neurons, skeletal muscle fibers, and their synapses. In a mouse model of ALS, they showed that deficiencies in miR-206 accelerate disease progression (121), which is likely due to the fact that miR-206 is required for efficient regeneration of neuromuscular synapses after injury (122). Further analysis of skeletal muscle also revealed interesting findings in mitochondrial genes, which are also known to be affected in ALS. Investigators identified several miRNAs—miR-23a, miR-29b, miR-206 and miR-455—all of which were upregulated in ALS patients compared to normal control subjects (123).

Not only has work been done on individual miRNAs (Table 11.3), there has also been recent attention to changes in the miRNA machinery. Dicer deletion, a major step in miRNA processing (reviewed in 124), resulted in progressive paralysis, axonopathy, and astrocytosis, which are all common features in the pathogenesis of ALS (125). Research into the drosha complex, another miRNA processing step, has also demonstrated that TDP-43 directly binds to the drosha complex, thereby inhibiting another very important miRNA processing step (126).

Seeking Answers in the Histone Code

Because histone tail modification is fundamental to the expression of all genes, it makes sense to screen candidate ALS-related genes for these epigenetic modifications. For this reason, investigators worldwide have screened a large number of pan-HDAC inhibitors in ALS, particularly class I and II inhibitors (e.g., valproic acid [VPA], sodium phenylbutyrate [SPB], and trichostatin A [TSA]), which have been tested in the SOD1 mouse model of ALS and in humans. In 2011, Yoo and Ko injected SOD1-G93A mice with TSA, a potent inhibitor of HDAC function, and found that inhibition led to motor neuron survival and protection from axonal degeneration. These studies also showed a reduction in gliosis, muscle atrophy, and an upregulation of the glutamate transporter in spinal tissue (127). Another study using sodium phenylbutyrate (SPB) injections showed extended survival and improved clinical and neuropathological features. The investigators attributed these changes to the SPB-induced upregulation of beta cell lymphoma 2 (bcl-2), which blocks cytochrome c and caspase activation, both of which have been shown to induce apoptosis in many neurodegenerative diseases including ALS (128). SPB has been used in a clinical ALS study of safety, tolerability, and efficacy in reducing global HDAC levels. The compound appears to be tolerable with doses of 9–21 g/day, and therapeutically efficient in increasing histone acetylation levels. However, efficacy in slowing or halting the ALS disease process has not been reported (129). VPA is another HDAC inhibitor that has been assessed in clinical trials for ALS, but did not exhibit a beneficial effect on survival or disease progression (130). Interestingly, in the SOD1 mouse model of ALS, VPA treatment did show neuroprotective affects, but, as in the human studies, there was no increase in mean survival rate (131).

ALS studies with class III HDACs (e.g., SIRT 1-SIRT7) have also been pursued. One study found that the upregulation of SIRT1 was neuroprotective in SOD1 G93A mice (132), and in a complimentary study investigators found a significant decrease in SIRT1 mRNA levels in the same model (133). These findings begin to suggest that a causal relationship may exist between SIRT1 levels and motor neuron degeneration.

AN EPIGENETIC PERSPECTIVE ON HUNTINGTON'S DISEASE

Huntington's disease (HD) is an inherited progressive neurodegenerative disorder. The genetic abnormality that causes HD is an expanded CAG trinucleotide repeat within the huntingtin gene (*HTT*). A "normal" CAG repeat level on the *HTT* gene has fewer than 36 repeats. The gene is considered expanded if it has 36 or more repeats, and more than 40 always causes HD (134). Offspring of an affected parent have a 50% chance of inheriting HD. Although sporadic forms of the disease do occur, they are rare (6%–8%). Clinically, HD patients exhibit many cognitive, motor, psychiatric, and metabolic problems (reviewed in 134). Classical HD symptoms include chorea, dystonia, loss of postural reflexes, rigidity, cognitive impairment, depression, and anxiety (134). Pathologically, HD is characterized by neuronal loss in the striatum and surrounding areas. The most affected neurons are the striatal medium spiny neurons, which show recurring dendrites and shape/size alterations of the dendritic spines (135). Other features include cortical volume loss, particularly affecting large pyramidal neurons in layers III, V, and VI (136), fibrillar astrogliosis (137), and intracellular inclusions of HTT protein aggregates (135). Although a host of cellular mechanisms have been proposed as targets for HD treatment, epigenetic mechanisms have been of great interest since the late 1980s (138, 139), reviewed in Table 11.4.

Global DNA Methylation Analysis

Unlike other neurodegenerative diseases discussed in this chapter, DNA methylation studies of HD have been ongoing for nearly three decades. The first hard evidence of methylation changes came from the work of Farrer and colleagues in 1992. These investigators explored the possibility that DNA methylation levels are important factors in early-onset HD, particularly because of the role DNA methylation has on other imprinting genes. Through the analysis of 1,764 patients, it was shown that three independent mechanisms influencing age of onset may be directly mitigated by DNA methylation levels (140). Further genome-wide studies analyzing intergenerational CAG repeats were completed to determine whether changes in methylation would result in trinucleotide repeat instability. Treatment with DNA methyltransferase inhibitors (5-aza-deoxycytidine)

showed a dramatic destabilizing effect on HD genes, indicating that changes in methylation patterns during development may trigger intergenerational repeats that lead to disease (141).

Because transcriptional changes are the earliest known alterations in HD (142), Christopher and colleagues sought to determine if DNA methylation levels affect the polyglutamine expansion of the huntingtin protein. Using reduced representation bisulfite sequencing, the investigators found that the majority of genes that show expression changes in the presence of the mutated form of *HTT* underwent significant changes in DNA methylation levels (143).

Because previous work had identified a significant reduction in the G-coupled, adenosine A2A receptor, A2AR (144), Villar-Menendez and colleagues analyzed its expression and methylation/hydroxymethylation levels. Using both HD mouse models and human HD cases, the investigators were able to identify an increase in 5meC levels and a reduction in 5hmC levels in the 5'UTR region of *ADORA2A* gene in the putamen of HD patients (145). These data indicate that methylation alterations in other non-disease-causing genes may be vital in addressing the multifactorial nature of the disease.

MicroRNAs

A growing body of evidence has linked miRNA alterations to the pathogenesis of HD. MiRNA array studies performed by Lee and colleagues revealed many downregulated miRNAs (miR-22, miR-29c, miR-128, miR-132, miR-138, miR-218, miR-222, miR-344, and miR-674) in the striatum in two strains of HD-mice (146). Similar to findings in ALS, the investigators also identified decreased levels of drosha, an integral step in miRNA processing (146). Likewise, Johnson and colleagues determined that pan-neuronal miRNAs were also decreased, altering the expression of HD-related genes (147). It was suggested that these alterations might be due to the aberrant nuclear localization of the transcriptional repressor (REST) (147). Another interesting finding regarding the REST hypothesis was found through the actions of miR-22. Namely, Jovicic and colleagues have identified a causal link between miR-22 and multiple predicted targets known to be affected in HD histone deacetylase 4 (HDAC4), REST corepresor 1 (Rcor1), and regulator of G-protein signaling 2 (Rgs2). In light of these findings, investigators increased miR-22 levels in primary striatal and cortical cultures exposed to a mutated human huntingtin fragment

(Htt171-82Q), and found that miR-22 was neuroprotective at many levels (148). These findings reinforce the hypothesis that miRNAs have the ability to affect multiple neurodegenerative processes through separate mechanisms.

Recent work by Ghose and colleagues investigated whether or not deregulated miRNAs and loss of function of transcription factors recruited to mutant *HTT* aggregates could lead to an HD-like transcriptional profile. This hypothesis stems from previous work in which Ghose and colleagues identified several miRNAs (miR-125b, miR-146a, and miR-150) that were downregulated in the STHdh^{Q111}/Hdh^{Q111}cell model for HD. Using the same cell model, they were able to show that disease-causing mutations in HD do in fact induce miRNA alterations that interact with various transcription factors, leading to an HD-like transcriptional profile (e.g., p53, NFkB) (149, 150).

Seeking Answers in the Histone Code

Although much effort has been directed at determining the effect of mutant huntingtin and its physiological role in neurodegeneration, the exact mechanism still remains elusive. Multiple studies in HD, including cellular and animal models, have shown that mutant huntingtin alters HAT activity (151) (Table 11.4). It has been believed for decades that creb-binding protein (CBP) functions as a HAT and plays a critical role in neurodegeneration (152). More important, CBP sequesteration due to mutant huntingtin has been shown to lead to neuronal dysfunction (153, 154) by hypomethylating/hypoacetylating a host of HD-related genes (155, 156). Other studies have implicated CBP function in other memory-associated neurodegenerative diseases (e.g., AD, PD), which may indicate that CBP alterations found in HD are a common phenomenon among neurodegenerative diseases. In fact, primary neurons transfected with mutant huntingtin exhibit significant deficits in CBP levels and consequently global histone acetylation (157).

Another cellular model carrying HD mutations that lead to expanded polyglutamine (148Q) repeats shows a significant deficit in HAT activity compared to wild-type. This decrease in HAT activity is directly correlated with a global decrease in histone acetylation levels (158). Although it has been reported that HDAC activity is retained in primary neurons carrying the expanded polyglutamine repeats, human studies indicate that, possibly, too much activity may be influencing these wide changes in histone acetylation levels (159).

Because of the general association with an overall decrease in HAT activity in HD models, recent

TABLE 11.4. ADDITIONAL EPIGENETIC MODIFICATION IN HUNTIGNTON'S DISEASE

	References
DNA Methylation	
(Hypo)methylation in HD brain/blood/model	(141, 143, 145, 342, 343)
(Hyper)methylation in HD brain/blood/model	(143, 145)
No change in methylation in HD brain/blood/model	(344)
Histone Alterations	
Histone alterations and related molecules (e.g., HDACs, HATs, methylation, phosphorylation) in HD brain/blood/model	(156, 158, 159, 161, 163, 345–374)
MicroRNA	
Upregulation of microRNAs in AD brain/blood/model	(146, 147, 150, 375–379)
Downregulation of microRNAs in HD brain/blood/model	(146–150, 378, 380, 381)
No change in microRNAs in HD brain/blood/model	(146, 150)

work has focused on defining a therapeutic role for histone deacetylase inhibitors in a number of HD models. For example, in an attempt to address the effectiveness of HDAC targets in a model of disease, Quinti and colleagues used R6/2 HD mice to determine the overall effect of HDAC levels. They determined by multiple means that there was an increase in the expression of HDAC1, as well as decreased HDAC4, HDAC 5, and HDAC 6. However, no changes in HDAC protein levels were reported (160). Subsequent studies addressing non-selective HDAC inhibitors (e.g., SAHA, sodium butyrate) in similar model systems, including cellular and fly models, have reported that these inhibitors may be protective (161, 162), although more recent work has focused on selective HDAC targets.

Thomas and colleagues have identified a selective HDAC inhibitor, HDACi 4b, that appears to ameliorate a wide range of motor and behavioral symptoms while adjusting transcriptional abnormalities associated with HD (163). This exciting work has led to subsequent mechanistic studies demonstrating that HDACi 4b preferentially inhibits HDAC3, followed by HDAC1 (164). The same investigators also showed that three separate

HD models of disease—fly, cell, and mice—all showed suppression of HD pathogenic symptoms with HDACi 4b treatment. Although these studies are extremely promising, HDAC enzymes are as complex and ubiquitous as histone proteins themselves, and much work will need to be done to bring this basic research to the clinic.

OVERARCHING MECHANISMS AMONG NEURODEGENERATIVE DISEASES

Many commonalities have been noted among the major neurodegenerative diseases. All of these disorders tend to be age-related and progressive, to have both familial and sporadic forms that typically present with highly similar if not identical characteristics in the clinic and at autopsy, and to have common and multifactorial pathogenic antecedents, including mitochondrial, inflammatory, protein-folding, caspase, apoptosis, and oxidative stress abnormalities. Yet these disorders manifest in entirely different neural systems: the neocortex and temporal lobes in AD, the substantia nigra pars compacta in PD, the striatum in HD, and the motor cortex and spinal cord in ALS. Such outcomes are difficult to explain given a set of identical genes for the cells in cortex, nigra, striatum, motor cortex, and spinal cord. They may be less difficult to explain, however, for epigenetic mechanisms, which are designed to take a fixed gene code and produce cells with different attributes.

Especially in aging, cells of the nervous system are continually challenged with statistically inevitable insults. There is a small but tangible risk in every protein-folding event, in every cell in the human body, potentially stimulating an unintentional response. Just as epigenetic mechanisms can dictate the differential morphology and function of various cells, it seems reasonable to suggest that, in the process, epigenetic mechanisms might inadvertently lead to differential responses to common pathogenetic mechanisms. Multiple studies have shown, for instance, that neurons of the substantia nigra are exquisitely sensitive to localized or nearby inflammation (165), resulting in Parkinson's-like dopamine neuron neurodegeneration and PD symptoms. Alterations in Aβ metabolism seem to be most prominent in the neocortex and temporal lobes, as is the pathology these alterations produce. Thus, it is possible that epigenetics could explain how common neurodegenerative mechanisms nonetheless manifest in different parts of the nervous system to produce different neurologic disorders.

At the same time, much recent research has shown that a wide range of the pathogenic mechanisms in AD, PD, HD, and ALS are subject to regulation by epigenetic mechanisms. This is certainly the case for CNS innate inflammatory responses (166), Aβ metabolism and tau processing, α-synuclein generation, huntingtin-gene/protein expression, and the other pathogenetic mechanisms reviewed in this chapter. As such, a viable hypothesis may be that epigenetics could mediate both specific pathogenetic mechanisms and specific vulnerabilities of different neural systems to those pathogenetic mechanisms.

Environmental Nutrition

Because the epigenome requires a constant recycling of nutrients and bioactive food components to function normally (167), there is a clear connection between epigenetic mechanisms and nutritional elements. To the extent that these epigenetic mechanisms play a role in neurodegenerative diseases, it follows that the nutritional substrates on which epigenetic mechanisms depend may also be implicated in CNS disorders. Although cell metabolism involves thousands of bioavailable molecules and pathways, a handful of key nutritional elements are consistently reduced in neurodegenerative diseases.

B-vitamin supplementation, for example, is by far the most common vitamin prescription in neurodegenerative diseases (168). In fact, B_{12} (cobalamin) deficiencies can cause overt dementia (169) and accelerated aging (170), as manifest by decreased brain volume to the lower limits of normal in otherwise healthy individuals (171). Deficiencies in other B vitamins, such as folate, thiamine, and B_6, have also been implicated in healthy aging and neurodegeneration (168).

The reason that B vitamins are so important is because of the one-carbon metabolic pathway. The one-carbon pathway maintains genomic stability by providing critical metabolites (e.g., S-adenosylmethionine [SAM]) that directly affect gene regulation through the actions of DNA methylation and histone modifications (reviewed in 52, 172). It is through these pathways that neurodegenerative diseases might ultimately unite into one common disease. The cofactor folate, for example, has been observed to be deficient in all four of the neurodegenerative disorders considered in this chapter (173–178) and decreases in folate bioavailability lead to two important processes that also appear to be affected in these disorders: an increase in the cytotoxic sulfur-containing amino acid, homocysteine (173, 176, 179–184), and a decrease in S-adenosylmethionine (51, 52, 174, 185–188), the crucial methyl donor for DNA methylation (reviewed in the first section of this chapter). Although many of these studies have been publicly available for decades, their connection to the epigenome and their involvement in neurodegeneration is just now being realized. These studies do not imply that B vitamin supplementation will reverse or cure neurodegeneration, which appears to begin as much as 30 years before clinical presentation (189), but they do suggest that B vitamin supplementation could be beneficial in slowing down disease progression if taken early enough.

Mitochondrial Function

In many neurodegenerative diseases, including the four major disorders covered in this chapter, impaired mitochondrial function appears to be an early, common, and intensely studied link (190). Mitochondria are the primary (but not sole) intracellular source of ATP, which powers a host of metabolic processes from cell signaling to calcium homeostasis (191). In addition to ATP, other energy-related molecules such as acetyl-Coenzyme A (acetyl-CoA), S-adenosylmethionine (SAM), and NADH are either generated or regenerated in mitochondria (192). As such, mitochondrial dysfunction would likely impact virtually all neurodegenerative processes, and this is equally true with respect to epigenetic mechanisms of disease, where ATP plays a key role in gene regulation (193) and the one-carbon metabolic pathway that generates methyl groups for DNA methylation (194). A sufficiency of mitochondria-derived ATP is obviously necessary to support the millions of epigenetic modifications that regulate the expression of both normal and disease-associated genes.

We have recently suggested that mitochondrial dysfunction could be an overarching mechanism leading to the epigenetic alterations of AD (195, 196). In this research we also describe the cellular effects of multifunctional free radical quenchers and their ability to reinvigorate failing mitochondria in a cellular model of AD. Namely, the antioxidants restored availability of epigenetic-modifying enzymes (e.g., KAT6b) that are essential for modulating the structure of chromatin and, consequently, gene expression (197).

FUTURE DIRECTIONS

Epigenetics currently sits in a very exciting, non-Mendelian, post-genomic era in which it is possible to begin to address the etiology of disease by examining the complex interplay of genes with their cellular, organ, whole body, and external environments. Because the field of epigenetics is relatively new to research in neurodegeneration, it is expected that many findings now appear to be less than clear, as is the continuing definition of epigenetics itself. Alternatively, despite decades of research, the antecedents of the major neurologic disorders also remain unclear and may demand epigenetic approaches to clarify them. Geneticists, for example, have a defined space, the genome, to work in, but are confronted by the fact that many people may have gene polymorphisms that confer high risk for neurodegenerative disorders, yet remain completely healthy. Having a virtually unlimited space, the interplay of the environment with the genome, epigeneticists may have a significant advantage in explaining such findings: the penetrance of many disease-risk genes may well trace back to epigenetics.

Epigenetics is also a pivotal or translational point between the genome and the cellular, organ, and whole animal environment in which a specific cell lies. It is the means by which stimuli at all these levels of environment can dictate specific beneficial or pathological responses in individual cells or whole classes of cells. Conversely, gene expression can change the environment to affect epigenetic mechanisms. Epigenetics and gene expression are inextricably linked feedback and feedforward mechanisms, the basic elements of which will be important for understanding both normal biological function and pathological dysfunction.

Finally, there are several important technical problems with epigenetic research into neurodegenerative diseases that need to be addressed in the near future. First among these is the issue of heterogeneity within samples, particularly as it relates to genome-wide studies wherein tissue samples are ground up and analyzed. Although it is true that specific genes expressed by specific cell classes can be pulled out, many genes are ubiquitously expressed (e.g., mitochondrial, epigenetic, inflammatory, and lysosomal genes) in every major cell class in the brain. In fact, even the same class of neurons can have dichotomous expression profiles depending on location or activity level. By contrast, it is well known that disease does not affect all cells equally, even though they may be immediately adjacent to each other. Future work therefore needs to focus on specific classes of cells identified by specific markers, obtained, for example, by laser-capture microdissection or other methods. These isolation techniques allow for more precise analysis of the cells in question and more precise definition among neurons and other resident cell classes, such as astrocytes, microglia, oligodendrocytes, and vascular cells.

In summary, the future of epigenetic research will rely heavily on understanding the ever-changing environment and its effect on the relatively static genome. The interplay between the two should continue to be highly informative with respect to neurodegenerative diseases.

ACKNOWLEDGMENTS

I want to thank Dr. Paul Coleman and Dr. Joseph Rogers for their guidance and their overwhelming support in making this a truly comprehensive review. I would like to acknowledge two funding sources that have allowed me the time to write this review, NIRG Alzheimer's Association Award NIRG-14-321390 and ABRC award ADH-080000.

REFERENCES

1. Riggs AD RV & Martienssen RA (1996). *Epigenetic mechanisms of gene regulation.* Plainview, NY: Cold Spring Harbor Laboratory Press.

2. Maeshima K, Imai R, Tamura S, & Nozaki T (2014). Chromatin as dynamic 10-nm fibers. *Chromosoma* 123(3):225–237.

3. van Steensel B (2011). Chromatin: constructing the big picture. *EMBO J* 30(10):1885–1895.

4. Crider KS, Yang TP, Berry RJ, & Bailey LB (2012). Folate and DNA methylation: a review of molecular mechanisms and the evidence for folate's role. *Adv Nutr* 3(1):21–38.

5. Clayton AL, Hazzalin CA, & Mahadevan LC (2006). Enhanced histone acetylation and transcription: a dynamic perspective. *Mol Cell* 23(3):289–296.

6. Ha M, Ng DW, Li WH, & Chen ZJ (2011). Coordinated histone modifications are associated with gene expression variation within and between species. *Genome Res* 21(4):590–598.

7. Ha M & Kim VN (2014). Regulation of microRNA biogenesis. *Nat Rev Mol Cell Biol* 15(8):509–524.

8. Treiber T, Treiber N, & Meister G (2012). Regulation of microRNA biogenesis and function. *Thromb Haemost* 107(4):605–610.

9. Li Y & Tollefsbol TO (2011). DNA methylation detection: bisulfite genomic sequencing analysis. *Methods Mol Biol* 791:11–21.

10. Herman JG, Graff JR, Myohanen S, Nelkin BD, & Baylin SB (1996). Methylation-specific PCR: a novel PCR assay for methylation status of CpG islands. *Proc Natl Acad Sci U S A* 93(18):9821–9826.

11. Tost J & Gut IG (2007). DNA methylation analysis by pyrosequencing. *Nat Protoc* 2(9):2265–2275.

12. Wong NC, et al. (2013). Exploring the utility of human DNA methylation arrays for profiling mouse genomic DNA. *Genomics* 102(1):38–46.

13. Masser DR, Stanford DR, & Freeman WM (2015). Targeted DNA methylation analysis by next-generation sequencing. *J Vis Exp* (96):e52488.

14. Hashimoto K, Kokubun S, Itoi E, & Roach HI (2007). Improved quantification of DNA methylation using methylation-sensitive restriction enzymes and real-time PCR. *Epigenetics* 2(2):86–91.

15. Mohn F, Weber M, Schubeler D, & Roloff TC (2009). Methylated DNA immunoprecipitation (MeDIP). *Methods Mol Biol* 507:55–64.

16. Booth MJ, et al. (2013). Oxidative bisulfite sequencing of 5-methylcytosine and 5-hydroxymethylcytosine. *Nat Protoc* 8(10):1841–1851.

17. Yu M, et al. (2012). Tet-assisted bisulfite sequencing of 5-hydroxymethylcytosine. *Nat Protoc* 7(12):2159–2170.

18. Salbert G & Weber M (2012). Tracking genomic hydroxymethylation by the base. *Nat Methods* 9(1):45–46.

19. Nelson JD, Denisenko O, & Bomsztyk K (2006). Protocol for the fast chromatin immunoprecipitation (ChIP) method. *Nat Protoc* 1(1): 179–185.

20. Raha D, Hong M, & Snyder M (2010). ChIP-Seq: a method for global identification of regulatory elements in the genome. *Curr Protoc Mol Biol* Chapter 21:Unit 21 19 21–14.

21. Buck MJ & Lieb JD (2004). ChIP-chip: considerations for the design, analysis, and application of genome-wide chromatin immunoprecipitation experiments. *Genomics* 83(3):349–360.

22. Ho JW, et al. (2011). ChIP-chip versus ChIP-seq: lessons for experimental design and data analysis. *BMC Genomics* 12:134.

23. Chen C, Tan R, Wong L, Fekete R, & Halsey J (2011). Quantitation of microRNAs by real-time RT-qPCR. *Methods Mol Biol* 687:113–134.

24. Liu CG, Calin GA, Volinia S, & Croce CM (2008). MicroRNA expression profiling using microarrays. *Nat Protoc* 3(4):563–578.

25. Eminaga S, Christodoulou DC, Vigneault F, Church GM, & Seidman JG (2013). Quantification of microRNA expression with next-generation sequencing. *Curr Protoc Mol Biol*, Chapter 4:Unit 4 17.

26. Git A, et al. (2010). Systematic comparison of microarray profiling, real-time PCR, and next-generation sequencing technologies for measuring differential microRNA expression. *RNA* 16(5):991–1006.

27. Rathmann KL & Conner CS (2007). Alzheimer's disease: clinical features, pathogenesis, and treatment. *Ann Pharmacother* 41(9):1499–1504.

28. Berdasco M & Esteller M (2012). Hot topics in epigenetic mechanisms of aging: 2011. *Aging Cell* 11(2):181–186.

29. Amouyel P, Brousseau T, Fruchart JC, & Dallongeville J (1993). Apolipoprotein E-epsilon 4 allele and Alzheimer's disease. *Lancet* 342(8882):1309.

30. Zubenko GS, et al. (1994). Association of the apolipoprotein E epsilon 4 allele with clinical subtypes of autopsy-confirmed Alzheimer's disease. *Am J Med Genet* 54(3):199–205.

31. Dunn BK (2003). Hypomethylation: one side of a larger picture. *Ann N Y Acad Sci* 983:28–42.

32. Mastroeni D, et al. (2010). Epigenetic changes in Alzheimer's disease: decrements in DNA methylation. *Neurobiol Aging* 31(12):2025–2037.

33. Mastroeni D, McKee A, Grover A, Rogers J, & Coleman PD (2009). Epigenetic differences in cortical neurons from a pair of monozygotic twins discordant for Alzheimer's disease. *PLoS One* 4(8):e6617.

34. Chouliaras L, et al. (2013). Consistent decrease in global DNA methylation and hydroxymethylation in the hippocampus of Alzheimer's disease patients. *Neurobiol Aging* 34(9):2091–2099.

35. Sung HY, Choi EN, Ahn Jo S, Oh S, & Ahn JH (2011). Amyloid protein-mediated differential DNA methylation status regulates gene expression in Alzheimer's disease model cell line. *Biochem Biophys Res Commun* 414(4):700–705.

36. Lashley T, et al. (2015). Alterations in global DNA methylation and hydroxymethylation are not detected in Alzheimer's disease. *Neuropathol Appl Neurobiol* 41(4):497–506.

37. Coppieters N, et al. (2014). Global changes in DNA methylation and hydroxymethylation in Alzheimer's disease human brain. *Neurobiol Aging* 35(6):1334–1344.

38. Yu L, et al. (2015). Association of Brain DNA methylation in SORL1, ABCA7, HLA-DRB5, SLC24A4, and BIN1 with pathological diagnosis of Alzheimer disease. *JAMA Neurol* 72(1):15–24.

39. De Jager PL, et al. (2014). Alzheimer's disease: early alterations in brain DNA methylation at ANK1, BIN1, RHBDF2 and other loci. *Nat Neurosci* 17(9):1156–1163.

40. Lunnon K, et al. (2014). Methylomic profiling implicates cortical deregulation of ANK1 in Alzheimer's disease. *Nat Neurosci* 17(9): 1164–1170.

41. Chen YA, et al. (2013). Discovery of cross-reactive probes and polymorphic CpGs in the Illumina Infinium Human Methylation 450 microarray. *Epigenetics* 8(2):203–209.

42. Harper KN, Peters BA, & Gamble MV (2013). Batch effects and pathway analysis: two potential perils in cancer studies involving DNA methylation array analysis. *Cancer Epidemiol Biomarkers Prev* 22(6):1052–1060.

43. Hardy JA & Higgins GA (1992). Alzheimer's disease: the amyloid cascade hypothesis. *Science* 256(5054):184–185.

44. Hardy J (2006). Alzheimer's disease: the amyloid cascade hypothesis: an update and reappraisal. *J Alzheimers Dis* 9(3 Suppl):151–153.

45. West RL, Lee JM, & Maroun LE (1995). Hypomethylation of the amyloid precursor protein gene in the brain of an Alzheimer's disease patient. *J Mol Neurosci* 6(2):141–146.

46. Hou Y, et al. (2013). Changes in methylation patterns of multiple genes from peripheral blood leucocytes of Alzheimer's disease patients. *Acta Neuropsychiatr* 25(2):66–76.

47. Guo X, Wu X, Ren L, Liu G, & Li L (2011). Epigenetic mechanisms of amyloid-beta production in anisomycin-treated SH-SY5Y cells. *Neuroscience* 194:272–281.

48. Iwata A, et al. (2014). Altered CpG methylation in sporadic Alzheimer's disease is associated with APP and MAPT dysregulation. *Hum Mol Genet* 23(3):648–656.

49. Barrachina M & Ferrer I (2009). DNA methylation of Alzheimer disease and tauopathy-related genes in postmortem brain. *J Neuropathol Exp Neurol* 68(8):880–891.

50. Brohede J, Rinde M, Winblad B, & Graff C (2010). A DNA methylation study of the amyloid precursor protein gene in several brain regions from patients with familial Alzheimer disease. *J Neurogenet* 24(4):179–181.

51. Fuso A, et al. (2012). S-adenosylmethionine reduces the progress of the Alzheimer-like features induced by B-vitamin deficiency in mice. *Neurobiol Aging* 33(7):1482 e1481–1416.

52. Fuso A, Seminara L, Cavallaro RA, D'Anselmi F, & Scarpa S (2005). S-adenosylmethionine/homocysteine cycle alterations modify DNA methylation status with consequent deregulation of PS1 and BACE and beta-amyloid production. *Mol Cell Neurosci* 28(1):195–204.

53. Chan A, Tchantchou F, Rogers EJ, & Shea TB (2009). Dietary deficiency increases presenilin expression, gamma-secretase activity, and Abeta levels: potentiation by ApoE genotype and alleviation by S-adenosyl methionine. *J Neurochem* 110(3):831–836.

54. Fuso A, et al. (2008). B-vitamin deprivation induces hyperhomocysteinemia and brain S-adenosylhomocysteine, depletes brain S-adenosylmethionine, and enhances PS1 and

BACE expression and amyloid-beta deposition in mice. *Mol Cell Neurosci* 37(4):731–746.

55. Choi JK & Kim SC (2007). Environmental effects on gene expression phenotype have regional biases in the human genome. *Genetics* 175(4):1607–1613.

56. Hou L, Zhang X, Wang D, & Baccarelli A (2012). Environmental chemical exposures and human epigenetics. *Int J Epidemiol* 41(1):79–105.

57. Litherland SA (2008). Immunopathogenic interaction of environmental triggers and genetic susceptibility in diabetes: is epigenetics the missing link? *Diabetes* 57(12):3184–3186.

58. Turner AJ, Isaac RE, & Coates D (2001). The neprilysin (NEP) family of zinc metalloendopeptidases: genomics and function. *Bioessays* 23(3):261–269.

59. Chen KL, et al. (2009). The epigenetic effects of amyloid-beta(1–40) on global DNA and neprilysin genes in murine cerebral endothelial cells. *Biochem Biophys Res Commun* 378(1):57–61.

60. Hafez D, et al. (2011). Neprilysin-2 is an important beta-amyloid degrading enzyme. *Am J Pathol* 178(1):306–312.

61. Mastroeni D, et al. (2011). Epigenetic mechanisms in Alzheimer's disease. *Neurobiol Aging* 32(7):1161–1180.

62. Tohgi H, et al. (1999). The methylation status of cytosines in a tau gene promoter region alters with age to downregulate transcriptional activity in human cerebral cortex. *Neurosci Lett* 275(2):89–92.

63. Mukaetova-Ladinska EB, Harrington CR, Roth M, & Wischik CM (1996). Alterations in tau protein metabolism during normal aging. *Dementia* 7(2):95–103.

64. Mastroeni D, et al. (2008). Epigenetic changes in Alzheimer's disease: Decrements in DNA methylation. *Neurobiol Aging* (12):2025–2037.

65. Zhou XW, Li X, Bjorkdahl C, Sjogren MJ, Alafuzoff I, Soininen H, Grundke-Iqbal I, Iqbal K, Winblad B, Pei JJ. (2006). Assessments of the accumulation severities of amyloid beta-protein and hyperphosphorylated tau in the medial temporal cortex of control and Alzheimer's brains. *Neurobiol Dis*. 22(3):657–668. Epub 2006 Mar 2.

66. Zhou XW, et al. (2008). Tau hyperphosphorylation correlates with reduced methylation of protein phosphatase 2A. *Neurobiol Dis*.

67. Yoon SY, et al. (2007). Methotrexate decreases PP2A methylation and increases tau phosphorylation in neuron. *Biochem Biophys Res Commun* 363(3):811–816.

68. Zhang CE, et al. (2008). Homocysteine induces tau phosphorylation by inactivating protein phosphatase 2A in rat hippocampus. *Neurobiol Aging* 29(11):1654–1665.

69. Wang Y, et al. (2015). Cross talk between PI3K-AKT-GSK-3beta and PP2A pathways determines

tau hyperphosphorylation. *Neurobiol Aging* 36(1):188–200.

70. Nicolia V, Fuso A, Cavallaro RA, Di Luzio A, & Scarpa S (2010). B vitamin deficiency promotes tau phosphorylation through regulation of GSK3beta and PP2A. *J Alzheimers Dis* 19(3):895–907.

71. Cohen JE, Lee PR, Chen S, Li W, & Fields RD (2011). MicroRNA regulation of homeostatic synaptic plasticity. *Proc Natl Acad Sci U S A* 108(28):11650–11655.

72. Hong J, Zhang H, Kawase-Koga Y, & Sun T (2013). MicroRNA function is required for neurite outgrowth of mature neurons in the mouse postnatal cerebral cortex. *Front Cell Neurosci* 7:151.

73. Serrano-Pozo A, Frosch MP, Masliah E, & Hyman BT (2011). Neuropathological alterations in Alzheimer disease. *Cold Spring Harb Perspect Med* 1(1):a006189.

74. Alexandrov PN, et al. (2012). microRNA (miRNA) speciation in Alzheimer's disease (AD) cerebrospinal fluid (CSF) and extracellular fluid (ECF). *Int J Biochem Mol Biol* 3(4):365–373.

75. Hebert SS, et al. (2008). Loss of microRNA cluster miR-29a/b-1 in sporadic Alzheimer's disease correlates with increased BACE1/beta-secretase expression. *Proc Natl Acad Sci U S A* 105(17):6415–6420.

76. Wang WX, et al. (2008). The expression of microRNA miR-107 decreases early in Alzheimer's disease and may accelerate disease progression through regulation of beta-site amyloid precursor protein-cleaving enzyme 1. *J Neurosci* 28(5):1213–1223.

77. Leidinger P, et al. (2013). A blood based 12-miRNA signature of Alzheimer disease patients. *Genome Biol* 14(7):R78.

78. Ogawa O, et al. (2003). Ectopic localization of phosphorylated histone H3 in Alzheimer's disease: a mitotic catastrophe? *Acta Neuropathol* 105(5):524–528.

79. Bolton SJ, Russelakis-Carneiro M, Betmouni S, & Perry VH (1999). Non-nuclear histone H1 is upregulated in neurones and astrocytes in prion and Alzheimer's diseases but not in acute neurodegeneration. *Neuropathol Appl Neurobiol* 25(5):425–432.

80. Duce JA, et al. (2006). Linker histone H1 binds to disease associated amyloid-like fibrils. *J Mol Biol* 361(3):493–505.

81. Love S, Barber R, & Wilcock GK (1999). Increased poly(ADP-ribosyl)ation of nuclear proteins in Alzheimer's disease. *Brain* 122 (Pt 2):247–253.

82. Francis YI, et al. (2009). Dysregulation of histone acetylation in the APP/PS1 mouse model of Alzheimer's disease. *J Alzheimers Dis*.

83. Fischer A, Sananbenesi F, Wang X, Dobbin M, & Tsai LH (2007). Recovery of learning and memory is associated with chromatin remodelling. *Nature* 447(7141):178–182.

84. Kilgore M, et al. (2010). Inhibitors of class 1 histone deacetylases reverse contextual memory deficits in a mouse model of Alzheimer's disease. *Neuropsychopharmacology* 35(4):870–880.

85. Su Y, et al. (2004). Lithium, a common drug for bipolar disorder treatment, regulates amyloid-beta precursor protein processing. *Biochemistry (Mosc).* 43(22):6899–6908.

86. Ricobaraza A, et al. (2009). Phenylbutyrate ameliorates cognitive deficit and reduces tau pathology in an Alzheimer's disease mouse model. *Neuropsychopharmacology* 34(7):1721–1732.

87. Rouaux C, et al. (2003). Critical loss of CBP/p300 histone acetylase activity by caspase-6 during neurodegeneration. *EMBO J* 22(24):6537–6549.

88. Lonze BE & Ginty DD (2002). Function and regulation of CREB family transcription factors in the nervous system. *Neuron* 35(4):605–623.

89. Zhang L, et al. (2014). Tubastatin A/ACY-1215 improves cognition in Alzheimer's disease transgenic mice. *J Alzheimers Dis* 41(4):1193–1205.

90. Selenica ML, et al. (2014). Histone deacetylase 6 inhibition improves memory and reduces total tau levels in a mouse model of tau deposition. *Alzheimers Res Ther* 6(1):12.

91. Sung YM, et al. (2013). Mercaptoacetamide-based class II HDAC inhibitor lowers Abeta levels and improves learning and memory in a mouse model of Alzheimer's disease. *Exp Neurol* 239:192–201.

92. Schneider SA & Obeso JA (2015). Clinical and pathological features of Parkinson's disease. *Curr Top Behav Neurosci* 22:205–220.

93. Gallegos S, Pacheco C, Peters C, Opazo CM, & Aguayo LG (2015). Features of alpha-synuclein that could explain the progression and irreversibility of Parkinson's disease. *Front Neurosci* 9:59.

94. Mullin S & Schapira A (2015). The genetics of Parkinson's disease. *Br Med Bull* 114(1):39–52.

95. Desplats P, et al. (2011). Alpha-synuclein sequesters Dnmt1 from the nucleus: a novel mechanism for epigenetic alterations in Lewy body diseases. *J Biol Chem* 286(11):9031–9037.

96. Mastroeni D, et al. (2013). Reduced RAN expression and disrupted transport between cytoplasm and nucleus; a key event in Alzheimer's disease pathophysiology. *PLoS One* 8(1):e53349.

97. Masliah E, Dumaop W, Galasko D, & Desplats P (2013). Distinctive patterns of DNA methylation associated with Parkinson disease: identification of concordant epigenetic changes in brain and peripheral blood leukocytes. *Epigenetics* 8(10):1030–1038.

98. Cai M, Tian J, Zhao GH, Luo W, & Zhang BR (2011). Study of methylation levels of parkin gene promoter in Parkinson's disease patients. *Int J Neurosci* 121(9):497–502.

99. Coppede F (2012). Genetics and epigenetics of Parkinson's disease. *Scientific World Journal* 2012:489830.

100. Chiba-Falek O, Lopez GJ, & Nussbaum RL (2006). Levels of alpha-synuclein mRNA in sporadic Parkinson disease patients. *Mov Disord* 21(10):1703–1708.

101. Pihlstrom L & Toft M (2011). Genetic variability in SNCA and Parkinson's disease. *Neurogenetics* 12(4):283–293.

102. Tan YY, et al. (2014). Methylation of alpha-synuclein and leucine-rich repeat kinase 2 in leukocyte DNA of Parkinson's disease patients. *Parkinsonism Relat Disord* 20(3):308–313.

103. Matsumoto L, et al. (2010). CpG demethylation enhances alpha-synuclein expression and affects the pathogenesis of Parkinson's disease. *PLoS One* 5(11):e15522.

104. Junn E, et al. (2009). Repression of alpha-synuclein expression and toxicity by microRNA-7. *Proc Natl Acad Sci U S A* 106(31):13052–13057.

105. Doxakis E (2010). Post-transcriptional regulation of alpha-synuclein expression by mir-7 and mir-153. *J Biol Chem* 285(17):12726–12734.

106. Fragkouli A & Doxakis E (2014). miR-7 and miR-153 protect neurons against MPP(+)-induced cell death via upregulation of mTOR pathway. *Front Cell Neurosci* 8:182.

107. Goers J, et al. (2003). Nuclear localization of alpha-synuclein and its interaction with histones. *Biochemistry* 42(28):8465–8471.

108. Kontopoulos E, Parvin JD, & Feany MB (2006). Alpha-synuclein acts in the nucleus to inhibit histone acetylation and promote neurotoxicity. *Hum Mol Genet* 15(20):3012–3023.

109. Monti B, et al. (2010). Valproic acid is neuroprotective in the rotenone rat model of Parkinson's disease: involvement of alpha-synuclein. *Neurotox Res* 17(2):130–141.

110. Donmez G & Outeiro TF (2013). SIRT1 and SIRT2: emerging targets in neurodegeneration. *EMBO Mol Med* 5(3):344–352.

111. Outeiro TF, et al. (2007). Sirtuin 2 inhibitors rescue alpha-synuclein-mediated toxicity in models of Parkinson's disease. *Science* 317(5837):516–519.

112. Jin H, et al. (2011). alpha-Synuclein negatively regulates protein kinase Cdelta expression to suppress apoptosis in dopaminergic neurons by reducing p300 histone acetyltransferase activity. *J Neurosci* 31(6):2035–2051.

113. Kanthasamy AG, Kitazawa M, Kanthasamy A, & Anantharam V (2003). Role of proteolytic

activation of protein kinase Cdelta in oxidative stress-induced apoptosis. *Antioxid Redox Signal* 5(5):609–620.

114. Brodie C & Blumberg PM (2003). Regulation of cell apoptosis by protein kinase c delta. *Apoptosis* 8(1):19–27.

115. Rowland LP & Shneider NA (2001). Amyotrophic lateral sclerosis. *N Engl J Med* 344(22): 1688–1700.

116. Chestnut BA, et al. (2011). Epigenetic regulation of motor neuron cell death through DNA methylation. *J Neurosci* 31(46):16619–16636.

117. Oates N & Pamphlett R (2007). An epigenetic analysis of SOD1 and VEGF in ALS. *Amyotroph Lateral Scler* 8(2):83–86.

118. Yang Y, Gozen O, Vidensky S, Robinson MB, & Rothstein JD (2010). Epigenetic regulation of neuron-dependent induction of astroglial synaptic protein GLT1. *Glia* 58(3):277–286.

119. Morahan JM, Yu B, Trent RJ, & Pamphlett R (2009). A genome-wide analysis of brain DNA methylation identifies new candidate genes for sporadic amyotrophic lateral sclerosis. *Amyotroph Lateral Scler* 10(5–6):418–429.

120. Figueroa-Romero C, et al. (2012). Identification of epigenetically altered genes in sporadic amyotrophic lateral sclerosis. *PLoS One* 7(12):e52672.

121. Williams AH, et al. (2009). MicroRNA-206 delays ALS progression and promotes regeneration of neuromuscular synapses in mice. *Science* 326(5959):1549–1554.

122. Williams R (2009). Robert Miller: a frontline fighter of amyotrophic lateral sclerosis. *Lancet Neurol* 8(7):608.

123. Russell AP, et al. (2013). Disruption of skeletal muscle mitochondrial network genes and miRNAs in amyotrophic lateral sclerosis. *Neurobiol Dis* 49:107–117.

124. He L & Hannon GJ (2004). MicroRNAs: small RNAs with a big role in gene regulation. *Nat Rev Genet* 5(7):522–531.

125. Haramati S, et al. (2010). miRNA malfunction causes spinal motor neuron disease. *Proc Natl Acad Sci U S A* 107(29):13111–13116.

126. Buratti E & Baralle FE (2010). The multiple roles of TDP-43 in pre-mRNA processing and gene expression regulation. *RNA Biol* 7(4):420–429.

127. Yoo YE & Ko CP (2011). Treatment with trichostatin A initiated after disease onset delays disease progression and increases survival in a mouse model of amyotrophic lateral sclerosis. *Exp Neurol* 231(1):147–159.

128. Ryu H, et al. (2005). Sodium phenylbutyrate prolongs survival and regulates expression of anti-apoptotic genes in transgenic amyotrophic lateral sclerosis mice. *J Neurochem* 93(5):1087–1098.

129. Cudkowicz ME, et al. (2009). Phase 2 study of sodium phenylbutyrate in ALS. *Amyotroph Lateral Scler* 10(2):99–106.

130. Piepers S, et al. (2009). Randomized sequential trial of valproic acid in amyotrophic lateral sclerosis. *Ann Neurol* 66(2):227–234.

131. Kim HY, et al. (2007). Clinical characteristics of familial amyotrophic lateral sclerosis with a Phe20Cys mutation in the SOD1 gene in a Korean family. *Amyotroph Lateral Scler* 8(2):73–78.

132. Markert CD, Kim E, Gifondorwa DJ, Childers MK, & Milligan CE (2010). A single-dose resveratrol treatment in a mouse model of amyotrophic lateral sclerosis. *J Med Food* 13(5):1081–1085.

133. Wang J, Zhang Y, Tang L, Zhang N, & Fan D (2011). Protective effects of resveratrol through the up-regulation of SIRT1 expression in the mutant hSOD1-G93A-bearing motor neuron-like cell culture model of amyotrophic lateral sclerosis. *Neurosci Lett* 503(3):250–255.

134. Novak MJ & Tabrizi SJ (2010). Huntington's disease. *BMJ* 340:c3109.

135. Rubinsztein DC & Carmichael J (2003). Huntington's disease: molecular basis of neurodegeneration. *Expert Rev Mol Med* 5(20):1–21.

136. Rosas HD, et al. (2002). Regional and progressive thinning of the cortical ribbon in Huntington's disease. *Neurology* 58(5):695–701.

137. Vonsattel JP & DiFiglia M (1998). Huntington disease. *J Neuropathol Exp Neurol* 57(5):369–384.

138. Wasmuth JJ, et al. (1988). A highly polymorphic locus very tightly linked to the Huntington's disease gene. *Nature* 332(6166):734–736.

139. Pritchard CA, Cox DR, & Myers RM (1989). Methylation at the Huntington disease-linked D4S95 locus. *Am J Hum Genet* 45(2):335–336.

140. Farrer LA, Cupples LA, Kiely DK, Conneally PM, & Myers RH (1992). Inverse relationship between age at onset of Huntington disease and paternal age suggests involvement of genetic imprinting. *Am J Hum Genet* 50(3):528–535.

141. Gorbunova V, Seluanov A, Mittelman D, & Wilson JH (2004). Genome-wide demethylation destabilizes CTG.CAG trinucleotide repeats in mammalian cells. *Hum Mol Genet* 13(23):2979–2989.

142. Hodges A, et al. (2006). Regional and cellular gene expression changes in human Huntington's disease brain. *Hum Mol Genet* 15(6):965–977.

143. Ng CW, et al. (2013). Extensive changes in DNA methylation are associated with expression of mutant huntingtin. *Proc Natl Acad Sci U S A* 110(6):2354–2359.

144. Blum D, Hourez R, Galas MC, Popoli P, & Schiffmann SN (2003). Adenosine receptors

and Huntington's disease: implications for pathogenesis and therapeutics. *Lancet Neurol* 2(6):366–374.

145. Villar-Menendez I, et al. (2013). Increased 5-methylcytosine and decreased 5-hydroxymethylcytosine levels are associated with reduced striatal A2AR levels in Huntington's disease. *Neuromolecular Med* 15(2):295–309.

146. Lee ST, et al. (2011). Altered microRNA regulation in Huntington's disease models. *Exp Neurol* 227(1):172–179.

147. Johnson R, et al. (2008). A microRNA-based gene dysregulation pathway in Huntington's disease. *Neurobiol Dis* 29(3):438–445.

148. Jovicic A, Zaldivar Jolissaint JF, Moser R, Silva Santos Mde F, & Luthi-Carter R (2013). MicroRNA-22 (miR-22) overexpression is neuroprotective via general anti-apoptotic effects and may also target specific Huntington's disease-related mechanisms. *PLoS One* 8(1):e54222.

149. Ghose J, Sinha M, Das E, Jana NR, & Bhattacharyya NP (2011). Regulation of miR-146a by RelA/NFkB and p53 in STHdh(Q111)/Hdh(Q111) cells, a cell model of Huntington's disease. *PLoS One* 6(8):e23837.

150. Sinha M, Ghose J, Das E, & Bhattarcharyya NP (2010). Altered microRNAs in STHdh(Q111)/Hdh(Q111) cells: miR-146a targets TBP. *Biochem Biophys Res Commun* 396(3):742–747.

151. Sadri-Vakili G & Cha JH (2006). Mechanisms of disease: histone modifications in Huntington's disease. *Nat Clin Pract Neurol* 2(6):330–338.

152. Valor LM, Viosca J, Lopez-Atalaya JP, & Barco A (2013). Lysine acetyltransferases CBP and p300 as therapeutic targets in cognitive and neurodegenerative disorders. *Curr Pharm Des* 19(28):5051–5064.

153. Chakraborty S, Senyuk V, Sitailo S, Chi Y, & Nucifora G (2001). Interaction of EVI1 with cAMP-responsive element-binding protein-binding protein (CBP) and p300/CBP-associated factor (P/CAF) results in reversible acetylation of EVI1 and in co-localization in nuclear speckles. *J Biol Chem* 276(48):44936–44943.

154. Choi YJ, et al. (2012). Suppression of aggregate formation of mutant huntingtin potentiates CREB-binding protein sequestration and apoptotic cell death. *Mol Cell Neurosci* 49(2):127–137.

155. Sadri-Vakili G, et al. (2007). Histones associated with downregulated genes are hypo-acetylated in Huntington's disease models. *Hum Mol Genet* 16(11):1293–1306.

156. McFarland KN, et al. (2012). Genome-wide histone acetylation is altered in a transgenic mouse model of Huntington's disease. *PLoS One* 7(7):e41423.

157. Jiang H, et al. (2006). Depletion of CBP is directly linked with cellular toxicity caused by mutant huntingtin. *Neurobiol Dis* 23(3):543–551.

158. Igarashi S, et al. (2003). Inducible PC12 cell model of Huntington's disease shows toxicity and decreased histone acetylation. *Neuroreport* 14(4):565–568.

159. Hoshino M, et al. (2003). Histone deacetylase activity is retained in primary neurons expressing mutant huntingtin protein. *J Neurochem* 87(1):257–267.

160. Quinti L, et al. (2010). Evaluation of histone deacetylases as drug targets in Huntington's disease models: study of HDACs in brain tissues from R6/2 and CAG140 knock-in HD mouse models and human patients and in a neuronal HD cell model. *PLoS Curr* 2. doi: 10.1371/currents.RRN1172.

161. Steffan JS, et al. (2001). Histone deacetylase inhibitors arrest polyglutamine-dependent neurodegeneration in Drosophila. *Nature* 413(6857):739–743.

162. Ryu H, et al. (2003). Histone deacetylase inhibitors prevent oxidative neuronal death independent of expanded polyglutamine repeats via an Sp1-dependent pathway. *Proc Natl Acad Sci U S A* 100(7):4281–4286.

163. Thomas EA, et al. (2008). The HDAC inhibitor 4b ameliorates the disease phenotype and transcriptional abnormalities in Huntington's disease transgenic mice. *Proc Natl Acad Sci U S A* 105(40):15564–15569.

164. Jia H, Kast RJ, Steffan JS, & Thomas EA (2012). Selective histone deacetylase (HDAC) inhibition imparts beneficial effects in Huntington's disease mice: implications for the ubiquitin-proteasomal and autophagy systems. *Hum Mol Genet* 21(24):5280–5293.

165. Rogers J, Mastroeni D, Leonard B, Joyce J, & Grover A (2007). Neuroinflammation in Alzheimer's disease and Parkinson's disease: are microglia pathogenic in either disorder? *Int Rev Neurobiol* 82:235–246.

166. Garden GA (2013). Epigenetics and the modulation of neuroinflammation. *Neurotherapeutics* 10(4):782–788.

167. Choi SW, Claycombe KJ, Martinez JA, Friso S, & Schalinske KL (2013). Nutritional epigenomics: a portal to disease prevention. *Adv Nutr* 4(5):530–532.

168. Nicolia V, Lucarelli M, & Fuso A (2014). Environment, epigenetics and neurodegeneration: focus on nutrition in Alzheimer's disease. *Exp Gerontol*.

169. Goebels N & Soyka M (2000). Dementia associated with vitamin B(12) deficiency: presentation of two cases and review of the literature. *J Neuropsychiatry Clin Neurosci* 12(3):389–394.

170. Selhub J, Troen A, & Rosenberg IH (2010). B vitamins and the aging brain. *Nutr Rev* 68 Suppl 2:S112–118.

171. Vogiatzoglou A, et al. (2008). Vitamin B12 status and rate of brain volume loss in community-dwelling elderly. *Neurology* 71(11):826–832.

172. Murray B, et al. (2014). Structure and function study of the complex that synthesizes S-adenosylmethionine. *IUCrJ* 1(Pt 4):240–249.

173. Duan W, et al. (2002). Dietary folate deficiency and elevated homocysteine levels endanger dopaminergic neurons in models of Parkinson's disease. *J Neurochem* 80(1):101–110.

174. Coppede F (2010). One-carbon metabolism and Alzheimer's disease: focus on epigenetics. *Curr Genomics* 11(4):246–260.

175. Mattson MP (2003). Gene-diet interactions in brain aging and neurodegenerative disorders. *Ann Intern Med* 139(5 Pt 2):441–444.

176. Mattson MP & Shea TB (2003). Folate and homocysteine metabolism in neural plasticity and neurodegenerative disorders. *Trends Neurosci* 26(3):137–146.

177. Yoshino Y (1984). Possible involvement of folate cycle in the pathogenesis of amyotrophic lateral sclerosis. *Neurochem Res* 9(3):387–391.

178. Brennan MJ, van der Westhuyzen J, Kramer S, & Metz J (1981). Neurotoxicity of folates: implications for vitamin B12 deficiency and Huntington's chorea. *Med Hypotheses* 7(7):919–929.

179. Clarke R, et al. (1998). Folate, vitamin B12, and serum total homocysteine levels in confirmed Alzheimer disease. *Arch Neurol* 55(11):1449–1455.

180. Kuhn W, Roebroek R, Blom H, van Oppenraaij D, & Muller T (1998). Hyperhomocysteinaemia in Parkinson's disease. *J Neurol* 245(12):811–812.

181. Valentino F, et al. (2010). Elevated cerebrospinal fluid and plasma homocysteine levels in ALS. *Eur J Neurol* 17(1):84–89.

182. Zoccolella S, et al. (2008). Elevated plasma homocysteine levels in patients with amyotrophic lateral sclerosis. *Neurology* 70(3):222–225.

183. Zoccolella S, Martino D, Defazio G, Lamberti P, & Livrea P (2006). Hyperhomocysteinemia in movement disorders: current evidence and hypotheses. *Curr Vasc Pharmacol* 4(3):237–243.

184. Andrich J, et al. (2004). Hyperhomocysteinaemia in treated patients with Huntington's disease homocysteine in HD. *Mov Disord* 19(2):226–228.

185. Fuso A, Nicolia V, Cavallaro RA, & Scarpa S (2011). DNA methylase and demethylase activities are modulated by one-carbon metabolism in Alzheimer's disease models. *J Nutr Biochem* 22(3):242–251.

186. Borro M, et al. (2010). One-carbon metabolism alteration affects brain proteome profile in a mouse model of Alzheimer's disease. *J Alzheimers Dis* 22(4):1257–1268.

187. Muller T, Woitalla D, Hauptmann B, Fowler B, & Kuhn W (2001). Decrease of methionine and S-adenosylmethionine and increase of homocysteine in treated patients with Parkinson's disease. *Neurosci Lett* 308(1):54–56.

188. Suchy J, Lee S, Ahmed A, & Shea TB (2010). Dietary supplementation with S-adenosyl methionine delays the onset of motor neuron pathology in a murine model of amyotrophic lateral sclerosis. *Neuromolecular Med* 12(1):86–97.

189. Braak H & Del Tredici K (2011). The pathological process underlying Alzheimer's disease in individuals under thirty. *Acta Neuropathol* 121(2):171–181.

190. Johri A & Beal MF (2012). Mitochondrial dysfunction in neurodegenerative diseases. *J Pharmacol Exp Ther* 342(3):619–630.

191. Papa S, et al. (2012). The oxidative phosphorylation system in mammalian mitochondria. *Adv Exper Med Biol* 942:3–37.

192. Wallace DC & Fan W (2010). Energetics, epigenetics, mitochondrial genetics. *Mitochondrion* 10(1):12–31.

193. Conaway RC & Conaway JW (1988). ATP activates transcription initiation from promoters by RNA polymerase II in a reversible step prior to RNA synthesis. *J Biol Chem* 263(6):2962–2968.

194. Klingenberg M (2008). The ADP and ATP transport in mitochondria and its carrier. *Biochim Biophys Acta* 1778(10):1978–2021.

195. Lewis PN, Lukiw WJ, De Boni U, & McLachlan DR (1981). Changes in chromatin structure associated with Alzheimer's disease. *J Neurochem* 37(5):1193–1202.

196. Mastroeni D, et al. (2008). Epigenetic changes in Alzheimer's disease: decrements in DNA methylation. *Neurobiol Aging* 31(12):2025–2037.

197. Mastroeni D, Khdour OM, Arce PM, Hecht SM, & Coleman PD (2015). Novel antioxidants protect mitochondria from the effects of oligomeric amyloid beta and contribute to the maintenance of epigenome function. *ACS Chem Neurosci* 6(4):588–598.

198. Bakulski KM, et al. (2012). Genome-wide DNA methylation differences between late-onset Alzheimer's disease and cognitively normal controls in human frontal cortex. *J Alzheimers Dis* 29(3):571–588.

199. Bihaqi SW, Huang H, Wu J, & Zawia NH (2011). Infant exposure to lead (Pb) and epigenetic modifications in the aging primate brain: implications for Alzheimer's disease. *J Alzheimers Dis* 27(4):819–833.

200. Bihaqi SW & Zawia NH (2012). Alzheimer's disease biomarkers and epigenetic intermediates

following exposure to Pb in vitro. *Curr Alzheimer Res* 9(5):555–562.

201. Briones A, et al. (2012). Stress-induced anhedonia is associated with an increase in Alzheimer's disease-related markers. *Br J Pharmacol* 165(4):897–907.

202. Cadena-del-Castillo C, et al. (2014). Age-dependent increment of hydroxymethylation in the brain cortex in the triple-transgenic mouse model of Alzheimer's disease. *J Alzheimers Dis* 41(3):845–854.

203. Condliffe D, et al. (2014). Cross-region reduction in 5-hydroxymethylcytosine in Alzheimer's disease brain. *Neurobiol Aging* 35(8):1850–1854.

204. D'Addario C, et al. (2012). Epigenetic regulation of fatty acid amide hydrolase in Alzheimer disease. *PLoS One* 7(6):e39186.

205. Fuso A, Cavallaro RA, Nicolia V, & Scarpa S (2012). PSEN1 promoter demethylation in hyperhomocysteinemic TgCRND8 mice is the culprit, not the consequence. *Curr Alzheimer Res* 9(5):527–535.

206. Guan JZ, Guan WP, Maeda T, & Makino N (2013). Analysis of telomere length and subtelomeric methylation of circulating leukocytes in women with Alzheimer's disease. *Aging Clin Exp Res* 25(1):17–23.

207. Kaut O, et al. (2014). DNA methylation of the TNF-alpha promoter region in peripheral blood monocytes and the cortex of human Alzheimer's disease patients. *Dement Geriatr Cogn Disord* 38(1–2):10–15.

208. Li YY, Chen T, Wan Y, & Xu SQ (2012). Lead exposure in pheochromocytoma cells induces persistent changes in amyloid precursor protein gene methylation patterns. *Environ Toxicol* 27(8):495–502.

209. Lin HC, Hsieh HM, Chen YH, & Hu ML (2009). S-Adenosylhomocysteine increases beta-amyloid formation in BV-2 microglial cells by increased expressions of beta-amyloid precursor protein and presenilin 1 and by hypomethylation of these gene promoters. *Neurotoxicology* 30(4):622–627.

210. Lin HC, Song TY, & Hu ML (2011). S-Adenosylhomocysteine enhances DNA damage through increased beta-amyloid formation and inhibition of the DNA-repair enzyme OGG1b in microglial BV-2 cells. *Toxicology* 290(2–3):342–349.

211. Miller AL (2003). The methionine-homocysteine cycle and its effects on cognitive diseases. *Altern Med Rev* 8(1):7–19.

212. Rao JS, Keleshian VL, Klein S, & Rapoport SI (2012). Epigenetic modifications in frontal cortex from Alzheimer's disease and bipolar disorder patients. *Transl Psychiatry* 2:e132.

213. Scarpa S, Fuso A, D'Anselmi F, & Cavallaro RA (2003). Presenilin 1 gene silencing by S-adenosylmethionine: a treatment for Alzheimer disease? *FEBS Lett* 541(1–3):145–148.

214. Shin J, Yu SB, Yu UY, Jo SA, & Ahn JH (2010). Swedish mutation within amyloid precursor protein modulates global gene expression towards the pathogenesis of Alzheimer's disease. *BMB Rep* 43(10):704–709.

215. Wang SC, Oelze B, & Schumacher A (2008). Age-specific epigenetic drift in late-onset Alzheimer's disease. *PLoS One* 3(7):e2698.

216. Wu J, et al. (2008). Alzheimer's disease (AD)-like pathology in aged monkeys after infantile exposure to environmental metal lead (Pb): evidence for a developmental origin and environmental link for AD. *J Neurosci* 28(1):3–9.

217. Zhu M, et al. (2014). Age-related brain expression and regulation of the chemokine CCL4/MIP-1beta in APP/PS1 double-transgenic mice. *J Neuropathol Exp Neurol* 73(4):362–374.

218. Bollati V, et al. (2011). DNA methylation in repetitive elements and Alzheimer disease. *Brain Behav Immun* 25(6):1078–1083.

219. Di Francesco A, et al. (2015). Global changes in DNA methylation in Alzheimer's disease peripheral blood mononuclear cells. *Brain Behav Immun* 45:139–144.

220. Pietrzak M, Rempala G, Nelson PT, Zheng JJ, & Hetman M (2011). Epigenetic silencing of nucleolar rRNA genes in Alzheimer's disease. *PLoS One* 6(7):e22585.

221. Sanchez-Mut JV, et al. (2014). Promoter hyper-methylation of the phosphatase DUSP22 mediates PKA-dependent TAU phosphorylation and CREB activation in Alzheimer's disease. *Hippocampus* 24(4):363–368.

222. Sung HY, Choi EN, Lyu D, Mook-Jung I, & Ahn JH (2014). Amyloid beta-mediated epigenetic alteration of insulin-like growth factor binding protein 3 controls cell survival in Alzheimer's disease. *PLoS One* 9(6):e99047.

223. Furuya TK, et al. (2012). Analysis of SNAP25 mRNA expression and promoter DNA methylation in brain areas of Alzheimer's disease patients. *Neuroscience* 220:41–46.

224. Grosser C, Neumann L, Horsthemke B, Zeschnigk M, & van de Nes J (2014). Methylation analysis of SST and SSTR4 promoters in the neocortex of Alzheimer's disease patients. *Neurosci Lett* 566:241–246.

225. Silva PN, et al. (2014). Analysis of HSPA8 and HSPA9 mRNA expression and promoter methylation in the brain and blood of Alzheimer's disease patients. *J Alzheimers Dis* 38(1):165–170.

226. Silva PN, et al. (2013). CNP and DPYSL2 mRNA expression and promoter methylation

levels in brain of Alzheimer's disease patients. *J Alzheimers Dis* 33(2):349–355.

227. Facchinetti P, et al. (2014). SET translocation is associated with increase in caspase cleaved amyloid precursor protein in CA1 of Alzheimer and Down syndrome patients. *Neurobiol Aging* 35(5):958–968.

228. Govindarajan N, Agis-Balboa RC, Walter J, Sananbenesi F, & Fischer A (2011). Sodium butyrate improves memory function in an Alzheimer's disease mouse model when administered at an advanced stage of disease progression. *J Alzheimers Dis* 26(1):187–197.

229. Graff J, et al. (2012). An epigenetic blockade of cognitive functions in the neurodegenerating brain. *Nature* 483(7388):222–226.

230. Lu X, et al. (2014). Histone acetyltransferase p300 mediates histone acetylation of PS1 and BACE1 in a cellular model of Alzheimer's disease. *PLoS One* 9(7):e103067.

231. Lukiw WJ, et al. (1992). Nuclear compartmentalization of aluminum in Alzheimer's disease (AD). *Neurobiol Aging* 13(1):115–121.

232. Marques SC, et al. (2012). Epigenetic regulation of BACE1 in Alzheimer's disease patients and in transgenic mice. *Neuroscience* 220:256–266.

233. Myung NH, et al. (2008). Evidence of DNA damage in Alzheimer disease: phosphorylation of histone H2AX in astrocytes. *Age (Dordr)* 30(4):209–215.

234. Narayan PJ, Lill C, Faull R, Curtis MA, & Dragunow M (2015). Increased acetyl and total histone levels in post-mortem Alzheimer's disease brain. *Neurobiol Dis* 74:281–294.

235. Sen A, Nelson TJ, & Alkon DL (2015). ApoE4 and Abeta oligomers reduce BDNF expression via HDAC nuclear translocation. *J Neurosci* 35(19):7538–7551.

236. Vincent I, Jicha G, Rosado M, & Dickson DW (1997). Aberrant expression of mitotic cdc2/cyclin B1 kinase in degenerating neurons of Alzheimer's disease brain. *J Neurosci* 17(10):3588–3598.

237. Walker MP, LaFerla FM, Oddo SS, & Brewer GJ (2013). Reversible epigenetic histone modifications and Bdnf expression in neurons with aging and from a mouse model of Alzheimer's disease. *Age (Dordr)* 35(3):519–531.

238. Wang Z, et al. (2014). Valproic acid reduces neuritic plaque formation and improves learning deficits in APP(Swe) /PS1(A246E) transgenic mice via preventing the prenatal hypoxia-induced down-regulation of neprilysin. *CNS Neurosci Ther* 20(3):209–217.

239. Muller M, et al. (2015). MicroRNA-29a is a candidate biomarker for Alzheimer's disease in cell-free cerebrospinal fluid. *Mol Neurobiol*.

240. Zhao ZB, et al. (2014). MicroRNA-922 promotes tau phosphorylation by downregulating ubiquitin carboxy-terminal hydrolase L1 (UCHL1) expression in the pathogenesis of Alzheimer's disease. *Neuroscience* 275:232–237.

241. Zhao Y, et al. (2014). Regulation of neurotropic signaling by the inducible, NF-kB-sensitive miRNA-125b in Alzheimer's disease (AD) and in primary human neuronal-glial (HNG) cells. *Mol Neurobiol* 50(1):97–106.

242. Zhang J, Hu M, Teng Z, Tang YP, & Chen C (2014). Synaptic and cognitive improvements by inhibition of 2-AG metabolism are through upregulation of microRNA-188–3p in a mouse model of Alzheimer's disease. *J Neurosci* 34(45):14919–14933.

243. Xu T, et al. (2014). MicroRNA-323–3p with clinical potential in rheumatoid arthritis, Alzheimer's disease and ectopic pregnancy. *Expert Opin Ther Targets* 18(2):153–158.

244. Tiribuzi R, et al. (2014). miR128 up-regulation correlates with impaired amyloid beta(1-42) degradation in monocytes from patients with sporadic Alzheimer's disease. *Neurobiol Aging* 35(2):345–356.

245. Tian N, Cao Z, & Zhang Y (2014). MiR-206 decreases brain-derived neurotrophic factor levels in a transgenic mouse model of Alzheimer's disease. *Neurosci Bull* 30(2):191–197.

246. Tan L, et al. (2014). Circulating miR-125b as a biomarker of Alzheimer's disease. *J Neurol Sci* 336(1–2):52–56.

247. Sun X, Wu Y, Gu M, & Zhang Y (2014). miR-342-5p decreases ankyrin G levels in Alzheimer's disease transgenic mouse models. *Cell Rep* 6(2):264–270.

248. Guedes JR, et al. (2014). Early miR-155 upregulation contributes to neuroinflammation in Alzheimer's disease triple transgenic mouse model. *Hum Mol Genet* 23(23):6286–6301.

249. Bhatnagar S, et al. (2014). Increased microRNA-34c abundance in Alzheimer's disease circulating blood plasma. *Front Mol Neurosci* 7:2.

250. Banzhaf-Strathmann J, et al. (2014). MicroRNA-125b induces tau hyperphosphorylation and cognitive deficits in Alzheimer's disease. *EMBO J* 33(15):1667–1680.

251. Villa C, et al. (2013). Expression of the transcription factor Sp1 and its regulatory hsa-miR-29b in peripheral blood mononuclear cells from patients with Alzheimer's disease. *J Alzheimers Dis* 35(3):487–494.

252. Hu YK, et al. (2013). MicroRNA-98 induces an Alzheimer's disease-like disturbance by targeting insulin-like growth factor 1. *Neurosci Bull* 29(6):745–751.

253. Absalon S, Kochanek DM, Raghavan V, & Krichevsky AM (2013). MiR-26b, upregulated in Alzheimer's disease, activates cell cycle entry, tau-phosphorylation, and apoptosis in postmitotic neurons. *J Neurosci* 33(37):14645–14659.
254. Liu W, et al. (2012). MicroRNA-16 targets amyloid precursor protein to potentially modulate Alzheimer's-associated pathogenesis in SAMP8 mice. *Neurobiol Aging* 33(3):522–534.
255. Fang M, et al. (2012). The miR-124 regulates the expression of BACE1/beta-secretase correlated with cell death in Alzheimer's disease. *Toxicol Lett* 209(1):94–105.
256. Li YY, et al. (2011). Increased expression of miRNA-146a in Alzheimer's disease transgenic mouse models. *Neurosci Lett* 487(1):94–98.
257. Wang H, et al. (2010). miR-106b aberrantly expressed in a double transgenic mouse model for Alzheimer's disease targets TGF-beta type II receptor. *Brain Res* 1357:166–174.
258. Wang X, et al. (2009). miR-34a, a microRNA upregulated in a double transgenic mouse model of Alzheimer's disease, inhibits bcl2 translation. *Brain Res Bull* 80(4–5):268–273.
259. Garza-Manero S, Arias C, Bermudez-Rattoni F, Vaca L, & Zepeda A (2015). Identification of age- and disease-related alterations in circulating miRNAs in a mouse model of Alzheimer's disease. *Front Cell Neurosci* 9:53.
260. Qi L, et al. (2012). A SNP site in pri-miR-124 changes mature miR-124 expression but no contribution to Alzheimer's disease in a Mongolian population. *Neurosci Lett* 515(1):1–6.
261. Zhu Y, Li C, Sun A, Wang Y, & Zhou S (2015). Quantification of microRNA-210 in the cerebrospinal fluid and serum: Implications for Alzheimer's disease. *Exp Ther Med* 9(3):1013–1017.
262. Lei X, Lei L, Zhang Z, Zhang Z, & Cheng Y (2015). Downregulated miR-29c correlates with increased BACE1 expression in sporadic Alzheimer's disease. *Int J Clin Exp Pathol* 8(2):1565–1574.
263. Liu CG, Wang JL, Li L, & Wang PC (2014). MicroRNA-384 regulates both amyloid precursor protein and beta-secretase expression and is a potential biomarker for Alzheimer's disease. *Int J Mol Med* 34(1):160–166.
264. Liu CG, Song J, Zhang YQ, & Wang PC (2014). MicroRNA-193b is a regulator of amyloid precursor protein in the blood and cerebrospinal fluid derived exosomal microRNA-193b is a biomarker of Alzheimer's disease. *Mol Med Rep* 10(5):2395–2400.
265. Zhu HC, et al. (2012). MicroRNA-195 downregulates Alzheimer's disease amyloid-beta production by targeting BACE1. *Brain Res Bull* 88(6):596–601.
266. Long JM & Lahiri DK (2011). MicroRNA-101 downregulates Alzheimer's amyloid-beta precursor protein levels in human cell cultures and is differentially expressed. *Biochem Biophys Res Commun* 404(4):889–895.
267. Geekiyanage H & Chan C (2011). MicroRNA-137/181c regulates serine palmitoyltransferase and in turn amyloid beta, novel targets in sporadic Alzheimer's disease. *J Neurosci* 31(41):14820–14830.
268. Nelson PT & Wang WX (2010). MiR-107 is reduced in Alzheimer's disease brain neocortex: validation study. *J Alzheimers Dis* 21(1):75–79.
269. Ai SX, et al. (2014). Hypomethylation of SNCA in blood of patients with sporadic Parkinson's disease. *J Neurol Sci* 337(1–2):123–128.
270. Coupland KG, et al. (2014). DNA methylation of the MAPT gene in Parkinson's disease cohorts and modulation by vitamin E in vitro. *Mov Disord* 29(13):1606–1614.
271. de Boni L, et al. (2011). Next-generation sequencing reveals regional differences of the alpha-synuclein methylation state independent of Lewy body disease. *Neuromolecular Med* 13(4):310–320.
272. Frieling H, et al. (2007). Global DNA hypomethylation and DNA hypermethylation of the alpha synuclein promoter in females with anorexia nervosa. *Mol Psychiatry* 12(3):229–230.
273. Jowaed A, Schmitt I, Kaut O, & Wullner U (2010). Methylation regulates alpha-synuclein expression and is decreased in Parkinson's disease patients' brains. *J Neurosci* 30(18):6355–6359.
274. Kaut O, Schmitt I, & Wullner U (2012). Genome-scale methylation analysis of Parkinson's disease patients' brains reveals DNA hypomethylation and increased mRNA expression of cytochrome P450 2E1. *Neurogenetics* 13(1):87–91.
275. Lin Q, et al. (2012). Promoter methylation analysis of seven clock genes in Parkinson's disease. *Neurosci Lett* 507(2):147–150.
276. Pieper HC, et al. (2008). Different methylation of the TNF-alpha promoter in cortex and substantia nigra: Implications for selective neuronal vulnerability. *Neurobiol Dis* 32(3):521–527.
277. Pihlstrom L, Berge V, Rengmark A, & Toft M (2015). Parkinson's disease correlates with promoter methylation in the alpha-synuclein gene. *Mov Disord* 30(4):577–580.
278. Richter J, et al. (2012). No evidence for differential methylation of alpha-synuclein in leukocyte DNA of Parkinson's disease patients. *Mov Disord* 27(4):590–591.
279. Song Y, et al. (2014). Pyrosequencing analysis of SNCA methylation levels in leukocytes from Parkinson's disease patients. *Neurosci Lett* 569:85–88.

280. Voutsinas GE, et al. (2010). Allelic imbalance of expression and epigenetic regulation within the alpha-synuclein wild-type and p.Ala53Thr alleles in Parkinson disease. *Hum Mutat* 31(6):685–691.

281. Kidd SK & Schneider JS (2010). Protection of dopaminergic cells from MPP+-mediated toxicity by histone deacetylase inhibition. *Brain Res* 1354:172–178.

282. Kidd SK & Schneider JS (2011). Protective effects of valproic acid on the nigrostriatal dopamine system in a 1-methyl-4-phenyl-1,2,3,6-tetrahydropyridine mouse model of Parkinson's disease. *Neuroscience* 194:189–194.

283. Liu L, et al. (2015). Protective role of SIRT5 against motor deficit and dopaminergic degeneration in MPTP-induced mice model of Parkinson's disease. *Behav Brain Res* 281:215–221.

284. Nicholas AP, et al. (2008). Striatal histone modifications in models of levodopa-induced dyskinesia. *J Neurochem* 106(1):486–494.

285. Patel VP & Chu CT (2014). Decreased SIRT2 activity leads to altered microtubule dynamics in oxidatively-stressed neuronal cells: implications for Parkinson's disease. *Exp Neurol* 257:170–181.

286. Song C, Kanthasamy A, Jin H, Anantharam V, & Kanthasamy AG (2011). Paraquat induces epigenetic changes by promoting histone acetylation in cell culture models of dopaminergic degeneration. *Neurotoxicology* 32(5):586–595.

287. Vartiainen S, Pehkonen P, Lakso M, Nass R, & Wong G (2006). Identification of gene expression changes in transgenic C. elegans overexpressing human alpha-synuclein. *Neurobiol Dis* 22(3):477–486.

288. Su M, et al. (2011). HDAC6 regulates aggresome-autophagy degradation pathway of alpha-synuclein in response to MPP+-induced stress. *J Neurochem* 117(1):112–120.

289. Wang H, et al. (2015). MiR-124 regulates apoptosis and autophagy process in MPTP model of Parkinson's disease by targeting to BIM. *Brain Pathol*. Mar;26(2):167–176.

290. Kim W, et al. (2014). miR-126 contributes to Parkinson's disease by dysregulating the insulin-like growth factor/phosphoinositide 3-kinase signaling. *Neurobiol Aging* 35(7):1712–1721.

291. Asci R, et al. (2013). Trasferrin receptor 2 gene regulation by microRNA 221 in SH-SY5Y cells treated with MPP(+) as Parkinson's disease cellular model. *Neurosci Res* 77(3):121–127.

292. Kabaria S, Choi DC, Chaudhuri AD, Mouradian MM, & Junn E (2015). Inhibition of miR-34b and miR-34c enhances alpha-synuclein expression in Parkinson's disease. *FEBS Lett* 589(3):319–325.

293. Zhao N, Jin L, Fei G, Zheng Z, & Zhong C (2014). Serum microRNA-133b is associated with low ceruloplasmin levels in Parkinson's disease. *Parkinsonism Relat Disord* 20(11):1177–1180.

294. Villar-Menendez I, et al. (2014). Increased striatal adenosine A2A receptor levels is an early event in Parkinson's disease-related pathology and it is potentially regulated by miR-34b. *Neurobiol Dis* 69:206–214.

295. Kanagaraj N, Beiping H, Dheen ST, & Tay SS (2014). Downregulation of miR-124 in MPTP-treated mouse model of Parkinson's disease and MPP iodide-treated MN9D cells modulates the expression of the calpain/cdk5 pathway proteins. *Neuroscience* 272:167–179.

296. Dorval V, et al. (2014). Gene and MicroRNA transcriptome analysis of Parkinson's related LRRK2 mouse models. *PLoS One* 9(1):e85510.

297. Cardo LF, et al. (2014). MiRNA profile in the substantia nigra of Parkinson's disease and healthy subjects. *J Mol Neurosci* 54(4):830–836.

298. Botta-Orfila T, et al. (2014). Identification of blood serum micro-RNAs associated with idiopathic and LRRK2 Parkinson's disease. *J Neurosci Res* 92(8):1071–1077.

299. Cho HJ, et al. (2013). MicroRNA-205 regulates the expression of Parkinson's disease-related leucine-rich repeat kinase 2 protein. *Hum Mol Genet* 22(3):608–620.

300. Minones-Moyano E, et al. (2011). MicroRNA profiling of Parkinson's disease brains identifies early downregulation of miR-34b/c which modulate mitochondrial function. *Hum Mol Genet* 20(15):3067–3078.

301. Gehrke S, Imai Y, Sokol N, & Lu B (2010). Pathogenic LRRK2 negatively regulates microRNA-mediated translational repression. *Nature* 466(7306):637–641.

302. Gillardon F, et al. (2008). MicroRNA and proteome expression profiling in early-symptomatic alpha-synuclein(A30P)-transgenic mice. *Proteomics Clin Appl* 2(5):697–705.

303. Schlaudraff F, et al. (2014). Orchestrated increase of dopamine and PARK mRNAs but not miR-133b in dopamine neurons in Parkinson's disease. *Neurobiol Aging* 35(10):2302–2315.

304. Haixia D, et al. (2012). Lack of association of polymorphism in miRNA-196a2 with Parkinson's disease risk in a Chinese population. *Neurosci Lett* 514(2):194–197.

305. de Mena L, et al. (2010). FGF20 rs12720208 SNP and microRNA-433 variation: no association with Parkinson's disease in Spanish patients. *Neurosci Lett* 479(1):22–25.

306. Bhusari SS, et al. (2010). Superoxide dismutase 1 knockdown induces oxidative stress and DNA methylation loss in the prostate. *Epigenetics* 5(5):402–409.

307. Tremolizzo L, et al. (2014). Whole-blood global DNA methylation is increased in amyotrophic lateral sclerosis independently of age of onset. *Amyotroph Lateral Scler Frontotemporal Degener* 15(1–2):98–105.

308. Belzil VV, et al. (2014). Characterization of DNA hypermethylation in the cerebellum of c9FTD/ALS patients. *Brain Res* 1584:15–21.

309. Xi Z, et al. (2013). Hypermethylation of the CpG island near the G4C2 repeat in ALS with a C9orf72 expansion. *Am J Hum Genet* 92(6):981–989.

310. Russ J, et al. (2015). Hypermethylation of repeat expanded C9orf72 is a clinical and molecular disease modifier. *Acta Neuropathol* 129(1):39–52.

311. Wong M, Gertz B, Chestnut BA, & Martin LJ (2013). Mitochondrial DNMT3A and DNA methylation in skeletal muscle and CNS of transgenic mouse models of ALS. *Front Cell Neurosci* 7:279.

312. Morahan JM, Yu B, Trent RJ, & Pamphlett R (2007). Are metallothionein genes silenced in ALS? *Toxicol Lett* 168(1):83–87.

313. Schmalbach S & Petri S (2010). Histone deacetylation and motor neuron degeneration. *CNS Neurol Disord Drug Targets* 9(3):279–284.

314. Zhang J, et al. (2006). Altered distributions of nucleocytoplasmic transport-related proteins in the spinal cord of a mouse model of amyotrophic lateral sclerosis. *Acta Neuropathol* 112(6):673–680.

315. Belzil VV, et al. (2013). Reduced C9orf72 gene expression in c9FTD/ALS is caused by histone trimethylation, an epigenetic event detectable in blood. *Acta Neuropathol* 126(6):895–905.

316. Bruneteau G, et al. (2013). Muscle histone deacetylase 4 upregulation in amyotrophic lateral sclerosis: potential role in reinnervation ability and disease progression. *Brain* 136(Pt 8):2359–2368.

317. Gal J, et al. (2013). HDAC6 regulates mutant SOD1 aggregation through two SMIR motifs and tubulin acetylation. *J Biol Chem* 288(21):15035–15045.

318. Janssen C, et al. (2010). Differential histone deacetylase mRNA expression patterns in amyotrophic lateral sclerosis. *J Neuropathol Exp Neurol* 69(6):573–581.

319. Kim SH, Shanware NP, Bowler MJ, & Tibbetts RS (2010). Amyotrophic lateral sclerosis-associated proteins TDP-43 and FUS/TLS function in a common biochemical complex to co-regulate HDAC6 mRNA. *J Biol Chem* 285(44):34097–34105.

320. Korner S, et al. (2013). Differential sirtuin expression patterns in amyotrophic lateral sclerosis (ALS) postmortem tissue: neuroprotective or neurotoxic properties of sirtuins in ALS? *Neurodegener Dis* 11(3):141–152.

321. Lagier-Tourenne C, et al. (2012). Divergent roles of ALS-linked proteins FUS/TLS and TDP-43 intersect in processing long pre-mRNAs. *Nat Neurosci* 15(11):1488–1497.

322. Petri S, et al. (2006). Additive neuroprotective effects of a histone deacetylase inhibitor and a catalytic antioxidant in a transgenic mouse model of amyotrophic lateral sclerosis. *Neurobiol Dis* 22(1):40–49.

323. Taes I, et al. (2013). Hdac6 deletion delays disease progression in the SOD1G93A mouse model of ALS. *Hum Mol Genet* 22(9):1783–1790.

324. Tibshirani M, et al. (2015). Cytoplasmic sequestration of FUS/TLS associated with ALS alters histone marks through loss of nuclear protein arginine methyltransferase 1. *Hum Mol Genet* 24(3):773–786.

325. Valle C, et al. (2014). Tissue-specific deregulation of selected HDACs characterizes ALS progression in mouse models: pharmacological characterization of SIRT1 and SIRT2 pathways. *Cell Death Dis* 5:e1296.

326. Wang WY, et al. (2013). Interaction of FUS and HDAC1 regulates DNA damage response and repair in neurons. *Nat Neurosci* 16(10):1383–1391.

327. Xia Q, Wang H, Zhang Y, Ying Z, & Wang G (2014). Loss of TDP-43 inhibits amyotrophic lateral sclerosis-linked mutant SOD1 aggresome formation in an HDAC6-dependent manner. *J Alzheimers Dis*.

328. Marcuzzo S, et al. (2015). Up-regulation of neural and cell cycle-related microRNAs in brain of amyotrophic lateral sclerosis mice at late disease stage. *Mol Brain* 8(1):5.

329. Butovsky O, et al. (2015). Targeting miR-155 restores abnormal microglia and attenuates disease in SOD1 mice. *Ann Neurol* 77(1):75–99.

330. Wakabayashi K, et al. (2014). Analysis of microRNA from archived formalin-fixed paraffin-embedded specimens of amyotrophic lateral sclerosis. *Acta Neuropathol Commun* 2(1):173.

331. Toivonen JM, et al. (2014). MicroRNA-206: a potential circulating biomarker candidate for amyotrophic lateral sclerosis. *PLoS One* 9(2):e89065.

332. Sumitha R, et al. (2014). Differential expression of microRNA-206 in the gastrocnemius and biceps brachii in response to CSF from sporadic

amyotrophic lateral sclerosis patients. *J Neurol Sci* 345(1–2):254–256.

333. Nolan K, et al. (2014). Increased expression of microRNA-29a in ALS mice: functional analysis of its inhibition. *J Mol Neurosci* 53(2):231–241.

334. De Felice B, et al. (2014). miR-338-3p is over-expressed in blood, CFS, serum and spinal cord from sporadic amyotrophic lateral sclerosis patients. *Neurogenetics* 15(4):243–253.

335. Zhou F, et al. (2013). miRNA-9 expression is upregulated in the spinal cord of G93A-SOD1 transgenic mice. *Int J Clin Exp Pathol* 6(9):1826–1838.

336. Parisi C, et al. (2013). Dysregulated microRNAs in amyotrophic lateral sclerosis microglia modulate genes linked to neuroinflammation. *Cell Death Dis* 4:e959.

337. Koval ED, et al. (2013). Method for widespread microRNA-155 inhibition prolongs survival in ALS-model mice. *Hum Mol Genet* 22(20):4127–4135.

338. Freischmidt A, Muller K, Ludolph AC, & Weishaupt JH (2013). Systemic dysregulation of TDP-43 binding microRNAs in amyotrophic lateral sclerosis. *Acta Neuropathol Commun* 1(1):42.

339. Kawahara Y & Mieda-Sato A (2012). TDP-43 promotes microRNA biogenesis as a component of the Drosha and Dicer complexes. *Proc Natl Acad Sci U S A* 109(9):3347–3352.

340. De Felice B, et al. (2012). A miRNA signature in leukocytes from sporadic amyotrophic lateral sclerosis. *Gene* 508(1):35–40.

341. Zhang Z, et al. (2013). Downregulation of microRNA-9 in iPSC-derived neurons of FTD/ALS patients with TDP-43 mutations. *PLoS One* 8(10):e76055.

342. Dion V, et al. (2008). Genome-wide demethylation promotes triplet repeat instability independently of homologous recombination. *DNA Repair (Amst)* 7(2):313–320.

343. Wang F, et al. (2013). Genome-wide loss of 5-hmC is a novel epigenetic feature of Huntington's disease. *Hum Mol Genet* 22(18): 3641–3653.

344. Reik W, Maher ER, Morrison PJ, Harding AE, & Simpson SA (1993). Age at onset in Huntington's disease and methylation at D4S95. *J Med Genet* 30(3):185–188.

345. Valdeolivas S, et al. (2015). Neuroprotective properties of cannabigerol in Huntington's disease: studies in R6/2 mice and 3-nitropropionate-lesioned mice. *Neurotherapeutics* 12(1):185–199.

346. Rawat V, Goux W, Piechaczyk M, & SR DM (2015). c-Fos protects neurons through a noncanonical mechanism involving HDAC3 interaction: identification of a 21-amino acid fragment with neuroprotective activity. *Mol Neurobiol.* 53(2):1165–1180.

347. Ratovitski T, Arbez N, Stewart JC, Chighladze E, & Ross CA (2015). PRMT5-mediated symmetric arginine dimethylation is attenuated by mutant huntingtin and is impaired in Huntington's Disease (HD). *Cell Cycle* 14(11):1716–1729.

348. Jia H, Morris CD, Williams RM, Loring JF, & Thomas EA (2015). HDAC inhibition imparts beneficial transgenerational effects in Huntington's disease mice via altered DNA and histone methylation. *Proc Natl Acad Sci U S A* 112(1): E56–64.

349. Thomas EA (2014). Involvement of HDAC1 and HDAC3 in the pathology of polyglutamine disorders: therapeutic implications for selective HDAC1/HDAC3 inhibitors. *Pharmaceuticals (Basel)* 7(6):634–661.

350. Smith MR, et al. (2014). A potent and selective Sirtuin 1 inhibitor alleviates pathology in multiple animal and cell models of Huntington's disease. *Hum Mol Genet* 23(11):2995–3007.

351. Mano T, Suzuki T, Tsuji S, & Iwata A (2014). Differential effect of HDAC3 on cytoplasmic and nuclear huntingtin aggregates. *PLoS One* 9(11):e111277.

352. Yeh HH, et al. (2013). Histone deacetylase class II and acetylated core histone immunohistochemistry in human brains with Huntington's disease. *Brain Res* 1504:16–24.

353. Vashishtha M, et al. (2013). Targeting H3K4 trimethylation in Huntington disease. *Proc Natl Acad Sci U S A* 110(32):E3027–3036.

354. Robinson R (2013). An HDAC in the cytoplasm, not the nucleus, plays a pathogenic role in Huntington's disease. *PLoS Biol* 11(11):e1001718.

355. Pena-Altamira LE, Polazzi E, & Monti B (2013). Histone post-translational modifications in Huntington's and Parkinson's diseases. *Curr Pharm Des* 19(28):5085–5092.

356. Mielcarek M, et al. (2013). HDAC4 reduction: a novel therapeutic strategy to target cytoplasmic huntingtin and ameliorate neurodegeneration. *PLoS Biol* 11(11):e1001717.

357. McFarland KN, et al. (2013). Genome-wide increase in histone H2A ubiquitylation in a mouse model of Huntington's disease. *J Huntingtons Dis* 2(3):263–277.

358. Lee J, et al. (2013). Epigenetic regulation of cholinergic receptor M1 (CHRM1) by histone H3K9me3 impairs Ca(2+) signaling in Huntington's disease. *Acta Neuropathol* 125(5):727–739.

359. Moumne L, Campbell K, Howland D, Ouyang Y, & Bates GP (2012). Genetic knock-down of

HDAC3 does not modify disease-related phenotypes in a mouse model of Huntington's disease. *PLoS One* 7(2):e31080. doi:10.1371/journal.pone.0031080

360. Konsoula Z & Barile FA (2012). Epigenetic histone acetylation and deacetylation mechanisms in experimental models of neurodegenerative disorders. *J Pharmacol Toxicol Methods* 66(3):215–220.

361. Jia H, et al. (2012). Histone deacetylase (HDAC) inhibitors targeting HDAC3 and HDAC1 ameliorate polyglutamine-elicited phenotypes in model systems of Huntington's disease. *Neurobiol Dis* 46(2):351–361.

362. Giralt A, et al. (2012). Long-term memory deficits in Huntington's disease are associated with reduced CBP histone acetylase activity. *Hum Mol Genet* 21(6):1203–1216.

363. Debacker K, et al. (2012). Histone deacetylase complexes promote trinucleotide repeat expansions. *PLoS Biol* 10(2):e1001257.

364. Bobrowska A, Donmez G, Weiss A, Guarente L, & Bates G (2012). SIRT2 ablation has no effect on tubulin acetylation in brain, cholesterol biosynthesis or the progression of Huntington's disease phenotypes in vivo. *PLoS One* 7(4):e34805.

365. Mielcarek M, et al. (2011). SAHA decreases HDAC 2 and 4 levels in vivo and improves molecular phenotypes in the R6/2 mouse model of Huntington's disease. *PLoS One* 6(11):e27746.

366. Lake F (2011). Hunting biomarkers for Huntington's disease: H2AFY. *Biomark Med* 5(6): 817–820.

367. Bobrowska A, Paganetti P, Matthias P, & Bates GP (2011). Hdac6 knock-out increases tubulin acetylation but does not modify disease progression in the R6/2 mouse model of Huntington's disease. *PLoS One* 6(6):e20696.

368. Bett JS, Benn CL, Ryu KY, Kopito RR, & Bates GP (2009). The polyubiquitin Ubc gene modulates histone H2A monoubiquitylation in the R6/2 mouse model of Huntington's disease. *J Cell Mol Med* 13(8B):2645–2657.

369. Benn CL, et al. (2009). Genetic knock-down of HDAC7 does not ameliorate disease pathogenesis in the R6/2 mouse model of Huntington's disease. *PLoS One* 4(6):e5747.

370. Pallos J, et al. (2008). Inhibition of specific HDACs and sirtuins suppresses pathogenesis in a Drosophila model of Huntington's disease. *Hum Mol Genet* 17(23):3767–3775.

371. Kim MO, et al. (2008). Altered histone monoubiquitylation mediated by mutant huntingtin induces transcriptional dysregulation. *J Neurosci* 28(15):3947–3957.

372. Yazawa I, Hazeki N, Nakase H, Kanazawa I, & Tanaka M (2003). Histone H3 is aberrantly phosphorylated in glutamine-repeat diseases. *Biochem Biophys Res Commun* 302(1): 144–149.

373. Cooper AJ, et al. (2000). Lysine-rich histone (H1) is a lysyl substrate of tissue transglutaminase: possible involvement of transglutaminase in the formation of nuclear aggregates in (CAG) (n)/Q(n) expansion diseases. *Dev Neurosci* 22(5–6):404–417.

374. Boutell JM, et al. (1999). Aberrant interactions of transcriptional repressor proteins with the Huntington's disease gene product, huntingtin. *Hum Mol Genet* 8(9):1647–1655.

375. Hoss AG, et al. (2015). miR-10b-5p expression in Huntington's disease brain relates to age of onset and the extent of striatal involvement. *BMC Med Genomics* 8(1):10.

376. Hoss AG, et al. (2014). MicroRNAs located in the Hox gene clusters are implicated in huntington's disease pathogenesis. *PLoS Genet* 10(2):e1004188.

377. Katta A, et al. (2013). Overload induced heat shock proteins (HSPs), MAPK and miRNA (miR-1 and miR133a) response in insulin-resistant skeletal muscle. *Cell Physiol Biochem* 31(2–3):219–229.

378. Jin J, et al. (2012). Interrogation of brain miRNA and mRNA expression profiles reveals a molecular regulatory network that is perturbed by mutant huntingtin. *J Neurochem* 123(4):477–490.

379. Gaughwin PM, et al. (2011). Hsa-miR-34b is a plasma-stable microRNA that is elevated in premanifest Huntington's disease. *Hum Mol Genet* 20(11):2225–2237.

380. Kocerha J, Xu Y, Prucha MS, Zhao D, & Chan AW (2014). microRNA-128a dysregulation in transgenic Huntington's disease monkeys. *Mol Brain* 7:46.

381. Cheng PH, et al. (2013). miR-196a ameliorates phenotypes of Huntington disease in cell, transgenic mouse, and induced pluripotent stem cell models. *Am J Hum Genet* 93(2):306–312.

12

Mitochondrial Changes and Bioenergetics in Neurodegenerative Diseases

ANDREW B. KNOTT AND ELLA BOSSY-WETZEL

INTRODUCTION

Mitochondria have long been recognized as important organelles for cellular survival and health, in large part because of their critical role in energy production. In addition to their function as cellular powerhouses, research in recent years has identified a multitude of other vital functions of mitochondria, including intracellular calcium handling, oxidative stress defense, signal transduction, and apoptosis. It is also becoming increasingly clear that—in stark contrast to the classical textbook representation of mitochondria as static, rod-shaped organelles—mitochondria are in fact highly dynamic, with the ability to move great distances, fuse, and divide. These dynamic properties of mitochondria are particularly important in neurons because of their unique morphology, including axonal processes that can extend long distances. More generally, central nervous system function is highly dependent on efficient mitochondrial function because neurons have high energy demands, which must be met almost entirely by mitochondrial oxidative phosphorylation.

Consistent with a central role for mitochondrial function in neuronal health, several rare mitochondrial diseases caused by mutations in either mitochondrial DNA (mtDNA) or nuclear DNA coding for mitochondrial proteins exhibit neurodegeneration as a central or secondary pathogenic feature[1–9] (Table 12.1). In addition, mutations in genes coding for proteins associated with mitochondria cause neurodegenerative diseases, such as Huntington's disease (HD),[10] and rare, familial forms of more common sporadic neurodegenerative diseases, such as Parkinson's disease (PD), Alzheimer's disease (AD), and amyotrophic lateral sclerosis (ALS)[11–21] (Table 12.2). Finally, multifaceted mitochondrial dysfunction has been observed in all of the most common neurodegenerative diseases, in both their familial and sporadic forms.[22]

This chapter highlights the overlapping and shared pathways of mitochondrial dysfunction in various neurodegenerative diseases. The chapter concludes by briefly summarizing current research in the development of therapeutics targeting mitochondria.

BIOENERGETIC FAILURE

Energy production is a defining role of mitochondria and one that is particularly important in neurons because of their high energy requirements. Multiple characteristics of neurodegenerative disease patients and cellular and animal models suggest that bioenergetic failure is a central and unifying feature of neurodegeneration. For example, early weight loss has been reported in PD, AD, and HD patients,[23–25] and diminished energy production has been documented by imaging studies of the diseased brain.[26–29] And while neurodegenerative diseases share many clinical features indicative of bioenergetic failure, molecular studies have revealed that the specific portions of the mitochondrial energy production mechanism that are affected differ in some cases.

Early studies of mitochondrial respiratory chain complex I inhibitors, such as 1-methyl-4-phenyl-1,2,3,6-tetrahydrodropyridine (MPTP) and rotenone, suggested a link between bioenergetic failure and PD. MPTP, a contaminant of the synthetic opioid 1-methyl-4-phenyl-4-propionoxypiperidine (MPPP), was found to cause PD-like symptoms in intravenous drug users and laboratory researchers exposed to the agent.[30,31] Similarly, rotenone was found to cause PD-like symptoms in animal models.[32] These early findings opened up the field of mitochondrial research in PD and paved the way for discovery of more direct evidence of bioenergetic defects

TABLE 12.1. MITOCHONDRIAL DISEASES WITH NEURODEGENERATIVE COMPONENTS

Disease	Mutated Gene(s)	Protein Function(s)	Phenotype
Autosomal dominant optic atrophy (ADOA)	OPA1 (n)	Mitochondrial fusion, cristae organization, apoptosis	Varying degrees of vision loss, accompanied by additional neurological symptoms
Charcot-Marie-Tooth hereditary neuropathy type 2A (CMT2A)	MFN2 (n)	Mitochondrial fusion	Peripheral neuropathy, muscle weakness, axonal degradation of sensory and motor neurons
Leber's hereditary optic neuropathy	ND1 (mt) ND2 (mt) ND4 (mt)	Complex I of the mitochondrial respiratory chain	Bilateral acute or sub-acute loss of central vision
Leigh syndrome	Multiple respiratory chain genes (mt and n)	Complexes I, II, IV, or V; succinate dehydrogenase; coenzyme Q10	Multi-systemic dysfunction, including extensive neurological pathogenesis
Pearson syndrome	Multiple genes (mt)	Mitochondrial polypeptide synthesis and respiratory chain	Anemia, marrow defects, and pancreatic fibrosis with neurological defects in some cases

Mt: mitochondrial; n: nuclear.

in the disease. For example, ATP levels were found to be decreased in the putamen and midbrain in early and advanced PD patients.[26] In addition, reduced protein expression of complex I proteins has been observed in the PD brain,[33,34] along with defective assembly and decreased activity in the substantia nigra and frontal cortex.[35-38] Finally,

TABLE 12.2. NEURODEGENERATIVE DISEASE-RELATED PROTEINS ASSOCIATED WITH MITOCHONDRIA

Protein	Properties	Disease
Aβ	Amyloid plaque component	AD
APP	Precursor of Aβ	AD
α-synuclein	Lewy body component	PD
DJ-1	ROS scavenger and sensor	PD
HTRA2	Apoptosis factor	PD
Huntingtin	Polyglutamine mutation causes disease	HD
LRRK2	Kinase	PD
Parkin	Ubiquitin E3 ligase	PD
PINK1	Mitochondrial kinase	PD
PS1/2	Components of γ-secretase that processes APP	AD
SOD1	Cu/Zn Superoxide dismutase	ALS

the alpha-ketoglutarate dehydrogenase complex, the rate-limiting enzyme of the TCA cycle, exhibits reduced staining in the PD brain.[39,40]

In AD, early PET imaging studies of patient brains revealed decreased glucose metabolism and metabolic failure.[27,28,32] Protein levels of complex I–IV subunits and complex IV activity have been reported to be decreased in the AD brain.[41-43] Finally, the activity of TCA cycle complexes, including pyruvate dehydrogenase, isocitrate dehydrogenase, and alpha-ketoglutarate, is impaired in the postmortem AD brain.[44,45]

Decreased glucose consumption in the HD brain and characteristic weight loss of HD patients are indicative of bioenergetic defects.[29] In addition, early in the disease, failure to upregulate ATP concentrations in the brain in response to increased energy demands has been noted.[46] Deficiencies in complex II and III, and to a lesser extent complex IV, have been reported in the HD brain.[29,47-49] Finally, the TCA cycle is also inhibited in HD, as evidenced by a large decrease in aconitase activity.[29,50]

Bioenergetic changes are also characteristic of ALS, though the nature of the changes remains somewhat unclear. Increased cortical activity of complexes I, II, and III has been reported in familial ALS with superoxide dismutase 1 (SOD1) mutations, but not sporadic ALS.[51] By contrast, an overall pattern of cortical motor-sensory hypo-metabolism has been observed in ALS patients[52] and decreased complex IV activity in spinal cord motor neurons of sporadic ALS patients has been reported.[53] Finally, multiple cellular models of ALS suggest an overall decrease in electron transport chain complex activity.[32,54]

INCREASED OXIDATIVE STRESS

Mitochondria release reactive oxygen species (ROS) as byproducts of energy production. While it was initially postulated that ROS had a uniformly negative effect on cellular health and life span, it is becoming increasingly clear that ROS, despite their potential toxicity, may play important roles in normal cellular physiology—for example, as signaling molecules and inducers of cytoprotective cell defense mechanisms.[55–57] These latter phenomena, which have collectively been given the name *mitohormesis*, may underlie some of the positive effects of ROS and the lack of positive effects and, in some cases, the negative effects of antioxidants that have been observed in research studies and clinical trials.[56,57] For example, the wide-ranging health benefits of physical exercise in a multitude of diseases—including neurodegenerative diseases such as AD[58]—are well-established despite (or perhaps because of) the transient increase in ROS that exercise produces.[57,59] Interestingly, antioxidant supplementation prior to workouts has been shown to counteract the health benefits of physical exercise.[60] Despite these more recent findings elucidating the beneficial effects of native ROS and induced, transient increases in ROS, persistent and large changes in ROS levels have the potential to disrupt the cellular milieu and contribute to pathology via increased oxidative stress, which can irreversibly damage lipids, proteins, and DNA.[61] In addition, oxidative damage of cellular components can facilitate protein misfolding and aggregation and mitochondrial dysfunction, which in turn stimulate ROS production even more, thus perpetuating a vicious cycle of dysfunction that ultimately culminates in cell death.

Oxidative damage to lipids is potentially important in neurodegenerative diseases because of the prevalence of polyunsaturated fatty acids in the lipid bilayer of the brain.[62] Lipid peroxidation is a pathological characteristic of PD, AD, HD, and ALS.[63] One particularly toxic lipid peroxidation product, 4-hydroxy-2-nonenal (HNE), is elevated in PD, AD, and HD and is often associated with characteristic inclusions and aggregates.[63]

Proteins are another important target of oxidative stress. Oxidative damage to proteins can contribute to the formation of highly cross-linked, undegradable protein aggregates.[62] For example, concentrations of liposfuscin—a hallmark of aging made up of oxidized proteins (30%–70%), lipids (20%–50%), sugar residues, and metals—increase with age, particularly in post-mitotic cells such as neurons.[64] Lipofuscin inhibits the degradation of oxidized proteins by disrupting lysosomal function and also contributes to increased ROS formation.[62,64] The rate of lipofuscin formation is increased in the superior frontal gyrus, but not superior temporal gyrus, of the AD brain,[65] and large amounts of lipofuscin have been observed in AD neurons containing amyloid.[66] More general markers of protein oxidation, such as carbonyl and 3-nitrotyrosine (3-NT) modifications and S-nitrosylation, are increased in AD, PD, HD, and ALS.[49,62,67–73]

Finally, oxidative damage to nuclear and mtDNA and diminished DNA repair capacity are thought to play an important role in neurodegeneration.[74] For example, elevated levels of oxidative lesions on DNA have been reported in neurons of ALS patients, and oxidative damage to mtDNA in PD is a well-established phenomenon.[74] Whether these oxidative changes to lipids, proteins, and DNA in neurodegenerative diseases are cause or consequence remains an open question and one that requires further examination.

MITOCHONDRIAL DNA MUTATIONS/DEFECTS

Mitochondria are unique among organelles because they contain their own genome, mtDNA, which includes 37 genes encoding 13 essential proteins of the oxidative phosphorylation system.[75] It has been hypothesized that mtDNA mutations might be particularly deleterious to neurons because of their high energy demands and post-mitotic state; however, the link between mtDNA damage and sporadic, age-related neurodegenerative diseases remains speculative.[76] MtDNA deletions and point mutations cause a multitude of genetic mitochondrial diseases, such as Pearson syndrome, Leber's heridetary optic neuropathy, and Leigh syndrome (Table 12.1). The nervous system is profoundly affected in many of these diseases, indicating that mtDNA stability is important in nerve cells and might play a role in neurodegenerative disease.[76]

Human postmortem studies have identified respiratory deficiency resulting from the accumulation of mtDNA deletions in the substantia nigra of samples from PD patients and age-matched controls,[75,77] suggesting that mtDNA deletions might play a role in both specific neurodegenerative diseases and aging in general. In addition, a recent study found that mtDNA mutation levels were significantly elevated in the substantia nigra of early PD and cases of incidental Lewy body disease.[78] Whether mtDNA damage is sufficient to cause PD symptoms remains controversial, although studies in animal models and the phenotype of patients with mitochondrial DNA polymerase gamma mutations hint at this possibility.[76] The potential role of mtDNA damage in AD is similarly unclear as different laboratories have reported varying results about the level of mtDNA mutations in the AD brain.[76] In HD, elevated levels of mtDNA deletions have been observed in the cerebral cortex of patients.[79] Finally, in ALS, mtDNA deletions are mildly increased in the brain,[76,80,81] and several mtDNA deletions have been associated with ALS-like pathologies.[76,82–85]

Studies utilizing cytoplasmic hybrid (cybrid) cells, whole cells fused with enucleated cells, and mutant mice with proofreading-deficient mitochondrial DNA polymerase gamma have attempted to elucidate further the contribution of mtDNA to neurodegenerative diseases. Cybrids containing mtDNA from PD patients have been shown, in general, to have reduced complex I activity, suggesting mtDNA encoded defects in PD.[32,86] Cybrid cell lines with mtDNA from AD patients replicate many of the pathological features observed in the AD brain, including increased Aβ secretion and decreased respiratory chain activity.[32,87,88] Finally, cybrids containing mtDNA from HD patients exhibited only mild mitochondrial changes and no significant modification of respiratory chain activity, but were more susceptible to apoptotic stimuli.[32,89] Mutant mice with proofreading-deficient mitochondrial DNA polymerase gamma readily accumulate mtDNA mutations and exhibit accelerated aging.[90,91] However, a recent study found that the accumulation of mtDNA mutations in dopaminergic neurons of these mutant mice to levels similar to those observed in PD patients were not toxic, but rather triggered a neuroprotective compensatory response at the mitochondrial level, suggesting that the tolerance threshold for mtDNA mutations in neurons is quite high.[92] As a whole, these cybrid and mutator mouse studies have largely mirrored the conflicting clinical observations, meaning that the significance of mtDNA damage in neurodegeneration remains an open question.

DEFECTIVE MITOCHONDRIAL CALCIUM HANDLING

Mitochondria serve as important buffers of calcium ions (Ca^{2+}), particularly in neurons in which Ca^{2+} is the primary second messenger linking membrane depolarization and synaptic activity.[93] The idea that defective Ca^{2+} handling by mitochondria could be a unifying feature of neurodegenerative diseases is gaining momentum. Altered Ca^{2+} homeostasis has been identified in PD, AD, HD, and ALS.[93]

Oligomers of α-synuclein, a protein that is mutated in some familial forms of PD and is believed to contribute to sporadic PD pathogenesis, was found to modulate Ca^{2+} influx in a dopaminergic cell line (SH-SY5Y),[94] possibly by forming pores in the plasma membrane or regulating Ca^{2+} membrane channels.[93,95,96] The relevance of Ca^{2+} level modulation by α-synuclein to PD remains unclear, and there have been conflicting data about the relationship between wild-type and mutant α-synuclein and Ca^{2+} homeostasis in different model systems and cell types.[93] However, several studies involving PTEN-induced putative kinase 1 (PINK1), a protein purported to be involved in PD pathogenesis, provide more compelling evidence for the involvement of Ca^{2+} dysfunction in PD.[93] For example, mutant PINK1 was found to exacerbate mitochondrial defects caused by mutant α-synuclein in a cellular model of PD, and the changes were mediated at least in part by the modulation of Ca^{2+} uptake.[97] Additional studies in cell lines and mice have yielded more controversial results; however, a potential relationship among PINK1, Ca^{2+} regulation, and disease pathogenesis is a possibility that warrants further investigation.[93]

Defective Ca^{2+} signaling has been reported in sporadic and familial AD.[93,98,99] Aβ oligomers can form ion-conducting channels by inserting into the plasma membrane, thus potentially causing increased Ca^{2+} influx and excitotoxicity.[100] Similarly in HD, Ca^{2+} overload and increased susceptibility to Ca^{2+}-induced permeability transition has been reported in lymphoblasts isolated from HD patients and animal models of HD.[93,101,102] However, the pathological significance of these phenomena remains unclear because increasing Ca^{2+} buffering capacity failed to improve disease progression in multiple studies.[93] Finally, in ALS, mitochondria from patients with sporadic and genetic forms of the disease exhibit Ca^{2+} handling deficiencies.[93] Supporting studies in mutant SOD1 mice also suggest that mitochondrial Ca^{2+} handling might contribute to ALS pathogenesis.[103]

IMPAIRED MITOCHONDRIAL DYNAMICS

Mitochondrial dynamics—the ability of mitochondria to divide, fuse, and move—are critical for cell function and survival, particularly in neurons. Mitochondria undergo regulated cycles of fission and fusion, and defects in these processes have been identified early in many neurodegenerative diseases.[104,105] When the balance between fission and fusion is disrupted, mitochondria can become fragmented or overly enlarged, resulting in many of the problems discussed earlier, including decreased energy production and increased oxidative stress.

The discovery of mutations in mitochondrial fission and fusion GTPases that resulted in inherited neurodegenerative diseases was the first clue that mitochondrial dynamics might play a vital role in neurological health. Specifically, mutations in mitofusin 2 (MFN2), a mitochondrial fusion protein, cause the peripheral neuropathy Charcot-Marie-Tooth subtype 2A (CMT2A), which is characterized by muscle weakness and degeneration of sensory and motor neurons.[4,106] In addition, mutations in the fusion protein optic atrophy 1 (OPA1) cause autosomal dominant optic atrophy (ADOA), which is characterized by progressive blindness and optic nerve degeneration.[1,2] Finally, a human patient case study reported a dominant negative mutation of the primary fission protein dynamin-related protein 1 (DRP1) that resulted in death of the neonate after just 37 days.[107] That mutations in these mitochondrial fission and fusion proteins affect neurological function suggested that mitochondrial dynamics might play an important role in the health of the nervous system in general and the development of neurodegenerative diseases in particular.

Indeed, it has become increasingly apparent that defects in mitochondrial fission and fusion are common features of age-related neurodegenerative disorders. Mitochondrial fragmentation has been observed in PD, AD, HD, and ALS.[108]

In PD, multiple proteins involved in the pathogenesis of both familial and sporadic forms of the disease, including PINK1, parkin, DJ-1, leucine-rich repeat kinase 2 (LRRK2), and α-synuclein, are involved in the regulation of mitochondrial dynamics.[104,109] In AD, an early study found that pathogenic Aβ peptide aggregates caused mitochondrial fragmentation in cultured cortical neurons.[110] More recently, studies of postmortem AD brain found that defects in mitochondrial dynamics increased with disease progression, and an overall pattern of increased mRNA and protein levels of mitochondrial fission genes and proteins—DRP1 and mitochondrial fission protein 1 (FIS1)—and decreased levels of fusion genes and proteins—MFN1/2 and OPA1—was reported.[111,112] Furthermore, abnormal interactions between DRP1 and Aβ/hyperphosphorylated tau were observed in the AD brain and were associated with increased mitochondrial fragmentation and disease progression.[111,113]

Similarly, in HD, increased expression of fission genes, *DRP1* and *FIS1*, and decreased expression of fusion genes, *MFN1/2* and *OPA1*, were observed in affected regions of the HD brain.[114] Mutant huntingtin protein also interacts with DRP1, increasing its enzymatic activity and stimulating mitochondrial fragmentation.[115,116] The dominant negative mutant of DRP1 (DRP1 K38A) was able to rescue mutant huntingtin-mediated mitochondrial fragmentation, mitochondrial transport defects, and neuronal cell death in mice.[115]

Finally, in ALS, the role of defects in mitochondrial dynamics is less clear, but several studies to date suggest that this shared mechanism of neurodegeneration might also be important in motor neuron disease. For example, in rat spinal cord neurons and co-cultured astrocytes carrying a mutation in the SOD protein (SODG93A), a protein mutated in some familial forms of ALS, fragmented mitochondria were observed.[117] Expression of dominant-negative DRP1 counteracted the fragmentation and restored cell viability.[117] In addition, decreased levels of OPA1 and increased levels of DRP1 were also observed.[118] Interestingly, a study of patients with frontotemporal dementia plus ALS implicated disrupted mitochondrial dynamics.[119] These patients had mutations in the coiled-coil-helix-coiled-coil-helix domain containing 10 gene (*CHCHD10*), which codes for a protein of unknown function that was shown to play a role in maintenance of the mitochondrial network.[119]

DEFECTIVE MITOPHAGY

Mitophagy is the autophagic mechanism by which cells selectively identify, degrade, and recycle defective and damaged mitochondria and mitochondrial components. The link between mitophagy and neurodegeneration was originally hypothesized because mutations in two genes that code for proteins in a major pathway of injury-induced mitophagy, PINK1 and parkin, are mutated in familial forms of PD.[120,121] In addition, because mitochondrial dysfunction and damage, originating from the various sources and involving the processes described here, is a well-established pathway of neurodegeneration, it is reasonable to hypothesize that mitochondrial quality control might be an important defense mechanism and one that is vulnerable to overload and dysfunction. Indeed, current research in neurodegeneration indicates that defects in mitochondrial quality control mechanisms, including mitophagy, are involved in multiple neurodegenerative diseases.[122]

PINK1 accumulates on damaged mitochondria and recruits parkin for ubiquitination and mitophagy.[16] The PINK1-parkin pathway promotes mitophagy and selective turnover of respiratory chain components in vivo.[17] Mutations in parkin and PINK1 reduce mitochondrial respiratory chain component turnover.[17] That mutations in parkin and PINK1 cause familial PD suggests that this protein clearance pathway is important in neurodegeneration and that impairment of this system could account for the bioenergetic defects observed in PD. In addition, further hinting at the importance of autophagy/mitophagy in PD pathogenesis, autophagy protein expression is reduced in the PD brain.[123] Furthermore, a study of induced pluripotent stem cells (iPSCs) derived from PINK1-mutated cells differentiated into dopaminergic neurons found that the differentiated neurons exhibited impaired recruitment of parkin to depolarized mitochondria, and increased mitochondrial copy number and upregulation of peroxisome proliferator-activated receptor gamma coactivator 1-alpha (PGC-1α), a key regulator of transcription of genes involved in mitochondrial biogenesis.[124] Introduction of wild-type PINK1 corrected these issues.[124]

While the link between mitochondrial quality control and neurodegeneration has been most closely studied in familial PD, several findings in patients and models of other neurodegenerative diseases are suggestive of a role for defective mitophagy in disease pathogenesis. For example, mitophagy is increased in mutant α-synuclein (A53T) mice, another model of PD.[11,125] In addition, a toxic, AD-linked fragment of human tau protein (NH2htau) adversely affects mitophagic efficiency.[126] Furthermore, aggregation of mutant SOD1 in familial ALS models is associated with activation of the PINK1 mitophagy pathway.[118,122] and loss of FUS or TDP-43, both of which contribute to ALS, results in decreased expression of parkin in adult mice.[127] Finally, retrograde transport of mitophagic vacuoles for fusion with lysosomes is an essential step in mitophagy, and mutant SOD1 impairs retrograde axonal transport in vivo and in vitro.[128,129]

MITOCHONDRIAL BIOGENESIS, TRANSCRIPTIONAL DYSREGULATION, AND PGC-1α

The antithesis of mitophagy is mitochondrial biogenesis, a complex process that involves significant crosstalk between the nucleus and mitochondria. Mitochondria are made up of more than 500 proteins, most of which are encoded by nuclear DNA.[130] Thus, efficient regulation of gene transcription is critical for maintenance of the mitochondrial network and bioenergetic functionality. The characterization of important regulators of transcription, such as PGC-1α, which is a primary regulator of most aspects of mitochondrial biogenesis, has established a link between mitochondrial dysfunction and transcriptional dysregulation in neurodegeneration.

PGC-1α is a ubiquitously expressed protein that regulates a wide range of transcription factors, including several that direct the transcription of nuclear-encoded mitochondrial proteins critical for mitochondrial biogenesis.[130,131] Predominantly localized to the cytoplasm, when phosphorylated, PGC-1α is retained in the nucleus to upregulate mitochondrial biogenesis.[130] It has also been found to localize to mitochondria.[132]

Impaired mitochondrial biogenesis has been reported in the AD brain.[133] In addition, decreased expression of PGC-1α and its downstream target proteins has been reported in PD,[130,134] AD,[130,133,135] and HD.[48,49,130] Evidence of PGC-1α involvement in ALS pathogenesis is less solid, but circumstantial links have been identified.[131]

Repression of PGC-1α and diminished mitochondrial biogenesis contribute to neurodegeneration in a mouse model of PD.[136] In addition, chronic MPP+ exposure resulted in decreased levels of PGC-1α.[137] Finally, a PGC-1α agonist, pioglitazone, was beneficial in multiple mouse models of PD.[131,138,139]

As mentioned earlier, impaired mitochondrial biogenesis has been observed in the human AD brain.[133] In addition, PGC-1α levels were decreased in the hippocampus of AD patients.[140] Supporting these findings in humans, in a mouse model of AD, levels of sirtuin 1 (SIRT1), a deacetylase that activates PGC-1α, were increased and acetylation levels of PGC-1α were decreased.[141]

The contribution of PGC-1α dysfunction to neurodegeneration has been most exhaustively studied in HD. HD mice lacking PGC-1α exhibit accelerated disease progression, while enhancement of function or expression can counteract disease progression, eliminating mutant huntingtin aggregation and ameliorating neurodegeneration.[142–145] In human HD patients, the haplotype of the gene coding for PGC-1α affects age of onset of disease.[146]

Similar to observations in AD mice, the PGC-1α agonist pioglitazone was beneficial in the mutant SOD1 mouse model of ALS.[147] In addition, increased levels of SIRT1 and decreased acetylation of PGC-1α were observed in SOD1 mutant mice, and upregulation of SIRT1 was protective.[141] Finally, overexpression of PGC-1α in SOD1 mutant mice increased motor function and survival.[148]

THERAPEUTICS FOR NEURODEGENERATIVE DISEASES TARGETING MITOCHONDRIAL DYSFUNCTION

Because evidence underscoring the central role of mitochondrial dysfunction in neurodegenerative diseases continues to grow and the overlapping and converging nature of the specific mechanisms involved in various diseases has been increasingly highlighted, agents that target mitochondrial defects are attractive prospects for the treatment of neurodegeneration. To date, several such agents that directly or indirectly act on mitochondria have been tested in animal models and clinical trials with varying degrees of success. Overall, initial success in animal models has yet to translate into similar success in human trials.

Coenzyme Q10

Coenzyme Q10 (CoQ10) is an electron transport chain substrate and antioxidant. Extensive studies in models of neurodegeneration have suggested a protective effect of CoQ10 against mitochondrial dysfunction and neurodegeneration.[32] For example, it protects against MPTP-mediated neurotoxicity,[149–151] and alone or in combination, increases survival, reduces mitochondrial dysfunction, and reverses pathology in ALS and HD mouse models.[152–155]

Despite these findings in model systems, clinical trials of CoQ10 have not, to date, indicated a significant neuroprotective effect. Multiple clinical trials in PD have provided conflicting results, but overall, findings have not supported a neuroprotective effect.[32] One HD clinical trial found only a mild effect on disease progression.[156] Finally, a phase II ALS trial did not find a significant effect of CoQ10, and progression to phase III was not recommended.[157]

Alpha-Lipoic Acid and Nicotinamide

Alpha-lipoic acid is a naturally occurring antioxidant found in mitochondria. Neuroprotective effects of alpha-lipoic acid, including increased survival, have been observed in mouse models of HD and ALS.[158,159] In combination with acetyl-L-carnitine, alpha-lipoic acid was also protective in a rotenone model of PD.[160] Nicotinamide, a complex I substrate, was shown to prevent MPTP-induced neurodegeneration in mice.[149]

PGC-1α, TORC1, and AMP Kinase

As highlighted earlier, mitochondrial biogenesis and gene transcription have garnered increasing attention in neurodegeneration, and because of its critical role in these processes, PGC-1α is widely considered to be a promising therapeutic target. Studies in cellular and animal models of PD suggest that PGC-1α might be protective against dopaminergic neuron loss.[134,136] Multiple studies in HD models (discussed in the preceding section) have suggested that PGC-1α might also be protective in HD.[32,144,145] Similarly, in the SOD1 mutant model of ALS, PGC-1α overexpression increased motor function and survival,[148] while expression only in muscle did not promote survival, but improved muscle function.[161] Early clinical trials for PGC-1α agonists, such as pioglitazone, are currently ongoing.[162]

Other proteins involved in PGC-1α pathways have also been investigated for therapeutic potential. For example, transducer of Creb-related binding protein 1 (TORC1) and AMP-activated protein kinase (AMPK) both seem to be involved in protective pathways present in HD models.[163,164] TORC1 regulates PGC-1α promoter activity and AMPK phosphorylates PGC-1α.[32]

Metformin and Metabolic Syndrome

Diabetes mellitus increases the risk of AD.[165,166] While the mechanisms underlying the association between diabetes and AD are unclear, a new study suggests a synergistic exacerbation of mitochondrial dysfunction and consequent learning and memory deficits in animal models (streptozotocin [STZ]-induced type 1 diabetes mice and transgenic AD mice overexpressing Aβ with diabetes).[167] Symptoms of mitochondrial dysfunction in these models include decreased complex I and IV activity and decreased respiratory rate.[167] Agents targeting the pathological intersection of metabolic syndrome and neurodegenerative diseases have become the focus of studies in animals and humans. For example, metformin, a diabetes drug that prevents hyperinsulinemia, has been extensively studied and has been found to have different effects in different settings. Ostensibly non-metabolic effects of metformin, including attenuation of the characteristic increase in tau phosphorylation and decrease in the synaptic protein synaptophysin, in a diabetes mouse model (db/db) suggested a beneficial effect against AD development.[168] However, a more recent study in a mouse model of AD found that metformin upregulated APP and presenilin-1 expression, increased Aβ levels, and contributed to mitochondrial dysfunction.[169] Insulin alleviated these negative effects, and co-administration of insulin and metformin restored physiological conditions.[169] Furthermore, metformin was reported to increase memory dysfunction in male AD mice, but improve memory function in female AD mice, suggesting gender-specific effects.[170] In humans with AD or mild cognitive impairment, metformin use was associated with poorer cognitive performance.[171] In sum, the potential of metformin as a therapeutic agent or target for cognitive impairment associated with AD remains uncertain (clinical trials are ongoing). The overlap between metabolic syndrome and neurodegenerative diseases and the contribution of mitochondrial dysfunction to both are promising areas for further investigation.

Creatine

Creatine is a guanidino compound involved in energy supply, and thus its therapeutic use targets bioenergetic dysfunction in general rather than a specific mitochondrial defect. In animal models of PD, AD, HD, and ALS, creatine has been shown to have both stand-alone and additive protective effects against neurodegeneration.[32] To date, trials in humans have provided mixed results. In PD trials, creatine was well tolerated and provided mild protective effects in some cases, including improvement in strength and endurance.[32,172–174] Larger, long-term trials are ongoing.[175] Creatine was similarly well tolerated in HD trials and more significant clinical outcomes, including slowing of cortical atrophy, were observed.[32,176,177] Finally, ALS clinical trials have yet to show substantial protective effects.[17]

Sirtuins

Sirtuins are NAD$^+$-dependent histone deacetylases known for their role in caloric restriction-mediated enhancement of health and longevity.[179] Of the seven sirtuin family proteins, only sirtuin 3 (SIRT3) is primarily localized to mitochondria, but because of their increasingly appreciated involvement in bioenergetics, including mitochondrial biogenesis via deacetylation of PGC-1α, sirtuins in general can be viewed as mitochondria-associated proteins. Numerous studies in model systems of neurodegeneration have shown largely positive results and are indicative of the neuroprotective qualities of caloric restriction, resveratrol, and sirtuin activation.[180] For example, caloric restriction and sirtuin 1 (SIRT1) supplementation had similar neuroprotective effects in the CK-p25 mouse model of neurodegeneration.[181] In regard to specific neurodegenerative diseases, SIRT2 inhibition was protective in a cellular and *Drosophila* model of PD,[182] while SIRT1 was neuroprotective in cellular models of ALS and AD and in the p25 mouse model of AD.[141] In addition, SIRT3, the mitochondrial sirtuin, was neuroprotective in the SOD1 mutant model of ALS.[117] Furthermore, caloric restriction was found to be protective in the PS1 mutant model of AD,[183] and resveratrol, a potent SIRT1 activator, was protective in the mutant APP mouse model of AD,[184] 3-NP model of HD,[185] and transgenic mouse model of HD.[186] Thus, cellular and animal studies evaluating sirtuins as potential therapeutics for neurodegeneration have generated generally positive results, but with some caveats and inconsistencies. Clinical trials seeking to confirm the efficacy and therapeutic potential of sirtuin manipulation are currently in progress or are inconclusive.[180]

CONCLUSION

Mitochondrial dysfunction has long been recognized as a shared feature of neurodegenerative diseases. More recently, research has elucidated some of the myriad pathways and mechanisms through which mitochondrial dysfunction operates to cause neuronal dysfunction and death. Further clarifying the relationships between these mechanisms and the proteins involved is a continuing challenge. The search for therapeutics that effectively target mitochondrial dysfunction in neurodegeneration is ongoing, and the continued development of technologies that allow more specific targeting of candidate therapeutic compounds will hopefully expedite the development process.

ACKNOWLEDGMENTS

This work is supported by NIH grant R01NS055193 (to EBW).

REFERENCES

1. Alexander, C., et al. OPA1, encoding a dynamin-related GTPase, is mutated in autosomal dominant optic atrophy linked to chromosome 3q28. *Nat. Genet.* **26**, 211–215 (2000).
2. Delettre, C., et al. Nuclear gene OPA1, encoding a mitochondrial dynamin-related protein, is mutated in dominant optic atrophy. *Nat. Genet.* **26**, 207–210 (2000).
3. Hudson, G., et al. Mutation of OPA1 causes dominant optic atrophy with external ophthalmoplegia, ataxia, deafness and multiple mitochondrial DNA deletions: a novel disorder of mtDNA maintenance. *Brain J. Neurol.* **131**, 329–337 (2008).
4. Kijima, K., et al. Mitochondrial GTPase mitofusin 2 mutation in Charcot-Marie-Tooth neuropathy type 2A. *Hum. Genet.* **116**, 23–27 (2005).
5. Züchner, S., et al. Axonal neuropathy with optic atrophy is caused by mutations in mitofusin 2. *Ann. Neurol.* **59**, 276–281 (2006).
6. Howell, N. Leber hereditary optic neuropathy: mitochondrial mutations and degeneration of the optic nerve. *Vision Res.* **37**, 3495–3507 (1997).
7. Finsterer, J. Leigh and Leigh-like syndrome in children and adults. *Pediatr. Neurol.* **39**, 223–235 (2008).
8. Pearson, H. A., et al. A new syndrome of refractory sideroblastic anemia with vacuolization of marrow precursors and exocrine pancreatic dysfunction. *J. Pediatr.* **95**, 976–984 (1979).
9. Santorelli, F. M., Barmada, M. A., Pons, R., Zhang, L. L., & DiMauro, S. Leigh-type neuropathology in Pearson syndrome associated with impaired ATP production and a novel mtDNA deletion. *Neurology* **47**, 1320–1323 (1996).
10. Bossy-Wetzel, E., Petrilli, A., & Knott, A. B. Mutant huntingtin and mitochondrial dysfunction. *Trends Neurosci.* **31**, 609–616 (2008).
11. Chinta, S. J., Mallajosyula, J. K., Rane, A., & Andersen, J. K. Mitochondrial α-synuclein accumulation impairs complex I function in dopaminergic neurons and results in increased mitophagy in vivo. *Neurosci. Lett.* **486**, 235–239 (2010).
12. Martin, L. J., et al. Parkinson's disease alpha-synuclein transgenic mice develop neuronal mitochondrial degeneration and cell death. *J. Neurosci. Off. J. Soc. Neurosci.* **26**, 41–50 (2006).
13. Irrcher, I., et al. Loss of the Parkinson's disease-linked gene DJ-1 perturbs mitochondrial dynamics. *Hum. Mol. Genet.* **19**, 3734–3746 (2010).
14. Strauss, K. M., et al. Loss of function mutations in the gene encoding Omi/HtrA2 in Parkinson's disease. *Hum. Mol. Genet.* **14**, 2099–2111 (2005).
15. Martin, I., Kim, J. W., Dawson, V. L., & Dawson, T. M. LRRK2 pathobiology in Parkinson's disease. *J. Neurochem.* **131**, 554–565 (2014).
16. Narendra, D. P., et al. PINK1 is selectively stabilized on impaired mitochondria to activate Parkin. *PLoS Biol.* **8**, e1000298 (2010).
17. Vincow, E. S., et al. The PINK1-Parkin pathway promotes both mitophagy and selective respiratory chain turnover in vivo. *Proc. Natl. Acad. Sci. U. S. A.* **110**, 6400–6405 (2013).
18. Anandatheerthavarada, H. K., & Devi, L. Amyloid precursor protein and mitochondrial dysfunction in Alzheimer's disease. *Neurosci. Rev. J. Bringing Neurobiol. Neurol. Psychiatry* **13**, 626–638 (2007).
19. De Strooper, B., Iwatsubo, T., & Wolfe, M. S. Presenilins and γ-secretase: structure, function, and role in Alzheimer disease. *Cold Spring Harb. Perspect. Med.* **2**, (2012).
20. Vijayvergiya, C., Beal, M. F., Buck, J., & Manfredi, G. Mutant superoxide dismutase 1 forms aggregates in the brain mitochondrial matrix of amyotrophic lateral sclerosis mice. *J. Neurosci. Off. J. Soc. Neurosci.* **25**, 2463–2470 (2005).
21. Rosen, D. R. Mutations in Cu/Zn superoxide dismutase gene are associated with familial amyotrophic lateral sclerosis. *Nature* **364**, 362 (1993).
22. Lin, M. T., & Beal, M. F. Mitochondrial dysfunction and oxidative stress in neurodegenerative diseases. *Nature* **443**, 787–795 (2006).
23. Chen, H., Zhang, S. M., Hernán, M. A., Willett, W. C., & Ascherio, A. Weight loss in Parkinson's disease. *Ann. Neurol.* **53**, 676–679 (2003).
24. Buchman, A. S., et al. Change in body mass index and risk of incident Alzheimer disease. *Neurology* **65**, 892–897 (2005).
25. Djoussé, L., et al. Weight loss in early stage of Huntington's disease. *Neurology* **59**, 1325–1330 (2002).
26. Hattingen, E., et al. Phosphorus and proton magnetic resonance spectroscopy demonstrates mitochondrial dysfunction in early and advanced Parkinson's disease. *Brain J. Neurol.* **132**, 3285–3297 (2009).
27. Rapoport, S. I. In vivo PET imaging and postmortem studies suggest potentially reversible and irreversible stages of brain metabolic failure in Alzheimer's disease. *Eur. Arch. Psychiatry Clin. Neurosci.* **249** Suppl 3, 46–55 (1999).
28. Mosconi, L., et al. Reduced hippocampal metabolism in MCI and AD: automated FDG-PET image analysis. *Neurology* **64**, 1860–1867 (2005).
29. Mochel, F., & Haller, R. G. Energy deficit in Huntington disease: why it matters. *J. Clin. Invest.* **121**, 493–499 (2011).
30. Langston, J. W., Ballard, P., Tetrud, J. W., & Irwin, I. Chronic Parkinsonism in humans due to a product of meperidine-analog synthesis. *Science* **219**, 979–980 (1983).
31. Burns, R. S., LeWitt, P. A., Ebert, M. H., Pakkenberg, H., & Kopin, I. J. The

clinical syndrome of striatal dopamine deficiency. Parkinsonism induced by 1-methyl-4-phenyl-1,2,3,6-tetrahydropyridine (MPTP). *N. Engl. J. Med.* **312**, 1418–1421 (1985).

32. Chaturvedi, R. K., & Flint Beal, M. Mitochondrial diseases of the brain. *Free Radic. Biol. Med.* **63**, 1–29 (2013).

33. Hattori, N., Tanaka, M., Ozawa, T., & Mizuno, Y. Immunohistochemical studies on complexes I, II, III, and IV of mitochondria in Parkinson's disease. *Ann. Neurol.* **30**, 563–571 (1991).

34. Mizuno, Y., et al. Deficiencies in complex I subunits of the respiratory chain in Parkinson's disease. *Biochem. Biophys. Res. Commun.* **163**, 1450–1455 (1989).

35. Keeney, P. M., Xie, J., Capaldi, R. A., & Bennett, J. P. Parkinson's disease brain mitochondrial complex I has oxidatively damaged subunits and is functionally impaired and misassembled. *J. Neurosci. Off. J. Soc. Neurosci.* **26**, 5256–5264 (2006).

36. Schapira, A. H., et al. Mitochondrial complex I deficiency in Parkinson's disease. *J. Neurochem.* **54**, 823–827 (1990).

37. Janetzky, B., et al. Unaltered aconitase activity, but decreased complex I activity in substantia nigra pars compacta of patients with Parkinson's disease. *Neurosci. Lett.* **169**, 126–128 (1994).

38. Parker, W. D., Parks, J. K., & Swerdlow, R. H. Complex I deficiency in Parkinson's disease frontal cortex. *Brain Res.* **1189**, 215–218 (2008).

39. Mizuno, Y., et al. An immunohistochemical study on alpha-ketoglutarate dehydrogenase complex in Parkinson's disease. *Ann. Neurol.* **35**, 204–210 (1994).

40. Gibson, G. E., et al. Deficits in a tricarboxylic acid cycle enzyme in brains from patients with Parkinson's disease. *Neurochem. Int.* **43**, 129–135 (2003).

41. Liang, W. S., et al. Alzheimer's disease is associated with reduced expression of energy metabolism genes in posterior cingulate neurons. *Proc. Natl. Acad. Sci. U. S. A.* **105**, 4441–4446 (2008).

42. Valla, J., Berndt, J. D., & Gonzalez-Lima, F. Energy hypometabolism in posterior cingulate cortex of Alzheimer's patients: superficial laminar cytochrome oxidase associated with disease duration. *J. Neurosci. Off. J. Soc. Neurosci.* **21**, 4923–4930 (2001).

43. Bosetti, F., et al. Cytochrome c oxidase and mitochondrial F1F0-ATPase (ATP synthase) activities in platelets and brain from patients with Alzheimer's disease. *Neurobiol. Aging* **23**, 371–376 (2002).

44. Bubber, P., Haroutunian, V., Fisch, G., Blass, J. P., & Gibson, G. E. Mitochondrial abnormalities in Alzheimer brain: mechanistic implications. *Ann. Neurol.* **57**, 695–703 (2005).

45. Shi, Q., et al. Inactivation and reactivation of the mitochondrial α-ketoglutarate dehydrogenase complex. *J. Biol. Chem.* **286**, 17640–17648 (2011).

46. Mochel, F., et al. Abnormal response to cortical activation in early stages of Huntington disease. *Mov. Disord. Off. J. Mov. Disord. Soc.* **27**, 907–910 (2012).

47. Benchoua, A., et al. Involvement of mitochondrial complex II defects in neuronal death produced by N-terminus fragment of mutated huntingtin. *Mol. Biol. Cell* **17**, 1652–1663 (2006).

48. Gu, M., et al. Mitochondrial defect in Huntington's disease caudate nucleus. *Ann. Neurol.* **39**, 385–389 (1996).

49. Browne, S. E., et al. Oxidative damage and metabolic dysfunction in Huntington's disease: selective vulnerability of the basal ganglia. *Ann. Neurol.* **41**, 646–653 (1997).

50. Tabrizi, S. J., et al. Biochemical abnormalities and excitotoxicity in Huntington's disease brain. *Ann. Neurol.* **45**, 25–32 (1999).

51. Browne, S. E., et al. Metabolic dysfunction in familial, but not sporadic, amyotrophic lateral sclerosis. *J. Neurochem.* **71**, 281–287 (1998).

52. Hatazawa, J., Brooks, R. A., Dalakas, M. C., Mansi, L., & Di Chiro, G. Cortical motor-sensory hypometabolism in amyotrophic lateral sclerosis: a PET study. *J. Comput. Assist. Tomogr.* **12**, 630–636 (1988).

53. Borthwick, G. M., Johnson, M. A., Ince, P. G., Shaw, P. J., & Turnbull, D. M. Mitochondrial enzyme activity in amyotrophic lateral sclerosis: implications for the role of mitochondria in neuronal cell death. *Ann. Neurol.* **46**, 787–790 (1999).

54. Menzies, F. M., et al. Mitochondrial dysfunction in a cell culture model of familial amyotrophic lateral sclerosis. *Brain J. Neurol.* **125**, 1522–1533 (2002).

55. Sena, L. A., & Chandel, N. S. Physiological roles of mitochondrial reactive oxygen species. *Mol. Cell* **48**, 158–167 (2012).

56. Yun, J., & Finkel, T. Mitohormesis. *Cell Metab.* **19**, 757–766 (2014).

57. Ristow, M. Unraveling the truth about antioxidants: mitohormesis explains ROS-induced health benefits. *Nat. Med.* **20**, 709–711 (2014).

58. Intlekofer, K. A., & Cotman, C. W. Exercise counteracts declining hippocampal function in aging and Alzheimer's disease. *Neurobiol. Dis.* **57**, 47–55 (2013).

59. Warburton, D. E. R., Nicol, C. W., & Bredin, S. S. D. Health benefits of physical activity: the evidence. *CMAJ Can. Med. Assoc. J. J. Assoc. Medicale Can.* **174**, 801–809 (2006).

60. Ristow, M., et al. Antioxidants prevent health-promoting effects of physical exercise in

humans. *Proc. Natl. Acad. Sci. U. S. A.* **106**, 8665–8670 (2009).

61. Nunnari, J., & Suomalainen, A. Mitochondria: in sickness and in health. *Cell* **148**, 1145–1159 (2012).

62. Thanan, R., et al. Oxidative stress and its significant roles in neurodegenerative diseases and cancer. *Int. J. Mol. Sci.* **16**, 193–217 (2014).

63. Reed, T. T. Lipid peroxidation and neurodegenerative disease. *Free Radic. Biol. Med.* **51**, 1302–1319 (2011).

64. Höhn, A., & Grune, T. Lipofuscin: formation, effects and role of macroautophagy. *Redox Biol.* **1**, 140–144 (2013).

65. Mountjoy, C. Q., Dowson, J. H., Harrington, C., Cairns, M. R., & Wilton-Cox, H. Characteristics of neuronal lipofuscin in the superior temporal gyrus in Alzheimer's disease do not differ from non-diseased controls: a comparison with disease-related changes in the superior frontal gyrus. *Acta Neuropathol. (Berl.)* **109**, 490–496 (2005).

66. Adamec, E., Mohan, P. S., Cataldo, A. M., Vonsattel, J. P., & Nixon, R. A. Up-regulation of the lysosomal system in experimental models of neuronal injury: implications for Alzheimer's disease. *Neuroscience* **100**, 663–675 (2000).

67. Reeg, S., & Grune, T. Protein oxidation in aging: does it play a role in aging progression? *Antioxid. Redox Signal.* **23**, 239–255 (2014).

68. Smith, C. D., et al. Excess brain protein oxidation and enzyme dysfunction in normal aging and in Alzheimer disease. *Proc. Natl. Acad. Sci. U. S. A.* **88**, 10540–10543 (1991).

69. Hensley, K., et al. Brain regional correspondence between Alzheimer's disease histopathology and biomarkers of protein oxidation. *J. Neurochem.* **65**, 2146–2156 (1995).

70. Picklo, M. J., Montine, T. J., Amarnath, V., & Neely, M. D. Carbonyl toxicology and Alzheimer's disease. *Toxicol. Appl. Pharmacol.* **184**, 187–197 (2002).

71. Túnez, I. et al. Important role of oxidative stress biomarkers in Huntington's disease. *J. Med. Chem.* **54**, 5602–5606 (2011).

72. Beal, M. F., et al. Increased 3-nitrotyrosine in both sporadic and familial amyotrophic lateral sclerosis. *Ann. Neurol.* **42**, 644–654 (1997).

73. Gu, Z., Nakamura, T., & Lipton, S. A. Redox reactions induced by nitrosative stress mediate protein misfolding and mitochondrial dysfunction in neurodegenerative diseases. *Mol. Neurobiol.* **41**, 55–72 (2010).

74. Madabhushi, R., Pan, L., & Tsai, L.-H. DNA damage and its links to neurodegeneration. *Neuron* **83**, 266–282 (2014).

75. Bender, A., et al. High levels of mitochondrial DNA deletions in substantia nigra neurons in aging and Parkinson disease. *Nat. Genet.* **38**, 515–517 (2006).

76. Pinto, M., & Moraes, C. T. Mitochondrial genome changes and neurodegenerative diseases. *Biochim. Biophys. Acta* **1842**, 1198–1207 (2014).

77. Kraytsberg, Y., et al. Mitochondrial DNA deletions are abundant and cause functional impairment in aged human substantia nigra neurons. *Nat. Genet.* **38**, 518–520 (2006).

78. Lin, M. T., et al. Somatic mitochondrial DNA mutations in early Parkinson and incidental Lewy body disease. *Ann. Neurol.* **71**, 850–854 (2012).

79. Horton, T. M., et al. Marked increase in mitochondrial DNA deletion levels in the cerebral cortex of Huntington's disease patients. *Neurology* **45**, 1879–1883 (1995).

80. Keeney, P. M., & Bennett, J. P., Jr. ALS spinal neurons show varied and reduced mtDNA gene copy numbers and increased mtDNA gene deletions. *Mol. Neurodegener.* **5**, 21 (2010).

81. Dhaliwal, G. K., & Grewal, R. P. Mitochondrial DNA deletion mutation levels are elevated in ALS brains. *Neuroreport* **11**, 2507–2509 (2000).

82. Comi, G. P., et al. Cytochrome c oxidase subunit I microdeletion in a patient with motor neuron disease. *Ann. Neurol.* **43**, 110–116 (1998).

83. Kirches, E., et al. Mitochondrial tRNA(Cys) mutation A5823G in a patient with motor neuron disease and temporal lobe epilepsy. *Pathobiol. J. Immunopathol. Mol. Cell. Biol.* **67**, 214–218 (1999).

84. Chen, Y., et al. Tumour suppressor SIRT3 deacetylates and activates manganese superoxide dismutase to scavenge ROS. *EMBO Rep.* **12**, 534–541 (2011).

85. Borthwick, G. M., et al. Motor neuron disease in a patient with a mitochondrial tRNAIle mutation. *Ann. Neurol.* **59**, 570–574 (2006).

86. Swerdlow, R. H. Does mitochondrial DNA play a role in Parkinson's disease? A review of cybrid and other supportive evidence. *Antioxid. Redox Signal.* **16**, 950–964 (2012).

87. Trimmer, P. A., et al. Mitochondrial abnormalities in cybrid cell models of sporadic Alzheimer's disease worsen with passage in culture. *Neurobiol. Dis.* **15**, 29–39 (2004).

88. Khan, S. M., et al. Alzheimer's disease cybrids replicate beta-amyloid abnormalities through cell death pathways. *Ann. Neurol.* **48**, 148–155 (2000).

89. Ferreira, I. L., et al. Mitochondrial-dependent apoptosis in Huntington's disease human cybrids. *Exp. Neurol.* **222**, 243–255 (2010).

90. Vermulst, M., et al. DNA deletions and clonal mutations drive premature aging in

mitochondrial mutator mice. *Nat. Genet.* **40**, 392–394 (2008).

91. Kujoth, G. C., et al. Mitochondrial DNA mutations, oxidative stress, and apoptosis in mammalian aging. *Science* **309**, 481–484 (2005).

92. Perier, C., et al. Accumulation of mitochondrial DNA deletions within dopaminergic neurons triggers neuroprotective mechanisms. *Brain J. Neurol.* **136**, 2369–2378 (2013).

93. Calì, T., Ottolini, D., & Brini, M. Mitochondrial Ca2+ and neurodegeneration. *Cell Calcium* **52**, 73–85 (2012).

94. Danzer, K. M., et al. Different species of alpha-synuclein oligomers induce calcium influx and seeding. *J. Neurosci. Off. J. Soc. Neurosci.* **27**, 9220–9232 (2007).

95. Lashuel, H. A., et al. Alpha-synuclein, especially the Parkinson's disease-associated mutants, forms pore-like annular and tubular protofibrils. *J. Mol. Biol.* **322**, 1089–1102 (2002).

96. Furukawa, K., et al. Plasma membrane ion permeability induced by mutant alpha-synuclein contributes to the degeneration of neural cells. *J. Neurochem.* **97**, 1071–1077 (2006).

97. Marongiu, R., et al. Mutant Pink1 induces mitochondrial dysfunction in a neuronal cell model of Parkinson's disease by disturbing calcium flux. *J. Neurochem.* **108**, 1561–1574 (2009).

98. Boada, M., et al. CALHM1 P86L polymorphism is associated with late-onset Alzheimer's disease in a recessive model. *J. Alzheimers Dis. JAD* **20**, 247–251 (2010).

99. Zatti, G., et al. The presenilin 2 M239I mutation associated with familial Alzheimer's disease reduces Ca2+ release from intracellular stores. *Neurobiol. Dis.* **15**, 269–278 (2004).

100. Demuro, A., et al. Calcium dysregulation and membrane disruption as a ubiquitous neurotoxic mechanism of soluble amyloid oligomers. *J. Biol. Chem.* **280**, 17294–17300 (2005).

101. Choo, Y. S., Johnson, G. V. W., MacDonald, M., Detloff, P. J., & Lesort, M. Mutant huntingtin directly increases susceptibility of mitochondria to the calcium-induced permeability transition and cytochrome c release. *Hum. Mol. Genet.* **13**, 1407–1420 (2004).

102. Gellerich, F. N., et al. Impaired regulation of brain mitochondria by extramitochondrial Ca2+ in transgenic Huntington disease rats. *J. Biol. Chem.* **283**, 30715–30724 (2008).

103. Barrett, E. F., Barrett, J. N., & David, G. Dysfunctional mitochondrial Ca(2+) handling in mutant SOD1 mouse models of fALS: integration of findings from motor neuron somata and motor terminals. *Front. Cell. Neurosci.* **8**, 184 (2014).

104. Knott, A. B., Perkins, G., Schwarzenbacher, R., & Bossy-Wetzel, E. Mitochondrial fragmentation in neurodegeneration. *Nat. Rev. Neurosci.* **9**, 505–518 (2008).

105. Burté, F., Carelli, V., Chinnery, P. F., & Yu-Wai-Man, P. Disturbed mitochondrial dynamics and neurodegenerative disorders. *Nat. Rev. Neurol.* **11**, 11–24 (2015).

106. Züchner, S., et al. Mutations in the mitochondrial GTPase mitofusin 2 cause Charcot-Marie-Tooth neuropathy type 2A. *Nat. Genet.* **36**, 449–451 (2004).

107. Waterham, H. R., et al. A lethal defect of mitochondrial and peroxisomal fission. *N. Engl. J. Med.* **356**, 1736–1741 (2007).

108. Reddy, P. H., et al. Dynamin-related protein 1 and mitochondrial fragmentation in neurodegenerative diseases. *Brain Res. Rev.* **67**, 103–118 (2011).

109. Wang, X., et al. LRRK2 regulates mitochondrial dynamics and function through direct interaction with DLP1. *Hum. Mol. Genet.* **21**, 1931–1944 (2012).

110. Barsoum, M. J., et al. Nitric oxide-induced mitochondrial fission is regulated by dynamin-related GTPases in neurons. *EMBO J.* **25**, 3900–3911 (2006).

111. Manczak, M., Calkins, M. J., & Reddy, P. H. Impaired mitochondrial dynamics and abnormal interaction of amyloid beta with mitochondrial protein Drp1 in neurons from patients with Alzheimer's disease: implications for neuronal damage. *Hum. Mol. Genet.* **20**, 2495–2509 (2011).

112. Wang, X., et al. Amyloid-beta overproduction causes abnormal mitochondrial dynamics via differential modulation of mitochondrial fission/fusion proteins. *Proc. Natl. Acad. Sci. U. S. A.* **105**, 19318–19323 (2008).

113. Manczak, M., & Reddy, P. H. Abnormal interaction between the mitochondrial fission protein Drp1 and hyperphosphorylated tau in Alzheimer's disease neurons: implications for mitochondrial dysfunction and neuronal damage. *Hum. Mol. Genet.* **21**, 2538–2547 (2012).

114. Shirendeb, U., et al. Abnormal mitochondrial dynamics, mitochondrial loss and mutant huntingtin oligomers in Huntington's disease: implications for selective neuronal damage. *Hum. Mol. Genet.* **20**, 1438–1455 (2011).

115. Song, W., et al. Mutant huntingtin binds the mitochondrial fission GTPase dynamin-related protein-1 and increases its enzymatic activity. *Nat. Med.* **17**, 377–382 (2011).

116. Shirendeb, U. P., et al. Mutant huntingtin's interaction with mitochondrial protein Drp1 impairs

mitochondrial biogenesis and causes defective axonal transport and synaptic degeneration in Huntington's disease. *Hum. Mol. Genet.* **21**, 406–420 (2012).

117. Song, W., Song, Y., Kincaid, B., Bossy, B., & Bossy-Wetzel, E. Mutant SOD1G93A triggers mitochondrial fragmentation in spinal cord motor neurons: neuroprotection by SIRT3 and PGC-1α. *Neurobiol. Dis.* **51**, 72–81 (2013).

118. Liu, W., et al. Mitochondrial fusion and fission proteins expression dynamically change in a murine model of amyotrophic lateral sclerosis. *Curr. Neurovasc. Res.* **10**, 222–230 (2013).

119. Bannwarth, S., et al. A mitochondrial origin for frontotemporal dementia and amyotrophic lateral sclerosis through CHCHD10 involvement. *Brain J. Neurol.* **137**, 2329–2345 (2014).

120. Kitada, T., et al. Mutations in the parkin gene cause autosomal recessive juvenile parkinsonism. *Nature* **392**, 605–608 (1998).

121. Valente, E. M., et al. PINK1 mutations are associated with sporadic early-onset parkinsonism. *Ann. Neurol.* **56**, 336–341 (2004).

122. Dupuis, L. Mitochondrial quality control in neurodegenerative diseases. *Biochimie* **100**, 177–183 (2014).

123. Schapira, A. H. V., Olanow, C. W., Greenamyre, J. T., & Bezard, E. Slowing of neurodegeneration in Parkinson's disease and Huntington's disease: future therapeutic perspectives. *Lancet* **384**, 545–555 (2014).

124. Seibler, P., et al. Mitochondrial parkin recruitment is impaired in neurons derived from mutant PINK1 induced pluripotent stem cells. *J. Neurosci.* **31**, 5970–5976 (2011).

125. Choubey, V., et al. Mutant A53T alpha-synuclein induces neuronal death by increasing mitochondrial autophagy. *J. Biol. Chem.* **286**, 10814–10824 (2011).

126. Amadoro, G., et al. AD-linked, toxic NH2 human tau affects the quality control of mitochondria in neurons. *Neurobiol. Dis.* **62**, 489–507 (2014).

127. Lagier-Tourenne, C., et al. Divergent roles of ALS-linked proteins FUS/TLS and TDP-43 intersect in processing long pre-mRNAs. *Nat. Neurosci.* **15**, 1488–1497 (2012).

128. Magrané, J., Sahawneh, M. A., Przedborski, S., Estévez, Á. G., & Manfredi, G. Mitochondrial dynamics and bioenergetic dysfunction is associated with synaptic alterations in mutant SOD1 motor neurons. *J. Neurosci. Off. J. Soc. Neurosci.* **32**, 229–242 (2012).

129. Magrané, J., Cortez, C., Gan, W.-B., & Manfredi, G. Abnormal mitochondrial transport and morphology are common pathological denominators in SOD1 and TDP43 ALS mouse models. *Hum. Mol. Genet.* **23**, 1413–1424 (2014).

130. Zhu, J., Wang, K. Z. Q., & Chu, C. T. After the banquet: mitochondrial biogenesis, mitophagy, and cell survival. *Autophagy* **9**, 1663–1676 (2013).

131. Róna-Vörös, K., & Weydt, P. The role of PGC-1α in the pathogenesis of neurodegenerative disorders. *Curr. Drug Targets* **11**, 1262–1269 (2010).

132. Aquilano, K., et al. Peroxisome proliferator-activated receptor gamma co-activator 1alpha (PGC-1alpha) and sirtuin 1 (SIRT1) reside in mitochondria: possible direct function in mitochondrial biogenesis. *J. Biol. Chem.* **285**, 21590–21599 (2010).

133. Sheng, B., et al. Impaired mitochondrial biogenesis contributes to mitochondrial dysfunction in Alzheimer's disease. *J. Neurochem.* **120**, 419–429 (2012).

134. Zheng, B., et al. PGC-1α, A potential therapeutic target for early intervention in Parkinson's disease. *Sci. Transl. Med.* **2**, 52ra73–52ra73 (2010).

135. Qin, W., et al. PGC-1alpha expression decreases in the Alzheimer disease brain as a function of dementia. *Arch. Neurol.* **66**, 352–361 (2009).

136. Shin, J.-H., et al. PARIS (ZNF746) repression of PGC-1α contributes to neurodegeneration in Parkinson's disease. *Cell* **144**, 689–702 (2011).

137. Zhu, J. H., et al. Impaired mitochondrial biogenesis contributes to depletion of functional mitochondria in chronic MPP+ toxicity: dual roles for ERK1/2. *Cell Death Dis.* **3**, e312 (2012).

138. Breidert, T., et al. Protective action of the peroxisome proliferator-activated receptor-gamma agonist pioglitazone in a mouse model of Parkinson's disease. *J. Neurochem.* **82**, 615–624 (2002).

139. Dehmer, T., Heneka, M. T., Sastre, M., Dichgans, J., & Schulz, J. B. Protection by pioglitazone in the MPTP model of Parkinson's disease correlates with I kappa B alpha induction and block of NF kappa B and iNOS activation. *J. Neurochem.* **88**, 494–501 (2004).

140. Helisalmi, S., et al. Genetic study between SIRT1, PPARD, PGC-1alpha genes and Alzheimer's disease. *J. Neurol.* **255**, 668–673 (2008).

141. Kim, D., et al. SIRT1 deacetylase protects against neurodegeneration in models for Alzheimer's disease and amyotrophic lateral sclerosis. *EMBO J.* **26**, 3169–3179 (2007).

142. Cui, L., et al. Transcriptional repression of PGC-1α by mutant huntingtin leads to mitochondrial dysfunction and neurodegeneration. *Cell* **127**, 59–69 (2006).

143. Weydt, P., et al. Thermoregulatory and metabolic defects in Huntington's disease transgenic

mice implicate PGC-1alpha in Huntington's disease neurodegeneration. *Cell Metab.* **4**, 349–362 (2006).

144. Johri, A., et al. Pharmacologic activation of mitochondrial biogenesis exerts widespread beneficial effects in a transgenic mouse model of Huntington's disease. *Hum. Mol. Genet.* **21**, 1124–1137 (2012).

145. Tsunemi, T., et al. PGC-1α rescues Huntington's disease proteotoxicity by preventing oxidative stress and promoting TFEB function. *Sci. Transl. Med.* **4**, 142ra97 (2012).

146. Weydt, P., et al. The gene coding for PGC-1alpha modifies age at onset in Huntington's Disease. *Mol. Neurodegener.* **4**, 3 (2009).

147. Schütz, B., et al. The oral antidiabetic pioglitazone protects from neurodegeneration and amyotrophic lateral sclerosis-like symptoms in superoxide dismutase-G93A transgenic mice. *J. Neurosci. Off. J. Soc. Neurosci.* **25**, 7805–7812 (2005).

148. Zhao, W., et al. Peroxisome proliferator activator receptor gamma coactivator-1alpha (PGC-1α) improves motor performance and survival in a mouse model of amyotrophic lateral sclerosis. *Mol. Neurodegener.* **6**, 51 (2011).

149. Schulz, J. B., Henshaw, D. R., Matthews, R. T., & Beal, M. F. Coenzyme Q10 and nicotinamide and a free radical spin trap protect against MPTP neurotoxicity. *Exp. Neurol.* **132**, 279–283 (1995).

150. Beal, M. F., Matthews, R. T., Tieleman, A., & Shults, C. W. Coenzyme Q10 attenuates the 1-methyl-4-phenyl-1,2,3,tetrahydropyridine (MPTP) induced loss of striatal dopamine and dopaminergic axons in aged mice. *Brain Res.* **783**, 109–114 (1998).

151. Cleren, C., et al. Therapeutic effects of coenzyme Q10 (CoQ10) and reduced CoQ10 in the MPTP model of Parkinsonism. *J. Neurochem.* **104**, 1613–1621 (2008).

152. Matthews, R. T., Yang, L., Browne, S., Baik, M., & Beal, M. F. Coenzyme Q10 administration increases brain mitochondrial concentrations and exerts neuroprotective effects. *Proc. Natl. Acad. Sci. U. S. A.* **95**, 8892–8897 (1998).

153. Ferrante, R. J., et al. Therapeutic effects of coenzyme Q10 and remacemide in transgenic mouse models of Huntington's disease. *J. Neurosci. Off. J. Soc. Neurosci.* **22**, 1592–1599 (2002).

154. Smith, K. M., et al. Dose ranging and efficacy study of high-dose coenzyme Q10 formulations in Huntington's disease mice. *Biochim. Biophys. Acta* **1762**, 616–626 (2006).

155. Stack, E. C., et al. Combination therapy using minocycline and coenzyme Q10 in R6/2

transgenic Huntington's disease mice. *Biochim. Biophys. Acta* **1762**, 373–380 (2006).

156. Huntington Study Group. A randomized, placebo-controlled trial of coenzyme Q10 and remacemide in Huntington's disease. *Neurology* **57**, 397–404 (2001).

157. Kaufmann, P., et al. Phase II trial of CoQ10 for ALS finds insufficient evidence to justify phase III. *Ann. Neurol.* **66**, 235–244 (2009).

158. Andreassen, O. A., Ferrante, R. J., Dedeoglu, A., & Beal, M. F. Lipoic acid improves survival in transgenic mouse models of Huntington's disease. *Neuroreport* **12**, 3371–3373 (2001).

159. Andreassen, O. A., et al. Effects of an inhibitor of poly(ADP-ribose) polymerase, desmethylselegiline, trientine, and lipoic acid in transgenic ALS mice. *Exp. Neurol.* **168**, 419–424 (2001).

160. Zhang, H., et al. Combined R-alpha-lipoic acid and acetyl-L-carnitine exerts efficient preventative effects in a cellular model of Parkinson's disease. *J. Cell. Mol. Med.* **14**, 215–225 (2010).

161. Da Cruz, S., et al. Elevated PGC-1α activity sustains mitochondrial biogenesis and muscle function without extending survival in a mouse model of inherited ALS. *Cell Metab.* **15**, 778–786 (2012).

162. Carta, A. R., & Simuni, T. Thiazolidinediones under preclinical and early clinical development for the treatment of Parkinson's disease. *Expert Opin. Investig. Drugs* **24**, 219–227 (2014).

163. Chaturvedi, R. K., et al. Transducer of regulated CREB-binding proteins (TORCs) transcription and function is impaired in Huntington's disease. *Hum. Mol. Genet.* **21**, 3474–3488 (2012).

164. Fu, J., et al. trans-(-)-ε-Viniferin increases mitochondrial sirtuin 3 (SIRT3), activates AMP-activated protein kinase (AMPK), and protects cells in models of Huntington Disease. *J. Biol. Chem.* **287**, 24460–24472 (2012).

165. Ott, A., et al. Diabetes mellitus and the risk of dementia: The Rotterdam Study. *Neurology* **53**, 1937–1942 (1999).

166. Alagiakrishnan, K., Sankaralingam, S., Ghosh, M., Mereu, L., & Senior, P. Antidiabetic drugs and their potential role in treating mild cognitive impairment and Alzheimer's disease. *Discov. Med.* **16**, 277–286 (2013).

167. Wang, Y., et al. Synergistic exacerbation of mitochondrial and synaptic dysfunction and resultant learning and memory deficit in a mouse model of diabetic Alzheimer's disease. *J. Alzheimers Dis. JAD* **43**, 451–463 (2015).

168. Li, J., Deng, J., Sheng, W., & Zuo, Z. Metformin attenuates Alzheimer's disease-like neuropathology in obese, leptin-resistant mice. *Pharmacol. Biochem. Behav.* **101**, 564–574 (2012).

169. Picone, P., et al. Metformin increases APP expression and processing via oxidative stress, mitochondrial dysfunction and NF-κB activation: use of insulin to attenuate metformin's effect. *Biochim. Biophys. Acta* **1853**, 1046–1059 (2015).

170. DiTacchio, K. A., Heinemann, S. F., & Dziewczapolski, G. Metformin treatment alters memory function in a mouse model of Alzheimer's disease. *J. Alzheimers Dis. JAD* **44**, 43–48 (2015).

171. Moore, E. M., et al. Increased risk of cognitive impairment in patients with diabetes is associated with metformin. *Diabetes Care* **36**, 2981–2987 (2013).

172. Bender, A., Samtleben, W., Elstner, M., & Klopstock, T. Long-term creatine supplementation is safe in aged patients with Parkinson disease. *Nutr. Res. N. Y. N* **28**, 172–178 (2008).

173. Hass, C. J., Collins, M. A., & Juncos, J. L. Resistance training with creatine monohydrate improves upper-body strength in patients with Parkinson disease: a randomized trial. *Neurorehabil. Neural Repair* **21**, 107–115 (2007).

174. NINDS NET-PD Investigators. A pilot clinical trial of creatine and minocycline in early Parkinson disease: 18-month results. *Clin. Neuropharmacol.* **31**, 141–150 (2008).

175. Elm, J. J., & NINDS NET-PD Investigators. Design innovations and baseline findings in a long-term Parkinson's trial: the National Institute of Neurological Disorders and Stroke Exploratory Trials in Parkinson's Disease Long-Term Study-1. *Mov. Disord. Off. J. Mov. Disord. Soc.* **27**, 1513–1521 (2012).

176. Hersch, S. M., et al. Creatine in Huntington disease is safe, tolerable, bioavailable in brain and reduces serum 8OH2'dG. *Neurology* **66**, 250–252 (2006).

177. Rosas, H. D., et al. PRECREST: a phase II prevention and biomarker trial of creatine in at-risk Huntington disease. *Neurology* **82**, 850–857 (2014).

178. Patel, B. P., & Hamadeh, M. J. Nutritional and exercise-based interventions in the treatment of amyotrophic lateral sclerosis. *Clin. Nutr. Edinb. Scotl.* **28**, 604–617 (2009).

179. Kincaid, B., & Bossy-Wetzel, E. Forever young: SIRT3 a shield against mitochondrial meltdown, aging, and neurodegeneration. *Front. Aging Neurosci.* **5**, 48 (2013).

180. Herskovits, A. Z., & Guarente, L. Sirtuin deacetylases in neurodegenerative diseases of aging. *Cell Res.* **23**, 746–758 (2013).

181. Gräff, J., et al. A dietary regimen of caloric restriction or pharmacological activation of SIRT1 to delay the onset of neurodegeneration. *J. Neurosci. Off. J. Soc. Neurosci.* **33**, 8951–8960 (2013).

182. Outeiro, T. F., et al. Sirtuin 2 inhibitors rescue α-synuclein-mediated toxicity in models of Parkinson's disease. *Science* **317**, 516–519 (2007).

183. Zhu, H., Guo, Q., & Mattson, M. P. Dietary restriction protects hippocampal neurons against the death-promoting action of a presenilin-1 mutation. *Brain Res.* **842**, 224–229 (1999).

184. Karuppagounder, S. S., et al. Dietary supplementation with resveratrol reduces plaque pathology in a transgenic model of Alzheimer's disease. *Neurochem. Int.* **54**, 111–118 (2009).

185. Kumar, P., Padi, S. S. V., Naidu, P. S., & Kumar, A. Effect of resveratrol on 3-nitropropionic acid-induced biochemical and behavioural changes: possible neuroprotective mechanisms. *Behav. Pharmacol.* **17**, 485–492 (2006).

186. Ho, D. J., Calingasan, N. Y., Wille, E., Dumont, M., & Beal, M. F. Resveratrol protects against peripheral deficits in a mouse model of Huntington's disease. *Exp. Neurol.* **225**, 74–84 (2010).

13

Cell Culture, iPS Cells and Neurodegenerative Diseases

ROXANA NAT AND ANDREAS EIGENTLER

INTRODUCTION

Neurodegenerative diseases (NDDs) comprise a large group of neurological disorders with heterogeneous clinical and pathological manifestations affecting specific sites within the nervous system. Until recently, the genetic basis for many NDDs was largely unknown. Thanks to intensive genome sequencing, candidate genes that underlie or predispose individuals to NDDs are now being discovered (reviewed in [1]). Although most NDDs are of multifactorial etiology, like idiopathic Parkinson's disease (PD) and Alzheimer's disease (AD), a subset of entities was found to be due to a defined genetic cause, which ranges from trinucleotide repeat expansions to point mutations following different traits of inheritance. However, even for well-understood monogenic disorders, such as Friedreich's ataxia (FRDA) or Huntington's disease (HD), the cellular and molecular links between causative mutations and the symptoms exhibited by affected patients are incompletely understood [2, 3].

A hallmark of NDDs is the chronic and progressive loss of specific types of neurons, such as cerebral cortex glutamatergic and basal forebrain cholinergic neurons in AD, midbrain dopaminergic neurons in PD, striatal GABAergic neurons in HD, motor neurons in amyotrophic lateral sclerosis (ALS) and spinal muscular atrophy (SMA), cerebellar and peripheral sensory neurons in ataxias, and others.

Obtaining information from the analysis of postmortem tissue regarding neuronal function and dysfunction in disease is limited, as it represents end-stage disease and does not allow conclusions regarding disease dynamics. The limitation to acquire patient neural tissue and generate primary neuronal cultures hampers the understanding of human pathophysiology.

Modeling NDDs in animals has led to important advances in the understanding and investigating of disease mechanisms and identifying candidate therapeutics. Cellular models have been widely used, in addition to *in vivo* models, in order to elucidate and investigate cell-type specific pathophysiologic features. All common and widely accepted disease mechanisms have been modeled and examined in primary neuronal cell cultures. The majority of those primary neuronal cultures have been derived from rodents. Here a large variety of neurons like motor neurons, hippocampal neurons, mesencephalic dopaminergic neurons, striatal neurons, cortical neurons, and cerebellar neurons have been cultured and investigated according to cell-type specific processes in the most affected neuronal subtypes in each disease.

However, translation of findings from rodent models into the human system proved to be problematic. The human nervous system differs significantly from rodents in its overall structure and cell type composition [4]. The human brain has a proportionately larger upper cortical layer and a better developed prefrontal and temporal cortex [5]. Differences in life span between humans and rodents may explain why animal models often fail to recapitulate key aspects of the pathology of late onset diseases like AD and PD [6]. Accordingly, many drugs that display efficacy in animal models have not translated successfully to humans [7].

Therefore, creating disease models using human neurons generated through the reprogramming of non-neural cells, easily available from patients (e.g., blood cells, skin fibroblasts), may offer improved insights into the molecular and cellular bases of neurologic disorders, including NDD. One very recent strategy for generating disease phenotypes in a dish includes direct lineage reprogramming (or transdifferentiation) of non-neural cells into neurons or neural stem cells. However, despite considerable progress, this

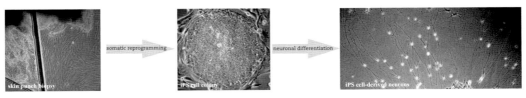

FIGURE 13.1. From patient non-neural cells to specific neurons in a dish via iPS cell technology.

technology has several limitations regarding the number and subtypes of the "instant" neurons (reviewed in [8, 9]).

Another more "classical" strategy is the reprograming of somatic cells via the induced pluripotent stem (iPS) cell technology depicted in Figure 13.1. Since the breakthrough discovery of Yamanaka in 2006 [10], followed by the derivation of patient-specific iPS cells one year later [11], considerable progress in reprogramming methods was achieved, including increasing efficiency, non-integrating approaches, and stoichiometry-controlled protocols [12, 13].

Human iPS cells share salient characteristics of embryonic stem (ES) cells, showing the capacity to self-renew and to differentiate *in vitro* and *in vivo* into the cell types that make up the human body. This includes the various types of mature neurons affected by NDDs. Stem cells allow, for the first time, the generation of large numbers of postmitotic human neurons, such as cortical pyramidal neurons, striatal interneurons, motor neurons, or dopaminergic neurons [14, 15], for preclinical research in cell culture. In particular, the iPS cell technology opens doors for intensified research on human iPS cell-derived neurons because, in comparison to human ES cells, ethical concerns can be dispelled.

The promise of iPS cells in disease models, drug discovery, and cell therapy was intensively reviewed [6, 16, 17]. In this chapter, we examine the progress in the human iPS cell systems related to common and rare NDDs, focusing on the pathophysiological features revealed in cell cultures, and the neuronal subtypes most affected in each NDD.

NDD AND iPS CELL CULTURES

To date, the reprogramming of patient somatic cells into iPS cell-based models has been achieved for the most common NDDs, such as AD and PD, but also for rare NDDs, especially for the monogenic types such as HD, SMA, and some ataxias like FRDA and spinocerebellar ataxias (SCAs).

We review here the pathophysiological findings in patient iPS cell-derived cultures related to these NDDs (Table 13.1).

Alzheimer's Disease

AD is the most common neurodegenerative disease. While the majority of AD cases are idiopathic (or sporadic), a few familial AD (FAD) cases follow an early-onset autosomal dominant trait, related to *APP* [18], *PRESENILIN1* and *2* (*PSEN1* and *PSEN2*) genes [19].

The modeling of AD via iPS cell technology was performed for both idiopathic and familial cases. The iPS cells derived from patients carrying mutations in *PSEN1* and *PSEN2* were successfully differentiated into neural cells, showing increased amyloid β42 secretion compared to the healthy controls [20]. iPS cells derived from patients carrying APP duplication showed an increased level of both Aβ (1-40) and phospho-tau in differentiated neurons in long-term neural cultures [21].

A recent report revealed endoplasmic reticulum (ER) and oxidative stress phenotypes associated with intracellular Aβ accumulation in iPS cell-derived cortical neurons from familial and sporadic AD patients [22]. Furthermore, some cortical neurons showed an improvement in stress responses to drugs like docosahexaenoic acid (DHA), which might be beneficial in a subset of patients.

Parkinson's Disease

PD is the second most common NDD. While PD is largely a late-onset idiopathic disease, 5%–10% cases are familial, transmitted in either an autosomal-dominant or autosomal recessive fashion [23]. The protein α-synuclein, the gene product of the *SNCA* gene, comprises the major component of Lewy bodies in sporadic and in some cases of autosomal dominant types and therefore appears to be central to PD pathophysiology [24, 25]. Genetic discoveries and cell culture systems of the last years have highlighted the importance of the ubiquitin proteasome system,

TABLE 13.1. HUMAN IPS CELLS AND NEURODEGENERATIVE DISEASES

Disease	Most Affected Neurons (N) and Histopathology (H)	Gene	Reported Disease-Related Phenotype	References
Alzheimer's disease (AD)	N: basal forebrain cholinergic neurons, glutamatergic neurons such as cortical pyramidal and hippocampal neurons	PSEN 1&2	Increased amyloid β42 secretion, response to γ-secretase inhibitor, increased Aβ42/40, gene expression changes	[20, 86]
	H: neurofibrillary tangles, amyloid plaques, loss of neurons and synapses	idiopathic, APP mutation	increased amyloid β(1–40) and phospho-tau levels, effect of β-secretase inhibitor	[21]
			Aβ oligomer accumulation, ER and oxidative stress	[22]
			increased Aβ42, Aβ38, and phospho-tau levels	[87]
		healthy controls	neurotoxicity of pre-fibrillary Aβ in iPS cell-derived glutamatergic neurons;	[88]
		APP; PSEN	3D model, phospho-tau and Aβ deposits, improvement after β- and γ-secretase inhibition	[82]
Parkinson's disease (PD)	N: midbrain nigro-striatal dopaminergic (DA) neurons	Idiopathic	Proof-of-concept	[26, 89]
	H: Lewy bodies, loss of DA neurons	LRRK2	Increased caspase-3 activation and DA neuron death with various cell stress conditions,	[29]
		PINK1	higher levels of mitochondrial damage, reversal upon ZFN-mediated repair	[35]
			ERK-dependent changes, genetic correction	[34]
			Impaired stress-induced mitochondrial translocation of parkin in DA neurons	[30]
		SCNA	Increased neural α-synuclein protein levels	[31]
			sensitivity to oxidative stress	[32]
		GBA	Increased neural α-synuclein protein levels, autophagic and lysosomal defects	[90]
		PARK2	Increased oxidative stress, abnormal mitochondrial morphology, Lewy body formation	[91]
		PINK1 and PARKIN	Pronounced dendrite degeneration, Lewy-body precursor inclusions, enlarged mitochondria,	[81]
		PINK1 and LRRK2	mitochondrial abnormalities, increased vulnerability	[33]

Disease	Features	Gene	Description	References
Huntington's disease (HD)	N: striatal GABAergic medium spiny neurons, cortical neurons; H: neural inclusion bodies, loss of striatal/cortical neurons	HTT	Proof-of-concept; Increase in lysosomal activity; Alterations in electrophysiology, cell vulnerability; Genetic correction; In vivo effects, transplantation	[38, 39] [40] [92] [41] [42, 43]
Amyotrophic lateral sclerosis (ALS)	N: upper and lower motor neurons (MN); H: ubiquitinated inclusion bodies, loss of (MN)	SOD1	Proof-of-concept; NF aggregation and neurite degeneration in MN, genetic modification with TALEN, initial hyperexcitability and reduced output of MN	[60, 93] [64]
		C9orf72	Accumulation of repeat-RNA foci > altered RNA metabolism	[94]
		TDP-43	Stress-dependent cellular defects	[95]
		Idiopathic	De-novo TDP-43 aggregation	[96]
		TDP-43 and C9orf72	Intrinsic membrane hyperexcitability and genetic correction of mutation, drug screening	[63, 65, 97] [61, 62]
Spinal muscular atrophy, type I (SMA)	N: spinal (MN); H: loss of anterior horn cells	SMN1 deletion	Reduced number of MN, decreased soma size, synaptic defects, different gene splicing profile; Inhibition of apoptosis; genetic correction	[48, 50] [49] [51]
Friedrich ataxia (FRDA)	N: dorsal root ganglia (DRG) peripheral neurons, cerebellar neurons; H: reduced number of DRG neurons, iron misdistribution	FXN	GAA repeat instability due to mismatch-repair; reduced ψm, delayed neuronal maturation, mitochondrial phenotype in cardiomyocytes,; differential frataxin dynamics during peripheral sensory neurogenesis	[69, 70] [72] [71]
Spinocerebellar ataxia, type 2 (SCA2)	N: cerebellar, striatal, and cortical neurons; H: intranuclear inclusion bodies, neuronal loss	ATAXIN2	Impaired neural rosette formation, reduced neuronal survival	[76]
Spinocerebellar ataxia, type 3 (SCA3)	N: cerebellar neurons, striatal and cortical neurons; H: intranuclear inclusion bodies, neuronal loss	ATAXIN 3	Excitation-induced cleavage and aggregation of Ataxin 3, reversal after inhibition of Ca^{2+} dependent calpain proteases	[77]

mitochondrial dysfunction, and oxidative stress in PD pathogenesis.

Soldner et al. derived iPS cells from idiopathic PD patients and subsequently differentiated them into dopaminergic neurons. They further accelerated PD-pathology related phenotypes *in vitro* with neurotoxins such as MPTP, or the overexpression of PD-related genes such as *SNCA* or *LRKK2* [26]. They were further able to manipulate patient-specific iPS cells from PD patients with mutations in the *SNCA* gene *via* zinc-finger nuclease (ZFN)–mediated genome editing. Using this technology, they not only generated isogenic control iPS cell lines, but also introduced the mutation in healthy stem cell lines [27].

Sanchez-Danes et al. generated PD iPS cells from idiopathic as well as genetic forms (LRRK2 mutation) [28]. Over long-term culture of iPS cell-derived dopaminergic neurons, morphological differences were found, such as a reduction in neurite arborization and an accumulation of autophagosomes, indicating an impairment of autophagosome clearance in patient neurons.

Regarding familiar PD, Nguyen et al. [29] found that iPS cell-derived dopaminergic neurons from patients carrying an *LRRK2* mutation had increased expression of oxidative stress response genes and α-synuclein protein. The mutant neurons were also more sensitive than the control neurons to caspase-3 activation and cell death caused by exposure to hydrogen peroxide, MG-132 (a proteasome inhibitor), and 6-hydroxydopamine. The finding of increased susceptibility to stress in patient-derived neurons provides insights into the pathogenesis of PD and a potential basis for a cellular screening.

Seibler et al. [30] generated iPS cells from PD patients carrying point mutations in the *PINK1* gene (Q456X; V170G). They compared the mitochondrial translocation of parkin in DA neurons under mitochondrial stress conditions, thereby making a step forward in PD pathogenesis *in vitro*.

Two recent studies focused on the iPS cell-derived models of PD carrying a triplication in the *SNCA* gene. Devine et al. showed that the levels of α-synuclein protein were increased in the dopaminergic population derived from patients, comparing with the healthy controls [31], while Byers et al. focused on the differences in sensitivity to oxidative stress correlated with this mutation [32].

Assessments of pharmacological substances on iPS cell-derived neurons from patients suffering from PD due to mutations in *LRRK2* and *PINK1* were performed by Cooper et al. They demonstrated a positive response on mitochondrial function with substances like coenzyme Q_{10}, rapamycin, and a LRRK2 kinase inhibitor [33].

Two additional studies regarding a successful genetic correction of familial PD-iPS cells due to LRRK2 mutations were reported recently. Again, target-specific ZFN were used to generate isogenic control. This approach revealed mutation-specific dysregulations of ERK-dependent gene expression contributing to neurodegeneration [34]. Sanders et al. [35] demonstrated the absence of mitochondrial DNA damage in ZFN-corrected LRRK2-iPS cell-derived neural progenitors and neurons.

Huntington's Disease

HD is an autosomal dominant neurodegenerative disorder resulting from an expanded CAG triplet repeat in the Huntingtin gene (*HTT*) [36]. Although the protein huntingtin is ubiquitously expressed in mammalian cells, mainly striatal GABAergic medium spiny neurons with a dopamine- and cyclic AMP-regulated phosphoprotein (DARPP-32)-positive phenotype are susceptible to neurodegeneration in HD [37].

The first HD-iPS cell lines were successfully generated by Park et al. from a patient with a 72 CAG repeat tract [38]. In a subsequent study, Zhang et al. differentiated these patient-specific iPS cells into striatal neurons. Besides a stable CAG repeat expansion in all patient-derived cells, an enhanced caspase 3/7 activity was found [39]. Camnasio et al. observed also an enhanced lysosomal activity in HD iPS cells and iPS cell-derived neurons [40].

A stable genetic correction during differentiation into DARPP-32 positive neurons was demonstrated after the exchange of mutated allele with a normal repeat allele by homologous recombination techniques applied to iPS cells. This was followed by a reversal of HD-related phenotypic features like cell death and mitochondrial alterations [41].

Going a step further, using *in vivo* approaches, the HD iPS cell-derived neural precursors were successfully transplanted into a HD rat model with striatal degeneration, showing survival migration and neuronal differentiation of transplanted cells into the lesion, as well as improvement of motor and behavioral functions [42, 43]. No aggregate formation was found at early time-points in the graft; however, after administration of a proteasome inhibitor and/or at later time points after grafting, HD typical pathology became manifest [43].

Motor Neuron Diseases

SMA is characterized by the selective degeneration of lower motor neurons (MNs) in the brainstem and spinal cord [44]. SMA is an autosomal recessive disorder caused by homozygous mutations in the Survival of Motor Neuron-1 (*SMN1*) gene [45, 46]. It remains to be clarified how a deficiency in SMN is responsible for the selective degeneration of lower MNs [47].

SMA iPS cells demonstrated a lack of SMN1 expression and reduced levels of the full-length protein compensated by SMN2 [48]. Significant differences regarding the number of MNs, as well as their soma size and synapse formation ability, could be observed between patient and control iPS cell-derived neuronal cultures, therefore reflecting disease-specific phenotypes. Furthermore, valproic acid and tobramycin, two drugs known to increase full-length SMN mRNA levels from the SMN2 locus, were tested in SMA iPS cells, showing an increase in SMN protein expression with a nuclear punctuate localization. In a subsequent experiment, Sareen et al. [49] found an increased apoptosis in SMA-specific cells, proposing the inhibition of apoptosis as another potential target for therapeutic intervention.

Rescue experiments in terms of ectopic expression of *SMN* via genome editing were recently performed in SMA iPS cells [50, 51], demonstrating the restoration of the impaired MN differentiation. Additionally, a single-stranded oligonucleotide approach was applied to convert *SMN2* into an *SMN1*-like gene. Furthermore, transplantation of corrected SMA-iPS cells into a SMA mouse model demonstrated an improvement of phenotype [51].

ALS is characterized by a progressive loss of both upper and lower MNs in the cerebral cortex, brainstem, and spinal cord. ALS has an idiopathic form and less common familial forms (FALS) [52], all characterized by the presence of inclusion bodies in lower MNs [53]. Mutations in the Cu/Zn superoxide dismutase 1 (*SOD1*) gene [54], in the transactive response DNA-binding protein 43 gene (*TDP-43*) [55], and in the fused in sarcoma gene (*FUS*) [56, 57] were identified in some FALS. More recently, a large repeat expansion mutation in the *C9orf72* gene was discovered and is thought to constitute the most common genetic cause of ALS [58, 59].

Dimos et al. [60] were the first to generate ALS-patient-specific iPS cells, subsequently differentiated into MNs and glia. Due to the fact that more than 90% of ALS cases are idiopathic,

patient-specific iPS cell models might overcome this drawback through the integration of the genetic as well as individual environmental background.

Egawa et al. [61] generated FALS-iPS cell-derived MNs and performed chemical compound testing. They demonstrated a beneficial effect of a histone deacetylase inhibitor on the MNs in culture. Yang et al. [62] performed a screening for small molecules and unraveled a kinase inhibitor, kenpaullone, as an MN survival-promoting substance.

New pathophysiological insights came from the electrophysiological studies on iPS cell-derived MNs from FALS and isogenic control lines [63], which revealed membrane hyperexcitability in FALS MNs. Application of a potassium channel blocker abolished the hyperexcitability and resulted in an increased survival of MNs.

Further investigation of SOD1 ALS-iPS cells and derived MNs revealed neurofilament aggregation due to the altered composition of neurofilament subunits [64], as well as the involvement of oxidative and ER stress, altered mitochondrial function, and subcellular transport [65] in ALS pathology. In addition, genetic correction of the mutations allowed the reversal of these phenotypes [64, 65].

Ataxias

The degenerative ataxias are a group of hereditary or idiopathic diseases that are characterized by the degeneration of cerebellar-brainstem structures and spinal pathways [66].

FRDA, an autosomal-recessive ataxia, is caused by a GAA triplet expansion in the first intron of the Frataxin (*FXN*) gene [67]. Major neuropathologic findings comprise a degeneration of dorsal root ganglia (DRG), with loss of large sensory neurons, followed by cerebellar degeneration [2, 68].

FRDA-iPS cell lines have been established [69–72]. Although a specific disease-related phenotype was not yet reported, FRDA iPS cells were able to recapitulate some of the molecular aspects of FRDA, including the phenomenon of repeat-length instability, epigenetic silencing of the *FXN* locus, and low levels of Frataxin expression [69]. MSH2, a critical component of the DNA mismatch repair (MMR) machinery important for mediating repeat-length instability, was highly expressed in FRDA-iPS cells relative to donor fibroblasts [69].

It remains to be shown whether FRDA iPS cell derivatives will present cell-type-specific expansions of GAA repeats. Given that FRDA-iPS cells can be directed to differentiate into sensory neurons [71], as well as cardiomyocytes [70, 72], the tissue-specific detection of FRDA hallmarks is the major focus of FRDA research. So far, no overt phenotype was observed in iPS-cell derived neurons in FRDA, in contrast to the reported mitochondrial phenotype in FRDA-iPS cell-derived cardiomyocytes [72, 73].

During the differentiation process of FRDA iPS cells to peripheral neurons via the generation of neural crest cells, a differential expression of the mutant protein was observed between control and FRDA iPS cells [71], with FRDA-specific cells lacking an upregulation found in control cells. A recent study [74] showed the capacity of FRDA-iPS cell-derived neurons to survive and integrate after transplantation into the cerebellum of an adult rodent brain.

Spinocerebellar ataxias (SCAs) comprise a clinically and pathophysiologically heterogeneous group of autosomal dominant NDDs. Spinocerebellar ataxia type 2 (SCA2) and type 3 (SCA3) belong to the group of CAG-triple repeat disorders, also known as polyQ-disorders due to abnormally long polyglutamine tracts within the corresponding protein. As in most of these polyglutamine diseases, patients with a repeat expansion above a critical threshold form neuronal intranuclear inclusion bodies [75]. Xia et al. [76] generated SCA2 iPS cells that demonstrated an abnormality during neural differentiation in neural rosette formation and reduced life span of terminally differentiated SCA2 iPS-cell derived neurons.

Koch et al. [77] investigated the formation of early aggregates and their behavior in time and demonstrated that SCA3-iPS cell-derived neurons constitute an appropriate cellular model in the study of aberrant human protein processing. Moreover, they concluded that neurons are able to cope, at least in the beginning, with the aggregated mutant material and cytotoxicity evolved over time. Besides, the key role of the protease calpain in ATXN3-aggregation formation suggested a therapeutic benefit of the calpain inhibitors.

For all NDDs described here, the iPS cell models proved the presence of disease-inherent phenotypes in iPS cells and/or the iPS cell-derived affected neurons. For some NDDs, the iPS cell models revealed new pathophysiological insights and promising candidate substance testing.

VALIDITY, LIMITATIONS, AND IMPROVEMENTS FOR iPS CELL-DERIVED NEURONAL CULTURES

During recent years the generation of iPS cell lines from human material has become routine. The proof-of-principle has already been achieved, but a number of issues still need to be resolved before the full potential of these cells can be exploited in clinical practice. These include deriving high-quality iPS cells using non-integrative methods and complete epigenetic resetting [12, 13, 78].

Regarding the *in vitro* differentiation of iPS cells toward specific neuronal phenotypes, the proof-of-principle has also been achieved. Numerous studies demonstrated that *in vitro* developmentally based human neuronal culture systems can reproduce a phenotype normally observed *in vivo* in adult life. A remaining major challenge is to guide *in vitro* differentiation of iPS cells into the defined and homogeneous neuronal populations, in order to faithfully and reproducibly recapitulate NDD pathologies. Protocols for subtypes of neurons with different degrees of heterogeneity are currently being used for modeling NDDs, such as for MNs [49, 61, 62], dopaminergic neurons [27, 28, 33] cortical neurons [22], striatal neurons [39, 41] and peripheral neurons [71].

To fully tap into the potential of the iPS technology and to progress toward a fundamental understanding of the causes of disease selectivity in the loss of neuron subtypes, it is necessary to establish reproducible and tailored protocols for the differentiation of iPS cells specifically into these neuronal subtypes *in vitro*. Alternatively, the relevant neuronal subtype needs to be sorted out or visualized using specific reporter genes [79].

Another limitation is related to late-onset NDDs, such as AD and PD. Most iPS cell-derived neurons seem to more closely resemble embryonic neurons than mature and aged neurons, as systematically showed in a recent time-course analysis of their electrophysiological properties [80]. Long-time cultures are required to model the late-onset disorders, and it may be necessary to devise protocols that favor aging- and degeneration-associated features [81].

The patient-derived *in vitro* cell models can potentially overcome the limitations of animal models, despite their own limitations. The 3D models seem to overcome some of these limitations [82]. The iPS cell derivatives can be additionally used to functionally analyze the specific cells after transplantation and differentiation in animal models, as was already shown for SMA and HD [42, 43, 51]. However, the NDD *in vitro* models should be complemented to NDD *in vivo* models in order to reflect defects involved in neural circuitry.

The most promising aspect of patient-derived cellular models is the idea of curing diseases *in vitro*. Hence, patient donor cells (like fibroblasts) could be genetically corrected, reprogrammed into iPS cells, and further differentiated into the desired progenitor cell. Another possibility is to generate isogenic iPS cell lines by genetic modifications through target specific ZFNs, TALENs, or CRISPR/Cas9 technologies [83, 84]. This aspect has already been proven by generating isogenic iPS cell lines for HD [41], PD [27, 34], SMA [50, 51], and ALS [65].

Better identification of a dysfunctional pathway in patients suffering from complex NDDs is the primary requirement for rational therapeutic drug development. The human iPS cell-derived models could have a positive impact on the screening of compound libraries and drug safety screens, and at the same time reduce the animal dependency of the current drug development pipeline. The proof-of-principle was already demonstrated for the iPS cell-derived models in AD [22], PD [33], SMN [49], and ALS [61, 62].

Finally, iPS cell technology will be an important driver of personalized medicine. Prior to treatment, patient-derived iPS cells or differentiated progenies can be used to tailor a particular drug type and dose according to the genetic and cellular profile.

CONCLUSION

In this chapter we have attempted to outline the revolutionary impact that iPS cell technologies have on NDD modeling and therapy. We have presented studies showing that it is now possible to differentiate patient-derived iPS cells into disease-susceptible cell phenotypes. Experiments have proved the presence of disease-inherent phenotypes in iPS cells and the iPS cell-derived affected neurons, and even have revealed new pathophysiological insights and promising candidate substance testing in some NDDs.

However, much work is still needed to optimize and integrate the specific differentiation protocols in the disease-related iPS cell models. Another approach is to generate appropriate control lines, which, in the case of genetic diseases, could be obtained via correction of the mutation and subsequent generation of isogenic lines from the same individual. Such approach would minimize the noise of one's individual genetic background, which might otherwise hamper comparability and corollaries [27, 85]. Patient iPS cell-derived neurons provide a unique opportunity to gain insights into the pathophysiology of NDDs, as well as for drug screening, cell therapy, and personalized medicine.

REFERENCES

1. Handel AE, Disanto G, Ramagopalan SV. Next-generation sequencing in understanding complex neurological disease. *Expert Rev Neurother* 2013; 13: 215–227.
2. Koeppen AH. Friedreich's ataxia: pathology, pathogenesis, and molecular genetics. *J Neurol Sci* 2011; 303: 1–12.
3. Perdomini M, Hick A, Puccio H, Pook MA. Animal and cellular models of Friedreich ataxia. *J Neurochemistry* 2013; 126: 65–79.
4. Hansen DV, Lui JH, Parker PR, Kriegstein AR. Neurogenic radial glia in the outer subventricular zone of human neocortex. *Nature* 2010; 464: 554–561.
5. Clowry G, Molnar Z, Rakic P. Renewed focus on the developing human neocortex. *J Anat* 2010; 217: 276–288.
6. Livesey FJ. Human stem cell models of dementia. *Hum Mol Genet* 2014; 23: R35–R39.
7. Dragunow M. The adult human brain in preclinical drug development. *Nat Rev Drug Discov* 2008; 7: 659–666.
8. Qiang L, Fujita R, Yamashita T, Angulo S, Rhinn H, Rhee D et al. Directed conversion of Alzheimer's disease patient skin fibroblasts into functional neurons. *Cell* 2011; 146: 359–371.
9. Ang CE, Wernig M. Induced neuronal reprogramming. *J Comp Neurol* 2014; 522: 2877–2886.
10. Takahashi K, Yamanaka S. Induction of pluripotent stem cells from mouse embryonic and adult fibroblast cultures by defined factors. *Cell* 2006; 126: 663–676.
11. Takahashi K, Tanabe K, Ohnuki M, Narita M, Ichisaka T, Tomoda K et al. Induction of pluripotent stem cells from adult human fibroblasts by defined factors. *Cell* 2007; 131: 861–872.
12. Yu J, Hu K, Smuga-Otto K, Tian S, Stewart R, Slukvin II et al. Human induced pluripotent stem cells free of vector and transgene sequences. *Science* 2009; 324: 797–801.
13. Okita K, Yamakawa T, Matsumura Y, Sato Y, Amano N, Watanabe A et al. An efficient nonviral method to generate integration-free human-induced pluripotent stem cells from cord blood and peripheral blood cells. *Stem Cells* 2013; 31: 458–466.

14. Zeng H, Guo M, Martins-Taylor K, Wang X, Zhang Z, Park JW et al. Specification of region-specific neurons including forebrain glutamatergic neurons from human induced pluripotent stem cells. *PLoS One* 2010; 5: e11853.

15. Liu H, Zhang SC. Specification of neuronal and glial subtypes from human pluripotent stem cells. *Cell Mol Life Sci* 2011; 68: 3995–4008.

16. Robinton DA, Daley GQ. The promise of induced pluripotent stem cells in research and therapy. *Nature* 2012; 481: 295–305.

17. Cao L, Tan L, Jiang T, Zhu XC, Yu JT. Induced pluripotent stem cells for disease modeling and drug discovery in neurodegenerative diseases. *Mol Neurobiol* 2014; 52: 244–255.

18. Chartier-Harlin MC, Crawford F, Houlden H, Warren A, Hughes D, Fidani L et al. Early-onset Alzheimer's disease caused by mutations at codon 717 of the [beta]-amyloid precursor protein gene. *Nature* 1991; 353: 844–846.

19. Tanzi RE, Kovacs DM, Kim TW, Moir RD, Guenette SY, Wasco W. The gene defects responsible for familial Alzheimer's disease. *Neurobiol Dis* 1996; 3: 159–168.

20. Yagi T, Ito D, Okada Y, Akamatsu W, Nihei Y, Yoshizaki T et al. Modeling familial Alzheimer's disease with induced pluripotent stem cells. *Hum Mol Genet* 2011; 20: 4530–4539.

21. Israel MA, Yuan SH, Bardy C, Reyna SM, Mu Y, Herrera C et al. Probing sporadic and familial Alzheimer's disease using induced pluripotent stem cells. *Nature* 2012.; 482: 216–220.

22. Kondo T, Asai M, Tsukita K, Kutoku Y, Ohsawa Y, Sunada Y et al. Modeling Alzheimer's disease with iPSCs reveals stress phenotypes associated with intracellular Abeta and differential drug responsiveness. *Cell Stem Cell* 2013; 12: 487–496.

23. Lesage S, Brice A. Parkinson's disease: from monogenic forms to genetic susceptibility factors. *Hum Mol Genet* 2009; 18: R48-R59.

24. Polymeropoulos MH, Lavedan C, Leroy E, Ide SE, Dehejia A, Dutra A, et al. Mutation in the α-synuclein gene identified in families with Parkinson's disease. *Science* 1997; 276: 2045–2047.

25. Singleton AB, Farrer M, Johnson J, Singleton A, Hague S, Kachergus J, et al. α-synuclein locus triplication causes Parkinson's disease. *Science* 2003; 302: 841.

26. Soldner F, Hockemeyer D, Beard C, Gao Q, Bell GW, Cook EG, et al. Parkinson's disease patient-derived induced pluripotent stem cells free of viral reprogramming factors. *Cell* 2009; 136: 964–977.

27. Soldner F, Laganiére Je, Cheng A, Hockemeyer D, Gao Q, Alagappan R, et al. Generation of isogenic pluripotent stem cells differing exclusively at two early onset Parkinson point mutations. *Cell* 2011; 146: 318–331.

28. Sanchez-Danes A, Richaud-Patin Y, Carballo-Carbajal I, Jimenez-Delgado S, Caig C, Mora S, et al. Disease-specific phenotypes in dopamine neurons from human iPS-based models of genetic and sporadic Parkinson's disease. *EMBO Mol Med* 2012; 4: 380–395.

29. Nguyen H, Byers B, Cord B, Shcheglovitov A, Byrne J, Gujar P, et al. LRRK2 Mutant iPSC-derived DA neurons demonstrate increased susceptibility to oxidative stress. *Cell Stem Cell* 2011; 8: 267–280.

30. Seibler P, Graziotto J, Jeong H, Simunovic F, Klein C, Krainc D. Mitochondrial parkin recruitment is impaired in neurons derived from mutant PINK1 induced pluripotent stem cells. *J Neuroscience* 2011; 31: 5970–5976.

31. Devine MJ, Ryten M, Vodicka P, Thomson AJ, Burdon T, Houlden H, et al. Parkinson's disease induced pluripotent stem cells with triplication of the α-synuclein locus. *Nat Commun* 2011; 2: 440.

32. Byers B, Cord B, Nguyen HN, Schüle B, Fenno L, Lee PC, et al. SNCA triplication Parkinson's patient's iPSC-derived DA neurons accumulate alpha-synuclein and are susceptible to oxidative stress. *PLoS One* 2011; 6: e26159.

33. Cooper O, Seo H, Andrabi S, Guardia-Laguarta C, Graziotto J, Sundberg M, et al. Pharmacological rescue of mitochondrial deficits in iPSC-derived neural cells from patients with familial Parkinson's disease. *Sci Transl Med* 2012; 4: 141ra90.

34. Reinhardt P, Schmid B, Burbulla LF, Schondorf DC, Wagner L, Glatza M, et al. Genetic correction of a LRRK2 mutation in human iPSCs links parkinsonian neurodegeneration to ERK-dependent changes in gene expression. *Cell Stem Cell* 2013; 12: 354–367.

35. Sanders LH, Laganiére Je, Cooper O, Mak SK, Vu BJ, Huang YA, et al. LRRK2 mutations cause mitochondrial DNA damage in iPSC-derived neural cells from Parkinson's disease patients: reversal by gene correction. *Neurobiol Dis* 2014; 62: 381–386.

36. The Huntington's Disease Collaborative Research Group. A novel gene containing a trinucleotide repeat that is expanded and unstable on Huntington's disease chromosomes. The Huntington's Disease Collaborative Research Group. *Cell* 1993; 72: 971–983.

37. Mitchell IJ, Cooper AJ, Griffiths MR. The selective vulnerability of striatopallidal neurons. *Prog Neurobiol* 1999; 59: 691–719.

38. Park IH, Arora N, Huo H, Maherali N, Ahfeldt T, Shimamura A, et al. Disease-specific induced pluripotent stem cells. *Cell* 2008; 134: 877–886.

39. Zhang N, An MC, Montoro D, Ellerby LM. Characterization of human Huntington's disease cell model from induced pluripotent stem cells. *PLoS Curr* 2010; 2: RRN1193.

40. Camnasio S, Carri AD, Lombardo A, Grad I, Mariotti C, Castucci A, et al. The first reported generation of several induced pluripotent stem cell lines from homozygous and heterozygous Huntington's disease patients demonstrates mutation related enhanced lysosomal activity. *Neurobiol Dis* 2012; 46: 41–51.

41. An MC, Zhang N, Scott G, Montoro D, Wittkop T, Mooney S, et al. Genetic correction of Huntington's disease phenotypes in induced pluripotent stem cells. *Cell Stem Cell* 2012; 11: 253–263.

42. Jeon I, Lee N, Li JY, Park IH, Park KS, Moon J et al. Neuronal properties, in vivo effects and pathology of a Huntington's disease patient-derived induced pluripotent stem cells. *Stem Cells* 2012; 30: 2054–2062.

43. Mu S, Wang J, Zhou G, Peng W, He Z, Zhao Z, et al. Transplantation of induced pluripotent stem cells improves functional recovery in Huntington's disease rat model. *PLoS One* 2014; 9: e101185.

44. Lefebvre S, Burglen L, Reboullet S, Clermont O, Burlet P, Viollet L, et al. Identification and characterization of a spinal muscular atrophy-determining gene. *Cell* 1995; 80: 155–165.

45. Lefebvre S, Burglen L, Frezal J, Munnich A, Melki J. The role of the SMN gene in proximal spinal muscular atrophy. *Hum Mol Gen*et 1998; 7: 1531–1536.

46. Coovert DD, Le TT, McAndrew PE, Strasswimmer J, Crawford TO, Mendell JR et al. The survival motor neuron protein in spinal muscular atrophy. *Hum Mol Genet* 1997; 6: 1205–1214.

47. Monani UR. Spinal muscular atrophy: a deficiency in a ubiquitous protein; a motor neuron-specific disease. *Neuron* 2005; 48: 885–895.

48. Ebert AD, Yu J, Rose FF, Mattis VB, Lorson CL, Thomson JA, et al. Induced pluripotent stem cells from a spinal muscular atrophy patient. *Nature* 2009; 457: 277–280.

49. Sareen D, Ebert AD, Heins BM, McGivern JV, Ornelas L, Svendsen CN. Inhibition of apoptosis blocks human motor neuron cell death in a stem cell model of spinal muscular atrophy. *PLoS One* 2012; 7: e39113.

50. Chang T, Zheng W, Tsark W, Bates S, Huang H, Lin RJ et al. Brief report: phenotypic rescue of induced pluripotent stem cell-derived motoneurons of a spinal muscular atrophy patient. *Stem Cells* 2011; 29: 2090–2093.

51. Corti S, Nizzardo M, Simone C, Falcone M, Nardini M, Ronchi D, et al. Genetic correction of human induced pluripotent stem cells from patients with spinal muscular atrophy. *Sci Transl Med* 2012; 4: 165ra162.

52. Bruijn LI, Miller TM, Cleveland DW. Unraveling the mechanisms involved in motor neuron degeneration in ALS. *Annu Rev Neurosci* 2004; 27: 723–749.

53. Lowe J. New pathological findings in amyotrophic lateral sclerosis. *J Neurol Sci* 1994; 124 Suppl: 38–51.

54. Rosen DR, Siddique T, Patterson D, Figlewicz DA, Sapp P, Hentati A, et al. Mutations in Cu/Zn superoxide dismutase gene are associated with familial amyotrophic lateral sclerosis. *Nature* 1993; 362: 59–62.

55. Sreedharan J, Blair IP, Tripathi VB, Hu X, Vance C, Rogelj B, et al. TDP-43 mutations in familial and sporadic amyotrophic lateral sclerosis. *Science* 2008; 319: 1668–1672.

56. Kwiatkowski TJ, Jr., Bosco DA, Leclerc AL, Tamrazian E, Vanderburg CR, Russ C, et al. Mutations in the FUS/TLS gene on chromosome 16 cause familial amyotrophic lateral sclerosis. *Science* 2009; 323: 1205–1208.

57. Vance C, Rogelj B, Hortobagyi T, De Vos KJ, Nishimura AL, Sreedharan J, et al. Mutations in FUS, an RNA processing protein, cause familial amyotrophic lateral sclerosis type 6. *Science* 2009; 323: 1208–1211.

58. DeJesus-Hernandez M, Mackenzie IR, Boeve BF, Boxer AL, Baker M, Rutherford NJ, et al. Expanded GGGGCC hexanucleotide repeat in noncoding region of C9ORF72 causes chromosome 9p-linked FTD and ALS. *Neuron* 2011; 72: 245–256.

59. Majounie E, Renton AE, Mok K, Dopper EG, Waite A, Rollinson S, et al. Frequency of the C9orf72 hexanucleotide repeat expansion in patients with amyotrophic lateral sclerosis and frontotemporal dementia: a cross-sectional study. *Lancet Neurol* 2012; 11: 323–330.

60. Dimos JT, Rodolfa KT, Niakan KK, Weisenthal LM, Mitsumoto H, Chung W, et al. Induced pluripotent stem cells generated from patients with ALS can be differentiated into motor neurons. *Science* 2008; 321: 1218–1221.

61. Egawa N, Kitaoka S, Tsukita K, Naitoh M, Takahashi K, Yamamoto T, et al. Drug screening for ALS using patient-specific induced pluripotent stem cells. *Sci Transl Med* 2012; 4: 145ra104.

62. Yang YM, Gupta SK, Kim KJ, Powers BE, Cerqueira A, Wainger BJ, et al. A small molecule screen in stem-cell-derived motor neurons identifies a kinase inhibitor as a candidate therapeutic for ALS. *Cell Stem Cell* 2013; 12: 713–726.

63. Wainger BJ, Kiskinis E, Mellin C, Wiskow O, Han SS, Sandoe J, et al. Intrinsic membrane

hyperexcitability of amyotrophic lateral scle-rosis patient-derived motor neurons. *Cell Rep* 2014; 7: 1–11.

64. Chen H, Qian K, Du Z, Cao J, Petersen A, Liu H, et al. Modeling ALS with iPSCs reveals that mutant SOD1 misregulates neurofilament balance in motor neurons. *Cell Stem Cell* 2014; 14: 796–809.

65. Kiskinis E, Sandoe J, Williams LA, Boulting GL, Moccia R, Wainger BJ, et al. Pathways disrupted in human ALS motor neurons identified through genetic correction of mutant SOD1. *Cell Stem Cell* 2014; 14: 781–795.

66. Harding AE. Classification of the hereditary atax-ias and paraplegias. *Lancet* 1983; 1: 1151–1155.

67. Campuzano V, Montermini L, Molto MD, Pianese L, Cossee M, Cavalcanti F, et al. Friedreich's ataxia: autosomal recessive disease caused by an intronic GAA triplet repeat expansion. *Science* 1996; 271: 1423–1427.

68. Pandolfo M. Friedreich ataxia: the clinical pic-ture. *J Neurol* 2009; 256 Suppl 1: 3–8.

69. Ku S, Soragni E, Campau E, Thomas EA, Altun G, Laurent LC, et al. Friedreich's ataxia induced pluripotent stem cells model intergenerational GAATTC triplet repeat instability. *Cell Stem Cell* 2010; 7: 631–637.

70. Liu J, Verma PJ, Evans-Galea MV, Delatycki MB, Michalska A, Leung J, et al. Generation of induced pluripotent stem cell lines from Friedreich ataxia patients. *Stem Cell Rev* 2011; 7: 703–713.

71. Eigentler A, Boesch S, Schneider R, Dechant G, Nat R. Induced pluripotent stem cells from Friedreich ataxia patients fail to upregulate frataxin during in vitro differentiation to peripheral sen-sory neurons. *Stem Cells Dev* 2013; 22: 3271–3282.

72. Hick A, Wattenhofer-Donze M, Chintawar S, Tropel P, Simard JP, Vaucamps N, et al. Neurons and cardiomyocytes derived from induced plu-ripotent stem cells as a model for mitochondrial defects in Friedreich's ataxia. *Dis Model Mech* 2013; 6: 608–621.

73. Lee YK, Ho PW, Schick R, Lau YM, Lai WH, Zhou T, et al. Modeling of Friedreich ataxia-related iron overloading cardiomyopathy using patient-specific-induced pluripotent stem cells. *Pflugers Arch* 2013; 466: 1831–1844.

74. Bird MJ, Needham K, Frazier AE, van RJ, Leung J, Hough S, et al. Functional characterization of Friedreich ataxia iPS-derived neuronal progeni-tors and their integration in the adult brain. *PLoS One* 2014; 9: e101718.

75. Paulson HL, Perez MK, Trottier Y, Trojanowski JQ, Subramony SH, Das SS, et al. Intranuclear inclusions of expanded polyglutamine protein in spinocerebellar ataxia type 3. *Neuron* 1997; 19: 333–344.

76. Xia G, Santostefano K, Hamazaki T, Liu J, Subramony SH, Terada N, et al. Generation of human-induced pluripotent stem cells to model spinocerebellar ataxia type 2 in vitro. *J Mol Neurosci* 2013; 51: 237–248.

77. Koch P, Breuer P, Peitz M, Jungverdorben J, Kesavan J, Poppe D, et al. Excitation-induced ataxin-3 aggregation in neurons from patients with Machado-Joseph disease. *Nature* 2011.; 480: 543–546.

78. Ma H, Morey R, O'Neil RC, He Y, Daughtry B, Schultz MD, et al. Abnormalities in human plu-ripotent cells due to reprogramming mecha-nisms. *Nature* 2014; 511: 177–183.

79. Pasca SP, Panagiotakos G, Dolmetsch RE. Generating human neurons in vitro and using them to understand neuropsychiatric disease. *Annu Rev Neurosci* 2014; 37: 479–501.

80. Pre D, Nestor MW, Sproul AA, Jacob S, Koppensteiner P, Chinchalongporn V, et al. A time course analysis of the electrophysiological properties of neurons differentiated from human induced pluripotent stem cells (iPSCs). *PLoS One* 2014; 9: e103418.

81. Miller JD, Ganat YM, Kishinevsky S, Bowman RL, Liu B, Tu EY, et al. Human iPSC-based modeling of late-onset disease via progerin-induced aging. *Cell Stem Cell* 2013; 13: 691–705.

82. Choi SH, Kim YH, Hebisch M, Sliwinski C, Lee S, D'Avanzo C, et al. A three-dimensional human neural cell culture model of Alzheimer's disease. *Nature* 2014; 515: 274–278.

83. Zou J, Maeder ML, Mali P, Pruett-Miller SM, Thibodeau-Beganny S, Chou BK, et al. Gene tar-geting of a disease-related gene in human induced pluripotent stem and embryonic stem cells. *Cell Stem Cell* 2009; 5: 97–110.

84. Lombardo A, Genovese P, Beausejour CM, Colleoni S, Lee YL, Kim KA, et al. Gene editing in human stem cells using zinc finger nucleases and integrase-defective lentiviral vector delivery. *Nat Biotech* 2007; 25: 1298–1306.

85. Han S, Williams L, Eggan K. Constructing and deconstructing stem cell models of neurological disease. *Neuron* 2011; 70: 626–644.

86. Sproul AA, Jacob S, Pre D, Kim SH, Nestor MW, Navarro-Sobrino M, et al. Characterization and molecular profiling of *PSEN1* familial Alzheimer's disease iPSC-derived neural progenitors. *PLoS One* 2014; 9: e84547.

87. Muratore CR, Rice HC, Srikanth P, Callahan DG, Shin T, Benjamin LNP, et al. The famil-ial Alzheimer's disease APPV717I mutation alters APP processing and Tau expression in iPSC-derived neurons. *Hum Mol Genet* 2014; 23: 3523–3536.

88. Vazin T, Ball KA, Lu H, Park H, Ataeijannati Y, Head-Gordon T, et al. Efficient derivation of cortical glutamatergic neurons from human pluripotent stem cells: a model system to study neurotoxicity in Alzheimer's disease. *Neurobiol Dis* 2014; 62: 62–72.

89. Hargus G, Cooper O, Deleidi M, Levy A, Lee K, Marlow E, et al. Differentiated Parkinson patient-derived induced pluripotent stem cells grow in the adult rodent brain and reduce motor asymmetry in Parkinsonian rats. *Proc Natl Acad Sci U S A* 2010; 107: 15921–15926.

90. Schöndorf DC, Aureli M, McAllister FE, Hindley CJ, Mayer F, Schmid B, et al. iPSC-derived neurons from GBA1-associated Parkinson's disease patients show autophagic defects and impaired calcium homeostasis. *Nat Commun* 2014; 5: 4028.

91. Imaizumi Y, Okada Y, Akamatsu W, Koike M, Kuzumaki N, Hayakawa H, et al. Mitochondrial dysfunction associated with increased oxidative stress and alpha-synuclein accumulation in PARK2 iPSC-derived neurons and postmortem brain tissue. *Mol Brain* 2012; 5: 35.

92. The HD iPSC Consortium. Induced pluripotent stem cells from patients with Huntington's disease show CAG-repeat-expansion-associated phenotypes. *Cell Stem Cell* 2012; 11: 264–278.

93. Boulting GL, Kiskinis E, Croft GF, Amoroso MW, Oakley DH, Wainger BJ, et al. A functionally characterized test set of human induced pluripotent stem cells. *Nat Biotech* 2011; 29: 279–286.

94. Sareen D, O'Rourke JG, Meera P, Muhammad AK, Grant S, Simpkinson M, et al. Targeting RNA foci in iPSC-derived motor neurons from ALS patients with a C9ORF72 repeat expansion. *Sci Transl Med* 2013; 5: 208ra149.

95. Zhang Z, Almeida S, Lu Y, Nishimura AL, Peng L, Sun D, et al. Downregulation of microRNA-9 in iPSC-derived neurons of FTD/ALS patients with TDP-43 mutations. *PLoS One* 2013; 8: e76055.

96. Burkhardt MF, Martinez FJ, Wright S, Ramos C, Volfson D, Mason M, et al. A cellular model for sporadic ALS using patient-derived induced pluripotent stem cells. *Mol Cell Neurosci* 2013; 56: 355–364.

97. Devlin AC, Burr K, Borooah S, Foster JD, Cleary EM, Geti I, et al. Human iPSC-derived motoneurons harbouring TARDBP or C9ORF72 ALS mutations are dysfunctional despite maintaining viability. *Nat Commun* 2015; 6: 5999.

14

Animal Models of Neurodegenerative Diseases

DAVID BAGLIETTO-VARGAS, RAHASSON R. AGER,
RODRIGO MEDEIROS, AND FRANK M. LAFERLA

ALZHEIMER DISEASE OVERVIEW

Clinical Features

Alzheimer's disease (AD) was described for the first time by the German psychiatrist Alois Alzheimer in 1906. In that report, Dr. Alzheimer described the clinicopathological examination of a woman, Auguste D, who presented severe symptoms of dementia at the early age of 51 years [1]. Currently, AD is clinically characterized by the appearance of gradual and progressive memory and cognitive impairment. Although the first characterized patient was in her early 50s, most AD cases appear in individuals 65 and older, with increased incidence in subsequent decades [2]. From a public health perspective, AD imposes a severe financial and social burden, with a current global estimated annual cost of ~$600 billion, which is projected to grow to $1.1 trillion by 2030 [2]. Alzheimer's Disease International (ADI) estimates that AD affects ~35 million people worldwide today, a figure that is expected to quadruple in the next 40 years, with one new case appearing every 33 seconds [3, 4].

Alzheimer's disease can be classified into two separate, but similar clinical types. Familial, or early-onset AD (FAD), represents a small fraction of AD cases (~2%), and is inheritable in a autosomal-dominant manner due to mutations in three genes: amyloid protein precursor (APP), presenilin-1 (PSEN1), and presenilin-2 (PSEN2) [5]. The majorities of AD cases (~98%) however, occur idiopathically, and are known as sporadic AD (SAD). The etiology underlying SAD is complex and multifactorial, resulting from a combination of genetic, epigenetic, and lifestyle factors. Furthermore, the majority of SAD patients are elder subjects who commonly suffer from a variety of comorbidities (e.g., stroke, stress, diabetes, seizures, osteoporosis, cancer, and renal disease), which can greatly add to the complexity underlying the pathogenesis of SAD [6, 7].

Neuropathology

The brains of AD patients are characterized pathologically by the accumulation of amyloid plaques, neurofibrillary tangles (NFTs), neuroinflammation, and extensive synaptic and neuronal loss [5]. The principal component of the amyloid plaque is the amyloid-β (Aβ) peptide, a 36- to 43-amino acid peptide. Aβ is produced by proteolysis of the amyloid-β protein precursor (APP) by the sequential action of two proteases: beta-site APP-cleaving enzyme 1 (BACE-1), or β-secretase, followed by the presenilin/γ-secretase complex [5, 8]. Once generated, the Aβ peptide can accumulate into neuritic deposits, which are surrounded by swollen and neurodegerative neurites, and activated glia [9]. In addition to accumulation within the brain, Aβ is also frequently found deposited in the walls of blood vessels [10]. Vascular Aβ accumulation can both accompany parenchymal brain Aβ and be found alone in a condition know as cerebral amyloid angiopathy (CAA), also a neurodegenerative disorder. Although early studies in AD focused on the neurotoxicity of amyloid plaques, accumulating evidence indicates that smaller, soluble aggregates of Aβ, such as oligomers and protofibrils, are more neurotoxic, with even minute quantities leading to impairments in long-term potentiation, synaptic dysfunction, neuronal loss, and consequently memory deficits [11].

AD is also defined by the predominantly intracellular accumulation of a second cardinal protein aggregate: neurofibrillary tangle (NFTs). These intracellular lesions are primarily composed of hyperphosphorylated forms of the microtubule-associate protein, tau. Under physiological conditions, tau is a highly soluble and natively unfolded protein that interacts with tubulin and plays a key role in the assemblage and stability of microtubules [12, 13]. In pathological conditions, such as AD, tau can be excessively phosphorylated, cleaved, glycosylated, and so on, causing disruption of microtubules, and altering the postsynaptic physiology, leading to synaptic dysfunction and cognitive deficits [5, 14, 15]. No mutations in the tau gene (or other tau-interacting proteins) have been found to be associated with FAD. However, mutations in tau are associated with frontotemporal dementia (FTD), providing a direct genetic link between tau accumulation, neurodegeneration, and dementia [16].

Synaptic and neuronal degeneration are key hallmarks of all neurodegenerative disorders, including AD. The degree of synaptic loss in the brain is the feature most robustly associated with the level of cognitive impairment found in AD patients [17]. Clinical and prospective population-based studies suggest that synaptic degeneration occurs early in AD pathogenesis, as it is observed in patients with mild cognitive impairment (MCI), a well-accepted precursor stage of AD [17, 18]. As the disease progresses, massive brain atrophy, due to selective neuronal degeneration, ensues. For example, areas of the limbic system are particularly vulnerable to AD pathogenesis, specifically the entorhinal cortex and hippocampus. Furthermore, several other cortical areas are affected in AD, such as the temporal, parietal, and frontal neocortex, as well as subcortical projections from the basal forebrain, or locus coeruleus [19].

The immune system has been found to contribute to the synaptic and neuronal loss associated with most neurodegenerative disorders, though the identification of the exact molecular mechanisms remains an area of active investigation [20–22]. Indeed, inflammation in AD is largely considered a major cofactor that actively contributes to disease progression [23–26]. Epidemiological studies show an association between the suppression of inflammation and reduced risk for AD [27–29]. Furthermore, reactive glial cells are a common feature in AD, with both microglia and astrocytes observed surrounding Aβ plaques [21]. The molecular mechanisms that mediate the immune response, associated with AD, are an intensive area of research, with several proinflammatory cytokines and chemokines (including interleukin-1β [IL-1β], interleukin-6, interleukin-12, interleukin-23, tumor necrosis factor-α [TNF-α], etc.) implicated as playing an important role in disease progression [24–26].

Genetics

The first genetic links to FAD were identified over 20 years ago [30]. Several groups of families with a strong history of high AD incidence were found to have mutations in genes that were inherited in an autosomal-dominant fashion. All known autosomal-dominant AD-associated mutations are present in three genes: APP, PSEN1, and PSEN2. Although these mutations represent a small fraction of AD cases (~2%), the discovery of these genes has greatly contributed to the understanding of AD pathogenesis, and has facilitated the development of transgenic AD animal models.

Amyloid Protein Precursor Mutation

APP is a transmembrane protein that plays an important role in axonal pruning, neuronal migration, and cognitive function [31–33]. The APP gene was the first gene described linked to autosomal dominant AD. The Aβ peptide was first identified by protein sequencing of amyloid plaque cores collected from AD and Down syndrome (trisomy 21) patients, leading to the hypothesis that the gene encoding the Aβ peptide would be located on chromosome 21 [34]. The hypothesis was corroborated when several groups identified the cDNA encoding APP on chromosome 21 [35–37]. Currently, ~20 APP mutations have been identified that either increase the production of Aβ, influence its conformation or resistance to proteolysis, or lead to preferential generation of longer Aβ species (primarily Aβ42), which are more prone to aggregation and more toxic [38–46].

Presenilin Mutations

The majority of autosomal-dominant AD-associated mutations (~200) are found in genes encoded for the presenilin proteins (PSEN1 and PSEN2) [47–49]. Presenilins comprise the catalytic subunit of the γ-secretase complex, which also includes nicastrin, presenilin enhancer 2 (PEN2), and anterior pharynx-defective 1 (APH1) [50, 51]. By virtue of its role in cleaving multiple type-1, single-pass, intramembranous proteins, γ-secretase also plays a key role in several important cellular and biological functions such as cell adhesion, calcium homeostasis, transport, trafficking, cell fate determination, and apoptosis [52]. In AD, mutations in PSEN genes induce a shift of the γ-secretase activity in APP processing that result in a selective overproduction of longer Aβ species, particularly Aβ42, resulting in an increase in the ratio of Aβ42 to shorter, more common variants, such as Aβ40 [53–55] (Box 14.1).

BOX 14.1 APP PROCESSING AND TAU PHOSPHORYLATION

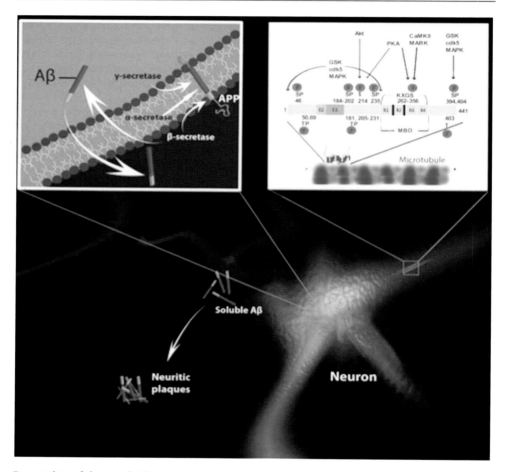

Processing of the amyloid precursor protein (APP) can be divided into a non-amyloidogenic pathway and an amyloidogenic pathway. In the more prevalent non-amyloidogenic pathway, APP is cleaved by α-secretase at a position 83 amino acids from the carboxy (C) terminus, producing a large amino (N)-terminal ectodomain (sAPPα), which is secreted into the extracellular medium [224]. The resulting 83-amino-acid C-terminal fragment (C83) is retained in the membrane and subsequently cleaved by the γ-secretase, producing a short fragment termed p3 [225] along with the APP intracellular domain (AICD). Importantly, cleavage by α-secretase occurs within the Aβ region, thereby precluding formation of Aβ. The amyloidogenic pathway is an alternative cleavage pathway for APP, which leads to Aβ generation. The initial proteolysis is mediated by β-secretase at a position located 99 amino acids from the C terminus. As a result, sAPPβ is released into the extracellular space, and leaves the 99-amino-acid C-terminal stub (C99) within the membrane, with the newly generated N-terminus corresponding to the first amino acid of Aβ. Subsequent cleavage of this fragment by the γ-secretase releases an intact Aβ peptide and the AICD [226].

The microtubule-associate protein tau (MAPT) is hyperphosphorylated in multiple sites, reducing its affinity to the microtubes, which leads to neuronal cytoskeleton destabilization and its aggregation. Serines and threonines are the majority of the putative phosphorylative sites on tau. Several important kinases and phosphatases regulate tau phosphorylation, including glycogen synthase kinase-3β (GSK3β), cyclin-dependent kinase-5 (CDK5), mitogen-activated protein kinases (MAPKs), microtubule affinity-regulating kinases (MARKs), protein kinase cAMP-dependent/B/C/N (PKA, PKB/Akt, PKC, PKN), and Ca^{2+}/calmodulin-dependent protein kinase II (CaMKII).

AD Risk Factor Genes

AD-linked mutations represent a small proportion of total AD cases (~2%), while the majority of AD cases are late-onset or sporadic in nature (SAD). In this regard, several genes have been described that increase the risk of SAD (http://www.alzforum.org/genetics). Among these, the gene coding for apolipoprotein E (APOE) confers the greatest risk for developing SAD (http://www.alzforum.org/genetics). There are three alleles for APOE in humans—ε2, ε3, and ε4—and they differ by amino acid substitutions at positions 112 or 158 [56]. The ε3 allele is the most common form, while ε4 increases the risk for AD, and ε2 is protective against AD [57, 58]. A single copy of ε4 increases AD risk by ~3–4-fold, whereas two copies increase risk by ~12-fold [59]. In addition, each copy of ε4 lowers the age of onset in both sporadic and familial AD [57, 60].

The use of genome-wide arrays have allowed researchers to identify new genetic risk factors associated with sporadic AD, including BIN1, CLU, ABCA7, CR1, PICALM, MS4AGA, CD33, MS4A4E and CD2AP [61, 62]. Although the genes identified in the genome-wide association studies (GWASs) have a smaller effect on the increased risk, with odds ratios (ORs) of 0.9 to 1.2, compared to the much larger effect of APOE4 (OR 3.7), further investigation of the impact of these genes in AD is expected to provide new insights into its pathogenesis [63].

MODELING AD USING TRANSGENIC ANIMALS

The discovery of AD-associated genes has provided a crucial tool for the development of AD animal models that better recapitulate the hallmark characteristics of the disease. Multiple transgenic animals have been developed over the past decade to study the pathological mechanisms underlying AD. The main animal species used to model AD and other neurodegenerative diseases are rodents, as they offer several important advantages over other species: they can be readily manipulated genetically, their brain physiology is similar to humans, and they are relatively inexpensive to house. Furthermore, rodent models develop pathology in a comparatively short period of time, which makes it possible to test the impact of interventions introduced at any stage of the disease, including well before the onset of pathology, something that would require decades in humans. Here, we describe and summarize the main classes of transgenic rodent models, primarily mice, that are used to study AD, as shown in Figure 14.1.

Amyloid Protein Precursor Transgenic Mouse Models

Overexpression of human APP harboring FAD-associated mutations has been the most common way to generate transgenic mouse models of AD, and is widely used in the field. Unlike humans, wildtype mice do not develop Aβ deposits during the course of normal aging, likely because of differences in three amino acids within the Aβ sequence between human and rodent [64]. Currently, there are over 50 different transgenic mouse models that overexpress human wildtype, or FAD-associated mutant APP, and that have been used in AD research (http://www.alzforum.org/research-models). The first transgenic mice only overexpressed wildtype human APP, and as such, these mice only developed mild neuropathological changes, without deposition of Aβ plaques, suggesting that wildtype APP overexpression may not recapitulate the human disease efficiently in mice [65–67]. In order to more robustly promote Aβ neuropathology in mouse models, APP containing one or more FAD-associated mutations was subsequently utilized. Of those, the PDAPP [68], Tg2576 [69], and APP23 [70] mouse models are the most commonly used in AD-related research. The PDAPP transgenic mouse model expresses the human "Indiana" mutation within an APP minigene (V717F, APPInd) under the control of the platelet-derived growth factor (PDGF) promoter [69, 71]. On the other hand, the Tg2576 and APP23 models both express human APP containing the "Swedish" mutation driven by the hamster prion protein (PrP) and murine Thy-1 promoter, respectively. In mice overexpressing mutant APP, age-dependent development and maturation of Aβ plaques in the brain are commonly detected. The age of the onset of Aβ plaque formation is highly dependent on the type of mutation and the promoter used for the transgene expression, as well as the resulting expression levels of the transgene in the brain. Notably, Aβ plaques found in the brains of AD transgenic mice are structurally similar to those found in the human brain; they initiate as diffuse plaques consisting mainly of Aβ42, develop a dense Aβ42 core, and then incorporate Aβ40, as well as numerous other non-Aβ components such as ubiquitin and α-synuclein [72]. As in the human brain, these plaques stain positive with both thioflavin and Congo red, and show similar fibrillar structures by microscopy. Many, but not all, of these mutant APP transgenic mice also exhibit an age-dependent cognitive impairment that mimics the human disease [68–70]. Other

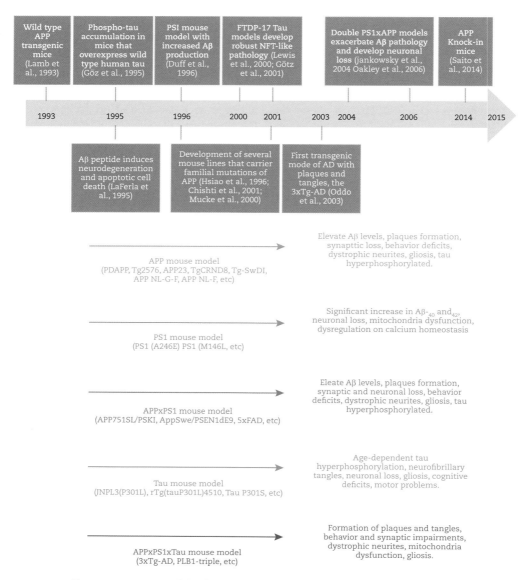

FIGURE 14.1. Transgenic mouse models of AD. Time line of the most relevant transgenic mouse models of AD (top). Main neuropathological features (below) that develop the current AD transgenic mouse model.

neuropathological hallmarks similar to human AD are observed, including dystrophic neurites, reactive astrocytes, and activated microglia, elevated innate immune and inflammatory responses, synaptic loss, and deficits in electrophysiological and neurochemical signals [73]. Almost all APP transgenic mice, however, do not exhibit robust neurodegeneration or NFT-like tau pathology in the brain, suggesting that even the expression of FAD-linked APP mutations are not sufficient to drive all pathological pathways in mice.

Presenilin Transgenic Mouse Models

The discovery of FAD mutations in the presenilin (PS) genes, which influence APP processing, opened the path for PS1 and PS2 transgenic mouse models. In contrast to APP transgenic mice, presenilin transgenic mice do not develop plaque pathology in the brain. This is also likely due to the differences in the mouse Aβ sequence as compared to that of humans, which greatly diminish the tendency of Aβ to aggregate [64]. This issue was solved by introducing human

APP into presenilin transgenic mice by crossing APP and presenilin transgenic lines, resulting in a double transgenic mouse with robust generation of Aβ42 and formation of Aβ plaques at much earlier ages than parental APP transgenic mice alone [54]. These double transgenic mice are now widely studied for amyloid pathology, and for the evaluation of anti-Aβ strategies. Single presenilin mutant mice, however, exhibit some aspects of AD pathology without aberrant accumulation of Aβ in the brain. For example, several PS1 mutant mice exhibit a sign of age-dependent neurodegeneration in the CA1 subregion, and synaptic loss in the stratum radiatum area of hippocampus [74–76]. Although no plaques are detected, a significant increase in intracellular accumulation of Aβ42, but not Aβ40, is also observed in PS1 (L286V) transgenic mice by 17–24 months of age [76]. In addition, certain PS1 mutations appear to facilitate NFT formation via the activation of GSK-3β in neurons. PS1 (I213T) knock-in mice exhibit phospho-tau deposits in the hippocampus as early as 7 months of age, and later develop Congo red-, thioflavin T-, and various phospho- and conformational-specific tau antibody-positive insoluble tau deposits in CA3 neurons by 14–16 months of age, even without apparent Aβ accumulation [77]. This observation is in part supported by clinical evidence from individuals who possess this unique PS1 mutation, and develop frontotemporal dementia (FTD)/Pick's disease with aberrant tau deposits but no Aβ pathology [78–80].

Tau Transgenic Mouse Models

In AD, no genetic mutations have been linked to the *MAPT* gene, suggesting that tau pathology in AD is downstream of Aβ pathology. To study the effects of aggregated tau, however, transgenic mice overexpressing human wildtype tau have been generated by several laboratories, and have exhibited age-dependent changes in tau pathology [81–85]. Götz and colleagues generated a transgenic mouse model overexpressing the longest form of human tau (tau40, 2N4R), under the control of Thy-1 promoter, and observed accumulation of PHF-1-positive phospho-tau in somatodendritic compartments by 3 months of age [85]. However, no NFT-like pathology was detected. Similarly, transgenic mice overexpressing the shortest form of human tau (0N3R) developed phospho-tau deposits in somatodendritic compartments, but no NFT-like structures were observed, even at 19 months of age [84]. On the other hand, in

another transgenic mouse model, overexpressing (N3R) tau, tau was observed to aggregate into straight filamentous structures in the spinal cord and brain stem by 6 months of age [83]. Although axonal degeneration was also observed in one of these models, the subsequent appearance of NFT formation and neuronal loss lay unresolved, limiting the usefulness of human wildtype tau transgenic mice as a disease model for AD.

This issue was somewhat resolved by generating mouse models overexpressing tau harboring mutations linked to FTDP-17. There are many studies addressing the pathological effects and functional consequences of human tau mutations, with the most commonly studied tau mutations being G272V, N279K, P301L, V337M, and R406W [86]. All these mutations markedly reduce the stability of the microtubules, presumably by promoting the hyperphosphorylation of tau, promoting their assemblage into filament aggregates. The identification of key kinases and phosphatases, which modulate pathological changes of tau in AD and related tauopathies, has been another major focus of research. The majority of these studies concentrated on the role that GSK-3β and CDK5 play in phosphorylating tau. Double transgenic mouse models have been developed for mutant tau and GSK-3β, or CDK5 [87, 88]. These bigenic models showed a dramatic increase in tau hyperphosphorylation and NFTs; moreover, the hippocampal atrophy observed in the GSK-3β single transgenic mice is accelerated in the tau/GSK-3β line [87]. Furthermore, crossing mice with mutants in the tau-phosphatase PP2A with mutant tau mice results in a remarkable increase in the number of the hippocampal neurons expressing hyperphosphorylated tau and NFTs [89]. Together, these data highlight the critical role that certain kinases and phosphatases play in triggering key modifications in tau, and also suggest that these enzymes may be valuable therapeutic targets.

Transgenic Mouse Models Developing Both Aβ and Tau Neuropathologies

Because NFTs represent the second hallmark feature of AD, creating mice that develop both Aβ and tau pathologies was an essential step in the process of investigating the molecular relationship between both lesions, and to better evaluate the therapeutic efficacy of anti-AD interventions. The first mouse model to successfully exhibit both hallmark pathologies was generated by crossing the two independent transgenic lines, Tg2576 and

JNPL3 mice [90]. Interestingly, while Aβ plaque pathology was developed in the same manner as the parental Tg2576 mice, the development of NFTs was significantly accelerated and increased versus the parental JNPL3 mice [90]. The double transgenic mice also develop NFTs in areas such as the subiculum and hippocampus, where the tangle pathology was rarely detected in JNPL3 mice, suggesting that Aβ potentiates tau pathology. The same phenomenon was observed by crossing JNPL3 mice with another APP transgenic mouse model, APP23, showing that the resulting double transgenic mice develop exacerbated tau pathology in areas with high Aβ plaques [91]. Similarly, Boutajangout and colleagues generated a transgenic mouse harboring only FAD-associated mutations, APP751 (Swedish/London) and PS1 (M146L), together with overexpression of human wildtype tau by crossing the three independent lines [92]. Although Aβ plaque pathology develops as early as 3–4 months of age in these mice, and phospho-tau deposits are associated with these Aβ plaques, these mice do not develop NFTs, even by 18 months of age. Rather than crossing independent mutant mouse lines, our lab generated a triple-transgenic model of AD (3xTg-AD), in which two transgenes (encoding mutant APP and mutant tau) were microinjected into single-cell embryos from homozygous mutant PS1 knock-in mice. The 3xTg-AD mouse model possesses the "Swedish" double mutation in APP (K670N/M671L), an FTDP-17-associated mutation in tau (P301L), and an FAD-associated mutation in PS1 (M146V) [93]. Both APP and tau transgenes are overexpressed in the forebrain region under the control of Thy1.2 promoter. A major advantage of this approach is the fact that the APP and tau transgenes integrated at the same genetic locus, which prevented segregation in subsequent generations. As a result, 3xTg-AD mice have much more cost-effective breeding requirements, and there is no mixing or altering of the genetic background. The 3xTg-AD model develops age-dependent Aβ and tau pathologies, with intracellular Aβ accumulation by 6 months of age, and Aβ plaques by 9–12 months of age; the accumulation of phospho-tau and NFT-like formation occurs at later ages [93]. Other hallmark pathologies, including astrogliosis, activated microglia, loss of synapses, and neurodegeneration, are also detected [94–96]. The 3xTg-AD mice also show age- and pathology-dependent cognitive decline that makes the model suitable for assessing the relationship between neuropathology and cognition [97]. The 3xTg-AD mouse model has helped to elucidate molecular interplay between Aβ and tau, as modulating Aβ42 levels directly influence tau pathology [97, 98]. Mechanistically, the ubiquitination of tau by carboxyl terminus Hsc70-interacting protein (CHIP) and subsequent degradation by proteasome are impaired by accumulation of Aβ [98–100]. Furthermore, Aβ oligomers, but not monomers, target the proteasome, thereby facilitating tau accumulation [101]. These findings support the amyloid cascade hypothesis, and imply the impairment of ubiquitin proteasome mechanisms in the pathogenesis of AD.

Overall, the development of these animal models has provided an important step forward in understanding key biological and molecular pathological mechanisms that occur in AD. In particular, the 3xTg-AD mouse model has successfully recapitulated several crucial AD neuropathological features observed in human cases (Figure 14.2), and has been a valuable tool in the field of AD research. With the creation of transgenic animal models, multiple preventive and disease-modifying therapeutics strategies have been developed and evaluated, and many are in various stages of preclinical and clinical development.

TRANSLATIONAL FINDINGS: FROM AD MODELS TO HUMAN

Aβ-Targeted Therapeutics

Introduced over two decades ago, the amyloid cascade hypothesis remains the most referenced hypothesis explaining the pathophysiology of AD [102]. The hypothesis originated, in part, from the overwhelming molecular and biochemical data obtained from the generation of transgenic animal models containing human mutated APP with or without human mutated PS1. The underlying assumption of the amyloid cascade hypothesis proposes that an imbalance between Aβ production, aggregation, and/or clearance initiates the neuropathology and clinical phenotype found in AD. Therefore, Aβ, as the hypothesized initiator of AD, has been the primary target of therapeutic development over the past two decades [103, 104]. Along with providing invaluable insight into the mechanism governing AD pathology, animal models have also been valuable tools in the development of therapeutic strategies to treat AD. In the following section, we will discuss some examples of therapeutic strategies that have entered clinical testing in AD patients after emerging from successful preclinical work in animal models.

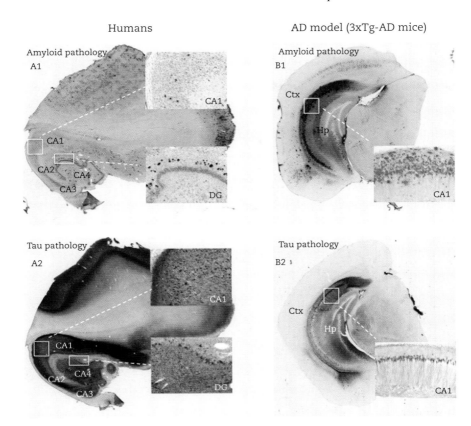

FIGURE 14.2. Aβ and tau pathology in humans and animal models. Light microscopic images from human cases (A1 and A2) and the 3xTg-AD animal model of AD (B1 and B2). Elevated numbers of plaques and intraneuronal tau accumulation are observed in the hippocampal area in an elderly human patient with AD. 3xTg-AD mice also exhibit a significant amount of plaques and intraneuronal tau pathology at 18 months of age.

Hp: hippocampus; Ctx: cortex.

Aβ Vaccines and Anti-Aβ Immunotherapy

With the amyloid hypothesis serving as their guide, researchers began targeting different forms of Aβ using immunotherapy in the late 1990's. By the start of the twenty-first century, immunization experiments using synthetic full-length Aβ1-42, had been conducted in transgenic AD model mice. In a groundbreaking study by Schenk et al., researchers found that immunization of [PDAPP] mice with full-length, aggregated Aβ1-42 prevented the deposition of extracellular Aβ as well as the formation of dystrophic neuritis and astrogliosis [105]. Additional research involving active immunization with Aβ1-42, using a variety of Aβ immunogens and routes of administration, successfully reduced cerebral Aβ burden, increased Aβ plasma levels, and improved cognitive performance in animal models of AD. The encouraging results from Aβ immunization studies observed in mouse models of AD were translated to a phase 1 safety trial using the AN1792 vaccine developed by Elan and Wyeth; however, the trial was halted in early 2002 because several patients began to show signs of meningoencephalitis and leukoencephalopathy [106]. Despite finding these adverse effects during the initial AN1792 vaccine trails, researchers have refined and identified several new Aβ-targeted vaccines using the data obtained from animal models, as we can observe in Table 14.1.

Of note, several high profile anti-Aβ immunotherapies successfully tested in mice—including bapineuzimab [107, 108] (Elan and Wyeth), solanezumab [109] (Eli Lilly), and IVIG [110] (Baxter Healthcare)—have entered clinical trials based on successes in the preclinical stage (Table 14.1). There have been several recent reviews that provide an in-depth account on the progress of Aβ immunotherapies in clinical trials [111, 112],

TABLE 14.1. LIST OF NOTABLE COMPOUNDS THAT DEMONSTRATED PRECLINICAL EFFICACY IN ANIMAL MODELS OF AD AND THEIR TRANSITIONS INTO CLINICAL TESTING

Compound	Intervention	Animal Model	Preclinical Assessment	Current or Completed Clinical Trial	References
Aβ vaccine (ANI 1792)	Anti-Aβ immunotherapy	PDAPP transgenic mice	Reduction of plaque load	Phase II, halted due to toxicity	Schenk et al., 1999
Bapineuzimab (3D6)	Anti-Aβ immunotherapy	PDAPP transgenic mice Tg2576 transgenic mice	Reduction of diffuse plaques and vascular Aβ	Phase III, no cognitive efficacy	Bacskai et al., 2002; Schroeter et al., 2008
Solanezumab	Anti-Aβ immunotherapy	PDAPP transgenic mice	Decreased plaque load	Phase III, recruiting	DeMattos et al., 2001
IVIG	Anti-Aβ immunotherapy	APP/PS transgenic mice	Reduction of plaque load	Phase III, no cognitive efficacy	Magga et al., 2010
LY2886721	β-Secretase inhibitor	PDAPP transgenic mice	Reduced brain Aβ, sAPP, and C99 levels	Phase II, halted due to liver toxicity	May et al., 2004
Semagacestat	γ-Secretase inhibitor	Tg2576 transgenic mice	Decreased Aβ levels in CSF and brain	Phase III, halted due to some cognitive worsening	Lanz et al., 2004
AADvac1	Anti-tau immunotherapy	Mutant tau transgenic rat	Reduced NFT pathology, and tau oligomers	Phase I, recruiting	Kontsekova et al., 2014
Vitamin E	Antioxidant	Tg2576 transgenic mice	Decreased brain lipid peroxidation levels, reduced Aβ load	Phase III, no cognitive efficacy	Conte et al., 2004; Sung et al., 2004
CHF5074	Immune modulator	Tg2576 transgenic mice	Decreased Aβ load and gliosis, and improved memory function	Phase II, awaiting safety results	Sivilia et al., 2013

and a more focused look at the mechanisms of immunotherapy in neurodegenerative diseases, including AD, will be presented in Chapter 17 of this volume.

β- and γ-Secretase Inhibitors

Another class of emerging therapeutics aimed at decreasing Aβ levels are the secretase inhibitors, which target APP processing [113]. As such, targeting BACE1, the rate-limiting first step in Aβ production, has received substantial attention as a possible prime drug target [114]. Transgenic mouse models deficient in BACE1 have been a valuable tool to demonstrate that blocking β-secretase activity eliminates CNS Aβ accumulation [115, 116]. Furthermore, by studying the phenotype of BACE1-deficient mice, researchers have been able to identify potential side effects of targeting BACE1 in human patients [117, 118].

The multitude of reported phenotypic alterations in BACE1-deficient mice are due to changes in the processing of BACE1 targets. Therefore, a BACE1 inhibitor for the treatment of AD should selectively target APP processing alone. For example, in a study by Fukumoto and colleagues, using the non-peptidic compound TAK-070 (a non-competitive BACE1 inhibitor), they observed a decreased in soluble Aβ levels and an increase in the soluble fragment of APP generated by non-amyloidogenic processing (sAPPα), demonstrating the effectiveness of selective BACE1 inhibition against AβPP while sparing enzymatic activity toward its other targets [119]. In addition, May et al. report that the compound LY2886721 can also selectively inhibit the hydrolytic activity of BACE1 to APP, with little toxic effect in animal studies [120]. As such, great strides in discovering more selective BACE1 inhibitors are being made. Several emerging compounds exhibit significant brain Aβ reduction in preclinical studies, and compounds including LY2886721 have entered early clinical trials, as shown in Table 14.1 [121].

In addition to BACE1 cleavage, proper γ-secretase function is also needed for the generation of Aβ. γ-secretase is a membrane-associated protease complex with a catalytic core composed of PS1 or PS2 [122], and has also been a hotly pursued therapeutic target for the treatment of AD [123]. As such, several γ-secretase inhibitors (GSIs) have been developed over the past several years, and critical proof of concept studies showing that chronic GSI treatment can decrease Aβ deposition have been conducted in various

animal models of AD [124, 125]. Of note is the GSI semagacestat (Eli Lilly), which was shown by Lanz and coworkers to reduce the acute levels of Aβ in brain, CSF, and plasma [126]. Unfortunately, semagacestat was halted in phase 3 clinical trials in 2011 for exacerbating cognitive deficits in some participants, potentially through off-target effects, as shown in Table 14.1 [127]. Like inhibitors of BACE1, GSI delivery is linked to unwanted side effects, which have also been identified through the analysis of phenotypic changes in preclinical mouse models [128].

The persuit of an effective inhibitor of γ-secretase activity has led to the production of γ-secretase modulators. In contrast to γ-secretase inhibition, which seek to block Aβ1-42 production altogether, γ-secretase modulators (GSMs) shift Aβ production away from Aβ1-42 toward shorter and less pathogenic species or selectively target APP processing while sparing other γ-secretase targets. Since their discovery, many GSMs have been developed and tested in preclinical animal models [129–131].

Non-Aβ-Targeted Therapeutics
Tau-Based Therapeutics

While the amyloid cascade hypothesis has driven the development of several amyloid-centric therapies over the past decade, researchers have successfully tested countless other therapeutic strategies in AD animal models, several classes of which have made their way to clinical testing [132]. Of particular interest are therapeutics targeted at the primary component of the NFT, the protein tau. Though historically an understudy relative to Aβ, tau and NFT load has a much better correlation with the severity of dementia in AD patients than Aβ burden [133]. Moreover, the discovery that mutations in tau can cause related forms of neurodegenerative disease—frontotemporal dementia (FTD) [134]—strongly suggested that aberrant forms of tau are the proximal cause of neurodegeneration. Additionally, when APP transgenic mouse models are crossed with tau knock-out mice, they demonstrate improved memory despite no changes in Aβ load [135], and studies in tau knock-out mice have found relatively subtle phenotypic changes, which suggest that targeting tau in humans could be relatively safe [136].

One proposed mechanism underlining tau pathogenesis in AD postulates that tau can diffuse from neuron to neuron in a prion-like manner. Indeed, such a mechanism would allow the opportunity to target tau via immunotherapy. Several groups of researchers have tested this hypothesis in various transgenic animal models. In a study by D'Abramo et al., using a passive immunization approach, the authors found that targeting tau with the MC1 antibody resulted in decreases in both detergent-soluble and insoluble tau in a tau-only transgenic mouse model [137]. In another study, by Boutajangout et al., immunization of tau transgenic mice with the PHF1 antibody led to better performance on the traverse beam task, and 58% less tau pathology in the hippocampus [138]. We have also conducted successful preclinical analysis using immunization against tau in our 3xTg-AD model [139]. Currently, the first clinical trials utilizing tau immunotherapy are just beginning. Of note is the active tau vaccine, AADvac1 (Axon Neuroscience). This active tau vaccine has been shown to effectively reduce tau load in a tau transgenic rat model [140], and the results of its use in human patients is eagerly awaited.

Antioxidants

A significant amount of evidence has shown that oxidative stress is a distinguishing factor between AD and cognitively normal patients [141, 142]. Indeed, elevated oxidative stress has also been reported in the brains of transgenic animal models of AD, where it can appear before the accumulation of overt Aβ pathology [143]. Over the years, researchers have used transgenic models to establish a clear relationship between Aβ and oxidative stress. For example, it has been shown that Aβ deposition and accumulation can lead to increase free radical generation [144], and that Aβ can also bind Aβ-binding alcohol dehydrogenase (ABAD) in the mitochondria, also resulting in increased free radicals [145]. Thus, different classes of antioxidant compounds have been tested for the treatment of AD, including some natural compounds known for their antioxidant properties, which have been shown to be effective cognitive modulators in transgenic AD models [146–148], and some, like vitamin E [147, 149], have transitioned into clinical testing [150].

Immune Modulators

Inflammation has long been associated with AD pathogenesis [151]. Activated glia and pro-inflammatory cytokines, including IL-1β, TNF-α, and IL-6, have been observed in both the brains of human AD patients and transgenic animal models. Additionally, epidemiological studies have determined that long-term use of non-steroidal anti-inflammatory drugs (NSAIDs) can reduce the risk of developing AD by 25%–40% [27, 152],

though conflicting reports have also been published [153–155]. Nevertheless, researchers continue to move forward, developing new NSAID derivatives for preclinical testing. One emerging candidate, CHF5074, has been shown to reduce Aβ load and gliosis in an APP transgenic mouse model [131]. In a second study by Sivilia et. al, the authors found that long-term treatment with CHF5074 also significantly reduces Aβ plaque burden, intraneuronal Aβ accumulation, and microglia activation [156]. The preclinical success of CHF5074 led to human trials of the drug in patients with MCI that saw some cognitive improvements over baseline during the duration of the study [157].

ANIMAL MODEL LIMITATIONS

Over the past few decades, animal models have provided invaluable and fundamental information toward the understanding of AD pathogenesis [158, 159]. Many transgenic and non-transgenic models have been used extensively to evaluate numerous potential therapeutic strategies, obtaining relevant and significant results, such as ameliorating cognitive deficits, and reducing AD-type neuropathology [160]. Despite the numerous successes of preclinical studies in animal models, none of these therapeutic interventions has been successfully translated to human patients over the past two decades, and no new therapeutic drugs have been approved for AD since the approval of the acetylcholine esterase inhibitors (i.e., Tacrine, Donepezil, etc.) and the N-methyl D-aspartate receptor antagonist, memantine (http://www.alz.org/research/science/alzheimers_disease_treatments.asp). This matter raises concern over why therapeutic interventions in animal models have not translated into effective therapies for human AD cases. Also, these therapeutic fails are leading researchers to question the predictability and reliability of current animal models of AD. Next, we discuss several of the most important discordances between humans and animal models that might explain the poor translational outcome of different therapeutic strategies.

A significant discrepancy between human AD and AD animal models is found among the composition of the amyloid aggregates. In animal models, Aβ plaques show a much more compact core, while in AD patients, plaque core density is lower and the morphology is more amorphous [161]. This disparity may be due to Aβ sequence differences in humans versus animal models, coupled with the fact that most animal model express both the human Aβ and their endogenous form [162]. In addition, animal models, specifically rodents, require a significantly higher expression of the APP transgene (5- to 12-fold) to generate Aβ plaques in their short life span. Besides the increased Aβ production, in the APP transgenic models, these animals also overproduce full-length APP and, therefore, more fragments of APP besides Aβ, including soluble ectodomains (sAPPα/β) and the APP intracellular domain (AICD), which may interfere with different biological functions and/ or might trigger artificial pathological phenotypes, potentially masking the toxic role of Aβ. To resolve these problems, researchers are developing novel models, such as the innovative APP knock-in mouse model, created by Saido and colleagues [163]. In this novel model, the mouse Aβ sequence is "humanized" and multiple FAD-linked mutations—the "Swedish" double mutation (KM670/671NL) and the Beyreuther/Iberian mutation (I716F)—are also introduced. This approach avoids the need to overexpress APP and its various metabolites, and it also eliminates the background of mouse Aβ [163]. This innovate model, together with other emerging knock-in models, will provide a better understanding of the underlying mechanisms driving AD pathology, by more closely recapitulating the pathological cascade of events that occurs in human AD patients [163–166].

Another important long-standing limitation of animal models of AD was the difficulty of recapitulating neurofibrillary tangles (NFTs), a cardinal and invariant pathological feature of AD. Even transgenic models that overexpress human wild-type tau—in the presence or absence of human Aβ—do not develop full-blown NFTs [81–85, 167, 168]. This problem was resolved through the introduction of mutations in the tau gene, which cause frontotemporal dementia with Parkinsonism linked to chromosome 17 (FTDP-17), thereby facilitating the development of tauopathies in transgenic animals [73, 134]. Although transgenic models harboring FTD-17-associated tau mutations have helped in unraveling disease processes associated with tau aggregation, it may present an incomplete perspective of AD pathology since mutations in tau are not observed in human AD cases.

One of the most significant points of contention is that the majority of animal models do not recapitulate the extensive neuronal loss found in human AD that consequently leads to cognitive and memory deficits. As we described previously, imaging and clinical studies in AD patients show that brain areas that comprise the limbic system,

including entorhinal cortex and hippocampus, are particularly vulnerable to AD pathogenesis [169–177]. In fact, notable neuronal loss is already present in the hippocampus and entorhinal cortex in mild-moderated AD cases [178, 179]. However, few animal models for AD show significant neuronal loss, particularly within the hippocampal formation [180–185]. The most likely reason that transgenic animals do not develop extensive neuronal loss, compared to human cases, is the short life span of these models, although other factors, such as background strain, may also play an important role [158]. Therefore, current animal models of AD may better mimic the earlier, presymptomatic phase of the disease, since most of them do not develop neuronal loss, and therefore results obtained during preclinical experimentation in these models may be better translated in the context of disease prevention instead of later stage treatments [186]. Hence, it is critical to design strategies to create relevant animal models that mimic the massive neuronal loss found in AD patients. In order to recapitulate the extensive neuronal degeneration that leads to cognitive deficits in AD patients, we have developed an innovative animal model of inducible neuronal loss [187–189]. This unique model, denominated CaM/Tet-DTA, uses the tetracycline–off system, under control of the Calmodulin kinase II promoter, to temporally and spatially regulate the expression of diphtheria toxin A-chain (DTA) in forebrain neurons, allowing for the ablation of neurons in regions that are significantly affected in AD, such as the CA1 area of the hippocampus [190]. Therefore, utilization of this model could be valuable when designing studies to identify therapeutic strategies that could improve or mitigate cognitive deficits related to overt neuronal loss.

Despite the importance of the factors described in the preceding, it is plausible that one of the most important discordance factors between animal models and human AD patients is that the majority of the existing AD models were created using the genetic mutations linked to familial AD (FAD), which, as we mentioned previously, represent a small fraction of total AD cases (~2%). As such, no existing AD animal model recapitulates the sporadic form of this disease, which represents the majority of AD cases (~98%), as is shown in more detail in Figure 14.3.

Although both types of AD (FAD and SAD) develop similar pathological phenotypes (e.g., plaques, tangles, synaptic impairments, and neuronal loss), the factors triggering the neurodegenerative process are completely different. In FAD, the pathological buildup is due to the presence of

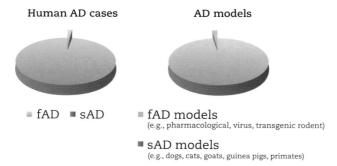

FIGURE 14.3. Human AD versus AD models. The majority of human AD cases (left) represent the sporadic form of the diseases (~98%), while a small fraction of AD cases correspond to the familial form (~2%). However, the vast majority of existing AD models (right) are developed using autosomal-dominant FAD-associated mutations in APP, PS1, and PS2. A small number of animal models, including dogs, cats, bears, goats, sheep, guinea pigs, and primates, spontaneously develop AD pathology and might model the SAD cases.

an autosomal-dominant mutation in the APP, PS1, or PS2 genes, while the etiology of the sporadic form is complex and multifactorial, likely combining genetic, epigenetic, and environmental factors. In addition, the majority of SAD patients are elderly subjects who commonly suffer from a variety of chronic medical conditions (comorbidity), including stroke, hypertension, anxiety, stress, diabetes, osteoporosis, sleep apnea, and renal disease. Epidemiological studies have shown that elderly AD patients have on average two to eight chronic conditions [7, 191–193]. Therefore, these studies suggest that comorbid conditions may play an important role in the clinical course of the disease.

In the past decade, multiple studies have been performed in animal models to understand the impact and relationship of these medical conditions on AD pathogenesis and cognitive impairment. Among these, one of the most important comorbid conditions that affect elderly people is cerebrovascular disease, which includes stroke, cerebral infarct, and traumatic brain injury. In fact, subjects who suffer vascular injury are two to five times more likely to develop AD, and the majority of AD cases show severe cerebrovascular lesions, suggesting a strong interaction between both disorders [194–197]. Studies in AD animal models have shown that vascular injury triggers Aβ and tau pathology, and causes rapid cognitive decline [198–201]. In addition, other vascular complications, such as hypertension and diabetes, are important risk factors for AD, and studies in AD animal models suggest that both hypertension and diabetes accelerate or trigger AD pathogenesis [202–209]. Furthermore, adverse lifestyle factors, such as stress and anxiety, are also considered important comorbid factors impacting in the

course of AD development [210–212]. In regard to stress, epidemiological studies have shown that AD patients have elevated levels of cortisol in both plasma and cerebrospinal fluid (CSF) due to potential alterations in the hypothalamic-pituitary-adrenal (HPA) axis [213–215]. Therefore, several groups have investigated the effect of acute and chronic stress, and stress hormones (GCs; cortisol in humans and corticosterone in rodents) and corticotrophin releasing hormone (CRH) on AD pathology *in vivo*, and found markedly increased Aβ and tau levels, and impaired cognition [216–221]. Together, these studies indicate an important role of comorbid medical conditions in the development of pathological and cognitive impairments in AD. The absence of these medical conditions in animal models suggests that these comorbid conditions may be important factors contributing to the lack of concordance between AD animal models and the human disease, which might be a significant factor as to the poor success of clinical trial interventions.

Finally, there are also markedly inherent differences in the physiology of animals versus humans, including the pharmacology of drug metabolism, neurotransmitter wiring, the lack of many relevant human functional genotypes, differences of readouts in cognitive states, and so on—all of which substantially contribute to the translational concern between animals and humans [222, 223].

Although there remains an important discordance between the current animal models and human AD patients, these models have provided important information in understanding key biological and molecular pathological mechanisms that occur in AD.

FUTURE DIRECTIONS AND CONCLUSION

One of the major challenges facing AD researchers over the course of the next decade will be the development of better tools with which to translate preclinical successes to clinical successes. Such developments will also serve to aid researchers in better understanding the underlying pathological mechanisms of neurodegenerative diseases such as AD. Animal models will play a key role in this important challenge, and it will be critical in particular to develop novel and innovative models that mimic the pathological cascade of the sporadic form of disease, rather than the familial. Additionally, it will be necessary to perform longitudinal studies in models that spontaneously develop pathological features of AD and other neurodegenerative disorders, such as primates, guinea pigs, and so on, in order to gain a better understanding of the aging effect on disease progression. These studies will require time and economic support. However, the discovery of factors associated with aging that are involved in the development and progress of the sporadic form of the disease is of critical importance to developing new strategies for the treatment and prevention of neurodegenerative disorders. In addition, it will be important to design animal models that replicate the human form of disease without the need to overexpress any human transgenes. Overall, these important steps will allow better translational concordance from model to humans, and will allow researchers to develop novel and innovative disease-modifying approaches to treat these devastating neurodegenerative diseases that are affecting the human population.

REFERENCES

1. Graeber, M. B., et al., Rediscovery of the case described by Alois Alzheimer in 1911: historical, histological and molecular genetic analysis. *Neurogenetics*, 1997. 1(1): 73–80.
2. 2014 Alzheimer's disease facts and figures. *Alzheimers Dement*, 2014. 10(2): e47–92.
3. 2012 Alzheimer's disease facts and figures. *Alzheimers Dement*, 2012. 8(2): 131–168.
4. Hebert, L. E., et al., Alzheimer disease in the US population: prevalence estimates using the 2000 census. *Arch Neurol*, 2003. 60(8): 1119–1122.
5. Querfurth, H. W., and F. M. LaFerla, Alzheimer's disease. *N Engl J Med*, 2010. 362(4): 329–344.
6. Magaki, S., et al., Comorbidity in dementia: update of an ongoing autopsy study. *J Am Geriatr Soc*, 2014. 62(9): 1722–1728.
7. Doraiswamy, P. M., et al., Prevalence and impact of medical comorbidity in Alzheimer's disease. *J Gerontol A Biol Sci Med Sci*, 2002. 57(3): M173–M177.
8. LaFerla, F. M., K. N. Green, and S. Oddo, Intracellular amyloid-beta in Alzheimer's disease. *Nat Rev Neurosci*, 2007. 8(7): 499–509.
9. Dickson, T. C., and J. C. Vickers, The morphological phenotype of beta-amyloid plaques and associated neuritic changes in Alzheimer's disease. *Neuroscience*, 2001. 105(1): 99–107.
10. Smith, E. E., and S. M. Greenberg, Beta-amyloid, blood vessels, and brain function. *Stroke*, 2009. 40(7): 2601–2606.
11. Walsh, D. M., and D. J. Selkoe, A beta oligomers: a decade of discovery. *J Neurochem*, 2007. 101(5): 1172–1184.
12. Avila, J., et al., Role of tau protein in both physiological and pathological conditions. *Physiol Rev*, 2004. 84(2): 361–384.
13. Weingarten, M. D., et al., A protein factor essential for microtubule assembly. *Proc Natl Acad Sci U S A*, 1975. 72(5): 1858–1862.
14. Ittner, L. M., et al., Dendritic function of tau mediates amyloid-beta toxicity in Alzheimer's disease mouse models. *Cell*, 2010. 142(3): 387–397.
15. Johnson, G. V., and W. H. Stoothoff, Tau phosphorylation in neuronal cell function and dysfunction. *J Cell Sci*, 2004. 117(Pt 24): 5721–5729.
16. Poorkaj, P., et al., Tau is a candidate gene for chromosome 17 frontotemporal dementia. *Ann Neurol*, 1998. 43(6): 815–825.
17. Selkoe, D. J., Alzheimer's disease is a synaptic failure. *Science*, 2002. 298(5594): 789–791.
18. Penzes, P., et al., Dendritic spine pathology in neuropsychiatric disorders. *Nat Neurosci*, 2011. 14(3): 285–293.
19. Brun, A., and E. Englund, Regional pattern of degeneration in Alzheimer's disease: neuronal loss and histopathological grading. *Histopathology*, 2002. 41(3A): 40–55.
20. Bettcher, B. M., and J. H. Kramer, Longitudinal inflammation, cognitive decline, and Alzheimer's disease: a mini-review. *Clin Pharmacol Ther*, 2014. 96(4): 464–469.
21. Lucin, K. M., and T. Wyss-Coray, Immune activation in brain aging and neurodegeneration: too much or too little? *Neuron*, 2009. 64(1): 110–122.
22. Wyss-Coray, T., and L. Mucke, Inflammation in neurodegenerative disease: a double-edged sword. *Neuron*, 2002. 35(3): 419–432.
23. Mosher, K. I., and T. Wyss-Coray, Microglial dysfunction in brain aging and Alzheimer's disease. *Biochem Pharmacol*, 2014. 88(4): 594–604.
24. Griffin, W. S., Neuroinflammatory cytokine signaling and Alzheimer's disease. *N Engl J Med*, 2013. 368(8): 770–771.

25. Heneka, M. T., et al., Neuroinflammatory processes in Alzheimer's disease. *J Neural Transm*, 2010. 117(8): 919–947.

26. Kitazawa, M., T. R. Yamasaki, and F. M. LaFerla, Microglia as a potential bridge between the amyloid beta-peptide and tau. *Ann N Y Acad Sci*, 2004. 1035: 85–103.

27. Szekely, C. A., et al., No advantage of A beta 42-lowering NSAIDs for prevention of Alzheimer dementia in six pooled cohort studies. *Neurology*, 2008. 70(24): 2291–2298.

28. in t' Veld, B. A., et al., Nonsteroidal antiinflammatory drugs and the risk of Alzheimer's disease. *N Engl J Med*, 2001. 345(21): 1515–1521.

29. Breitner, J. C., et al., Inverse association of anti-inflammatory treatments and Alzheimer's disease: initial results of a co-twin control study. *Neurology*, 1994. 44(2): 227–232.

30. Tanzi, R. E., and L. Bertram, New frontiers in Alzheimer's disease genetics. *Neuron*, 2001. 32(2): 181–184.

31. Young-Pearse, T. L., et al., Biochemical and functional interaction of disrupted-in-schizophrenia 1 and amyloid precursor protein regulates neuronal migration during mammalian cortical development. *J Neurosci*, 2010. 30(31): 10431–10440.

32. Wei, W., et al., Amyloid beta from axons and dendrites reduces local spine number and plasticity. *Nat Neurosci*, 2010. 13(2): 190–196.

33. Nikolaev, A., et al., APP binds DR6 to trigger axon pruning and neuron death via distinct caspases. *Nature*, 2009. 457(7232): 981–989.

34. Masters, C. L., et al., Amyloid plaque core protein in Alzheimer disease and Down syndrome. *Proc Natl Acad Sci U S A*, 1985. 82(12): 4245–4249.

35. Goldgaber, D., et al., Characterization and chromosomal localization of a cDNA encoding brain amyloid of Alzheimer's disease. *Science*, 1987. 235(4791): 877–880.

36. Tanzi, R. E., et al., Amyloid beta protein gene: cDNA, mRNA distribution, and genetic linkage near the Alzheimer locus. *Science*, 1987. 235(4791): 880–884.

37. Kang, J., et al., The precursor of Alzheimer's disease amyloid A4 protein resembles a cell-surface receptor. *Nature*, 1987. 325(6106): 733–736.

38. Nilsberth, C., et al., The "Arctic" APP mutation (E693G) causes Alzheimer's disease by enhanced Abeta protofibril formation. *Nat Neurosci*, 2001. 4(9): 887–893.

39. Grabowski, T. J., et al., Novel amyloid precursor protein mutation in an Iowa family with dementia and severe cerebral amyloid angiopathy. *Ann Neurol*, 2001. 49(6): 697–705.

40. Murrell, J. R., et al., Early-onset Alzheimer disease caused by a new mutation (V717L) in the amyloid precursor protein gene. *Arch Neurol*, 2000. 57(6): 885–887.

41. Mullan, M., et al., A pathogenic mutation for probable Alzheimer's disease in the APP gene at the N-terminus of beta-amyloid. *Nat Genet*, 1992. 1(5): 345–347.

42. Hendriks, L., et al., Presenile dementia and cerebral haemorrhage linked to a mutation at codon 692 of the beta-amyloid precursor protein gene. *Nat Genet*, 1992. 1(3): 218–221.

43. Chartier-Harlin, M. C., et al., Early-onset Alzheimer's disease caused by mutations at codon 717 of the beta-amyloid precursor protein gene. *Nature*, 1991. 353(6347): 844–846.

44. Murrell, J., et al., A mutation in the amyloid precursor protein associated with hereditary Alzheimer's disease. *Science*, 1991. 254(5028): 97–99.

45. Goate, A., et al., Segregation of a missense mutation in the amyloid precursor protein gene with familial Alzheimer's disease. *Nature*, 1991. 349(6311): 704–706.

46. Levy, E., et al., Mutation of the Alzheimer's disease amyloid gene in hereditary cerebral hemorrhage, Dutch type. *Science*, 1990. 248(4959): 1124–1126.

47. Rogaev, E. I., et al., Familial Alzheimer's disease in kindreds with missense mutations in a gene on chromosome 1 related to the Alzheimer's disease type 3 gene. *Nature*, 1995. 376(6543): 775–778.

48. Levy-Lahad, E., et al., Candidate gene for the chromosome 1 familial Alzheimer's disease locus. *Science*, 1995. 269(5226): 973–977.

49. Sherrington, R., et al., Cloning of a gene bearing missense mutations in early-onset familial Alzheimer's disease. *Nature*, 1995. 375(6534): 754–760.

50. Van Gassen, G. and W. Annaert, Amyloid, presenilins, and Alzheimer's disease. *Neuroscientist*, 2003. 9(2): 117–126.

51. Sisodia, S. S., and P. H. St George-Hyslop, gamma-Secretase, Notch, Abeta and Alzheimer's disease: where do the presenilins fit in? *Nat Rev Neurosci*, 2002. 3(4): 281–290.

52. Green, K. N., and F. M. LaFerla, Linking calcium to Abeta and Alzheimer's disease. *Neuron*, 2008. 59(2): 190–194.

53. Holcomb, L., et al., Accelerated Alzheimer-type phenotype in transgenic mice carrying both mutant amyloid precursor protein and presenilin 1 transgenes. *Nat Med*, 1998. 4(1): 97–100.

54. Borchelt, D. R., et al., Accelerated amyloid deposition in the brains of transgenic mice coexpressing mutant presenilin 1 and amyloid precursor proteins. *Neuron*, 1997. 19(4): 939–945.

55. Scheuner, D., et al., Secreted amyloid beta-protein similar to that in the senile plaques of Alzheimer's

disease is increased in vivo by the presenilin 1 and 2 and APP mutations linked to familial Alzheimer's disease. *Nat Med*, 1996. 2(8): 864–870.

56. Fan, J., J. Donkin, and C. Wellington, Greasing the wheels of Abeta clearance in Alzheimer's disease: the role of lipids and apolipoprotein E. *Biofactors*, 2009. 35(3): 239–248.

57. Corder, E. H., et al., Gene dose of apolipoprotein E type 4 allele and the risk of Alzheimer's disease in late onset families. *Science*, 1993. 261(5123): 921–923.

58. Strittmatter, W. J., et al., Apolipoprotein E: high-avidity binding to beta-amyloid and increased frequency of type 4 allele in late-onset familial Alzheimer disease. *Proc Natl Acad Sci U S A*, 1993. 90(5): 1977–1981.

59. Bales, K. R., et al., Apolipoprotein E, amyloid, and Alzheimer disease. *Mol Interv*, 2002. 2(6): 363–375, 339.

60. Pastor, P., et al., Apolipoprotein Eepsilon4 modifies Alzheimer's disease onset in an E280A PS1 kindred. *Ann Neurol*, 2003. 54(2): 163–169.

61. Naj, A. C., et al., Common variants at MS4A4/MS4A6E, CD2AP, CD33 and EPHA1 are associated with late-onset Alzheimer's disease. *Nat Genet*, 2011. 43(5): 436–441.

62. Hollingworth, P., et al., Common variants at ABCA7, MS4A6A/MS4A4E, EPHA1, CD33 and CD2AP are associated with Alzheimer's disease. *Nat Genet*, 2011. 43(5): 429–435.

63. Karch, C. M., and A. M. Goate, Alzheimer's disease risk genes and mechanisms of disease pathogenesis. *Biol Psychiatry*, 2015. 77(1): 43–51.

64. Dyrks, T., et al., Amyloidogenicity of rodent and human beta A4 sequences. *FEBS Lett*, 1993. 324(2): 231–236.

65. Mucke, L., et al., High-level neuronal expression of abeta 1–42 in wild-type human amyloid protein precursor transgenic mice: synaptotoxicity without plaque formation. *J Neurosci*, 2000. 20(11): 4050–4058.

66. Buxbaum, J. D., et al., Expression of APP in brains of transgenic mice containing the entire human APP gene. *Biochem Biophys Res Commun*, 1993. 197(2): 639–645.

67. Lamb, B. T., et al., Introduction and expression of the 400 kilobase amyloid precursor protein gene in transgenic mice [corrected]. *Nat Genet*, 1993. 5(1): 22–30.

68. Games, D., et al., Alzheimer-type neuropathology in transgenic mice overexpressing V717F beta-amyloid precursor protein. *Nature*, 1995. 373(6514): 523–527.

69. Hsiao, K., et al., Correlative memory deficits, Abeta elevation, and amyloid plaques in transgenic mice. *Science*, 1996. 274(5284): 99–102.

70. Sturchler-Pierrat, C., et al., Two amyloid precursor protein transgenic mouse models with Alzheimer disease-like pathology. *Proc Natl Acad Sci U S A*, 1997. 94(24): 13287–13292.

71. Rockenstein, E. M., et al., Levels and alternative splicing of amyloid beta protein precursor (APP) transcripts in brains of APP transgenic mice and humans with Alzheimer's disease. *J Biol Chem*, 1995. 270(47): 28257–28267.

72. Yang, F., et al., Plaque-associated alpha-synuclein (NACP) pathology in aged transgenic mice expressing amyloid precursor protein. *Brain Res*, 2000. 853(2): 381–383.

73. Kitazawa, M., R. Medeiros, and F. M. Laferla, Transgenic mouse models of Alzheimer disease: developing a better model as a tool for therapeutic interventions. *Curr Pharm Des*, 2012. 18(8): 1131–1147.

74. Rutten, B. P., et al., Age-related loss of synaptophysin immunoreactive presynaptic boutons within the hippocampus of APP751SL, PS1M146L, and APP751SL/PS1M146L transgenic mice. *Am J Pathol*, 2005. 167(1): 161–173.

75. Sadowski, M., et al., Amyloid-beta deposition is associated with decreased hippocampal glucose metabolism and spatial memory impairment in APP/PS1 mice. *J Neuropathol Exp Neurol*, 2004. 63(5): 418–428.

76. Chui, D. H., et al., Transgenic mice with Alzheimer presenilin 1 mutations show accelerated neurodegeneration without amyloid plaque formation. *Nat Med*, 1999. 5(5): 560–564.

77. Tanemura, K., et al., Formation of tau inclusions in knock-in mice with familial Alzheimer disease (FAD) mutation of presenilin 1 (PS1). *J Biol Chem*, 2006. 281(8): 5037–5041.

78. Dermaut, B., et al., A novel presenilin 1 mutation associated with Pick's disease but not beta-amyloid plaques. *Ann Neurol*, 2004. 55(5): 617–626.

79. Amtul, Z., et al., A presenilin 1 mutation associated with familial frontotemporal dementia inhibits gamma-secretase cleavage of APP and notch. *Neurobiol Dis*, 2002. 9(2): 269–273.

80. Gomez-Isla, T., et al., The impact of different presenilin 1 andpresenilin 2 mutations on amyloid deposition, neurofibrillary changes and neuronal loss in the familial Alzheimer's disease brain: evidence for other phenotype-modifying factors. *Brain*, 1999. **122 (Pt 9)**: 1709–1719.

81. Duff, K., et al., Characterization of pathology in transgenic mice over-expressing human genomic and cDNA tau transgenes. *Neurobiol Dis*, 2000. 7(2): 87–98.

82. Spittaels, K., et al., Prominent axonopathy in the brain and spinal cord of transgenic mice over-expressing four-repeat human tau protein. *Am J Pathol*, 1999. 155(6): 2153–2165.

83. Ishihara, T., et al., Age-dependent emergence and progression of a tauopathy in transgenic mice overexpressing the shortest human tau isoform. *Neuron*, 1999. 24(3): 751–762.

84. Brion, J. P., G. Tremp, and J. N. Octave, Transgenic expression of the shortest human tau affects its compartmentalization and its phosphorylation as in the pretangle stage of Alzheimer's disease. *Am J Pathol*, 1999. 154(1): 255–270.

85. Gotz, J., et al., Somatodendritic localization and hyperphosphorylation of tau protein in transgenic mice expressing the longest human brain tau isoform. *EMBO J*, 1995. 14(7): 1304–1313.

86. Goedert, M., and M. Hasegawa, The tauopathies: toward an experimental animal model. *Am J Pathol*, 1999. 154(1): 1–6.

87. Engel, T., et al., Cooexpression of FTDP-17 tau and GSK-3beta in transgenic mice induce tau polymerization and neurodegeneration. *Neurobiol Aging*, 2006. 27(9): 1258–1268.

88. Noble, W., et al., Cdk5 is a key factor in tau aggregation and tangle formation in vivo. *Neuron*, 2003. 38(4): 555–565.

89. Deters, N., L. M. Ittner, and J. Gotz, Substrate-specific reduction of PP2A activity exaggerates tau pathology. *Biochem Biophys Res Commun*, 2009. 379(2): 400–405.

90. Lewis, J., et al., Enhanced neurofibrillary degeneration in transgenic mice expressing mutant tau and APP. *Science*, 2001. 293(5534): 1487–1491.

91. Bolmont, T., et al., Induction of tau pathology by intracerebral infusion of amyloid-beta-containing brain extract and by amyloid-beta deposition in APP x Tau transgenic mice. *Am J Pathol*, 2007. 171(6): 2012–2020.

92. Boutajangout, A., et al., Characterisation of cytoskeletal abnormalities in mice transgenic for wild-type human tau and familial Alzheimer's disease mutants of APP and presenilin-1. *Neurobiol Dis*, 2004. 15(1): 47–60.

93. Oddo, S., et al., Triple-transgenic model of Alzheimer's disease with plaques and tangles: intracellular Abeta and synaptic dysfunction. *Neuron*, 2003. 39(3): 409–421.

94. Medeiros, R., et al., Calpain inhibitor A-705253 mitigates Alzheimer's disease-like pathology and cognitive decline in aged 3xTgAD mice. *Am J Pathol*, 2012. 181(2): 616–625.

95. Blurton-Jones, M., et al., Neural stem cells improve cognition via BDNF in a transgenic model of Alzheimer disease. *Proc Natl Acad Sci U S A*, 2009. 106(32): 13594–13599.

96. Kitazawa, M., et al., Lipopolysaccharide-induced inflammation exacerbates tau pathology by a cyclin-dependent kinase 5-mediated pathway in a transgenic model of Alzheimer's disease. *J Neurosci*, 2005. 25(39): 8843–8853.

97. Billings, L. M., et al., Intraneuronal Abeta causes the onset of early Alzheimer's disease-related cognitive deficits in transgenic mice. *Neuron*, 2005. 45(5): 675–688.

98. Oddo, S., et al., Blocking Abeta42 accumulation delays the onset and progression of tau pathology via the C terminus of heat shock protein70-interacting protein: a mechanistic link between Abeta and tau pathology. *J Neurosci*, 2008. 28(47): 12163–12175.

99. Dickey, C. A., et al., The high-affinity HSP90-CHIP complex recognizes and selectively degrades phosphorylated tau client proteins. *J Clin Invest*, 2007. 117(3): 648–658.

100. Dickey, C. A., et al., Deletion of the ubiquitin ligase CHIP leads to the accumulation, but not the aggregation, of both endogenous phospho- and caspase-3-cleaved tau species. *J Neurosci*, 2006. 26(26): 6985–6996.

101. Tseng, B. P., et al., Abeta inhibits the proteasome and enhances amyloid and tau accumulation. *Neurobiol Aging*, 2008. 29(11): 1607–1618.

102. Hardy, J., and D. J. Selkoe, The amyloid hypothesis of Alzheimer's disease: progress and problems on the road to therapeutics. *Science*, 2002. 297(5580): 353–356.

103. Jang, H., et al., Alzheimer's disease: which type of amyloid-preventing drug agents to employ? *Phys Chem Chem Phys*, 2013. 15(23): 8868–8877.

104. Citron, M., Strategies for disease modification in Alzheimer's disease. *Nat Rev Neurosci*, 2004. 5(9): 677–685.

105. Schenk, D., et al., Immunization with amyloid-beta attenuates Alzheimer-disease-like pathology in the PDAPP mouse. *Nature*, 1999. 400(6740): 173–177.

106. Orgogozo, J. M., et al., Subacute meningoencephalitis in a subset of patients with AD after Abeta42 immunization. *Neurology*, 2003. 61(1): 46–54.

107. Schroeter, S., et al., Immunotherapy reduces vascular amyloid-beta in PDAPP mice. *J Neurosci*, 2008. 28(27): 6787–6793.

108. Bacskai, B. J., et al., Non-Fc-mediated mechanisms are involved in clearance of amyloid-beta in vivo by immunotherapy. *J Neurosci*, 2002. 22(18): 7873–7878.

109. DeMattos, R. B., et al., Peripheral anti-A beta antibody alters CNS and plasma A beta clearance and decreases brain A beta burden in a mouse model of Alzheimer's disease. *Proc Natl Acad Sci U S A*, 2001. 98(15): 8850–8855.

110. Magga, J., et al., Human intravenous immunoglobulin provides protection against Abeta toxicity by multiple mechanisms in a mouse model

of Alzheimer's disease. *J Neuroinflammation*, 2010. 7: 90.

111. Goure, W. F., et al., Targeting the proper amyloid-beta neuronal toxins: a path forward for Alzheimer's disease immunotherapeutics. *Alzheimers Res Ther*, 2014. 6(4): 42.

112. Prins, N. D., and P. Scheltens, Treating Alzheimer's disease with monoclonal antibodies: current status and outlook for the future. *Alzheimers Res Ther*, 2013. 5(6): 56.

113. Chow, V. W., et al., An overview of APP processing enzymes and products. *Neuromolecular Med*, 2010. 12(1): 1–12.

114. Cole, S. L., and R. Vassar, BACE1 structure and function in health and Alzheimer's disease. *Curr Alzheimer Res*, 2008. 5(2): 100–120.

115. Cai, H., et al., BACE1 is the major beta-secretase for generation of Abeta peptides by neurons. *Nat Neurosci*, 2001. 4(3): 233–234.

116. Luo, Y., et al., Mice deficient in BACE1, the Alzheimer's beta-secretase, have normal phenotype and abolished beta-amyloid generation. *Nat Neurosci*, 2001. 4(3): 231–232.

117. Hu, X., et al., BACE1 deficiency causes altered neuronal activity and neurodegeneration. *J Neurosci*, 2010. 30(26): 8819–8829.

118. Harrison, S. M., et al., BACE1 (beta-secretase) transgenic and knockout mice: identification of neurochemical deficits and behavioral changes. *Mol Cell Neurosci*, 2003. 24(3): 646–655.

119. Fukumoto, H., et al., A noncompetitive BACE1 inhibitor TAK-070 ameliorates Abeta pathology and behavioral deficits in a mouse model of Alzheimer's disease. *J Neurosci*, 2010. 30(33): 11157–11166.

120. May, P. C., et al., Robust central reduction of amyloid-beta in humans with an orally available, non-peptidic beta-secretase inhibitor. *J Neurosci*, 2011. 31(46): 16507–16516.

121. Yan, R. and R. Vassar, Targeting the beta secretase BACE1 for Alzheimer's disease therapy. *Lancet Neurol*, 2014. 13(3): 319–329.

122. Steiner, H., The catalytic core of gamma-secretase: presenilin revisited. *Curr Alzheimer Res*, 2008. 5(2): p. 147–157.

123. Wolfe, M. S., Inhibition and modulation of gamma-secretase for Alzheimer's disease. *Neurotherapeutics*, 2008. 5(3): 391–398.

124. Abramowski, D., et al., Dynamics of Abeta turnover and deposition in different beta-amyloid precursor protein transgenic mouse models following gamma-secretase inhibition. *J Pharmacol Exp Ther*, 2008. 327(2): 411–424.

125. Dovey, H. F., et al., Functional gamma-secretase inhibitors reduce beta-amyloid peptide levels in brain. *J Neurochem*, 2001. 76(1): 173–181.

126. Lanz, T. A., et al., Studies of Abeta pharmacodynamics in the brain, cerebrospinal fluid, and plasma in young (plaque-free) Tg2576 mice using the gamma-secretase inhibitor N2-[(2S)-2-(3,5-difluorophenyl)-2-hydroxy-ethanoyl]-N1-[(7S)-5-methyl-6-oxo-6,7-dihydro-5H-dibenzo[b,d]azepin-7-yl]-L-alaninamide (LY-411575). *J Pharmacol Exp Ther*, 2004. 309(1): 49–55.

127. Doody, R. S., et al., A phase 3 trial of semagacestat for treatment of Alzheimer's disease. *N Engl J Med*, 2013. 369(4): 341–350.

128. Wong, G. T., et al., Chronic treatment with the gamma-secretase inhibitor LY-411,575 inhibits beta-amyloid peptide production and alters lymphopoiesis and intestinal cell differentiation. *J Biol Chem*, 2004. 279(13): 12876–12882.

129. Van Broeck, B., et al., Chronic treatment with a novel gamma-secretase modulator, JNJ-40418677, inhibits amyloid plaque formation in a mouse model of Alzheimer's disease. *Br J Pharmacol*, 2011. 163(2): 375–389.

130. Kounnas, M. Z., et al., Modulation of gamma-secretase reduces beta-amyloid deposition in a transgenic mouse model of Alzheimer's disease. *Neuron*, 2010. 67(5): 769–780.

131. Imbimbo, B. P., et al., CHF5074, a novel gamma-secretase modulator, attenuates brain beta-amyloid pathology and learning deficit in a mouse model of Alzheimer's disease. *Br J Pharmacol*, 2009. 156(6): 982–993.

132. Schneider, L. S., et al., Clinical trials and late-stage drug development for Alzheimer's disease: an appraisal from 1984 to 2014. *J Intern Med*, 2014. 275(3): 251–283.

133. Nelson, P. T., et al., Correlation of Alzheimer disease neuropathologic changes with cognitive status: a review of the literature. *J Neuropathol Exp Neurol*, 2012. 71(5): 362–381.

134. Medeiros, R., D. Baglietto-Vargas, and F. M. LaFerla, The role of tau in Alzheimer's disease and related disorders. *CNS Neurosci Ther*, 2011. 17(5): 514–524.

135. Roberson, E. D., et al., Reducing endogenous tau ameliorates amyloid beta-induced deficits in an Alzheimer's disease mouse model. *Science*, 2007. 316(5825): 750–754.

136. Denk, F., and R. Wade-Martins, Knock-out and transgenic mouse models of tauopathies. *Neurobiol Aging*, 2009. 30(1): 1–13.

137. d'Abramo, C., et al., Tau passive immunotherapy in mutant P301L mice: antibody affinity versus specificity. *PLoS One*, 2013. 8(4): e62402.

138. Boutajangout, A., et al., Passive immunization targeting pathological phospho-tau protein in a mouse model reduces functional

decline and clears tau aggregates from the brain. *J Neurochem*, 2011. 118(4): 658–667.

139. Walls, K. C., et al., p-Tau immunotherapy reduces soluble and insoluble tau in aged 3xTg-AD mice. *Neurosci Lett*, 2014. 575: 96–100.

140. Kontsekova, E., et al., First-in-man tau vaccine targeting structural determinants essential for pathological tau-tau interaction reduces tau oligomerisation and neurofibrillary degeneration in an Alzheimer's disease model. *Alzheimers Res Ther*, 2014. 6(4): 44.

141. Gabbita, S. P., M. A. Lovell, and W. R. Markesbery, Increased nuclear DNA oxidation in the brain in Alzheimer's disease. *J Neurochem*, 1998. 71(5): 2034–2040.

142. Sayre, L. M., et al., 4-Hydroxynonenal-derived advanced lipid peroxidation end products are increased in Alzheimer's disease. *J Neurochem*, 1997. 68(5): 2092–2097.

143. Resende, R., et al., Brain oxidative stress in a triple-transgenic mouse model of Alzheimer disease. *Free Radic Biol Med*, 2008. 44(12): 2051–2057.

144. Cutler, R. G., et al., Involvement of oxidative stress-induced abnormalities in ceramide and cholesterol metabolism in brain aging and Alzheimer's disease. *Proc Natl Acad Sci U S A*, 2004. 101(7): 2070–2075.

145. Takuma, K., et al., ABAD enhances Abeta-induced cell stress via mitochondrial dysfunction. *FASEB J*, 2005. 19(6): 597–598.

146. Murakami, K., et al., Vitamin C restores behavioral deficits and amyloid-beta oligomerization without affecting plaque formation in a mouse model of Alzheimer's disease. *J Alzheimers Dis*, 2011. 26(1): 7–18.

147. Sung, S., et al., Early vitamin E supplementation in young but not aged mice reduces Abeta levels and amyloid deposition in a transgenic model of Alzheimer's disease. *FASEB J*, 2004. 18(2): 323–325.

148. Lim, G. P., et al., The curry spice curcumin reduces oxidative damage and amyloid pathology in an Alzheimer transgenic mouse. *J Neurosci*, 2001. 21(21): 8370–8377.

149. Conte, V., et al., Vitamin E reduces amyloidosis and improves cognitive function in Tg2576 mice following repetitive concussive brain injury. *J Neurochem*, 2004. 90(3): 758–764.

150. Farina, N., et al., Vitamin E for Alzheimer's dementia and mild cognitive impairment. *Cochrane Database Syst Rev*, 2012. 11: CD002854.

151. Akiyama, H., et al., Inflammation and Alzheimer's disease. *Neurobiol Aging*, 2000. 21(3): 383–421.

152. Szekely, C.A., et al., Nonsteroidal anti-inflammatory drugs for the prevention of Alzheimer's disease: a systematic review. *Neuroepidemiology*, 2004. 23(4): 159–169.

153. Jaturapatporn, D., et al., Aspirin, steroidal and non-steroidal anti-inflammatory drugs for the treatment of Alzheimer's disease. *Cochrane Database Syst Rev*, 2012. 2: CD006378.

154. Breitner, J. C., et al., Extended results of the Alzheimer's disease anti-inflammatory prevention trial. *Alzheimers Dement*, 2011. 7(4): 402–411.

155. Breitner, J. C., et al., Risk of dementia and AD with prior exposure to NSAIDs in an elderly community-based cohort. *Neurology*, 2009. 72(22): 1899–1905.

156. Sivilia, S., et al., Multi-target action of the novel anti-Alzheimer compound CHF5074: in vivo study of long term treatment in Tg2576 mice. *BMC Neurosci*, 2013. 14: 44.

157. Ross, J., et al., CHF5074 reduces biomarkers of neuroinflammation in patients with mild cognitive impairment: a 12-week, double-blind, placebo-controlled study. Curr Alzheimer Res, 2013. 10(7): 742–753.

158. LaFerla, F. M., and K. N. Green, Animal models of Alzheimer disease. *Cold Spring Harb Perspect Med*, 2012. 2(11): 1–13.

159. Ashe, K. H., and K. R. Zahs, Probing the biology of Alzheimer's disease in mice. *Neuron*, 2010. 66(5): 631–45.

160. Van Dam, D., and P. P. De Deyn, Drug discovery in dementia: the role of rodent models. *Nat Rev Drug Discov*, 2006. 5(11): 956–70.

161. Roher, A. E., and T. A. Kokjohn, Of mice and men: the relevance of transgenic mice Abeta immunizations to Alzheimer's disease. *J Alzheimers Dis*, 2002. 4(5): 431–434.

162. Balducci, C., and G. Forloni, APP transgenic mice: their use and limitations. *Neuromolecular Med*, 2011. 13(2): 117–137.

163. Saito, T., et al., Single App knock-in mouse models of Alzheimer's disease. *Nat Neurosci*, 2014. 17(5): 661–663.

164. Plucinska, K., et al., Knock-in of human BACE1 cleaves murine APP and reiterates Alzheimer-like phenotypes. *J Neurosci*, 2014. 34(32): 10710–10728.

165. Ryan, D., et al., Spatial learning impairments in PLB1Triple knock-in Alzheimer mice are task-specific and age-dependent. *Cell Mol Life Sci*, 2013. 70(14): 2603–2619.

166. Siman, R., et al., Presenilin-1 P264L knock-in mutation: differential effects on abeta production, amyloid deposition, and neuronal vulnerability. *J Neurosci*, 2000. 20(23): 8717–8726.

167. Chabrier, M. A., et al., Synergistic effects of amyloid-beta and wild-type human tau on dendritic spine loss in a floxed double transgenic model of Alzheimer's disease. *Neurobiol Dis*, 2014. 64: 107–117.

168. Dickstein, D. L., et al., Changes in dendritic complexity and spine morphology in transgenic mice expressing human wild-type tau. *Brain Struct Funct*, 2010. 214(2–3): 161–179.

169. Franko, E., and O. Joly, Evaluating Alzheimer's disease progression using rate of regional hippocampal atrophy. *PLoS One*, 2013. 8(8): e71354.

170. Erten-Lyons, D., et al., Neuropathologic basis of age-associated brain atrophy. *JAMA Neurol*, 2013. 70(5): 616–622.

171. Pievani, M., et al., APOE4 is associated with greater atrophy of the hippocampal formation in Alzheimer's disease. *Neuroimage*, 2011. 55(3): 909–919.

172. Frisoni, G. B., et al., Mapping local hippocampal changes in Alzheimer's disease and normal ageing with MRI at 3 Tesla. *Brain*, 2008. 131(Pt 12): 3266–3276.

173. West, M. J., et al., Hippocampal neurons in preclinical Alzheimer's disease. *Neurobiol Aging*, 2004. 25(9): 1205–1212.

174. Kril, J. J., et al., Neuron loss from the hippocampus of Alzheimer's disease exceeds extracellular neurofibrillary tangle formation. *Acta Neuropathol*, 2002. 103(4): 370–376.

175. Bobinski, M., et al., Neurofibrillary pathology: correlation with hippocampal formation atrophy in Alzheimer disease. *Neurobiol Aging*, 1996. 17(6): 909–919.

176. West, M. J., et al., Differences in the pattern of hippocampal neuronal loss in normal ageing and Alzheimer's disease. *Lancet*, 1994. 344(8925): 769–772.

177. Ball, M. J., Neuronal loss, neurofibrillary tangles and granulovacuolar degeneration in the hippocampus with ageing and dementia: a quantitative study. *Acta Neuropathol*, 1977. 37(2): 111–118.

178. Scheff, S. W., et al., Hippocampal synaptic loss in early Alzheimer's disease and mild cognitive impairment. *Neurobiol Aging*, 2006. 27(10): 1372–1384.

179. Gomez-Isla, T., et al., Profound loss of layer II entorhinal cortex neurons occurs in very mild Alzheimer's disease. *J Neurosci*, 1996. 16(14): 4491–500.

180. Trujillo-Estrada, L., et al., Early neuronal loss and axonal/presynaptic damage is associated with accelerated amyloid-beta accumulation in AbetaPP/PS1 Alzheimer's disease mice subiculum. *J Alzheimers Dis*, 2014. 42(2): 521–541.

181. Baglietto-Vargas, D., et al., Calretinin interneurons are early targets of extracellular amyloid-beta pathology in PS1/AbetaPP Alzheimer mice hippocampus. *J Alzheimers Dis*, 2010. 21(1): 119–132.

182. Moreno-Gonzalez, I., et al., Extracellular amyloid-beta and cytotoxic glial activation induce significant entorhinal neuron loss in young PS1(M146L)/APP(751SL) mice. *J Alzheimers Dis*, 2009. 18(4): 755–776.

183. Oakley, H., et al., Intraneuronal beta-amyloid aggregates, neurodegeneration, and neuron loss in transgenic mice with five familial Alzheimer's disease mutations: potential factors in amyloid plaque formation. *J Neurosci*, 2006. 26(40): 10129–10140.

184. Ramos, B., et al., Early neuropathology of somatostatin/NPY GABAergic cells in the hippocampus of a PS1xAPP transgenic model of Alzheimer's disease. *Neurobiol Aging*, 2006. 27(11): 1658–1672.

185. Casas, C., et al., Massive CA1/2 neuronal loss with intraneuronal and N-terminal truncated Abeta42 accumulation in a novel Alzheimer transgenic model. *Am J Pathol*, 2004. 165(4): 1289–1300.

186. Zahs, K. R., and K. H. Ashe, "Too much good news": are Alzheimer mouse models trying to tell us how to prevent, not cure, Alzheimer's disease? *Trends Neurosci*, 2010. 33(8): 381–389.

187. Myczek, K., et al., Hippocampal adaptive response following extensive neuronal loss in an inducible transgenic mouse model. *PLoS One*, 2014. 9(9): e106009.

188. Yeung, S. T., et al., Impact of hippocampal neuronal ablation on neurogenesis and cognition in the aged brain. *Neuroscience*, 2014. 259: 214–222.

189. Yamasaki, T. R., et al., Neural stem cells improve memory in an inducible mouse model of neuronal loss. *J Neurosci*, 2007. 27(44): 11925–11933.

190. Price, J. L., et al., Neuron number in the entorhinal cortex and CA1 in preclinical Alzheimer disease. *Arch Neurol*, 2001. 58(9): 1395–1402.

191. Clodomiro, A., et al., Somatic comorbidities and Alzheimer's disease treatment. *Neurol Sci*, 2013. 34(9): 1581–1589.

192. Schubert, C. C., et al., Comorbidity profile of dementia patients in primary care: are they sicker? *J Am Geriatr Soc*, 2006. 54(1): 104–109.

193. Sanderson, M., et al., Co-morbidity associated with dementia. *Am J Alzheimers Dis Other Demen*, 2002. 17(2): 73–78.

194. Cumming, T. B., and A. Brodtmann, Can stroke cause neurodegenerative dementia? *Int J Stroke*, 2011. 6(5): 416–424.

195. Johnson, V. E., W. Stewart, and D. H. Smith, Traumatic brain injury and amyloid-beta pathology: a link to Alzheimer's disease? *Nat Rev Neurosci*, 2010. 11(5): 361–370.

196. Kalaria, R. N., The role of cerebral ischemia in Alzheimer's disease. *Neurobiol Aging*, 2000. 21(2): 321–330.

197. Kalaria, R. N., et al., The amyloid precursor protein in ischemic brain injury and chronic hypoperfusion. *Ann N Y Acad Sci*, 1993. 695: 190–193.

198. Koike, M. A., et al., Oligemic hypoperfusion differentially affects tau and amyloid-{beta}. *Am J Pathol*, 2010. 177(1): 300–310.

199. Uryu, K., et al., Multiple proteins implicated in neurodegenerative diseases accumulate in axons after brain trauma in humans. *Exp Neurol*, 2007. 208(2): 185–192.

200. Tesco, G., et al., Depletion of GGA3 stabilizes BACE and enhances beta-secretase activity. *Neuron*, 2007. 54(5): 721–737.

201. Zhang, X., et al., Hypoxia-inducible factor 1alpha (HIF-1alpha)-mediated hypoxia increases BACE1 expression and beta-amyloid generation. *J Biol Chem*, 2007. 282(15): 10873–10880.

202. Thorin, E., Hypertension and Alzheimer disease: another brick in the wall of awareness. *Hypertension*, 2015. 65(1): 36–38.

203. Cifuentes, D., et al., Hypertension accelerates the progression of Alzheimer-like pathology in a mouse model of the disease. *Hypertension*, 2015. 65(1): 218–224.

204. Son, S. J., et al., Effect of hypertension on the resting-state functional connectivity in patients with Alzheimer's disease (AD). *Arch Gerontol Geriatr*, 2015. 60(1): 210–216.

205. Abbondante, S., et al., *Genetic ablation of tau mitigates cognitive impairment induced by type 1 diabetes. Am J Pathol*, 2014. 184(3): 819–826.

206. Devi, L., et al., Mechanisms underlying insulin deficiency-induced acceleration of beta-amyloidosis in a mouse model of Alzheimer's disease. *PLoS One*, 2012. 7(3): e32792.

207. Takeda, S., et al., Diabetes-accelerated memory dysfunction via cerebrovascular inflammation and Abeta deposition in an Alzheimer mouse model with diabetes. *Proc Natl Acad Sci U S A*, 2010. 107(15): 7036–7041.

208. Jolivalt, C. G., et al., Type 1 diabetes exaggerates features of Alzheimer's disease in APP transgenic mice. *Exp Neurol*, 2010. 223(2): 422–431.

209. Freitag, M. H., et al., Midlife pulse pressure and incidence of dementia: the Honolulu-Asia Aging Study. *Stroke*, 2006. 37(1): 33–37.

210. Pardon, M. C., Therapeutic potential of some stress mediators in early Alzheimer's disease. *Exp Gerontol*, 2011. 46(2–3): 170–173.

211. Rothman, S. M., and M. P. Mattson, Adverse stress, hippocampal networks, and Alzheimer's disease. *Neuromolecular Med*, 2010. 12(1): 56–70.

212. Starkstein, S. E., et al., The construct of generalized anxiety disorder in Alzheimer disease. *Am J Geriatr Psychiatry*, 2007. 15(1): 42–49.

213. Popp, J., et al., Cerebrospinal fluid cortisol and clinical disease progression in MCI and dementia of Alzheimer's type. *Neurobiol Aging*, 2015. 36(2): 601–607.

214. Huang, C. W., et al., Elevated basal cortisol level predicts lower hippocampal volume and cognitive decline in Alzheimer's disease. *J Clin Neurosci*, 2009. 16(10): 1283–1286.

215. Csernansky, J. G., et al., Plasma cortisol and progression of dementia in subjects with Alzheimer-type dementia. *Am J Psychiatry*, 2006. 163(12): 2164–2169.

216. Cuadrado-Tejedor, M., et al., Chronic mild stress accelerates the onset and progression of the Alzheimer's disease phenotype in Tg2576 mice. *J Alzheimers Dis*, 2012. 28(3): 567–578.

217. Rothman, S. M., et al., 3xTgAD mice exhibit altered behavior and elevated Abeta after chronic mild social stress. *Neurobiol Aging*, 2012. 33(4): 830, e1–12.

218. Sotiropoulos, I., et al., Stress acts cumulatively to precipitate Alzheimer's disease-like tau pathology and cognitive deficits. *J Neurosci*, 2011. 31(21): 7840–7847.

219. Catania, C., et al., The amyloidogenic potential and behavioral correlates of stress. *Mol Psychiatry*, 2009. 14(1): 95–105.

220. Green, K. N., et al., Glucocorticoids increase amyloid-beta and tau pathology in a mouse model of Alzheimer's disease. *J Neurosci*, 2006. 26(35): 9047–9056.

221. Jeong, Y. H., et al., Chronic stress accelerates learning and memory impairments and increases amyloid deposition in APPV717I-CT100 transgenic mice, an Alzheimer's disease model. *FASEB J*, 2006. 20(6): 729–731.

222. Warren, H. S., et al., Mice are not men. *Proc Natl Acad Sci U S A*, 2015. 112(4): E345.

223. Geerts, H., Of mice and men: bridging the translational disconnect in CNS drug discovery. *CNS Drugs*, 2009. 23(11): 915–926.

224. Kojro, E., and F. Fahrenholz, The non-amyloidogenic pathway: structure and function of alpha-secretases. *Subcell Biochem*, 2005. 38: 105–127.

225. Haass, C., et al., beta-Amyloid peptide and a 3-kDa fragment are derived by distinct cellular mechanisms. *J Biol Chem*, 1993. 268(5): 3021–3024.

226. Jarrett, J. T., E. P. Berger, and P. T. Lansbury, Jr., The carboxy terminus of the beta amyloid protein is critical for the seeding of amyloid formation: implications for the pathogenesis of Alzheimer's disease. *Biochemistry*, 1993. 32(18): 4693–4697.

15

Metal-Protein Attenuating Compounds in Neurodegenerative Diseases

PENG LEI, SCOTT AYTON, AND ASHLEY I. BUSH

INTRODUCTION

Neurodegenerative disorders, including Alzheimer's disease (AD), Parkinson's disease (PD), Huntington's disease (HD), and amyotrophic lateral sclerosis (ALS), are progressive, incurable diseases of the aging population. The pathogenesis of these disorders has been investigated extensively in last three decades; however, the precise causes of the diseases remain elusive. One common feature of these diseases is the involvement of proteins that appear to dysfunction and misfold. These proteins include β-amyloid and tau of AD, α-synuclein in PD, huntingtin in HD, superoxide dismutase 1 (SOD1), and transactive response DNA-binding protein (TDP-43) in ALS (1). Since these proteins were identified in the pathology of each disease, it is hypothesized that misfolded protein aggregates are responsible for the neurotoxicity that ultimately causes the diseases. However, the failures of multiple clinical trials that targeted aggregating proteins (2, 3) suggest that the protein themselves may not be the most appropriate drug target.

We and others discovered that some transitional metals (e.g., zinc, copper, and iron) are enriched in the various pathologies of the neurodegenerative disorders. We propose that fatigue of metal homeostasis in the brain during the aging process causes deleterious metallic reactions in the brain, including the aggregation of neurodegenerative disease-linked proteins. Aggregation leads to loss of soluble, functional proteins, which, in turn, further impairs metal homeostasis. Therefore it is feasible to target this vicious circle using metal-protein attenuating compounds (MPACs); here we will discuss the evidences that support this therapeutic strategy and the progress toward a new therapy for neurodegenerative disorders. This chapter will provide an overview of the roles of metals in the brain before reviewing the evidence for impaired metal homeostasis in neurodegeneration and associated therapeutic opportunities.

PHYSIOLOGICAL ROLES OF METALS IN THE BRAIN

Zinc

Zinc is an element required by all living organisms; it plays essential roles as a cofactor to structurally stabilize proteins and to facilitate enzymatic catalysis. In the brain, zinc is concentrated in gray matter (4), highlighting its possible physiological roles in both postsynaptic and presynaptic activities. In fact, glutamatergic vesicular zinc represents 20%–30% of brain zinc (5), and the concentration of exchangeable zinc in the synapses is estimated to be 100–300 μM (6–8).

Synaptic zinc can inhibit the N-methyl-D-aspartate (NMDA) receptor at both low- and high-affinity binding sites (9, 10). It was demonstrated that presynaptic vesicular zinc release is needed for presynaptic plasticity that causes mossy-fiber long-term potentiation (LTP), since LTP was inhibited in the hippocampal CA3 region by zinc (11). A number of transactivation targets for synaptically-release zinc have been identified, including TrkB (12), GPR39 (13, 14), and the K+/Cl− co-transporter-2 (KCC2) (15).

Copper

Copper participates in a range of brain metabolic processes, and is a required cofactor for proteins termed *cuproteins*. Copper can shift between the cuprous (Cu^+) and the cupric (Cu^{2+}) states by accepting and donating electrons; this chemistry can be utilized to catalyze varies biological reactions. The major copper-enzymes include

Ceruloplasmin (Cp), SOD1, Lysyl oxidase, and Cytochrome *c* oxidase (16). The same ability to exchange electrons also enables the generation of free radicals in redox reactions, which may be potentially harmful to the brain. This will be discussed in the context of diseases later in the chapter.

In synapses, copper can transiently achieve a high concentration of 100µM (reviewed in 17) upon NMDA receptor activation (18, 19). It was released from activated synaptosomes (20) in a Ca^{2+}-dependent manner (21), and only can be freely exchanged in glutamatergic synapse. Copper treatment to cultured neurons attenuates the responses of NMDA, AMPA, glycine and GABA receptors (22–24); however, the physiological relevance of these findings is not yet proven. Interestingly, copper may have bi-phasic effects on neuronal activity depending on its concentration. Low copper levels (1 µM) have been shown to suppress long-term potentiation (LTP) in rat hippocampal slices (25); however, higher concentration (10 µM) promotes LTP activity through the AMPA receptor (GluR1 subunit) by markedly increasing PSD-95 (26). It was suggested that copper interacts with PrPc, which interacts with the NMDA receptor complex that mediates the effects (27).

Iron

Iron is found in both white and gray matter of the brain (28), and is utilized in a wide range of cellular processes, including neurotransmitter synthesis, myelination of neurons, and mitochondrial function. Although only 2% of body weight, the brain consumes 20% of the oxygen utilized by the body at rest (29); a high level of iron is therefore needed to meet the high energy requirement of the brain, making it the most abundant transition metal in the human brain, weighing about 60 mg (29). Compared with astrocytes and microglia, neurons and oligodendrocytes contain relatively higher amounts of iron due to their needs (30); of the various regions of the brain, the basal ganglia (especially substantia nigra, SN) contains the highest amount of iron (31).

Iron participates in the synthesis of monoamines, including dopamine, noradrenalin, and adrenaline, which makes the levels of monoamines sensitive to brain iron changes (32, 33). The activity of enzymes involved in the synthesis process are dependent on iron, such as tyrosine hydroxylase (34, 35), tryptophan hydroxylase (36), and phenylalanine hydroxylase (37).

Myelin is enriched in iron (38), and iron is required for myelination and oligodendrocyte biology. It was observed that iron deficiency can lead to deficient myelination, suggesting its importance in myelin synthesis. In a human study, 6-month-old iron-deficient infants had increased latency of auditory brainstem potentials and visual evoked potentials (an indirect marker of hypo-myelination) compared to normal controls (39). Restriction of iron during the early post-natal period in rats (a model of iron deficiency) resulted in a decrease in myelin proteins (40), which also indicates the involvement of iron in myelin synthesis.

In addition, several components of the electron transport chain rely on iron-proteins, including iron-sulphur clusters, heme-containing cytochromes, and co-enzyme cytochrome *c* (41), which makes iron a vital factor in mitochondrial function.

METAL HOMEOSTASIS IN THE BRAIN

Zinc

Zinc transport in cells is mediated by two families of zinc transporters, ZIP (Zrt-, Irt-like protein, SLC39A family) and ZnT (vertebrate cation diffusion facilitator family proteins, SLC30A family). ZIP family proteins are responsible for zinc import, and ZnT family proteins facilitate zinc export. Within the cell, zinc can be utilized by zinc-binding proteins, or can be exchanged between lumen of intracellular organelles and cytosol mediated by ZIPs and ZnTs (42).

There are 14 ZIP proteins (ZIP1-14) that have been identified (42). ZIPs are expressed in various tissues and cell types including neurons, but their function as zinc importers (43) or exchange mediators (44) depends on cell type. ZIPs contain eight transmembrane domains (TMDs) with both the amino- and carboxyl- termini exposed to the extracellular side of the membrane, and a histidine-rich amino acid sequence (3-5 His residues) located in a large cytosolic loop between TMDs 3 and 4 (45). It was predicted that the histidine-rich amino acid sequence is required for zinc binding; however, mutations of the region in ZIP1 do not inhibit zinc uptake (46). ZIP1 was the first identified human ZIP family member, and was discovered by its sequence homology to the yeast high-affinity divalent metal transporters (47). In the brain, ZIP1 and ZIP3 were found to be responsible for the majority of zinc uptake in neurons, and mice lacking these transporters are protected from drug-induced seizure by preventing zinc uptake (48). Interestingly, the same animal model also exhibited higher susceptibility to a seizure-induced drug, suggesting that zinc is mediating drug-induced toxicity (48). ZIP4, which gene involved in acrodermatitis enteropathica (a disease of zinc deficiency) (49), was reported to regulate zinc influx in hippocampus of mice, and can be regulated by tissue plasminogen activator under zinc replete conditions (50). Other ZIPs have also been implicated in the brain, including ZIP2, 6–8, 10, 12–14, but without clear functional relevance (51).

The ZnT protein family has 10 members (ZnT1–10), and ZnT1, 3, 4, 6, 9, and 10 are the main ZnT proteins that are expressed in the brain (51). Typically, ZnTs consist of six TMD with cytosolic amino- and carboxyl- termini (45). Between TMD 4 and 5, ZnTs have a histindine-rich putative metal-binding domain (45). In particular, ZnT1 is expressed on the plasma memberane of neurons and glia, and is responsible for zinc exportation (4). Evidence from ischemia research suggests that ZnT1 is necessary for zinc homeostasis (52), and ZnT1 may be able to protect from ischemia-induced neurotoxicity by promoting zinc export (53, 54). ZnT3 is neuron specific and is mainly presented in the synaptic vesicles in the hippocampus, cortex, and olfactory bulb (55); reduction of ZnT3 resulted in synaptic zinc depletion and age-dependent neurodegeneration (56). ZnT4 is responsible for endosomal/lysosomal zinc translocation (57, 58), similar to ZnT2 (59). ZnTs 6 and 10 transport zinc between cytoplasm and the Golgi apparatus (60, 61), which was found to be reduced in AD brains and an animal model of AD (62).

Copper

Copper content in human brains is at the range of low µg/g (wet weight) (63, 64), which is very similar to that of the mouse brain (65). The distribution of copper in the brain is not even; gray matter contains higher copper (~5µg/g) than the white matter (~2µg/g) (66, 67). As previously discussed, the redox activity of copper is utilized by a number of neuronal processes; however, excess copper may cause oxidation of proteins and DNA as well as lipid peroxidation, which can be harmful for neurons (68). Therefore, the brain copper metabolism is tightly regulated, leaving almost no free copper within the cytosol (69).

Copper is primarily imported by copper transporter 1 (Ctr1; SLC31A1) for most cell types (70). Human Ctr1 is a 190–amino acid protein that can bind to copper with high affinity (68). It contains three TMDs and an extracellular N terminus where the copper-binding domain of 19–amino acid motif, rich in serine and methionine, is located (71–73). The importance of Ctr1 in copper transport was demonstrated by the homozygous mCtr1-/- mice, where knock-out of Ctr1 caused embryonic lethality resultant from severe developmental deficits (74, 75). It was proposed that Ctr1 modulates copper uptake by endocytosis at the cell surface (76, 77), and is regulated by the extracellular copper level (78, 79). However, such observation may be cell-type dependent (72, 80), and therefore the precise mechanism of copper influx is yet to be defined.

A putative copper reductase is required on the cell surface to reduce copper from Cu^{2+} to $^{1+}$ for Ctr1 to pick up. Candidates, including Steap proteins (81) and Dcytb (82), have been identified. The intracellular copper then will be delivered to cupro-enzymes by copper chaperones, or will be bound by glutathione (83) or metallothionein (MT) (84). Major copper chaperones include Atox1, Ccs, and Cox17. Ccs is responsible for delivering copper to SOD1 (85). Ccs levels are increased in copper-deficient tissue (86), and deletion of the Ccs gene significantly reduces SOD1 activity, mimicking the SOD1 knock-out phenotype (87). Cox17 is a small 8-kDa protein that is required for cytochrome c oxidase function (88). It is found in both cytoplasm and the mitochondrial intermembrane to deliver copper cytochrome c oxidase accessory proteins Sco1 and Cox11 (89). Knock-out of Cox11 resulted in fetal death in utero (90), highlighting the importance of this protein.

Atox1 (also known as HAH1) is a 68–amino acid protein that is responsible for delivering copper for export (91). It chaperones copper for P-type ATPases, ATP7a and ATP7b, which mediate copper efflux in an energy-dependent process (92). Both ATP7a and 7b consist of eight TMDs, six metal-binding motifs (MXCXXC) in the cytoplasmic amino-terminal domain, and an ATP binding domain (93). ATP7a is ubiquitously expressed all over the body, but ATP7b is only expressed in the brain, liver, kidneys, and eyes (94). Both ATP7a and ATP7b are implicated in cellular Cu efflux; however, due to spatially divergent expression in tissues, the roles they play in maintaining body Cu homeostasis are quite different. Mutations in ATP7a can impair copper absorption in the small intestine, and result in systematic copper deficiency in infants, which is a lethal genetic disease called Menkes disease (95). On the other hand, mutations in ATP7b affect the incorporation of copper into ceruloplasmin (Cp), and cause cooper accumulation in the liver and brain, which is a severe metabolic disorder named Wilson's disease (96).

Iron

As previously discussed, the high demand for iron in the brain requires a tightly controlled mechanism to regulate iron and prevents spontaneous reaction with oxygen. As is the case for peripheral iron transport, brain iron is trafficked into neurons by transferrin (Tf) (97), which is synthesized in oligodendrocytes (30) and expressed throughout the brain (98). Tf selectively binds up to two ferric ions (10^{23} M^{-1} at pH 7.4) (99, 100); and holo-Tf is recognized by transferrin receptor 1 (TfR1) and 2 (TfR2) on the extracellular surface of brain cells. The binding affinity between holo-Tf and TfR1/2 is much higher than apo-Tf and TfR1/2 at pH7.4, which ensures a selective binding for iron uptake (101). The functional distinction between TfR1 and TfR2 in the brain is still unclear, but accumulating evidence suggests that they may have different roles in iron regulation. For example, the expression of TfR1 and TfR2 are regulated differently, where only TfR1 expression is affected by cellular iron status (102–104). In addition, TfR2 overexpression cannot compensate for the loss of TfR1, demonstrated by the early death of TfR1 knock-out mice (105). It is possible that TfR2 has a more specialized role, such as import iron into the mitochondria (106).

After binding to TfR, the complex is transported into the neurons via endocytosis. Since the pH of the endosome is lowered to pH 5.5 (107), Tf can no longer bind to iron, and ferric iron is reduced by a ferrireductase to ferrous state for transmembrane delivery into the cytosol. A number of proteins were found to have ferrireductase activity, including duodenal cytochrome B (108), cytochrome P450 reductase (109), NADH-dependent quinoid dihydropteridine reductase (110), and six-transmembrane epithelial antigen of the prostate protein 1–4 (111). However, these proteins are not highly expressed in neurons (112, 113). Apo-Tf and TfRs are recycled back to the cell surface for reuse. The binding between apo-Tf and TfR is enhanced at the low pH in the cytosol, which prevents Tf from being deposited in the lysosome as the endosome transits back to the cell surface. The complex between Apo-Tf and TfR1 is

destabilized at the neutral pH of the extracellular space, which allows for the release and recycling of Tf (101).

While Tf is recycled in the endosome trafficking apparatus, iron is removed from Tf and deposited within the cytosol. In its ferrous state, iron in the endosome can be transported across the membrane by divalent metal ion transporter 1 (DMT1) (114, 115). DMT1 can also transport other metals, such as copper (116), manganese (117), and cadmium (118).

After releasing from the endosome, iron can then be stored in the iron storage protein, ferritin (119), or can be utilized by proteins that require iron. Ferritin consists of heavy- (H-) and light- (L-) chain isoforms, which form a macromolecule of approximately 450 kDa (120). This macromolecule can bind up to 4,500 atoms of iron (120), stabilizing the ferric iron from oxidation (121, 122). Ferritin expression is differentially regulated: H-chain ferritin is expressed in neurons and oligodendrocytes, and L-chain ferritin is expressed in microglia and oligodendrocytes (30, 123). However, further studies are required to understand the reason for this differentiation. In addition to ferritin, neuromelannin also can store iron in the cell. Neuromelannin is a dark pigment usually expressed in the SN and locus coeruleus of the brain, made by metabolites of monoamine neurotransmitters including dopamine and norepinephrine (124).

Iron is exported by ferroportin (Fpn), which is the only known pathway in mammalian cells (125). Fpn transports ferrous iron out of the cell (126, 127), and ferrous iron is converted into ferric iron and picked up by apo-Tf. Fpn-mediated iron export is regulated by hepcidin (128, 129), since hepcidin binds to Fpn, which causes Fpn internalization and degradation (128, 130). We, and others, recently found that APP acts to stabilize Fpn to facilitate iron export in neurons (131–134), and overexpression of APP resulted in decreasing iron level *in vivo* (135), consistent with the hypothesis that APP acts as an iron-export agent. Iron export by ferroportin is also facilitated by a ferroxidase, such as ceruloplasmin (Cp) (136, 137). Cp is expressed by astrocytes in the brain (138, 139), and can bind to the cell surface via a glycosylphosphatidylinositol-anchor (140). The surface Cp therefore can also stabilize Fpn (141), and oxidizes iron for export. Rare mutations to Cp cause the genetic disorder Aceruloplasminemia (142), where iron accumulation occurs in peripheral tissue and brain (141, 143, 144). In oligodendrocytes, hephaestin also has ferroxidase activity (145).

METAL DYSHOMEOSTASIS IN ALZHEIMER'S DISEASE

Zinc

Zinc content in postmortem AD tissues has been detected by multiple groups using multiple methods (146–150), but neocortex zinc levels were not consistently changed (151). It was suggested that the detection of zinc can be affected by various methods of sample preparation (e.g., variability in fixation) (151) and therefore may not correctly reflect the pathological role of zinc in AD.

A number of ZnTs were altered in AD brain tissues, including ZnT1, 4, 6 (152), 3 (56), and 10 (62). The mRNA of ZnT1, 4, and 6 also increases in AD and is associated with disease progression using Braak stage (153), suggesting zinc dyshomeostasis in the disease. It was found that zinc deficiency can cause zinc accumulation in the brain by reducing the expression of ZnT1 (154, 155), which explains the increase of amyloid plaques in the brains of APP/PS1 transgenic mice with dietary zinc deficiency (156). In addition, 4-hydroxynonenal, a zinc export inhibitor, was found to be increased in AD brains induced by elevation of oxidative stress (157), which may also contribute to zinc dyshomeostasis in AD brains.

In contrast to the inconsistent report on total zinc content in AD brains, zinc level in the extracellular plaques of AD patients was found to be 1,055 µM using microparticle-induced-X ray emission (PIXE) analysis (150), suggesting the possibility of zinc's participation in Aβ aggregation. Zinc binds Aβ residues 6–28 (158, 159), which results in rapid aggregation (milliseconds) (160) and precipitation of the peptide (159) that can be reversed by metal chelators (161). Depending on the concentration ratio between zinc and Aβ, zinc induces different aggregates of Aβ. At substoichiometric concentrations, zinc promotes fibrillar, β-sheet enriched aggregates (162), in contrast to non-fibrillar and α-helical aggregates at stoichiometric concentrations (161, 163, 164). The zinc-induced Aβ aggregates are toxic (165), and are immune-active with A11 antibody, a marker of toxic Aβ form (166). These zinc-Aβ complexes are also resistant to proteolysis by zinc-dependent matrix metalloproteases (167, 168).

ADAM10, the α-secretase involved in the physiological processing of APP, is a zinc-dependent enzyme, and therefore zinc increases APP proteolysis (169). A separate report also found that zinc can inhibit γ-secretase activity (170). Zinc also increases presenilin 1 expression, and presenilin protein also facilitates cellular zinc uptake (171).

Zinc might also be involved in tangle formation and tau-mediated neurotoxicity in AD. It has been shown that zinc induces tau aggregation in micro-molar concentration (172–174), and is concentrated in neurons with neurofibrillary tangle pathology (175). A number of cell culture and animal studies have demonstrated that excess zinc is able to alter tau translation and phosphorylation, via upregulation of kinases of tau phosphorylation including GSK-3β, protein kinase B, ERK1/2, and c-Jun N-terminal kinase (176–178). Interestingly, a recent study using *Drosophila* hTauR406W model demonstrated that zinc can also directly bind to tau protein to promote tau-mediated neurotoxicity, in addition to its effect on tau phosphorylation (174).

Copper

Total intracellular copper levels are decreased in AD patients and animal models of AD (151, 179), but the levels of copper in the plaques is elevated (180). The remaining tissue copper is poorly ligated, which may contribute to the increased oxidative stress present in AD brains (181). The presence of redox-active copper (Cu^{2+}) promotes apoptosis via X-linked inhibitor of apoptosis protein or mitogen-activated protein kinase kinase 1/ Extracellular signal-regulated kinases pathways (182, 183).

Copper deficiency in neurons can impair the copper-dependent enzymes that are important for physiological cellular activities. Indeed, the activities of some copper-dependent enzymes, such as Cu/Zn-superoxide dismutase-1 (SOD1), cytochrome c oxidase, and peptidylglycine α-amidating monooxygenase, were shown to be decreased in AD brains (184, 185), which may cause the energy metabolism deficits also found in AD brains (186). In addition, it was shown that reduction in copper level deactivated the PI3K/ Akt/GSK3 pathway (187), which may promote tau hyperphosphorylation (178). Decreased copper can also promote amyloidogenic pathways of APP processing (188, 189), resulting in an enriched copper environment in lipid rafts with Aβ (190).

The interaction between copper and Aβ is well characterized. Copper binds to Aβ and promotes Aβ fibril aggregation under mildly acidic conditions at substoichiometric concentrations (162, 191–194). However, at neutral pH, copper induces the formation of dimer or oligomer (159, 195–197). Co-administration of Aβ and copper is toxic to cells (164, 198–200), which can be prevented by copper chelation (201, 202). Oxidative stress is likely involved in the cytotoxicity induced by Aβ-copper complex, since the complex catalytically generates hydrogen peroxide (198, 203, 204). The oxidation products include thiols, ascorbate, lipid or Aβ itself (205–210). Oxidation of Aβ itself may result in a cross-linked dimer by tyrosine 10, which is resistant to proteolytic degradation and prone to aggregation (206, 211, 212). In *Drosophila* with Aβ1-42 overexpression, manipulation of copper (by copper chelation, suppression of copper importers Ctr1B and Ctr1C, and overexpression of copper exporter DmATP7) significantly reduced Aβ oligomer formation and oxidative stress, enhanced motor ability, and prolonged the life span of these flies (213).

Copper also interacts with tau (214), which promotes its aggregation *in vitro* (215–217). In AD brains, copper-containing tangles were demonstrated as a source of oxidative stress (218), and *in vitro* experiments showed that hydrogen peroxide was produced by copper and a fragment of tau protein (219). In transgenic mice overexpressing mutant APP, presenilin, and tau, copper exposure accelerates tau hyperphosphorylation (220). However, in mice that overexpress only APP and presenilin, copper delivery drugs have been shown to reduce tau phosphorylation via inhibition of GSK-3β (221).

Iron

Iron accumulation in AD brains was first shown in 1953 (222), and subsequently was validated by a number of groups (28, 131, 223–229). The brain regions that accumulate iron in AD overlay with those regions affected by AD pathology, namely the cortex and hippocampus. Iron accumulation is not observed in regions without AD pathology, such as the cerebellum (131, 228, 230). Hippocampal iron deposition in AD patients correlates with the Mini-Mental State Examination (MMSE) score, as well as the disease duration (231, 232), indicating that iron is involved in the progression of the disease.

We were the first to calculate the impact of iron on longitudinal AD outcomes (233). Using ferritin (the major iron-binding protein) levels in CSF as an index, we showed that high brain-iron load was associated with poorer cognition and brain atrophy in a cohort of cognitively normal ($n = 91$), mild cognitive impairment ($n = 144$), and AD ($n = 67$) subjects over a 6–7-year period. The magnitude of impact of CSF ferritin on these and other AD-outcomes is comparable to the tau/Aβ$_{42}$ ratio—the best diagnostic CSF biomarker for AD. CSF ferritin independently predicted conversion to AD and improved the predictive potential of the tau/Aβ$_{42}$ ratio. Each 1 ng/ml increase in CSF ferritin brought forward diagnosis by 3 months. This study therefore introduced the utility of CSF iron reporters in predicting both cognitive deterioration and atrophy along the pathway to AD.

Iron also interacts with disease-related proteins Aβ and tau. Iron was shown to co-localize with both plaques and tangles in histological sections (223, 226, 229), where it was elevated three times compared to the neuropil level (180). *In vitro* experiments suggested that Aβ binds to iron and results in a more rapid aggregation (162, 234). The iron-Aβ aggregates are cytotoxic (235–239), possibly due to the oxidative stress induced by the reduction of iron (240). Tau protein can bind to iron as well (241, 242), and some *in vitro* evidence suggested that iron promotes Aβ aggregation (243), which may explain the co-localization between iron and tangles in AD (229). In addition, tau phosphorylation, a post-translational modification that is suggested to be involved in AD, can be altered by iron (244–247), which could be another source of neurotoxicity.

As previously discussed, iron is redox active and needs to be tightly regulated in the brain. Iron elevation in AD likely contributes to oxidative stress observed in affected brain regions (248). The downstream neurotoxic events induced by iron include activation of apoptotic signaling pathways (249), and damage of proteins and lipids such as Ca^{2+}-ATPase (250–253) and glutamate transporter (254–256), which leads to synaptic dysfunction and neuronal cell death (257). In addition, iron was recently found to be involved in a new cell death pathway termed *ferroptosis* (258), which is RAS-related and apoptosis independent. Ferroptosis can be prevented by iron chelation or iron uptake inhibition (259, 260). While ferroptosis has not yet been explored in AD, this cell death pathway may represent a new therapeutic target for AD.

The precise mechanism of how iron accumulates in AD brains is still unknown. However, among the complicated machinery of iron regulation, we found that APP binds to ferroportin in the neuronal membrane and facilitates iron export of neurons (131–134), which is neuroprotective (261). The expression of APP is regulated by iron, since APP has a 5'UTR iron responsive element (262). When iron accumulates, APP expression is elevated to facilitate the exportation of iron. However, iron elevation also increases the processing of APP, resulting in an elevated level of Aβ (263, 264), leading to accelerated degeneration in a mouse model of AD (265). On the other hand, total tau level is decreased in the AD cortex (266–269), and we found that loss of tau expression causes iron- and age-dependent cognitive loss and cortical atrophy in mice (270–272). Further, we found that tau mediates APP trafficking to the neuronal membrane (270), which is required for iron exportation. Therefore we hypothesized that the interaction between iron, APP, and tau forms a vicious cycle that collectively contributes to the pathogenesis of AD.

Metal Dyshomeostasis in Parkinson's DiseaseIron

Iron accumulation in the SN, as a pathological finding of PD, was described as early as 1924 (273). The observation has since been quantified using a range of techniques, including inductively coupled plasma mass spectrometry (ICPMS) (270, 274–276), X-ray fluorescence (277), and magnetic resonance imaging (MRI) (278). It has been consistently reported that the total iron content in SN of PD was increased about 50% (279). In addition, PD familial mutations in genes encoding LRRK2 (280), parkin (281), α-synuclein (282), PINK1 (283), and DJ-1 (282) all showed SN iron accumulation. Further evidences suggested that mutations in a number of iron-related proteins have been shown to be associated with the risk of PD, including Tf (284), IRP2 (285), ferritin (286), and DMT1 (287). Iron elevation to the nigra is itself a risk factor for PD (288, 289). However, the pathogenic relevance of iron in PD is constantly debated.

Iron accumulation in SN of PD could be a consequence of the failures of multiple iron-regulatory proteins. Loss of either tau (270, 271) or APP (276) proteins prevents iron export of neurons. In mice, loss of these proteins resulted in age-dependent iron elevation, nigral neuron loss, and motor impairment—symptoms that were prevented by chronic iron chelation (270–272, 276). Age-dependent motor deficits in tau knock-out mice have since been replicated independently (290). The original report of APP knock-out mice characterized motor impairment (291), but this had not previously been explained. The discovery that lowering of tau and APP proteins leads

to disease manifestation in mice is important because we found that both tau (270) and APP (276) protein levels were depleted in human PD substantia nigra neurons (independent of cell loss), thus engendering iron accumulation in disease. These biochemical mechanisms might explain how mutations in tau (MAPT) (292, 293) and APP (294) genes increase the risk for PD and Lewy body deposition (295).

Cp, a protein involved in iron exportation by its ferroxidase activity, is also implicated in PD. The specific activity of Cp is decreased ~80% in the SN of PD, possibly related to a marked drop in copper levels in the tissue (275). Similar to tau and APP (both implicated in iron export), Cp knockout mice also develop parkinsonism with elevated nigral iron, and can be rescued by iron chelation (275, 296).

Iron may serve as a disease predictor for PD. The observation that relaxation rate from T_2-weighted MRI can be used as an indication for iron content has allowed for a window into iron content in living human brains (278, 297, 298). Iron elevation in PD, shown by MRI, correlated with the disease susceptibility (299), severity (300, 301), and duration of PD (302, 303). Iron accumulation was also shown to be an early event in PD (278, 304), which might have utility as a biomarker.

Transcranial sonography (TCS) is another technique that can measure iron levels in the SN. Increased echogenicity of ultrasounds is indicative of iron accumulation (305–309). Control individuals with increased echogenicity by TCS have 17 times the risk of developing PD over the following 3 years (289). It is thought that PD progresses slowly, with biological changes occurring well before symptom onset. The early rise in iron, measured by TCS and MRI, supports a role for iron in the pathogenicity of PD.

Several iron chelation approaches have been reported as salutary in PD rodent models (310–313). One of the agents that has successfully reduced iron levels and improved motor function in animal models of PD is M30 [5-(N-methyl-N-propargylaminomethyl)-8-hydroxyquinoline] (314). This compound is reported to be multifunctional, combining the chelating ability of the 8-hydroxyquinoline moiety with the ability to inhibit monoamine oxidase through the propargyl moiety.

The strongest evidence to date that iron impacts on the progression of PD is obtained from a recent phase II clinical trial of the iron chelator, deferiprone for PD (315). Deferiprone lowered nigral iron content (as measured by MRI) and improved motor symptoms (Unified Parkinson's Diease Rating Scale) in a clinical trial of 18 months that employed a delayed-start paradigm of 6 months and withdrawal phase of 6 months. In this trial design, half the cohort started on the drug at the beginning of the trial, and the other half started on placebo; after 6 months the placebo group also began receiving the drug. The trial participants were then administered placebo for a following 6 months. Patients experienced improved motor symptoms while on deferiprone, and worsening motor symptoms when they were on placebo.

In an animal model of PD, deferiprone increases tyrosine hydroxylase–positive cells in the SN and motor performance. These functional improvements were likely the result of reduced iron load and reduced oxidative stress burden, which is the likely mechanism of action for the improvement observed in patients (315).

Copper

Low copper levels have been observed in surviving neurons within the SN of PD patients (316), which may be a result of copper's interaction with α-synuclein. It was shown that copper binds to α-synuclein in two sites (317), one of which is located in the N-terminal region (318–322). Using nuclear magnetic resonance (NMR) spectroscopy, a complex of Cu(I) and α-synuclein was identified, which contains an α-helical secondary structure and has restricted motility (323). Copper then can oxidize α-synuclein (324), resulting in a redox active complex (325–327). This complex directly enhances α-synuclein amyloid formation (328, 329), and induces toxic amorphous aggregates (327) instead of long fibrils generated by α-synuclein alone (330). The toxicity of α-synuclein requires the presence of copper (331), and excess copper induces a nontoxic level of α-synuclein to exhibit neurotoxicity (332). Restriction in cellular copper level limits the presence of α-synuclein aggregates and toxicity (333).

Interestingly, DJ-1 binds to copper and forms a homodimer (334), which may be required for its antioxidative activity (335). DJ-1 therefore can protect against copper-induced cytotoxicity (336), where the disease-related mutant impaired this function (335).

Zinc

Elevated nigral zinc was reported in PD patients, indicating a possible pathological involvement of zinc in PD (337), which is supported by recent biochemistry evidence. Excess of zinc directly causes nigro-striatal dopaminergic neurodegeneration, which can be attenuated by zinc chelation, inhibition of microglial activation (338), or NADPH oxidase inhibition (339). Further studies suggested that zinc modulates the activity of dopaminergic neurons via modulating the gating properties of a transient A-type K(+) (K(A)) channel (340). Mitochondrial inhibitor models of PD, such as 1-methyl-4-phenyl-1,2,3,6-tetrahydropyridine (MPTP) intoxication and 6-OHDA intoxication, can be blocked by zinc chelation (341), supports the notion that zinc accumulation could contribute to the pathogenesis of PD. The intracellular accumulation of zinc in PD may be explained by the PARK9 mutation of ATP13A2, a cause of juvenile-onset PD, which was recently shown to impair zinc homeostasis and consequently contributes to lysosomal dysfunction, impaired mitochondrial metabolism, and the accumulation of α-synuclein (342–344). Interestingly, zinc was also found to bind with DJ-1 (345).

METAL DYSHOMEOSTASIS IN HUNTINGTON'S DISEASE

Huntington's disease (HD) is a fatal autosomal dominant neurodegenerative disorder resulting from an expanded polyglutamine tract in the gene encoding huntingtin (Htt) (346). The mutant form of huntingtin (mHtt) is prone to aggregation, which propels the selective dysfunction, and eventual death, of medium spiny neurons (MSNs) within the striatum, manifesting in chorea motor symptoms that characterize the disease symptomatically (347, 348). Motor symptoms are progressive and are accompanied by dementia (including memory, attention, executive function, and cognitive flexibility deficits) (349); there is currently no disease-modifying treatment.

While it is known that mHtt is the principal driver of neuronal toxicity in HD, the molecular pathways activated by mHtt to elicit cell dysfunction and death have yet to be established. Dysregulated metal homeostasis could contribute to neuronal demise in HD. Iron and copper have been shown to be elevated in putamen from autopsy HD subjects (350). More recently, iron elevation has been characterized in living patients by MRI. Iron elevation in putamen and cadueate are elevated in presymptomatic patients, and this is exacerbated in manifest HD (351, 352). Cortical iron levels have also been shown to be elevated by MRI at more advanced disease stages. The cortical regions affected include superior frontal, left middle frontal, and bilaterally anterior cingulate, paracentral and precuneus, while no changes were observed in the thalamus, hippocampus, or amygdala. Iron levels across multiple brain regions have been observed to correlate with CAG triplet repeat length, and iron accumulation has also been shown to correlate with disease severity (352).

Brain copper and iron elevation has also been observed in the CAG140 and R6/2 mouse models of HD. Iron elevation in R6/2 brains is characterized by increased labile iron pool and deposition of iron in lysosomes (353). Decreased amyloid precursor protein (APP) accompanied iron elevation in the R6/2 mouse striatal and cortical tissue (353), which may explain copper and iron deposition, since APP promotes both the export of copper (354) and iron (131, 270). Iron accumulation in this model likely accumulates to disease progression since the iron chelator, desferrioxamine, improved motor function and ameliorated brain atrophy in the R6/2 model (355).

Targeting copper has also shown to confer benefit to HD models—both genetic and dietary interventions slow disease progression in an HTT exon 1 *Drosophila* model of HD (356). Copper interaction with mutant HTT was shown to propel toxicity in this model, since the copper-induced cell death was rescued by substituting key copper-coordinating residues, Met8 and His82, on Htt (356). The copper and zinc ionophores Cq and PBT2 have also been shown to extend life span and improve multiple behavioral, neuroanatomical, and biochemical phenotypes of the R6/2 mouse model of HD (353, 357, 358). PBT2 was recently shown to improve cognitive symptoms in a 26-week phase II clinical trial of 106 subjects (359).

It is not known what causes metal levels to change in HD; it is possible that Htt directly binds metals to alter their regulation. *In vitro* studies have revealed a putative reductase domain in the amino-terminal 171 residues of Htt that reduce Cu^{2+} to Cu^+, and Fe^{3+} to Fe^{2+} (353, 360), but the physiological or pathophysiological implications of this chemistry are unknown. Metals can pathologically interact with Htt by promoting its aggregation. Copper promotes the aggregation of Htt—an effect that can be abolished by the metal complexing agents EDTA and clioquinol (353).

METAL DYSHOMEOSTASIS IN AMYOTROPHIC LATERAL SCLEROSIS

Spinal cord and cortical motor neurons selectively degenerate in amyotrophic lateral sclerosis (ALS), which manifests as progressive motor impairment, paralysis, and eventual death. Riluzole, an inhibitor of tetrodotoxin-sensitive sodium channels, is the only therapy currently available for ALS, and it confers a modest improvement to life span by 2–3 months (361). The cause of sporadic ALS is unknown, but approximately 10% of ALS cases have identified genetic causes. ALS-causing genes include *TARDBP* (362), *FUS* (363), *C9orf72* (364, 365), and *Sod1* (366). The encoded proteins (respectively, TDP-43, FUS, C9ORF72, and SOD1) are observed in aggregated deposits within the brains of carriers (367). It is unknown how these distinct proteins accumulate in disease and propagate neuronal loss.

Mutations in *Sod1* (of which there are over 100) were the first identified causes of familial ALS and the most widely studied. While it is unknown how these mutations confer toxicity, it is likely that mutant SOD confers a toxic gain of function rather than a loss of SOD activity (368). Inclusions of SOD1 decorate the spinal cord in sporadic cases as well as familial cases with mutations in *Sod1* (368, 369); however, it is unclear whether the SOD1 proteopathy is itself the toxic species. SOD1 is a copper-containing protein, and copper is a redox-active metal that could contribute to the oxidative damage in ALS. In support of a role for copper in ALS, spinal cord copper levels have been shown to be elevated in transgenic mice carrying the SOD1G93A mutant (370–372), and lowering copper by both copper chelation and genetic manipulation rescues the ALS phenotype in mutant SOD1 transgenic mouse models (373–378). However, ablation of CCS1, the copper chaperone of SOD1, did not impact on the ALS phenotype of mutant SOD1 transgenic mice, suggesting that if copper is involved in ALS pathogenesis, the insertion of copper in SOD might not be the toxic step (379, 380). However, the moderate copper ionophore and nitric oxide scavenger, copper(II) diacetylbis(N(4)-methylthiosemicarbazonato) (CuII(ATSM)), loads copper into the active site of SOD1, and ameliorates the phenotype, suggesting that copper bound to SOD is indeed not toxic, and might protect against disease pathogenesis (381). However, copper might bind to allosteric sites on mutant SOD1, which are revealed by oxidation of the disulphide bridge required to maintain tertiary structure and stabilize dimeric SOD1 (382, 383). Recent findings have shown that transgenic models of ALS expressing SOD1 with mutations that disrupt copper binding at the active site still demonstrate a marked age-dependent rise in spinal cord copper levels in tissue fractions outside of SOD1 (384), which supports the role for allosteric copper binding to SOD1 in the pathogenic mechanism.

SOD1 also binds zinc, which has also implicated this metal in ALS. Although mutations in SOD1 can be found throughout the structure of the protein, they often result in reduced affinity of zinc binding (385). Zinc-deficient SOD1 might also be implicated in sporadic ALS, since loss of zinc in wild-type SOD1 destabilizes the native homodimer structure of SOD1, which could engender its aggregation (386).

Iron elevation may exacerbate ALS pathology since patients with hemochromatosis (characterized by iron deposition, particularly in the peripheral tissues) are at increased risk of ALS (387). ALS patients also have elevated serum ferritin, which reports elevated body iron stores (388).

METAL-PROTEIN ATTENUATING COMPOUNDS AS A THERAPEUTIC STRATEGY

Clioquinol and PBT2

Clioquinol (5-chloro-7-iodo-quinolin-8-ol) was indicated for parasitic infection but was withdrawn from sale because of a speculated side effect, subacute myelo-optico-neuropathy (SMON) observed in Japanese patients (389). However, this side effect has been questioned (390) because no subsequent clinical trials have observed SMON in participants treated with clioquinol, and the side effect has not been observed in any other country, which might suggest ethnic-specific effects. Clioquinol binds to metals, with a moderate affinity for iron, copper, and zinc (Kd_{Cu} is 1.2×10^{-10} M, Kd_{Zn} is 7×10^{-8} M) (391), and although it was initially considered a chelator (392–395), it has since been discovered that clioquinol has ionophore properties for zinc and copper (390, 396–400). Clioquinol is still considered a moderate iron chelator and not an ionophore since clioquinol lowers iron levels in animal models of iron overload (238, 270, 401–404), and does not cause uptake of iron in cellular assays testing for ionophore activity.

Given the unique properties of clioquinol to both redistribute copper and zinc into cellular compartments and remove excess iron, we hypothesized that this drug might correct metal mis-compartmentalization in AD. Clioquinol might have the multiple benefits of (1) preventing zinc and copper from interacting with Aβ to precipitate its aggregation, (2) redistributing zinc and copper into neurons that are deficient in these metals in AD, and (3) lowering pro-oxidant iron overload of neurons. Indeed, clioquinol was shown to inhibit Aβ oligomer formation (405, 406) and to protect against cell loss in an Aβ-injection model (407), and in transgenic models of AD, clioquinol lowered plaque burden (390) and improved cognitive performance (408). Importantly, in a phase II clinical trial of 32 patients, clioquinol prevented cognitive deterioration (ADAS-Cog) and lowered plasma Aβ42 levels over 36 weeks (409). Despite these promising findings, the development of clioquinol as a therapy for AD was abandoned due to complications with the large-scale (GMP) manufacturing of the compound, which made it unviable.

PBT2 is a second-generation 8-hydroxyquinoline based on the clioquinol chemical scaffold. PBT2 has demonstrated greater efficacy than clioquinol in preclinical models by improving cognitive function after only 11 days in a mouse model of AD (397). In a human phase IIa clinical trial of 78 AD patients, PBT2 treatment over 12 weeks caused a dose-dependent lowering of CSF Aβ and at the highest doses used in the study (250 mg), PBT2 improved executive function (410, 411). In follow-up phase IIb clinical trial, PBT2 did not improve cognitive or amyloid (PET imaging) outcomes. While the phase IIb study was of longer duration than the original phase IIa trial (1 year compared to 12 weeks), the number of trial participants was less; indeed, there were only 15 patients allocated to the placebo group in the study. The study was also complicated by the fact that the placebo group had a confounding reduction in amyloid burden in the brain, which was the primary endpoint of the phase IIb trial. Further clinical testing is required to determine the efficacy of PBT2 for Alzheimer's disease.

In addition to AD, PBT2 has also shown promising preclinical and clinical effects for HD. In a mouse model of HD, PBT2 increased life span, prevented loss of body weight, and improved motor performance (rotarod and clasping) (357). This study prompted a phase II double-blind, placebo controlled clinical trial of 109 HD patients treated with PBT2 (100 and 250 mg) or placebo over 26 weeks. The highest dose improved executive function in HD subjects; however, it did not affect motor disability. A phase II study of PBT2 for HD is planned.

Bis(thiosemicarbazone) Ligands

Copper-containing bis(thiosemicarbazone) compounds such as $Cu^{II}GTSM$ and $Cu^{II}ATSM$ act, in part, by delivering copper to cells. These scaffolds have also been explored in neurodegenerative diseases since the mechanism of action of PBT2 includes copper delivery to neurons. In a cell culture model, $Cu^{II}GTSM$ treatment lowered $A\beta$ levels, GSK3β activity, and phosphorylated tau levels in cell culture (412), which was recapitulated in a mouse model of AD, where cognitive performance was also improved by $Cu^{II}GTSM$(221). $Cu^{II}ATSM$ is a nitric oxide scavenger and donates copper to cells to a lesser degree than $Cu^{II}GTSM$; the ATSM analog did not improve cognitive outcomes in a mouse model for AD, but was neuroprotective in four animal models of PD (413).

IRON CHELATORS

Lowering elevated iron in AD is also a promising therapeutic target given that it was recently shown that high brain iron content (as reflected in CSF ferritin levels) worsened longitudinal cognitive performance and brain atrophy (233). Indeed, an iron chelator was first shown to improve cognitive outcomes in a phase II clinical trial for AD performed in 1991 (414). A single-blind study of 48 AD patients over 2 years showed that the iron chelator, desferrioxamine, improved cognitive outcomes in patients. While the drug is a strong iron chelator, it also binds aluminum, and it was initially hypothesized that the therapeutic benefit of desferrioxamine was imparted by lowering brain aluminium content. But the high binding affinity of iron and the orders of magnitude greater iron content in the brain compared to aluminum have led to a reinterpretation of this finding. Despite these promising findings, a follow-up trial was never performed. However, recently, a phase II clinical trial of the iron chelator deferiprone demonstrated lowered nigral iron content in subjects with PD, and improved their motor symptoms over 18 months (315), which also supports the exploration of iron chelators in clinical trials for AD.

CONCLUSIONS

The prevalence and associated societal and economic costs of neurodegenerative diseases are set to increase in line with the aging demographics of developed nations. However, neurodegenerative diseases remain therapeutically intractable diseases. We have outlined the complex changes in transition metals in AD, PD, HD, and ALS. While perturbations in metal homeostasis are not likely the ultimate cause of any of these diseases, increasing evidence demonstrates that metal dyshomeostasis impacts on neuronal dysfunction and symptom progression. Therefore, targeting metals pharmacologically could be an effective way of altering the trajectory of decline in patients. Moreover, since there are some common changes to metals in neurodegenerative disease (e.g., iron elevation), it is likely that the effective demonstration of a metal-targeting drug for one disease might also prove to have utility for other neurodegenerative diseases. Several phase II clinical trials of metal-targeting drugs have shown promise for various neurodegenerative diseases; we believe the timing is now right for large phase III clinical trials for confirmation of the therapeutic benefit of these drugs.

ACKNOWLEDGMENTS

Supported by funds from the National Health & Medical Research Council, Australian Research Council, Alzheimer's Australia Dementia Research Foundation, and the Cooperative Research Center for Mental Health. The Florey Institute acknowledges the funding support from the Victorian Government's Operational Infrastructure Support program.

REFERENCES

1. Chiti F, Dobson CM. Protein misfolding, functional amyloid, and human disease. *Annu Rev Biochem*. 2006;75:333–366.
2. Doody RS, Thomas RG, Farlow M, Iwatsubo T, Vellas B, Joffe S, et al. Phase 3 trials of solanezumab for mild-to-moderate Alzheimer's disease. *N Engl J Med*. 2014;370(4):311–321.
3. Salloway S, Sperling R, Fox NC, Blennow K, Klunk W, Raskind M, et al. Two phase 3 trials of bapineuzumab in mild-to-moderate Alzheimer's disease. *N Engl J Med*. 2014;370(4):322–333.
4. Sensi SL, Paoletti P, Bush AI, Sekler I. Zinc in the physiology and pathology of the CNS. *Nat Rev Neurosci*. 2009;10(11):780–791.
5. Danscher G, Stoltenberg M. Zinc-specific autometallographic in vivo selenium methods: tracing of zinc-enriched (ZEN) terminals, ZEN pathways, and pools of zinc ions in a multitude of other ZEN cells. *J Histochem Cytochem*. 2005;53(2):141–153.
6. Howell GA, Welch MG, Frederickson CJ. Stimulation-induced uptake and release of zinc in hippocampal slices. *Nature*. 1984;308(5961):736–738.

7. Assaf SY, Chung SH. Release of endogenous Zn2+ from brain tissue during activity. *Nature*. 1984;308(5961):734–736.

8. Vogt K, Mellor J, Tong G, Nicoll R. The actions of synaptically released zinc at hippocampal mossy fiber synapses. *Neuron*. 2000;26(1):187–196.

9. Paoletti P, Ascher P, Neyton J. High-affinity zinc inhibition of NMDA NR1-NR2A receptors. *J Neurosci*. 1997;17(15):5711–5725.

10. Mony L, Kew JN, Gunthorpe MJ, Paoletti P. Allosteric modulators of NR2B-containing NMDA receptors: molecular mechanisms and therapeutic potential. *Br J Pharmacol*. 2009;157(8):1301–1317.

11. Pan E, Zhang XA, Huang Z, Krezel A, Zhao M, Tinberg CE, et al. Vesicular zinc promotes presynaptic and inhibits postsynaptic long-term potentiation of mossy fiber-CA3 synapse. *Neuron*. 2011;71(6):1116–1126.

12. Huang YZ, Pan E, Xiong ZQ, McNamara JO. Zinc-mediated transactivation of TrkB potentiates the hippocampal mossy fiber-CA3 pyramid synapse. *Neuron*. 2008;57(4):546–558.

13. Besser L, Chorin E, Sekler I, Silverman WF, Atkin S, Russell JT, et al. Synaptically released zinc triggers metabotropic signaling via a zinc-sensing receptor in the hippocampus. *J Neurosci*. 2009;29(9):2890–2901.

14. Perez-Rosello T, Anderson CT, Schopfer FJ, Zhao Y, Gilad D, Salvatore SR, et al. Synaptic Zn2+ inhibits neurotransmitter release by promoting endocannabinoid synthesis. *J Neurosci*. 2013;33(22):9259–9272.

15. Hershfinkel M, Kandler K, Knoch ME, Dagan-Rabin M, Aras MA, Abramovitch-Dahan C, et al. Intracellular zinc inhibits KCC2 transporter activity. *Nat Neurosci*. 2009;12(6):725–727.

16. Scheiber IF, Mercer JF, Dringen R. Metabolism and functions of copper in brain. *Prog Neurobiol*. 2014;116:33–57.

17. Gaier ED, Eipper BA, Mains RE. Copper signaling in the mammalian nervous system: synaptic effects. *J Neurosci Res*. 2013;91(1):2–19.

18. Schlief ML, Craig AM, Gitlin JD. NMDA receptor activation mediates copper homeostasis in hippocampal neurons. *J Neurosci*. 2005;25(1):239–246.

19. Schlief ML, West T, Craig AM, Holtzman DM, Gitlin JD. Role of the Menkes copper-transporting ATPase in NMDA receptor-mediated neuronal toxicity. *Proc Natl Acad Sci U S A*. 2006; 103(40):14919–14924.

20. Hopt A, Korte S, Fink H, Panne U, Niessner R, Jahn R, et al. Methods for studying synaptosomal copper release. *J Neurosci Methods*. 2003;128(1–2):159–172.

21. Dodani SC, Domaille DW, Nam CI, Miller EW, Finney LA, Vogt S, et al. Calcium-dependent copper redistributions in neuronal cells revealed by a fluorescent copper sensor and X-ray fluorescence microscopy. *Proc Natl Acad Sci U S A*. 2011;108(15):5980–5985.

22. Vlachova V, Zemkova H, Vyklicky L, Jr. Copper modulation of NMDA responses in mouse and rat cultured hippocampal neurons. *Eur J Neurosci*. 1996;8(11):2257–2264.

23. Trombley PQ, Shepherd GM. Differential modulation by zinc and copper of amino acid receptors from rat olfactory bulb neurons. *J Neurophysiol*. 1996;76(4):2536–2546.

24. Weiser T, Wienrich M. The effects of copper ions on glutamate receptors in cultured rat cortical neurons. *Brain Res*. 1996;742(1–2):211–218.

25. Doreulee N, Yanovsky Y, Haas HL. Suppression of long-term potentiation in hippocampal slices by copper. *Hippocampus*. 1997;7(6):666–669.

26. Peters C, Munoz B, Sepulveda FJ, Urrutia J, Quiroz M, Luza S, et al. Biphasic effects of copper on neurotransmission in rat hippocampal neurons. *J Neurochem*. 2011;119(1):78–88.

27. You H, Tsutsui S, Hameed S, Kannanayakal TJ, Chen L, Xia P, et al. Aβ neurotoxicity depends on interactions between copper ions, prion protein, and N-methyl-D-aspartate receptors. *Proc Natl Acad Sci U S A*. 2012;109(5):1737–1742.

28. Connor JR, Snyder BS, Beard JL, Fine RE, Mufson EJ. Regional distribution of iron and iron-regulatory proteins in the brain in aging and Alzheimer's disease. *J Neurosci Res*. 1992;31(2): 327–335.

29. Halliwell B. Oxidative stress and neurodegeneration: where are we now? *J Neurochem*. 2006;97(6):1634–1658.

30. Connor JR, Menzies SL, St Martin SM, Mufson EJ. Cellular distribution of transferrin, ferritin, and iron in normal and aged human brains. *J Neurosci Res*. 1990;27(4):595–611.

31. Roskams AJ, Connor JR. Iron, transferrin, and ferritin in the rat brain during development and aging. *J Neurochem*. 1994;63(2):709–716.

32. Adhami VM, Husain R, Seth PK. Influence of iron deficiency and lead treatment on behavior and cerebellar and hippocampal polyamine levels in neonatal rats. *Neurochem Res*. 1996;21(8):915–922.

33. Kwik-Uribe CL, Gietzen D, German JB, Golub MS, Keen CL. Chronic marginal iron intakes during early development in mice result in persistent changes in dopamine metabolism and myelin composition. *J Nutr*. 2000;130(11):2821–2830.

34. Ramsey AJ, Hillas PJ, Fitzpatrick PF. Characterization of the active site iron in tyrosine hydroxylase: redox states of the iron. *J Biol Chem*. 1996;271(40):24395–24400.

35. Ramsey AJ, Daubner SC, Ehrlich JI, Fitzpatrick PF. Identification of iron ligands in tyrosine hydroxylase by mutagenesis of conserved histidinyl residues. *Protein Sci.* 1995;4(10):2082–2086.

36. Kuhn DM, Ruskin B, Lovenberg W. Tryptophan hydroxylase. The role of oxygen, iron, and sulfhydryl groups as determinants of stability and catalytic activity. *J Biol Chem.* 1980;255(9): 4137–4143.

37. Gottschall DW, Dietrich RF, Benkovic SJ, Shiman R. Phenylalanine hydroxylase. Correlation of the iron content with activity and the preparation and reconstitution of the apoenzyme. *J Biol Chem.* 1982;257(2):845–849.

38. LeVine SM. Oligodendrocytes and myelin sheaths in normal, quaking and shiverer brains are enriched in iron. *J Neurosci Res.* 1991;29(3):413–419.

39. Roncagliolo M, Garrido M, Walter T, Peirano P, Lozoff B. Evidence of altered central nervous system development in infants with iron deficiency anemia at 6 mo: delayed maturation of auditory brainstem responses. *Am J Clin Nutr.* 1998;68(3):683–690.

40. Ortiz E, Pasquini JM, Thompson K, Felt B, Butkus G, Beard J, et al. Effect of manipulation of iron storage, transport, or availability on myelin composition and brain iron content in three different animal models. *J Neurosci Res.* 2004;77(5):681–689.

41. Gille G, Reichmann H. Iron-dependent functions of mitochondria--relation to neurodegeneration. *J Neural Transm.* 2011;118(3):349–359.

42. Frederickson CJ, Koh JY, Bush AI. The neurobiology of zinc in health and disease. *Nature Rev Neurosci.* 2005;6(6):449–462.

43. Gaither LA, Eide DJ. The human ZIP1 transporter mediates zinc uptake in human K562 erythroleukemia cells. *J Biol Chem.* 2001;276(25):22258–22264.

44. Milon B, Dhermy D, Pountney D, Bourgeois M, Beaumont C. Differential subcellular localization of hZip1 in adherent and non-adherent cells. *FEBS Lett.* 2001;507(3):241–246.

45. Lichten LA, Cousins RJ. Mammalian zinc transporters: nutritional and physiologic regulation. *Ann Rev Nutr.* 2009;29:153–176.

46. Gitan RS, Shababi M, Kramer M, Eide DJ. A cytosolic domain of the yeast Zrt1 zinc transporter is required for its post-translational inactivation in response to zinc and cadmium. *J Biol Chem.* 2003;278(41):39558–39564.

47. Lioumi M, Ferguson CA, Sharpe PT, Freeman T, Marenholz I, Mischke D, et al. Isolation and characterization of human and mouse ZIRTL, a member of the IRT1 family of transporters, mapping within the epidermal differentiation complex. *Genomics.* 1999;62(2):272–280.

48. Qian J, Xu K, Yoo J, Chen TT, Andrews G, Noebels JL. Knockout of Zn transporters Zip-1 and Zip-3 attenuates seizure-induced CA1 neurodegeneration. *J Neurosci.* 2011;31(1):97–104.

49. Kury S, Dreno B, Bezieau S, Giraudet S, Kharfi M, Kamoun R, et al. Identification of SLC39A4, a gene involved in acrodermatitis enteropathica. *Nature Genet.* 2002;31(3):239–240.

50. Emmetsberger J, Mirrione MM, Zhou C, Fernandez-Monreal M, Siddiq MM, Ji K, et al. Tissue plasminogen activator alters intracellular sequestration of zinc through interaction with the transporter ZIP4. *J Neurosci.* 2010;30(19): 6538–6547.

51. Marger L, Schubert CR, Bertrand D. Zinc: an underappreciated modulatory factor of brain function. *Biochem Pharmacol.* 2014;91(4):426–435.

52. Tsuda M, Imaizumi K, Katayama T, Kitagawa K, Wanaka A, Tohyama M, et al. Expression of zinc transporter gene, ZnT-1, is induced after transient forebrain ischemia in the gerbil. *J Neurosci.* 1997;17(17):6678–6684.

53. Nolte C, Gore A, Sekler I, Kresse W, Hershfinkel M, Hoffmann A, et al. ZnT-1 expression in astroglial cells protects against zinc toxicity and slows the accumulation of intracellular zinc. *Glia.* 2004;48(2):145–155.

54. Kim AH, Sheline CT, Tian M, Higashi T, McMahon RJ, Cousins RJ, et al. L-type Ca(2+) channel-mediated Zn(2+) toxicity and modulation by ZnT-1 in PC12 cells. *Brain Res.* 2000; 886(1–2):99–107.

55. Palmiter RD, Cole TB, Quaife CJ, Findley SD. ZnT-3, a putative transporter of zinc into synaptic vesicles. *Proc Natl Acad Sci U S A.* 1996;93(25): 14934–14939.

56. Adlard PA, Parncutt JM, Finkelstein DI, Bush AI. Cognitive loss in zinc transporter-3 knock-out mice: a phenocopy for the synaptic and memory deficits of Alzheimer's disease? *J Neurosci.* 2010;30(5):1631–1636.

57. Huang L, Gitschier J. A novel gene involved in zinc transport is deficient in the lethal milk mouse. *Nature Genet.* 1997;17(3):292–297.

58. Kukic I, Lee JK, Coblentz J, Kelleher SL, Kiselyov K. Zinc-dependent lysosomal enlargement in TRPML1-deficient cells involves MTF-1 transcription factor and ZnT4 (Slc30a4) transporter. *Biochem J.* 2013;451(2):155–163.

59. Palmiter RD, Cole TB, Findley SD. ZnT-2, a mammalian protein that confers resistance to zinc by facilitating vesicular sequestration. *EMBO J.* 1996;15(8):1784–1791.

60. Huang L, Kirschke CP, Gitschier J. Functional characterization of a novel mammalian zinc

transporter, ZnT6. *J Biol Chem*. 2002;277(29): 26389–26395.

61. Bosomworth HJ, Thornton JK, Coneyworth LJ, Ford D, Valentine RA. Efflux function, tissue-specific expression and intracellular trafficking of the Zn transporter ZnT10 indicate roles in adult Zn homeostasis. *Metallomics*. 2012;4(8):771–779.

62. Bosomworth HJ, Adlard PA, Ford D, Valentine RA. Altered expression of ZnT10 in Alzheimer's disease brain. *PLoS ONE*. 2013;8(5):e65475.

63. Rahil-Khazen R, Bolann BJ, Myking A, Ulvik RJ. Multi-element analysis of trace element levels in human autopsy tissues by using inductively coupled atomic emission spectrometry technique (ICP-AES). *J Trace Elem Med Biol*. 2002;16(1):15–25.

64. Davies KM, Hare DJ, Cottam V, Chen N, Hilgers L, Halliday G, et al. Localization of copper and copper transporters in the human brain. *Metallomics*. 2013;5(1):43–51.

65. Waggoner DJ, Drisaldi B, Bartnikas TB, Casareno RL, Prohaska JR, Gitlin JD, et al. Brain copper content and cuproenzyme activity do not vary with prion protein expression level. *J Biol Chem*. 2000;275(11):7455–7458.

66. Dobrowolska J, Dehnhardt M, Matusch A, Zoriy M, Palomero-Gallagher N, Koscielniak P, et al. Quantitative imaging of zinc, copper and lead in three distinct regions of the human brain by laser ablation inductively coupled plasma mass spectrometry. *Talanta*. 2008;74(4):717–723.

67. Becker JS, Zoriy MV, Pickhardt C, Palomero-Gallagher N, Zilles K. Imaging of copper, zinc, and other elements in thin section of human brain samples (hippocampus) by laser ablation inductively coupled plasma mass spectrometry. *Anal Chem*. 2005;77(10):3208–3216.

68. Kaplan JH, Lutsenko S. Copper transport in mammalian cells: special care for a metal with special needs. *J Biol Chem*. 2009;284(38):25461–25465.

69. Rae TD, Schmidt PJ, Pufahl RA, Culotta VC, O'Halloran TV. Undetectable intracellular free copper: the requirement of a copper chaperone for superoxide dismutase. *Science*. 1999;284(5415):805–808.

70. Sharp PA. Ctr1 and its role in body copper homeostasis. *Int J Biochem Cell Biol*. 2003;35(3): 288–291.

71. Dancis A, Haile D, Yuan DS, Klausner RD. The Saccharomyces cerevisiae copper transport protein (Ctr1p): biochemical characterization, regulation by copper, and physiologic role in copper uptake. *J Biol Chem*. 1994;269(41): 25660–25667.

72. Eisses JF, Kaplan JH. The mechanism of copper uptake mediated by human CTR1: a mutational analysis. *J Biol Chem*. 2005;280(44):37159–37168.

73. Puig S, Lee J, Lau M, Thiele DJ. Biochemical and genetic analyses of yeast and human high affinity copper transporters suggest a conserved mechanism for copper uptake. *J Biol Chem*. 2002;277(29):26021–26030.

74. Kuo YM, Zhou B, Cosco D, Gitschier J. The copper transporter CTR1 provides an essential function in mammalian embryonic development. *Proc Natl Acad Sci U S A*. 2001;98(12):6836–6841.

75. Lee J, Prohaska JR, Thiele DJ. Essential role for mammalian copper transporter Ctr1 in copper homeostasis and embryonic development. *Proc Natl Acad Sci U S A*. 2001;98(12):6842–6847.

76. Molloy SA, Kaplan JH. Copper-dependent recycling of hCTR1, the human high affinity copper transporter. *J Biol Chem*. 2009; 284(43): 29704–29713.

77. Nose Y, Wood LK, Kim BE, Prohaska JR, Fry RS, Spears JW, et al. Ctr1 is an apical copper transporter in mammalian intestinal epithelial cells in vivo that is controlled at the level of protein stability. *J Biol Chem*. 2010;285(42):32385–32392.

78. Petris MJ, Smith K, Lee J, Thiele DJ. Copper-stimulated endocytosis and degradation of the human copper transporter, hCtr1. *J Biol Chem*. 2003;278(11):9639–9646.

79. Guo Y, Smith K, Petris MJ. Cisplatin stabilizes a multimeric complex of the human Ctr1 copper transporter: requirement for the extracellular methionine-rich clusters. *J Biol Chem*. 2004;279(45): 46393–46399.

80. Klomp AE, Tops BB, Van Denberg IE, Berger R, Klomp LW. Biochemical characterization and subcellular localization of human copper transporter 1 (hCTR1). *Biochem J*. 2002;364(Pt 2): 497–505.

81. Knutson MD. Steap proteins: implications for iron and copper metabolism. *Nutrition Rev*. 2007;65(7):335–340.

82. Wyman S, Simpson RJ, McKie AT, Sharp PA. Dcytb (Cybrd1) functions as both a ferric and a cupric reductase in vitro. *FEBS Lett*. 2008;582(13):1901–1906.

83. Freedman JH, Ciriolo MR, Peisach J. The role of glutathione in copper metabolism and toxicity. *J Biol Chem*. 1989;264(10):5598–5605.

84. Freedman JH, Peisach J. Resistance of cultured hepatoma cells to copper toxicity. Purification and characterization of the hepatoma metallothionein. *Biochim Biophys Acta*. 1989; 992(2): 145–154.

85. Culotta VC, Klomp LW, Strain J, Casareno RL, Krems B, Gitlin JD. The copper chaperone for superoxide dismutase. *J Biol Chem*. 1997;272(38): 23469–23472.

86. Bertinato J, L'Abbe MR. Copper modulates the degradation of copper chaperone for Cu,Zn superoxide dismutase by the 26 S proteosome. *J Biol Chem.* 2003;278(37):35071–35078.

87. Wong PC, Waggoner D, Subramaniam JR, Tessarollo L, Bartnikas TB, Culotta VC, et al. Copper chaperone for superoxide dismutase is essential to activate mammalian Cu/Zn superoxide dismutase. *Proc Natl Acad Sci U S A.* 2000; 97(6):2886–2891.

88. Glerum DM, Shtanko A, Tzagoloff A. Characterization of COX17, a yeast gene involved in copper metabolism and assembly of cytochrome oxidase. *J Biol Chem.* 1996;271(24):14504–14509.

89. Horng YC, Cobine PA, Maxfield AB, Carr HS, Winge DR. Specific copper transfer from the Cox17 metallochaperone to both Sco1 and Cox11 in the assembly of yeast cytochrome C oxidase. *J Biol Chem.* 2004;279(34):35334–35340.

90. Takahashi Y, Kako K, Kashiwabara S, Takehara A, Inada Y, Arai H, et al. Mammalian copper chaperone Cox17p has an essential role in activation of cytochrome C oxidase and embryonic development. *Mol Cell Biol.* 2002;22(21):7614–7621.

91. Klomp LW, Lin SJ, Yuan DS, Klausner RD, Culotta VC, Gitlin JD. Identification and functional expression of HAH1, a novel human gene involved in copper homeostasis. *J Biol Chem.* 1997;272(14):9221–9226.

92. Wang Y, Hodgkinson V, Zhu S, Weisman GA, Petris MJ. Advances in the understanding of mammalian copper transporters. *Adv Nutr.* 2011; 2(2): 129–137.

93. La Fontaine S, Ackland ML, Mercer JF. Mammalian copper-transporting P-type ATPases, ATP7A and ATP7B: emerging roles. *Int J Biochem Cell Biol.* 2010;42(2):206–209.

94. Vulpe C, Levinson B, Whitney S, Packman S, Gitschier J. Isolation of a candidate gene for Menkes disease and evidence that it encodes a copper-transporting ATPase. *Nature Genet.* 1993; 3(1): 7–13.

95. Danks DM, Stevens BJ, Campkell PE, Cartwright EC, Gillespie JM, Townley RR, et al. Menkes kinky-hair syndrome: an inherited defect in the intestinal absorption of copper with widespread effects. *Birth Defects.* 1974;10(10):132–137.

96. Wu J, Forbes JR, Chen HS, Cox DW. The LEC rat has a deletion in the copper transporting ATPase gene homologous to the Wilson disease gene. *Nature Genet.* 1994;7(4):541–545.

97. Swaiman KF, Machen VL. Iron uptake by mammalian cortical neurons. *Ann Neurol.* 1984;16(1):66–70.

98. Connor JR, Fine RE. The distribution of transferrin immunoreactivity in the rat central nervous system. *Brain Res.* 1986;368(2):319–328.

99. Harris WR. Estimation of the ferrous-transferrin binding constants based on thermodynamic studies of nickel(II)-transferrin. *J Inorg Biochem.* 1986;27(1):41–52.

100. He QY, Mason AB, Woodworth RC, Tam BM, MacGillivray RT, Grady JK, et al. Inequivalence of the two tyrosine ligands in the N-lobe of human serum transferrin. *Biochemistry.* 1997;36(48):14853–14860.

101. Dautry-Varsat A, Ciechanover A, Lodish HF. pH and the recycling of transferrin during receptor-mediated endocytosis. *Proc Natl Acad Sci U S A.* 1983;80(8):2258–2262.

102. Fleming RE, Migas MC, Holden CC, Waheed A, Britton RS, Tomatsu S, et al. Transferrin receptor 2: continued expression in mouse liver in the face of iron overload and in hereditary hemochromatosis. *Proc Natl Acad Sci U S A.* 2000;97(5):2214–2219.

103. Kawabata H, Germain RS, Ikezoe T, Tong X, Green EM, Gombart AF, et al. Regulation of expression of murine transferrin receptor 2. *Blood.* 2001;98(6):1949–1954.

104. Kawabata H, Nakamaki T, Ikonomi P, Smith RD, Germain RS, Koeffler HP. Expression of transferrin receptor 2 in normal and neoplastic hematopoietic cells. *Blood.* 2001;98(9):2714–2719.

105. Levy JE, Jin O, Fujiwara Y, Kuo F, Andrews NC. Transferrin receptor is necessary for development of erythrocytes and the nervous system. *Nature Genet.* 1999;21(4):396–399.

106. Mastroberardino PG, Hoffman EK, Horowitz MP, Betarbet R, Taylor G, Cheng D, et al. A novel transferrin/TfR2-mediated mitochondrial iron transport system is disrupted in Parkinson's disease. *Neurobiol Dis.* 2009;34(3):417–431.

107. Cheng Y, Zak O, Aisen P, Harrison SC, Walz T. Structure of the human transferrin receptor-transferrin complex. *Cell.* 2004;116(4):565–576.

108. McKie AT, Barrow D, Latunde-Dada GO, Rolfs A, Sager G, Mudaly E, et al. An iron-regulated ferric reductase associated with the absorption of dietary iron. *Science.* 2001;291(5509):1755–1759.

109. Lesuisse E, Casteras-Simon M, Labbe P. Cytochrome P-450 reductase is responsible for the ferrireductase activity associated with isolated plasma membranes of Saccharomyces cerevisiae. *FEMS Microbiol Lett.* 1997;156(1):147–152.

110. Lee PL, Halloran C, Cross AR, Beutler E. NADH-ferric reductase activity associated with dihydropteridine reductase. *Biochem Biophys Res Commun.* 2000;271(3):788–795.

111. Ohgami RS, Campagna DR, Greer EL, Antiochos B, McDonald A, Chen J, et al. Identification of a

ferrireductase required for efficient transferrin-dependent iron uptake in erythroid cells. *Nature Genet.* 2005;37(11):1264–1269.

112. Gunshin H, Starr CN, Direnzo C, Fleming MD, Jin J, Greer EL, et al. Cybrd1 (duodenal cytochrome b) is not necessary for dietary iron absorption in mice. *Blood.* 2005;106(8):2879–2883.

113. Gunshin H, Fujiwara Y, Custodio AO, Direnzo C, Robine S, Andrews NC. Slc11a2 is required for intestinal iron absorption and erythropoiesis but dispensable in placenta and liver. *J Clin Invest.* 2005;115(5):1258–1266.

114. Gunshin H, Mackenzie B, Berger UV, Gunshin Y, Romero MF, Boron WF, et al. Cloning and characterization of a mammalian proton-coupled metal-ion transporter. *Nature.* 1997;388(6641):482–488.

115. Fleming MD, Trenor CC, 3rd, Su MA, Foernzler D, Beier DR, Dietrich WF, et al. Microcytic anaemia mice have a mutation in Nramp2, a candidate iron transporter gene. *Nature Genet.* 1997;16(4):383–386.

116. Arredondo M, Munoz P, Mura CV, Nunez MT. DMT1, a physiologically relevant apical Cu1+ transporter of intestinal cells. *Am J Physiol Cell Physiol.* 2003;284(6):C1525–1530.

117. Wang X, Li GJ, Zheng W. Upregulation of DMT1 expression in choroidal epithelia of the blood-CSF barrier following manganese exposure in vitro. *Brain Res.* 2006;1097(1):1–10.

118. Picard V, Govoni G, Jabado N, Gros P. Nramp 2 (DCT1/DMT1) expressed at the plasma membrane transports iron and other divalent cations into a calcein-accessible cytoplasmic pool. *J Biol Chem.* 2000;275(46):35738–35745.

119. Granick S, Michaelis L. Ferritin and Apoferritin. *Science.* 1942;95(2469):439–440.

120. Harrison PM, Arosio P. The ferritins: molecular properties, iron storage function and cellular regulation. *Biochim Biophys Acta.* 1996;1275(3):161–203.

121. Lawson DM, Treffry A, Artymiuk PJ, Harrison PM, Yewdall SJ, Luzzago A, et al. Identification of the ferroxidase centre in ferritin. *FEBS Lett.* 1989;254(1–2):207–210.

122. Broxmeyer HE, Cooper S, Levi S, Arosio P. Mutated recombinant human heavy-chain ferritins and myelosuppression in vitro and in vivo: a link between ferritin ferroxidase activity and biological function. *Proc Natl Acad Sci U S A.* 1991;88(3):770–774.

123. Kaneko Y, Kitamoto T, Tateishi J, Yamaguchi K. Ferritin immunohistochemistry as a marker for microglia. *Acta Neuropathol.* 1989; 79(2): 129–136.

124. Sulzer D, Bogulavsky J, Larsen KE, Behr G, Karatekin E, Kleinman MH, et al. Neuromelanin biosynthesis is driven by excess cytosolic catecholamines not accumulated by synaptic vesicles. *Proc Natl Acad Sci U S A.* 2000;97(22):11869–11874.

125. Ganz T. Cellular iron: ferroportin is the only way out. *Cell Metab.* 2005;1(3):155–157.

126. Donovan A, Lima CA, Pinkus JL, Pinkus GS, Zon LI, Robine S, et al. The iron exporter ferroportin/Slc40a1 is essential for iron homeostasis. *Cell Metab.* 2005;1(3):191–200.

127. Thomas C, Oates PS. Differences in the uptake of iron from Fe(II) ascorbate and Fe(III) citrate by IEC-6 cells and the involvement of ferroportin/IREG-1/MTP-1/SLC40A1. *Pflugers Arch.* 2004;448(4):431–437.

128. Nemeth E, Tuttle MS, Powelson J, Vaughn MB, Donovan A, Ward DM, et al. Hepcidin regulates cellular iron efflux by binding to ferroportin and inducing its internalization. *Science.* 2004;306(5704):2090–2093.

129. Rivera S, Nemeth E, Gabayan V, Lopez MA, Farshidi D, Ganz T. Synthetic hepcidin causes rapid dose-dependent hypoferremia and is concentrated in ferroportin-containing organs. *Blood.* 2005;106(6):2196–2199.

130. Ramey G, Deschemin JC, Durel B, Canonne-Hergaux F, Nicolas G, Vaulont S. Hepcidin targets ferroportin for degradation in hepatocytes. *Haematologica.* 2010;95(3):501–504.

131. Duce JA, Tsatsanis A, Cater MA, James SA, Robb E, Wikhe K, et al. Iron-export ferroxidase activity of β-amyloid precursor protein is inhibited by zinc in Alzheimer's disease. *Cell.* 2010;142(6):857–867.

132. Wong BX, Ayton S, Lam LQ, Lei P, Adlard PA, Bush AI, et al. A comparison of ceruloplasmin to biological polyanions in promoting the oxidation of Fe under physiologically relevant conditions. *Biochim Biophys Acta.* 2014;1840(12): 3299–3310.

133. Wong BX, Tsatsanis A, Lim LQ, Adlard PA, Bush AI, Duce JA. beta-Amyloid precursor protein does not possess ferroxidase activity but does stabilize the cell surface ferrous iron exporter ferroportin. *PLoS ONE.* 2014;9(12):e114174.

134. McCarthy RC, Park YH, Kosman DJ. sAPP modulates iron efflux from brain microvascular endothelial cells by stabilizing the ferrous iron exporter ferroportin. *EMBO Rep.* 2014;15(7):809–815.

135. Wan L, Nie G, Zhang J, Zhao B. Overexpression of human wild-type amyloid-beta protein precursor decreases the iron content and increases the oxidative stress of neuroblastoma SH-SY5Y cells. *J Alzheimers Dis.* 2012;30(3):523–530.

136. Osaki S. Kinetic studies of ferrous ion oxidation with crystalline human ferroxidase (ceruloplasmin). *J Biol Chem*. 1966;241(21):5053–5059.

137. Patel BN, Dunn RJ, Jeong SY, Zhu Q, Julien J-P, David S. Ceruloplasmin regulates iron levels in the CNS and prevents free radical injury. *J Neurosci*. 2002;22(15):6578–6586.

138. Klomp LW, Gitlin JD. Expression of the ceruloplasmin gene in the human retina and brain: implications for a pathogenic model in aceruloplasminemia. *Human Mol Genet*. 1996;5(12):1989–1996.

139. Klomp LW, Farhangrazi ZS, Dugan LL, Gitlin JD. Ceruloplasmin gene expression in the murine central nervous system. *J Clin Invest*. 1996;98(1):207–215.

140. Patel BN, Dunn RJ, David S. Alternative RNA splicing generates a glycosylphosphatidylinositol-anchored form of ceruloplasmin in mammalian brain. *J Biol Chem*. 2000;275(6):4305–4310.

141. Kono S, Yoshida K, Tomosugi N, Terada T, Hamaya Y, Kanaoka S, et al. Biological effects of mutant ceruloplasmin on hepcidin-mediated internalization of ferroportin. *Biochim Biophys Acta*. 2010;1802(11):968–975.

142. Harris ZL, Takahashi Y, Miyajima H, Serizawa M, MacGillivray RT, Gitlin JD. Aceruloplasminemia: molecular characterization of this disorder of iron metabolism. *Proc Natl Acad Sci U S A*. 1995;92(7):2539–2543.

143. Olivieri S, Conti A, Iannaccone S, Cannistraci CV, Campanella A, Barbariga M, et al. Ceruloplasmin oxidation, a feature of Parkinson's disease CSF, inhibits ferroxidase activity and promotes cellular iron retention. *J Neurosci*. 2011;31(50):18568–18577.

144. Persichini T, De Francesco G, Capone C, Cutone A, Bonaccorsi di Patti MC, Colasanti M, et al. Reactive oxygen species are involved in ferroportin degradation induced by ceruloplasmin mutant Arg701Trp. *Neurochem Int*. 2012;60(4):360–364.

145. Qian ZM, Chang YZ, Zhu L, Yang L, Du JR, Ho KP, et al. Development and iron-dependent expression of hephaestin in different brain regions of rats. *J Cell Biochem*. 2007;102(5):1225–1233.

146. Danscher G, Jensen KB, Frederickson CJ, Kemp K, Andreasen A, Juhl S, et al. Increased amount of zinc in the hippocampus and amygdala of Alzheimer's diseased brains: a proton-induced X-ray emission spectroscopic analysis of cryostat sections from autopsy material. *J Neurosci Methods*. 1997;76(1):53–59.

147. Panayi AE, Spyrou NM, Iversen BS, White MA, Part P. Determination of cadmium and zinc in

Alzheimer's brain tissue using inductively coupled plasma mass spectrometry. *J Neurol Sci*. 2002;195(1):1–10.

148. Samudralwar DL, Diprete CC, Ni BF, Ehmann WD, Markesbery WR. Elemental imbalances in the olfactory pathway in Alzheimer's disease. *J Neurol Sci*. 1995;130(2):139–145.

149. Deibel MA, Ehmann WD, Markesbery WR. Copper, iron, and zinc imbalances in severely degenerated brain regions in Alzheimer's disease: possible relation to oxidative stress. *J Neurol Sci*. 1996;143(1–2):137–142.

150. Religa D, Strozyk D, Cherny RA, Volitaskis I, Haroutunian V, Winblad B, et al. Elevated cortical zinc in Alzheimer disease. *Neurology*. 2006;67(1):69–75.

151. Schrag M, Mueller C, Oyoyo U, Smith MA, Kirsch WM. Iron, zinc and copper in the Alzheimer's disease brain: a quantitative meta-analysis. Some insight on the influence of citation bias on scientific opinion. *Prog Neurobiol*. 2011;94(3):296–306.

152. Lyubartseva G, Smith JL, Markesbery WR, Lovell MA. Alterations of zinc transporter proteins ZnT-1, ZnT-4 and ZnT-6 in preclinical Alzheimer's disease brain. *Brain Pathol (Zurich, Switzerland)*. 2010;20(2):343–350.

153. Beyer N, Coulson DT, Heggarty S, Ravid R, Hellemans J, Irvine GB, et al. Zinc transporter mRNA levels in Alzheimer's disease postmortem brain. *J Alzheimers Dis*. 2012;29(4):863–873.

154. Takeda A, Minami A, Takefuta S, Tochigi M, Oku N. Zinc homeostasis in the brain of adult rats fed zinc-deficient diet. *J Neurosci Res*. 2001;63(5):447–452.

155. Chowanadisai W, Kelleher SL, Lonnerdal B. Zinc deficiency is associated with increased brain zinc import and LIV-1 expression and decreased ZnT-1 expression in neonatal rats. *J Nutr*. 2005;135(5):1002–1007.

156. Stoltenberg M, Bush AI, Bach G, Smidt K, Larsen A, Rungby J, et al. Amyloid plaques arise from zinc-enriched cortical layers in APP/PS1 transgenic mice and are paradoxically enlarged with dietary zinc deficiency. *Neuroscience*. 2007;150(2):357–369.

157. Smith JL, Xiong S, Lovell MA. 4-Hydroxynonenal disrupts zinc export in primary rat cortical cells. *Neurotoxicology*. 2006;27(1):1–5.

158. Bush AI, Multhaup G, Moir RD, Williamson TG, Small DH, Rumble B, et al. A novel zinc(II) binding site modulates the function of the beta A4 amyloid protein precursor of Alzheimer's disease. *J Biol Chem*. 1993;268(22):16109–16112.

159. Bush AI, Pettingell WH, Multhaup G, d Paradis M, Vonsattel JP, Gusella JF, et al. Rapid induction of Alzheimer A beta amyloid formation by zinc. *Science*. 1994;265(5177):1464–1467.

160. Noy D, Solomonov I, Sinkevich O, Arad T, Kjaer K, Sagi I. Zinc-amyloid beta interactions on a millisecond time-scale stabilize non-fibrillar Alzheimer-related species. *J Am Chem Soc*. 2008;130(4):1376–1383.

161. Huang X, Atwood CS, Moir RD, Hartshorn MA, Vonsattel JP, Tanzi RE, et al. Zinc-induced Alzheimer's Abeta1–40 aggregation is mediated by conformational factors. *J Biol Chem*. 1997;272(42):26464–26470.

162. Huang X, Atwood CS, Moir RD, Hartshorn MA, Tanzi RE, Bush AI. Trace metal contamination initiates the apparent auto-aggregation, amyloidosis, and oligomerization of Alzheimer's Abeta peptides. *J Biol Inorg Chem*. 2004;9(8): 954–960.

163. Yoshiike Y, Tanemura K, Murayama O, Akagi T, Murayama M, Sato S, et al. New insights on how metals disrupt amyloid beta-aggregation and their effects on amyloid-beta cytotoxicity. *J Biol Chem*. 2001;276(34):32293–32299.

164. Sharma AK, Pavlova ST, Kim J, Finkelstein D, Hawco NJ, Rath NP, et al. Bifunctional compounds for controlling metal-mediated aggregation of the abeta42 peptide. *J Am Chem Soc*. 2012;134(15):6625–6636.

165. Solomonov I, Korkotian E, Born B, Feldman Y, Bitler A, Rahimi F, et al. Zn2+-Abeta40 complexes form metastable quasi-spherical oligomers that are cytotoxic to cultured hippocampal neurons. *J Biol Chem*. 2012;287(24):20555–20564.

166. Chen WT, Liao YH, Yu HM, Cheng IH, Chen YR. Distinct effects of Zn2+, Cu2+, Fe3+, and Al3+ on amyloid-beta stability, oligomerization, and aggregation: amyloid-beta destabilization promotes annular protofibril formation. *J Biol Chem*. 2011;286(11):9646–9656.

167. Bush AI, Pettingell WH, Paradis MD, Tanzi RE. Modulation of A beta adhesiveness and secretase site cleavage by zinc. *J Biol Chem*. 1994;269(16):12152–12158.

168. Crouch PJ, Tew DJ, Du T, Nguyen DN, Caragounis A, Filiz G, et al. Restored degradation of the Alzheimer's amyloid-beta peptide by targeting amyloid formation. *J Neurochem*. 2009;108(5):1198–1207.

169. Lammich S, Kojro E, Postina R, Gilbert S, Pfeiffer R, Jasionowski M, et al. Constitutive and regulated alpha-secretase cleavage of Alzheimer's amyloid precursor protein by a disintegrin metalloprotease. *Proc Natl Acad Sci U S A*. 1999;96(7):3922–3927.

170. Hoke DE, Tan JL, Ilaya NT, Culvenor JG, Smith SJ, White AR, et al. In vitro gamma-secretase cleavage of the Alzheimer's amyloid precursor protein correlates to a subset of presenilin complexes and is inhibited by zinc. *FEBS J*. 2005;272(21):5544–5557.

171. Greenough MA, Volitaskis I, Li Q-X, Laughton KM, Evin G, Ho M, et al. Presenilins promote the cellular uptake of copper and zinc and maintain copper chaperone of SOD1-dependent copper/zinc superoxide dismutase activity. *J Biol Chem*. 2011;286(11):9776–9786.

172. Boom A, Authelet M, Dedecker R, Frédérick C, Van Heurck R, Daubie V, et al. Bimodal modulation of tau protein phosphorylation and conformation by extracellular Zn2+ in human-tau transfected cells. *Biochim Biophys Acta*. 2009;1793(6):1058–1067.

173. Mo Z-Y, Zhu Y-Z, Zhu H-L, Fan J-B, Chen J, Liang Y. Low micromolar zinc accelerates the fibrillization of human tau via bridging of Cys-291 and Cys-322. *J Biol Chem*. 2009;284(50):34648–34657.

174. Huang Y, Wu Z, Cao Y, Lang M, Lu B, Zhou B. Zinc binding directly regulates tau toxicity independent of tau hyperphosphorylation. *Cell Rep*. 2014.

175. Suh SW, Jensen KB, Jensen MS, Silva DS, Kesslak PJ, Danscher G, et al. Histochemically-reactive zinc in amyloid plaques, angiopathy, and degenerating neurons of Alzheimer's diseased brains. *Brain Res*. 2000;852(2):274–278.

176. An W-L, Bjorkdahl C, Liu R, Cowburn RF, Winblad B, Pei J-J. Mechanism of zinc-induced phosphorylation of p70 S6 kinase and glycogen synthase kinase 3beta in SH-SY5Y neuroblastoma cells. *J Neurochem*. 2005;92(5): 1104–1115.

177. Pei J-J, An W-L, Zhou X-W, Nishimura T, Norberg J, Benedikz E, et al. P70 S6 kinase mediates tau phosphorylation and synthesis. *FEBS Lett*. 2006;580(1):107–114.

178. Lei P, Ayton S, Bush AI, Adlard PA. GSK-3 in neurodegenerative diseases. *Int J Alz Dis*. 2011;2011:189246.

179. Barnham KJ, Bush AI. Biological metals and metal-targeting compounds in major neurodegenerative diseases. *Chem Soc Rev*. 2014;43(19):6727–6749.

180. Lovell MA, Robertson JD, Teesdale WJ, Campbell JL, Markesbery WR. Copper, iron and zinc in Alzheimer's disease senile plaques. *J Neurol Sci*. 1998;158(1):47–52.

181. James SA, Volitakis I, Adlard PA, Duce JA, Masters CL, Cherny RA, et al. Elevated labile Cu is associated with oxidative pathology

in Alzheimer disease. *Free Radic Biol Med.* 2012;52(2):298–302.

182. Brady DC, Crowe MS, Turski ML, Hobbs GA, Yao X, Chaikuad A, et al. Copper is required for oncogenic BRAF signalling and tumorigenesis. *Nature.* 2014;509(7501):492–496.

183. Daniel AG, Peterson EJ, Farrell NP. The bioinorganic chemistry of apoptosis: potential inhibitory zinc binding sites in caspase-3. *Angew Chem Int Ed Engl.* 2014;53(16):4098–4101.

184. Maurer I, Zierz S, Moller HJ. A selective defect of cytochrome c oxidase is present in brain of Alzheimer disease patients. *Neurobiol Aging.* 2000;21(3):455–462.

185. Bayer TA, Schafer S, Simons A, Kemmling A, Kamer T, Tepest R, et al. Dietary Cu stabilizes brain superoxide dismutase 1 activity and reduces amyloid Abeta production in APP23 transgenic mice. *Proc Natl Acad Sci U S A.* 2003;100(24):14187–14192.

186. McGeer EG, McGeer PL, Harrop R, Akiyama H, Kamo H. Correlations of regional postmortem enzyme activities with premortem local glucose metabolic rates in Alzheimer's disease. *J Neurosci Res.* 1990;27(4):612–619.

187. Malm TM, Iivonen H, Goldsteins G, Keksa-Goldsteine V, Ahtoniemi T, Kanninen K, et al. Pyrrolidine dithiocarbamate activates Akt and improves spatial learning in APP/PS1 mice without affecting beta-amyloid burden. *J Neurosci.* 2007;27(14):3712–3721.

188. Borchardt T, Camakaris J, Cappai R, Masters CL, Beyreuther K, Multhaup G. Copper inhibits beta-amyloid production and stimulates the non-amyloidogenic pathway of amyloid-precursor-protein secretion. *Biochem J.* 1999; 344 Pt 2: 461–467.

189. Cater MA, McInnes KT, Li Q-X, Volitaskis I, La Fontaine S, Mercer JFB, et al. Intracellular copper deficiency increases amyloid-beta secretion by diverse mechanisms. *Biochem J.* 2008; 412(1): 141–152.

190. Hung YH, Robb EL, Volitakis I, Ho M, Evin G, Li Q-X, et al. Paradoxical condensation of copper with elevated beta-amyloid in lipid rafts under cellular copper deficiency conditions: implications for Alzheimer disease. *J Biol Chem.* 2009;284(33):21899–21907.

191. Atwood CS, Moir RD, Huang X, Scarpa RC, Bacarra NM, Romano DM, et al. Dramatic aggregation of Alzheimer abeta by Cu(II) is induced by conditions representing physiological acidosis. *J Biol Chem.* 1998;273(21):12817–12826.

192. Faller P, Hureau C, Berthoumieu O. Role of metal ions in the self-assembly of the Alzheimer's amyloid-beta peptide. *Inorg Chem.* 2013;52(21):12193–12206.

193. Sarell CJ, Wilkinson SR, Viles JH. Substoichiometric levels of Cu2+ ions accelerate the kinetics of fiber formation and promote cell toxicity of amyloid-{beta} from Alzheimer disease. *J Biol Chem.* 2010;285(53):41533–41540.

194. Pedersen JT, Ostergaard J, Rozlosnik N, Gammelgaard B, Heegaard NH. Cu(II) mediates kinetically distinct, non-amyloidogenic aggregation of amyloid-beta peptides. *J Biol Chem.* 2011;286(30):26952–26963.

195. Jiao Y, Han DX, Yang P. Molecular modeling of the inhibitory mechanism of copper(II) on aggregation of amyloid beta-peptide. *Sci China Ser B.* 2005;48(6):580–590.

196. Jiao Y, Yang P. Mechanism of copper(II) inhibiting Alzheimer's amyloid beta-peptide from aggregation: a molecular dynamics investigation. *J Phys Chem B.* 2007;111(26):7646–7655.

197. Tõugu V, Karafin A, Zovo K, Chung RS, Howells C, West AK, et al. Zn(II)- and Cu(II)-induced non-fibrillar aggregates of amyloid-beta (1–42) peptide are transformed to amyloid fibrils, both spontaneously and under the influence of metal chelators. *J Neurochem.* 2009;110(6):1784–1795.

198. Huang X, Cuajungco MP, Atwood CS, Hartshorn MA, Tyndall JD, Hanson GR, et al. Cu(II) potentiation of alzheimer abeta neurotoxicity: correlation with cell-free hydrogen peroxide production and metal reduction. *J Biol Chem.* 1999;274(52):37111–37116.

199. Cuajungco MP, Goldstein LE, Nunomura A, Smith MA, Lim JT, Atwood CS, et al. Evidence that the beta-amyloid plaques of Alzheimer's disease represent the redox-silencing and entombment of abeta by zinc. *J Biol Chem.* 2000;275(26):19439–19442.

200. Choi JS, Braymer JJ, Nanga RP, Ramamoorthy A, Lim MH. Design of small molecules that target metal-A{beta} species and regulate metal-induced A{beta} aggregation and neurotoxicity. *Proc Natl Acad Sci U S A.* 2010;107(51):21990–21995.

201. Wu W-h, Lei P, Liu Q, Hu J, Gunn AP, Chen M-s, et al. Sequestration of copper from beta-amyloid promotes selective lysis by cyclen-hybrid cleavage agents. *J Biol Chem.* 2008;283(46):31657–31664.

202. Perrone L, Mothes E, Vignes M, Mockel A, Figueroa C, Miquel M-C, et al. Copper transfer from Cu-Abeta to human serum albumin inhibits aggregation, radical production and reduces Abeta toxicity. *Chem Bio Chem.* 2010;11(1):110–118.

203. Huang X, Atwood CS, Hartshorn MA, Multhaup G, Goldstein LE, Scarpa RC, et al. The A beta peptide of Alzheimer's disease directly produces hydrogen peroxide through metal ion reduction. *Biochemistry.* 1999;38(24): 7609–7616.

204. Jiang D, Men L, Wang J, Zhang Y, Chickenyen S, Wang Y, et al. Redox reactions of copper complexes formed with different beta-amyloid peptides and their sneuropathological [correction of neuropathalogical] relevance. *Biochemistry.* 2007;46(32):9270–9282.

205. Barnham KJ, Cappai R, Cherny RA, Bush AI, Masters CL. Redox-mediated A beta neurotoxicity. *J Neurochem.* 2004;88 Suppl 1:4.

206. Barnham KJ, Haeffner F, Ciccotosto GD, Curtain CC, Tew DJ, Mavros C, et al. Tyrosine gated electron transfer is key to the toxic mechanism of Alzheimer's disease beta-amyloid. *FASEB J.* 2004;18(12):1427–1429.

207. Barnham KJ, Ciccotosto GD, Tickler AK, Ali FE, Smith DG, Williamson NA, et al. Neurotoxic, redox-competent Alzheimer's beta-amyloid is released from lipid membrane by methionine oxidation. *J Biol Chem.* 2003;278(44):42959–42965.

208. Lauderback CM, Hackett JM, Keller JN, Varadarajan S, Szweda L, Kindy M, et al. Vulnerability of synaptosomes from apoE knock-out mice to structural and oxidative modifications induced by A beta(1–40): implications for Alzheimer's disease. *Biochemistry.* 2001; 40(8): 2548–2554.

209. Puglielli L, Friedlich AL, Setchell KDR, Nagano S, Opazo C, Cherny RA, et al. Alzheimer disease beta-amyloid activity mimics cholesterol oxidase. *J Clin Invest.* 2005;115(9):2556–2563.

210. Turnbull S, Tabner BJ, El-Agnaf OM, Twyman LJ, Allsop D. New evidence that the Alzheimer beta-amyloid peptide does not spontaneously form free radicals: an ESR study using a series of spin-traps. *Free Radic Biol Med.* 2001;30(10):1154–1162.

211. Atwood CS, Perry G, Zeng H, Kato Y, Jones WD, Ling K-Q, et al. Copper mediates dityrosine cross-linking of Alzheimer's amyloid-beta. *Biochemistry.* 2004;43(2):560–568.

212. Smith DP, Ciccotosto GD, Tew DJ, Fodero-Tavoletti MT, Johanssen T, Masters CL, et al. Concentration dependent Cu2+ induced aggregation and dityrosine formation of the Alzheimer's disease amyloid-beta peptide. *Biochemistry.* 2007;46(10):2881–2891.

213. Lang M, Fan Q, Wang L, Zheng Y, Xiao G, Wang X, et al. Inhibition of human high-affinity copper importer Ctr1 orthologous in the nervous system of Drosophila ameliorates Abeta42-induced Alzheimer's disease-like symptoms. *Neurobiol Aging.* 2013;34(11):2604–2612.

214. Soragni A, Zambelli B, Mukrasch MD, Biernat J, Jeganathan S, Griesinger C, et al. Structural characterization of binding of Cu(II) to tau protein. *Biochemistry.* 2008;47(41):10841–10851.

215. Ma QF, Li YM, Du JT, Kanazawa K, Nemoto T, Nakanishi H, et al. Binding of copper (II) ion to an Alzheimer's tau peptide as revealed by MALDI-TOF MS, CD, and NMR. *Biopolymers.* 2005;79(2):74–85.

216. Ma Q, Li Y, Du J, Liu H, Kanazawa K, Nemoto T, et al. Copper binding properties of a tau peptide associated with Alzheimer's disease studied by CD, NMR, and MALDI-TOF MS. *Peptides.* 2006;27(4):841–849.

217. Zhou LX, Du JT, Zeng ZY, Wu WH, Zhao YF, Kanazawa K, et al. Copper (II) modulates in vitro aggregation of a tau peptide. *Peptides.* 2007;28(11):2229–2234.

218. Sayre LM, Perry G, Harris PL, Liu Y, Schubert KA, Smith MA. In situ oxidative catalysis by neurofibrillary tangles and senile plaques in Alzheimer's disease: a central role for bound transition metals. *J Neurochem.* 2000;74(1): 270–279.

219. Su XY, Wu WH, Huang ZP, Hu J, Lei P, Yu CH, et al. Hydrogen peroxide can be generated by tau in the presence of Cu(II). *Biochem Biophys Res Commun.* 2007;358(2):661–665.

220. Kitazawa M, Cheng D, Laferla FM. Chronic copper exposure exacerbates both amyloid and tau pathology and selectively dysregulates cdk5 in a mouse model of AD. *J Neurochem.* 2009;108(6):1550–1560.

221. Crouch PJ, Hung LW, Adlard PA, Cortes M, Lal V, Filiz G, et al. Increasing Cu bioavailability inhibits Abeta oligomers and tau phosphorylation. *Proc Natl Acad Sci U S A.* 2009;106(2): 381–386.

222. Goodman L. Alzheimer's disease: a clinicopathologic analysis of twenty-three cases with a theory on pathogenesis. *J Nerv Mental Dis.* 1953;118(2):97–130.

223. Connor JR, Menzies SL, St Martin SM, Mufson EJ. A histochemical study of iron, transferrin, and ferritin in Alzheimer's diseased brains. *J Neurosci Res.* 1992;31(1):75–83.

224. Collingwood JF, Mikhaylova A, Davidson M, Batich C, Streit WJ, Terry J, et al. In situ characterization and mapping of iron compounds in Alzheimer's disease tissue. *J Alzheimers Dis.* 2005;7(4):267–272.

225. Baltes C, Princz-Kranz F, Rudin M, Mueggler T. Detecting amyloid-beta plaques in Alzheimer's disease. *Methods Mol Biol.* 2011;711:511–533.

226. Meadowcroft MD, Connor JR, Smith MB, Yang QX. MRI and histological analysis of beta-amyloid plaques in both human Alzheimer's disease and APP/PS1 transgenic mice. *JMRI.* 2009;29(5):997–1007.
227. Collingwood JF, Chong RK, Kasama T, Cervera-Gontard L, Dunin-Borkowski RE, Perry G, et al. Three-dimensional tomographic imaging and characterization of iron compounds within Alzheimer's plaque core material. *J Alzheimers Dis.* 2008;14(2):235–245.
228. Andrasi E, Farkas E, Scheibler H, Reffy A, Bezur L. Al, Zn, Cu, Mn and Fe levels in brain in Alzheimer's disease. *Arch Gerontol Geriatr.* 1995;21(1):89–97.
229. Smith MA, Harris PL, Sayre LM, Perry G. Iron accumulation in Alzheimer disease is a source of redox-generated free radicals. *Proc Natl Acad Sci U S A.* 1997;94(18):9866–9868.
230. Antharam V, Collingwood JF, Bullivant JP, Davidson MR, Chandra S, Mikhaylova A, et al. High field magnetic resonance microscopy of the human hippocampus in Alzheimer's disease: quantitative imaging and correlation with iron. *NeuroImage.* 2012; 59(2): 1249–1260.
231. Ding B, Chen KM, Ling HW, Sun F, Li X, Wan T, et al. Correlation of iron in the hippocampus with MMSE in patients with Alzheimer's disease. *JMRI.* 2009;29(4):793–798.
232. Zhu WZ, Zhong WD, Wang W, Zhan CJ, Wang CY, Qi JP, et al. Quantitative MR phase-corrected imaging to investigate increased brain iron deposition of patients with Alzheimer disease. *Radiology.* 2009; 253(2): 497–504.
233. Ayton S, Faux NG, Bush AI. Ferritin levels in the cerebrospinal fluid predict Alzheimer's disease outcomes and are regulated by APOE. *Nat Commun.* 2015;6:6760.
234. Mantyh PW, Ghilardi JR, Rogers S, DeMaster E, Allen CJ, Stimson ER, et al. Aluminum, iron, and zinc ions promote aggregation of physiological concentrations of beta-amyloid peptide. *J Neurochem.* 1993;61(3):1171–1174.
235. Schubert D, Chevion M. The role of iron in beta amyloid toxicity. *Biochem Biophys Res Commun.* 1995;216(2):702–707.
236. Liu B, Moloney A, Meehan S, Morris K, Thomas SE, Serpell LC, et al. Iron promotes the toxicity of amyloid beta peptide by impeding its ordered aggregation. *J Biol Chem.* 2011;286(6):4248–4256.
237. Rottkamp CA, Raina AK, Zhu XW, Gaier E, Bush AI, Atwood CS, et al. Redox-active iron mediates amyloid-beta toxicity. *Free Radic Biol Med.* 2001;30(4):447–450.
238. Rival T, Page RM, Chandraratna DS, Sendall TJ, Ryder E, Liu B, et al. Fenton chemistry and oxidative stress mediate the toxicity of the beta-amyloid peptide in a Drosophila model of Alzheimer's disease. *Eur J Neurosci.* 2009;29(7):1335–1347.
239. Kuperstein F, Yavin E. Pro-apoptotic signaling in neuronal cells following iron and amyloid beta peptide neurotoxicity. *J Neurochem.* 2003;86(1):114–125.
240. Everett J, Cespedes E, Shelford LR, Exley C, Collingwood JF, Dobson J, et al. Evidence of redox-active iron formation following aggregation of ferrihydrite and the Alzheimer's disease peptide beta-amyloid. *Inorg Chem.* 2014;53(6):2803–2809.
241. García de Ancos J, Correas I, Avila J. Differences in microtubule binding and self-association abilities of bovine brain tau isoforms. *J Biol Chem.* 1993;268(11):7976–7982.
242. Ledesma MD, Avila J, Correas I. Isolation of a phosphorylated soluble tau fraction from Alzheimer's disease brain. *Neurobiol Aging.* 1995;16(4):515–522.
243. Yamamoto A, Shin R-W, Hasegawa K, Naiki H, Sato H, Yoshimasu F, et al. Iron (III) induces aggregation of hyperphosphorylated tau and its reduction to iron (II) reverses the aggregation: implications in the formation of neurofibrillary tangles of Alzheimer's disease. *J Neurochem.* 2002; 82(5): 1137–1147.
244. Lovell MA, Xiong S, Xie C, Davies PL, Markesbery WR. Induction of hyperphosphorylated tau in primary rat cortical neuron cultures mediated by oxidative stress and glycogen synthase kinase-3. *J Alzheimers Dis.* 2004;6(6):659–71; discussion 73–81.
245. Chan A, Shea TB. Dietary and genetically-induced oxidative stress alter tau phosphorylation: influence of folate and apolipoprotein E deficiency. *J Alzheimers Dis.* 2006;9(4):399–405.
246. Huang X, Dai J, Huang C, Zhang Q, Bhanot O, Pelle E. Deferoxamine synergistically enhances iron-mediated AP-1 activation: a showcase of the interplay between extracellular-signal-regulated kinase and tyrosine phosphatase. *Free Radical Res.* 2007;41(10):1135–1142.
247. Muñoz P, Zavala G, Castillo K, Aguirre P, Hidalgo C, Nuñez MT. Effect of iron on the activation of the MAPK/ERK pathway in PC12 neuroblastoma cells. *Biol Res.* 2006;39(1):189–190.
248. Hare D, Ayton S, Bush A, Lei P. A delicate balance: Iron metabolism and diseases of the brain. *Front Aging Neurosci.* 2013;5:34.

249. Salvador GA, Uranga RM, Giusto NM. Iron and mechanisms of neurotoxicity. Int *J Alzheimers Dis.* 2010;2011:720658.

250. Mark RJ, Hensley K, Butterfield DA, Mattson MP. Amyloid beta-peptide impairs ion-motive ATPase activities: evidence for a role in loss of neuronal Ca2+ homeostasis and cell death. *J Neurosci.* 1995;15(9):6239–6249.

251. Ahuja RP, Borchman D, Dean WL, Paterson CA, Zeng J, Zhang Z, et al. Effect of oxidation on Ca2+ -ATPase activity and membrane lipids in lens epithelial microsomes. *Free Radic Biol Med.* 1999;27(1–2):177–185.

252. Moreau VH, Castilho RF, Ferreira ST, Carvalho-Alves PC. Oxidative damage to sarcoplasmic reticulum Ca2+-ATPase AT submicromolar iron concentrations: evidence for metal-catalyzed oxidation. *Free Radic Biol Med.* 1998;25(4–5):554–560.

253. Kaplan P, Matejovicova M, Mezesova V. Iron-induced inhibition of Na+, K(+)-ATPase and Na+/Ca2+ exchanger in synaptosomes: protection by the pyridoindole stobadine. *Neurochem Res.* 1997;22(12):1523–1529.

254. Gnana-Prakasam JP, Thangaraju M, Liu K, Ha Y, Martin PM, Smith SB, et al. Absence of iron-regulatory protein Hfe results in hyperproliferation of retinal pigment epithelium: role of cystine/glutamate exchanger. *Biochem J.* 2009;424(2):243–252.

255. Yu J, Guo Y, Sun M, Li B, Zhang Y, Li C. Iron is a potential key mediator of glutamate excitotoxicity in spinal cord motor neurons. *Brain Res.* 2009;1257:102–107.

256. Mitchell RM, Lee SY, Simmons Z, Connor JR. HFE polymorphisms affect cellular glutamate regulation. *Neurobiol Aging.* 2011;32(6):1114–1123.

257. Mattson MP. Metal-catalyzed disruption of membrane protein and lipid signaling in the pathogenesis of neurodegenerative disorders. *Ann N Y Acad Sci.* 2004;1012:37–50.

258. Dixon SJ, Lemberg KM, Lamprecht MR, Skouta R, Zaitsev EM, Gleason CE, et al. Ferroptosis: an iron-dependent form of nonapoptotic cell death. *Cell.* 2012;149(5):1060–1072.

259. Yagoda N, von Rechenberg M, Zaganjor E, Bauer AJ, Yang WS, Fridman DJ, et al. RAS-RAF-MEK-dependent oxidative cell death involving voltage-dependent anion channels. *Nature.* 2007;447(7146):864–868.

260. Yang WS, Stockwell BR. Synthetic lethal screening identifies compounds activating iron-dependent, nonapoptotic cell death in oncogenic-RAS-harboring cancer cells. *Chem Biol.* 2008;15(3):234–245.

261. Ayton S, Zhang M, Roberts BR, Lam LQ, Lind M, McLean C, et al. Ceruloplasmin and beta-amyloid precursor protein confer neuroprotection in traumatic brain injury and lower neuronal iron. *Free Radic Biol Med.* 2014;69:331–337.

262. Rogers JT, Randall JD, Cahill CM, Eder PS, Huang X, Gunshin H, et al. An iron-responsive element type II in the 5'-untranslated region of the Alzheimer's amyloid precursor protein transcript. *J Biol Chem.* 2002;277(47):45518–45528.

263. Li X, Liu Y, Zheng Q, Yao G, Cheng P, Bu G, et al. Ferritin light chain interacts with PEN-2 and affects gamma-secretase activity. *Neurosci Lett.* 2013;548:90–94.

264. Guo LY, Alekseev O, Li Y, Song Y, Dunaief JL. Iron increases APP translation and amyloid-beta production in the retina. *Exp Eye Res.* 2014;129:31–37.

265. Becerril-Ortega J, Bordji K, Freret T, Rush T, Buisson A. Iron overload accelerates neuronal amyloid-beta production and cognitive impairment in transgenic mice model of Alzheimer's disease. *Neurobiol Aging.* 2014;35(10):2288–2301.

266. Ksiezak-Reding H, Binder LI, Yen S-HC. Immunochemical and biochemical characterization of tau proteins in normal and Alzheimer's disease brains with Alz 50 and Tau-1. *J Biol Chem.* 1988;263(17):7948–7953.

267. Khatoon S, Grundke-Iqbal I, Iqbal K. Levels of normal and abnormally phosphorylated tau in different cellular and regional compartments of Alzheimer disease and control brains. *FEBS Lett.* 1994;351(1):80–84.

268. Zhukareva V, Sundarraj S, Mann D, Sjogren M, Blenow K, Clark CM, et al. Selective reduction of soluble tau proteins in sporadic and familial frontotemporal dementias: an international follow-up study. *Acta Neuropathol.* 2003;105(5):469–476.

269. van Eersel J, Bi M, Ke YD, Hodges JR, Xuereb JH, Gregory GC, et al. Phosphorylation of soluble tau differs in Pick's disease and Alzheimer's disease brains. *J Neural Transm.* 2009;116(10):1243–1251.

270. Lei P, Ayton S, Finkelstein DI, Spoerri L, Ciccotosto GD, Wright DK, et al. Tau deficiency induces parkinsonism with dementia by impairing APP-mediated iron export. *Nat Med.* 2012;18(2):291–295.

271. Lei P, Ayton S, Moon S, Zhang Q, Volitakis I, Finkelstein DI, et al. Motor and cognitive deficits in aged tau knockout mice in two background strains. *Mol Neurodegener.* 2014;9(1):29.

272. Lei P, Ayton S, Appukuttan AT, Volitakis I, Adlard PA, Finkelstein DI, et al. Clioquinol rescues Parkinsonism and dementia phenotypes of the tau knockout mouse. *Neurobiol Dis.* 2015.

273. Lhermitte J, Kraus WM, McAlpine D. Original papers: on the occurrence of abnormal deposits of iron in the brain in parkinsonism with special reference to its localisation. *J Neurol Psychopathol.* 1924;5(19):195–208.

274. Dexter DT, Wells FR, Lees AJ, Agid F, Agid Y, Jenner P, et al. Increased nigral iron content and alterations in other metal ions occurring in brain in Parkinson's disease. *J Neurochem.* 1989;52(6):1830–1836.

275. Ayton S, Lei P, Duce JA, Wong BX, Sedjahtera A, Adlard PA, et al. Ceruloplasmin dysfunction and therapeutic potential for Parkinson disease. *Ann Neurol.* 2013;73(4):554–559.

276. Ayton S, Lei P, Hare DJ, Duce JA, George JL, Adlard PA, et al. Parkinson's disease iron deposition caused by nitric oxide-induced loss of beta-amyloid precursor protein. *J Neurosci.* 2015;35(8):3591–3597.

277. Popescu BF, George MJ, Bergmann U, Garachtchenko AV, Kelly ME, McCrea RP, et al. Mapping metals in Parkinson's and normal brain using rapid-scanning x-ray fluorescence. *Phys Med Biol.* 2009;54(3):651–663.

278. Bartzokis G, Cummings JL, Markham CH, Marmarelis PZ, Treciokas LJ, Tishler TA, et al. MRI evaluation of brain iron in earlier- and later-onset Parkinson's disease and normal subjects. *Magn Reson Imaging.* 1999;17(2):213–222.

279. Ayton S, Lei P. Nigral iron elevation is an invariable feature of Parkinson's disease and is a sufficient cause of neurodegeneration. *BioMed Res Int.* 2014;2014:581256.

280. Bruggemann N, Hagenah J, Stanley K, Klein C, Wang C, Raymond D, et al. Substantia nigra hyperechogenicity with LRRK2 G2019S mutations. *Mov Disord.* 2011;26(5):885–888.

281. Hagenah JM, Konig IR, Becker B, Hilker R, Kasten M, Hedrich K, et al. Substantia nigra hyperechogenicity correlates with clinical status and number of Parkin mutated alleles. *J Neurol.* 2007;254(10):1407–1413.

282. Schweitzer KJ, Brussel T, Leitner P, Kruger R, Bauer P, Woitalla D, et al. Transcranial ultrasound in different monogenetic subtypes of Parkinson's disease. *J Neurol.* 2007;254(5):613–616.

283. Hagenah JM, Becker B, Bruggemann N, Djarmati A, Lohmann K, Sprenger A, et al. Transcranial sonography findings in a large family with homozygous and heterozygous PINK1 mutations. *J Neurol Neurosurg Psychiatry.* 2008;79(9):1071–1074.

284. Borie C, Gasparini F, Verpillat P, Bonnet AM, Agid Y, Hetet G, et al. Association study between iron-related genes polymorphisms and Parkinson's disease. *J Neurol.* 2002;249(7):801–804.

285. Deplazes J, Schobel K, Hochstrasser H, Bauer P, Walter U, Behnke S, et al. Screening for mutations of the IRP2 gene in Parkinson's disease patients with hyperechogenicity of the substantia nigra. *J Neural Transm.* 2004;111(4):515–521.

286. Foglieni B, Ferrari F, Goldwurm S, Santambrogio P, Castiglioni E, Sessa M, et al. Analysis of ferritin genes in Parkinson disease. *CCLM / FESCC.* 2007;45(11):1450–1456.

287. He Q, Du T, Yu X, Xie A, Song N, Kang Q, et al. DMT1 polymorphism and risk of Parkinson's disease. *Neurosci Lett.* 2011;501(3):128–31.

288. Peng J, Peng L, Stevenson FF, Doctrow SR, Andersen JK. Iron and paraquat as synergistic environmental risk factors in sporadic Parkinson's disease accelerate age-related neurodegeneration. *J Neurosci.* 2007; 27(26): 6914–6922.

289. Berg D, Seppi K, Behnke S, Liepelt I, Schweitzer K, Stockner H, et al. Enlarged substantia nigra hyperechogenicity and risk for Parkinson disease: a 37-month 3-center study of 1847 older persons. *Arch Neurol.* 2011; 68(7): 932–937.

290. Ma QL, Zuo X, Yang F, Ubeda OJ, Gant DJ, Alaverdyan M, et al. Loss of MAP function leads to hippocampal synapse loss and deficits in the Morris Water Maze with aging. *J Neurosci.* 2014;34(21):7124–7136.

291. Zheng H, Jiang M, Trumbauer ME, Sirinathsinghji DJ, Hopkins R, Smith DW, et al. beta-Amyloid precursor protein-deficient mice show reactive gliosis and decreased locomotor activity. *Cell.* 1995;81(4):525–531.

292. Simón-Sánchez J, Schulte C, Bras JM, Sharma M, Gibbs JR, Berg D, et al. Genome-wide association study reveals genetic risk underlying Parkinson's disease. *Nature Genet.* 2009;41(12):1308–1312.

293. Edwards TL, Scott WK, Almonte C, Burt A, Powell EH, Beecham GW, et al. Genome-wide association study confirms SNPs in SNCA and the MAPT region as common risk factors for Parkinson disease. *Ann Hum Genet.* 2010;74(2):97–109.

294. Schulte EC, Fukumori A, Mollenhauer B, Hor H, Arzberger T, Perneczky R, et al. Rare variants in beta-Amyloid precursor protein (APP) and Parkinson's disease. *Eur J Hum Genet.* 2015.

295. Sieczkowski E, Milenkovic I, Venkataramani V, Giera R, Strobel T, Hoftberger R, et al. I716F AbetaPP mutation associates with the deposition of oligomeric pyroglutamate amyloid-beta

and alpha-synucleinopathy with Lewy bodies. *J Alzheimers Dis.* 2015;44(1):103–114.

296. Ayton S, Lei P, Adlard PA, Volitakis I, Cherny RA, Bush AI, et al. Iron accumulation confers neurotoxicity to a vulnerable population of nigral neurons: implications for Parkinson's disease. *Mol Neurodegener.* 2014;9:27.

297. Bartzokis G, Beckson M, Hance DB, Marx P, Foster JA, Marder SR. MR evaluation of age-related increase of brain iron in young adult and older normal males. *Magn Reson Imaging.* 1997;15(1):29–35.

298. Bartzokis G, Cummings J, Perlman S, Hance DB, Mintz J. Increased basal ganglia iron levels in Huntington disease. *Arch Neurol.* 1999;56(5):569–574.

299. Baudrexel S, Nurnberger L, Rub U, Seifried C, Klein JC, Deller T, et al. Quantitative mapping of T1 and T2* discloses nigral and brainstem pathology in early Parkinson's disease. *NeuroImage.* 2010;51(2):512–520.

300. Wallis LI, Paley MN, Graham JM, Grunewald RA, Wignall EL, Joy HM, et al. MRI assessment of basal ganglia iron deposition in Parkinson's disease. *JMRI.* 2008;28(5):1061–1067.

301. Atasoy HT, Nuyan O, Tunc T, Yorubulut M, Unal AE, Inan LE. T2-weighted MRI in Parkinson's disease; substantia nigra pars compacta hypointensity correlates with the clinical scores. *Neurology India.* 2004;52(3):332–337.

302. Zhang J, Zhang Y, Wang J, Cai P, Luo C, Qian Z, et al. Characterizing iron deposition in Parkinson's disease using susceptibility-weighted imaging: an in vivo MR study. *Brain Res.* 2010;1330:124–130.

303. Kosta P, Argyropoulou MI, Markoula S, Konitsiotis S. MRI evaluation of the basal ganglia size and iron content in patients with Parkinson's disease. *J Neurol.* 2006;253(1):26–32.

304. Martin WR, Wieler M, Gee M. Midbrain iron content in early Parkinson disease: a potential biomarker of disease status. *Neurology.* 2008;70(16 Pt 2):1411–1417.

305. Berg D, Grote C, Rausch WD, Maurer M, Wesemann W, Riederer P, et al. Iron accumulation in the substantia nigra in rats visualized by ultrasound. *Ultrasound Med Biol.* 1999;25(6):901–904.

306. Berg D, Roggendorf W, Schroder U, Klein R, Tatschner T, Benz P, et al. Echogenicity of the substantia nigra: association with increased iron content and marker for susceptibility to nigrostriatal injury. *Arch Neurol.* 2002;59(6):999–1005.

307. Berg D. In vivo detection of iron and neuromelanin by transcranial sonography--a new approach for early detection of substantia nigra damage. *J Neural Transm.* 2006;113(6):775–780.

308. Zecca L, Berg D, Arzberger T, Ruprecht P, Rausch WD, Musicco M, et al. In vivo detection of iron and neuromelanin by transcranial sonography: a new approach for early detection of substantia nigra damage. *Mov Disord.* 2005;20(10):1278–1285.

309. Hochstrasser H, Bauer P, Walter U, Behnke S, Spiegel J, Csoti I, et al. Ceruloplasmin gene variations and substantia nigra hyperechogenicity in Parkinson disease. *Neurology.* 2004;63(10):1912–1917.

310. Youdim MB, Fridkin M, Zheng H. Novel bifunctional drugs targeting monoamine oxidase inhibition and iron chelation as an approach to neuroprotection in Parkinson's disease and other neurodegenerative diseases. *J Neural Transm.* 2004;111(10–11):1455–1471.

311. Gal S, Zheng H, Fridkin M, Youdim MB. Novel multifunctional neuroprotective iron chelator-monoamine oxidase inhibitor drugs for neurodegenerative diseases. In vivo selective brain monoamine oxidase inhibition and prevention of MPTP-induced striatal dopamine depletion. *J Neurochem.* 2005;95(1):79–88.

312. Zheng H, Gal S, Weiner LM, Bar-Am O, Warshawsky A, Fridkin M, et al. Novel multifunctional neuroprotective iron chelator-monoamine oxidase inhibitor drugs for neurodegenerative diseases: in vitro studies on antioxidant activity, prevention of lipid peroxide formation and monoamine oxidase inhibition. *J Neurochem.* 2005;95(1):68–78.

313. Febbraro F, Andersen KJ, Sanchez-Guajardo V, Tentillier N, Romero-Ramos M. Chronic intranasal deferoxamine ameliorates motor defects and pathology in the alpha-synuclein rAAV Parkinson's model. *Exp Neurol.* 2013;247: 45–58.

314. Avramovich-Tirosh Y, Amit T, Bar-Am O, Zheng H, Fridkin M, Youdim MB. Therapeutic targets and potential of the novel brain- permeable multifunctional iron chelator-monoamine oxidase inhibitor drug, M-30, for the treatment of Alzheimer's disease. *J Neurochem.* 2007;100(2):490–502.

315. Devos D, Moreau C, Devedjian JC, Kluza J, Petrault M, Laloux C, et al. Targeting chelatable iron as a therapeutic modality in Parkinson's disease. *Antioxidants Redox Signal.* 2014;21(2):195–210.

316. Davies KM, Bohic S, Carmona A, Ortega R, Cottam V, Hare DJ, et al. Copper pathology in vulnerable brain regions in Parkinson's disease. *Neurobiol Aging.* 2014;35(4):858–866.

317. Dudzik CG, Walter ED, Millhauser GL. Coordination features and affinity of the Cu(2)+

site in the alpha-synuclein protein of Parkinson's disease. *Biochemistry*. 2011;50(11):1771–1777.

318. Ahmad A, Burns CS, Fink AL, Uversky VN. Peculiarities of copper binding to alpha-synuclein. *J Biomol Struct Dyn*. 2012;29(4):825–842.

319. Bortolus M, Bisaglia M, Zoleo A, Fittipaldi M, Benfatto M, Bubacco L, et al. Structural characterization of a high affinity mononuclear site in the copper(II)-alpha-synuclein complex. *J Am Chem Soc*. 2010;132(51):18057–18066.

320. Lee JC, Gray HB, Winkler JR. Copper(II) binding to alpha-synuclein, the Parkinson's protein. *J Am Chem Soc*. 2008;130(22):6898–6899.

321. Binolfi A, Valiente-Gabioud AA, Duran R, Zweckstetter M, Griesinger C, Fernandez CO. Exploring the structural details of Cu(I) binding to alpha-synuclein by NMR spectroscopy. *J Am Chem Soc*. 2011; 133(2):194–196.

322. Binolfi A, Lamberto GR, Duran R, Quintanar L, Bertoncini CW, Souza JM, et al. Site-specific interactions of Cu(II) with alpha and beta-synuclein: bridging the molecular gap between metal binding and aggregation. *J Am Chem Soc*. 2008;130(35):11801–11812.

323. Miotto MC, Valiente-Gabioud AA, Rossetti G, Zweckstetter M, Carloni P, Selenko P, et al. Copper binding to the N-terminally acetylated, naturally occurring form of alpha-synuclein induces local helical folding. *J Am Chem Soc*. 2015; 137(20):6444–6447.

324. Dell'Acqua S, Pirota V, Anzani C, Rocco MM, Nicolis S, Valensin D, et al. Reactivity of copper-alpha-synuclein peptide complexes relevant to Parkinson's disease. *Metallomics*. 2015; 7(7):1091–1102.

325. Davies P, Wang X, Sarell CJ, Drewett A, Marken F, Viles JH, et al. The synucleins are a family of redox-active copper binding proteins. *Biochemistry*. 2011; 50(1):37–47.

326. Lucas HR, Debeer S, Hong MS, Lee JC. Evidence for copper-dioxygen reactivity during alpha-synuclein fibril formation. *J Am Chem Soc*. 2010;132(19):6636–6766.

327. Wang C, Liu L, Zhang L, Peng Y, Zhou F. Redox reactions of the alpha-synuclein-Cu(2+) complex and their effects on neuronal cell viability. *Biochemistry*. 2010;49(37):8134–8142.

328. Binolfi A, Rodriguez EE, Valensin D, D'Amelio N, Ippoliti E, Obal G, et al. Bioinorganic chemistry of Parkinson's disease: structural determinants for the copper-mediated amyloid formation of alpha-synuclein. *Inorg Chem*. 2010;49(22):10668–10679.

329. Paik SR, Shin HJ, Lee JH, Chang CS, Kim J. Copper(II)-induced self-oligomerization of alpha-synuclein. *Biochem J*. 1999;340 (Pt 3): 821–828.

330. Bharathi, Indi SS, Rao KSJ. Copper- and iron-induced differential fibril formation in alpha-synuclein: TEM study. *Neurosci Lett*. 2007;424(2):78–82.

331. Wright JA, Wang X, Brown DR. Unique copper-induced oligomers mediate alpha-synuclein toxicity. *FASEB J*. 2009;23(8):2384–2893.

332. Anandhan A, Rodriguez-Rocha H, Bohovych I, Griggs AM, Zavala-Flores L, Reyes-Reyes EM, et al. Overexpression of alpha-synuclein at nontoxic levels increases dopaminergic cell death induced by copper exposure via modulation of protein degradation pathways. *Neurobiol Dis*. 2015; 81:76–92.

333. Wang X, Moualla D, Wright JA, Brown DR. Copper binding regulates intracellular alpha-synuclein localisation, aggregation and toxicity. *J Neurochem*. 2010;113(3):704–714.

334. Puno MR, Patel NA, Moller SG, Robinson CV, Moody PC, Odell M. Structure of Cu(I)-bound DJ-1 reveals a biscysteinate metal binding site at the homodimer interface: insights into mutational inactivation of DJ-1 in Parkinsonism. *J Am Chem Soc*. 2013;135(43):15974–15977.

335. Girotto S, Cendron L, Bisaglia M, Tessari I, Mammi S, Zanotti G, et al. DJ-1 is a copper chaperone acting on SOD1 activation. *J Biol Chem*. 2014;289(15):10887–10899.

336. Bjorkblom B, Adilbayeva A, Maple-Grodem J, Piston D, Okvist M, Xu XM, et al. Parkinson disease protein DJ-1 binds metals and protects against metal-induced cytotoxicity. *J Biol Chem*. 2013;288(31):22809–22820.

337. Dexter DT, Carayon A, Javoy-Agid F, Agid Y, Wells FR, Daniel SE, et al. Alterations in the levels of iron, ferritin and other trace metals in Parkinson's disease and other neurodegenerative diseases affecting the basal ganglia. *Brain*. 1991;114 (Pt 4):1953–1975.

338. Kumar V, Singh BK, Chauhan AK, Singh D, Patel DK, Singh C. Minocycline rescues from zinc-induced nigrostriatal dopaminergic neurodegeneration: biochemical and molecular interventions. *Mol Neurobiol*. 2015; 53(5):2761–2777.

339. Kumar A, Singh BK, Ahmad I, Shukla S, Patel DK, Srivastava G, et al. Involvement of NADPH oxidase and glutathione in zinc-induced dopaminergic neurodegeneration in rats: similarity with paraquat neurotoxicity. *Brain Res*. 2012;1438:48–64.

340. Noh J, Chang SY, Wang SY, Chung JM. Dual function of Zn2+ on the intrinsic excitability of dopaminergic neurons in rat substantia nigra. *Neuroscience*. 2011;175:85–92.

341. Sheline CT, Zhu J, Zhang W, Shi C, Cai AL. Mitochondrial inhibitor models of Huntington's disease and Parkinson's disease induce zinc accumulation and are attenuated by inhibition of zinc neurotoxicity in vitro or in vivo. *Neurodegen Dis.* 2013;11(1):49–58.

342. Tsunemi T, Krainc D. Zn(2)(+) dyshomeostasis caused by loss of ATP13A2/PARK9 leads to lysosomal dysfunction and alpha-synuclein accumulation. *Hum Mol Genet.* 2014;23(11):2791–2801.

343. Park JS, Koentjoro B, Veivers D, Mackay-Sim A, Sue CM. Parkinson's disease-associated human ATP13A2 (PARK9) deficiency causes zinc dyshomeostasis and mitochondrial dysfunction. *Hum Mol Genet.* 2014;23(11):2802–2815.

344. Kong SM, Chan BK, Park JS, Hill KJ, Aitken JB, Cottle L, et al. Parkinson's disease-linked human PARK9/ATP13A2 maintains zinc homeostasis and promotes alpha-Synuclein externalization via exosomes. *Hum Mol Genet.* 2014;23(11):2816–2833.

345. Tashiro S, Caaveiro JM, Wu CX, Hoang QQ, Tsumoto K. Thermodynamic and structural characterization of the specific binding of Zn(II) to human protein DJ-1. *Biochemistry.* 2014;53(14):2218–2220.

346. MacDonald ME, Barnes G, Srinidhi J, Duyao MP, Ambrose CM, Myers RH, et al. Gametic but not somatic instability of CAG repeat length in Huntington's disease. *J Med Genet.* 1993;30(12):982–986.

347. Vonsattel JP, Myers RH, Stevens TJ, Ferrante RJ, Bird ED, Richardson EP, Jr. Neuropathological classification of Huntington's disease. *J Neuropath Exper Neurol.* 1985;44(6):559–577.

348. Graveland GA, Williams RS, DiFiglia M. Evidence for degenerative and regenerative changes in neostriatal spiny neurons in Huntington's disease. *Science.* 1985;227(4688):770–773.

349. Brandt J, Folstein SE, Folstein MF. Differential cognitive impairment in Alzheimer's disease and Huntington's disease. *Ann Neurol.* 1988;23(6):555–561.

350. Bartzokis G, Lu PH, Tishler TA, Fong SM, Oluwadara B, Finn JP, et al. Myelin breakdown and iron changes in Huntington's disease: pathogenesis and treatment implications. *Neurochem Res.* 2007;32(10):1655–1664.

351. Sanchez-Castaneda C, Squitieri F, Di Paola M, Dayan M, Petrollini M, Sabatini U. The role of iron in gray matter degeneration in Huntington's disease: a magnetic resonance imaging study. *Hum Brain Mapping.* 2015;36(1):50–66.

352. Rosas HD, Chen YI, Doros G, Salat DH, Chen NK, Kwong KK, et al. Alterations in brain transition metals in Huntington disease: an

353. Fox JH, Kama JA, Lieberman G, Chopra R, Dorsey K, Chopra V, et al. Mechanisms of copper ion mediated Huntington's disease progression. *PLoS ONE.* 2007;2(3):e334.

354. Bellingham SA, Lahiri DK, Maloney B, La Fontaine S, Multhaup G, Camakaris J. Copper depletion down-regulates expression of the Alzheimer's disease amyloid-beta precursor protein gene. *J Biol Chem.* 2004;279(19):20378–20386.

355. Chen J, Marks E, Lai B, Zhang Z, Duce JA, Lam LQ, et al. Iron accumulates in Huntington's disease neurons: protection by deferoxamine. *PLoS ONE.* 2013;8(10):e77023.

356. Xiao G, Fan Q, Wang X, Zhou B. Huntington disease arises from a combinatory toxicity of polyglutamine and copper binding. *Proc Natl Acad Sci U S A.* 2013;110(37):14995–5000.

357. Cherny RA, Ayton S, Finkelstein DI, Bush AI, McColl G, Massa SM. PBT2 reduces toxicity in a C. elegans model of polyQ aggregation and extends lifespan, reduces striatal atrophy and improves motor performance in the R6/2 mouse model of Huntington's disease. *J Huntingtons Dis.* 2012;1(2):211–219.

358. Nguyen T, Hamby A, Massa SM. Clioquinol down-regulates mutant huntingtin expression in vitro and mitigates pathology in a Huntington's disease mouse model. *Proc Natl Acad Sci U S A.* 2005;102(33):11840–11845.

359. Huntington Study Group Reach2HD Investigators. Safety, tolerability, and efficacy of PBT2 in Huntington's disease: a phase 2, randomised, double-blind, placebo-controlled trial. *Lancet Neurol.* 2015;14(1):39–47.

360. Fox JH, Connor T, Stiles M, Kama J, Lu Z, Dorsey K, et al. Cysteine oxidation within N-terminal mutant huntingtin promotes oligomerization and delays clearance of soluble protein. *J Biol Chem.* 2011;286(20):18320–18330.

361. Lacomblez L, Bensimon G, Leigh PN, Guillet P, Meininger V. Dose-ranging study of riluzole in amyotrophic lateral sclerosis. Amyotrophic Lateral Sclerosis/Riluzole Study Group II. *Lancet.* 1996;347(9013):1425–1431.

362. Sreedharan J, Blair IP, Tripathi VB, Hu X, Vance C, Rogelj B, et al. TDP-43 mutations in familial and sporadic amyotrophic lateral sclerosis. *Science.* 2008;319(5870):1668–1672.

363. Robberecht W, Philips T. The changing scene of amyotrophic lateral sclerosis. *Nat Rev Neurosci.* 2013;14(4):248–264.

364. DeJesus-Hernandez M, Mackenzie IR, Boeve BF, Boxer AL, Baker M, Rutherford NJ, et al.

evolving and intricate story. *Arch Neurol.* 2012;69(7):887–893.

Expanded GGGGCC hexanucleotide repeat in noncoding region of C9ORF72 causes chromosome 9p-linked FTD and ALS. *Neuron.* 2011;72(2):245–256.

365. Renton AE, Majounie E, Waite A, Simon-Sanchez J, Rollinson S, Gibbs JR, et al. A hexanucleotide repeat expansion in C9ORF72 is the cause of chromosome 9p21-linked ALS-FTD. *Neuron.* 2011;72(2):257–268.

366. Rosen DR, Siddique T, Patterson D, Figlewicz DA, Sapp P, Hentati A, et al. Mutations in Cu/Zn superoxide dismutase gene are associated with familial amyotrophic lateral sclerosis. *Nature.* 1993;362(6415):59–62.

367. Turner MR, Hardiman O, Benatar M, Brooks BR, Chio A, de Carvalho M, et al. Controversies and priorities in amyotrophic lateral sclerosis. *Lancet Neurol.* 2013;12(3):310–322.

368. Shaw BF, Valentine JS. How do ALS-associated mutations in superoxide dismutase 1 promote aggregation of the protein? *Trends Biochem Sci.* 2007;32(2):78–85.

369. Bosco DA, Morfini GA, Karabacak NM, Song Y, Gros-Louis F, Pasinelli P, et al. Wild-type and mutant SOD1 share an aberrant conformation and a common pathogenic pathway in ALS. *Nat Neurosci.* 2010;13(11):1396–1403.

370. Ahtoniemi T, Goldsteins G, Keksa-Goldsteine V, Malm T, Kanninen K, Salminen A, et al. Pyrrolidine dithiocarbamate inhibits induction of immunoproteasome and decreases survival in a rat model of amyotrophic lateral sclerosis. *Mol Pharmacol.* 2007;71(1):30–37.

371. Li QX, Mok SS, Laughton KM, McLean CA, Volitakis I, Cherny RA, et al. Overexpression of Abeta is associated with acceleration of onset of motor impairment and superoxide dismutase 1 aggregation in an amyotrophic lateral sclerosis mouse model. *Aging Cell.* 2006;5(2):153–165.

372. Tokuda E, Ono S, Ishige K, Naganuma A, Ito Y, Suzuki T. Metallothionein proteins expression, copper and zinc concentrations, and lipid peroxidation level in a rodent model for amyotrophic lateral sclerosis. *Toxicology.* 2007;229(1–2):33–41.

373. Hottinger AF, Fine EG, Gurney ME, Zurn AD, Aebischer P. The copper chelator d-penicillamine delays onset of disease and extends survival in a transgenic mouse model of familial amyotrophic lateral sclerosis. *Eur J Neurosci.* 1997;9(7):1548–1551.

374. Kiaei M, Bush AI, Morrison BM, Morrison JH, Cherny RA, Volitakis I, et al. Genetically decreased spinal cord copper concentration prolongs life in a transgenic mouse model of amyotrophic lateral sclerosis. *J Neurosci.* 2004;24(36):7945–7950.

375. Nagano S, Fujii Y, Yamamoto T, Taniyama M, Fukada K, Yanagihara T, et al. The efficacy of trientine or ascorbate alone compared to that of the combined treatment with these two agents in familial amyotrophic lateral sclerosis model mice. *Exp Neurol.* 2003;179(2):176–180.

376. Nagano S, Ogawa Y, Yanagihara T, Sakoda S. Benefit of a combined treatment with trientine and ascorbate in familial amyotrophic lateral sclerosis model mice. *Neurosci Lett.* 1999;265(3):159–162.

377. Tokuda E, Ono S, Ishige K, Watanabe S, Okawa E, Ito Y, et al. Ammonium tetrathiomolybdate delays onset, prolongs survival, and slows progression of disease in a mouse model for amyotrophic lateral sclerosis. *Exp Neurol.* 2008;213(1):122–128.

378. Petri S, Calingasan NY, Alsaied OA, Wille E, Kiaei M, Friedman JE, et al. The lipophilic metal chelators DP-109 and DP-460 are neuroprotective in a transgenic mouse model of amyotrophic lateral sclerosis. *J Neurochem.* 2007;102(3):991–1000.

379. Beckman JS, Esetvez AG, Barbeito L, Crow JP. CCS knockout mice establish an alternative source of copper for SOD in ALS. *Free Radic Biol Med.* 2002;33(10):1433–1435.

380. Bush AI, Tanzi RE. The galvanization of beta-amyloid in Alzheimer's disease. *Proc Natl Acad Sci U S A.* 2002;99(11):7317–7319.

381. McAllum EJ, Lim NK, Hickey JL, Paterson BM, Donnelly PS, Li QX, et al. Therapeutic effects of CuII(atsm) in the SOD1-G37R mouse model of amyotrophic lateral sclerosis. *ALS Frontotemp Degen.* 2013;14(7–8):586–590.

382. Kishigami H, Nagano S, Bush AI, Sakoda S. Monomerized Cu, Zn-superoxide dismutase induces oxidative stress through aberrant Cu binding. *Free Radic Biol Med.* 2010;48(7):945–952.

383. Watanabe S, Nagano S, Duce J, Kiaei M, Li QX, Tucker SM, et al. Increased affinity for copper mediated by cysteine 111 in forms of mutant superoxide dismutase 1 linked to amyotrophic lateral sclerosis. *Free Radic Biol Med.* 2007;42(10):1534–1542.

384. Tokuda E, Okawa E, Watanabe S, Ono S, Marklund SL. Dysregulation of intracellular copper homeostasis is common to transgenic mice expressing human mutant superoxide dismutase-1s regardless of their copper-binding abilities. *Neurobiol Dis.* 2013;54:308–319.

385. Sheng Y, Chattopadhyay M, Whitelegge J, Valentine JS. SOD1 aggregation and ALS: role of metallation states and disulfide status. *Curr Top Med Chem.* 2012;12(22):2560–2572.

386. Roberts BR, Tainer JA, Getzoff ED, Malencik DA, Anderson SR, Bomben VC, et al. Structural characterization of zinc-deficient human superoxide dismutase and implications for ALS. *J Mol Biol.* 2007;373(4):877–990.

387. Goodall EF, Greenway MJ, van Marion I, Carroll CB, Hardiman O, Morrison KE. Association of the H63D polymorphism in the hemochromatosis gene with sporadic ALS. *Neurology.* 2005;65(6):934–937.

388. Nadjar Y, Gordon P, Corcia P, Bensimon G, Pieroni L, Meininger V, et al. Elevated serum ferritin is associated with reduced survival in amyotrophic lateral sclerosis. *PLoS ONE.* 2012;7(9):e45034.

389. Tateishi J. Subacute myelo-optico-neuropathy: clioquinol intoxication in humans and animals. *Neuropathology.* 2000;20 Suppl:S20–24.

390. Cherny RA, Atwood CS, Xilinas ME, Gray DN, Jones WD, McLean CA, et al. Treatment with a copper-zinc chelator markedly and rapidly inhibits beta-amyloid accumulation in Alzheimer's disease transgenic mice. *Neuron.* 2001;30(3):665–676.

391. Di Vaira M, Bazzicalupi C, Orioli P, Messori L, Bruni B, Zatta P. Clioquinol, a drug for Alzheimer's disease specifically interfering with brain metal metabolism: structural characterization of its zinc(II) and copper(II) complexes. *Inorg Chem.* 2004;43(13):3795–3797.

392. Treiber C, Simons A, Strauss M, Hafner M, Cappai R, Bayer TA, et al. Clioquinol mediates copper uptake and counteracts copper efflux activities of the amyloid precursor protein of Alzheimer's disease. *J Biol Chem.* 2004;279(50):51958–51964.

393. Raman B, Ban T, Yamaguchi K-i, Sakai M, Kawai T, Naiki H, et al. Metal ion-dependent effects of clioquinol on the fibril growth of an amyloid {beta} peptide. *J Biol Chem.* 2005;280(16):16157–16162.

394. Priel T, Aricha-Tamir B, Sekler I. Clioquinol attenuates zinc-dependent beta-cell death and the onset of insulitis and hyperglycemia associated with experimental type I diabetes in mice. *Eur J Pharmacol.* 2007;565(1–3):232–239.

395. Barrea RA, Chen D, Irving TC, Dou QP. Synchrotron X-ray imaging reveals a correlation of tumor copper speciation with Clioquinol's anticancer activity. *J Cell Biochem.* 2009;108(1):96–105.

396. Nitzan YB, Sekler I, Frederickson CJ, Coulter DA, Balaji RV, Liang SL, et al. Clioquinol effects on tissue chelatable zinc in mice. *J Mol Med (Berl).* 2003;81(10):637–644.

397. Adlard PA, Cherny RA, Finkelstein DI, Gautier E, Robb E, Cortes M, et al. Rapid restoration of cognition in Alzheimer's transgenic mice with 8-hydroxy quinoline analogs is associated with decreased interstitial Abeta. *Neuron.* 2008;59(1):43–55.

398. Li C, Wang J, Zhou B. The metal chelating and chaperoning effects of clioquinol: insights from yeast studies. *J Alzheimers Dis.* 2010;21(4):1249–1262.

399. Park MH, Lee SJ, Byun HR, Kim Y, Oh YJ, Koh JY, et al. Clioquinol induces autophagy in cultured astrocytes and neurons by acting as a zinc ionophore. *Neurobiol Dis.* 2011;42(3):242–251.

400. Crouch PJ, Savva MS, Hung LW, Donnelly PS, Mot AI, Parker SJ, et al. The Alzheimer's therapeutic PBT2 promotes amyloid-beta degradation and GSK3 phosphorylation via a metal chaperone activity. *J Neurochem.* 2011;119(1):220–230.

401. Atamna H, Frey WH. A role for heme in Alzheimer's disease: heme binds amyloid beta and has altered metabolism. *Proc Natl Acad Sci U S A.* 2004;101(30):11153–11158.

402. Choi SM, Choi KO, Park YK, Cho H, Yang EG, Park H. Clioquinol, a Cu(II)/Zn(II) chelator, inhibits both ubiquitination and asparagine hydroxylation of hypoxia-inducible factor-1alpha, leading to expression of vascular endothelial growth factor and erythropoietin in normoxic cells. *J Biol Chem.* 2006;281(45):34056–34063.

403. Felkai S, Ewbank JJ, Lemieux J, Labbe JC, Brown GG, Hekimi S. CLK-1 controls respiration, behavior and aging in the nematode Caenorhabditis elegans. *EMBO J.* 1999;18(7):1783–1792.

404. Kaur D, Yantiri F, Rajagopalan S, Kumar J, Mo JQ, Boonplueang R, et al. Genetic or pharmacological iron chelation prevents MPTP-induced neurotoxicity in vivo: a novel therapy for Parkinson's disease. *Neuron.* 2003;37(6):899–909.

405. LeVine H, 3rd, Ding Q, Walker JA, Voss RS, Augelli-Szafran CE. Clioquinol and other hydroxyquinoline derivatives inhibit Abeta(1–42) oligomer assembly. *Neurosci Lett.* 2009;465(1):99–103.

406. Mancino AM, Hindo SS, Kochi A, Lim MH. Effects of clioquinol on metal-triggered amyloid-beta aggregation revisited. *Inorg Chem.* 2009;48(20):9596–9598.

407. Stoppelkamp S, Bell HS, Palacios-Filardo J, Shewan DA, Riedel G, Platt B. In vitro modelling of Alzheimer's disease: degeneration and cell death induced by viral delivery of amyloid and tau. *Exp Neurol.* 2011;229(2):226–237.

408. Grossi C, Francese S, Casini A, Rosi MC, Luccarini I, Fiorentini A, et al. Clioquinol decreases amyloid-beta burden and reduces

working memory impairment in a transgenic mouse model of Alzheimer's disease. *J Alzheimers Dis.* 2009;17(2):423–440.

409. Ritchie CW, Bush AI, Mackinnon A, Macfarlane S, Mastwyk M, MacGregor L, et al. Metal-protein attenuation with iodochlorhydroxyquin (clioquinol) targeting Abeta amyloid deposition and toxicity in Alzheimer disease: a pilot phase 2 clinical trial. *Arch Neurol.* 2003;60(12):1685–1691.

410. Lannfelt L, Blennow K, Zetterberg H, Batsman S, Ames D, Harrison J, et al. Safety, efficacy, and biomarker findings of PBT2 in targeting Abeta as a modifying therapy for Alzheimer's disease: a phase IIa, double-blind, randomised, placebo-controlled trial. *Lancet Neurol.* 2008;7(9):779–786.

411. Faux NG, Ritchie CW, Gunn AP, Rembach A, Tsatsanis A, Bedo J, et al. PBT2 rapidly improves cognition in Alzheimer's disease: additional

phase II analyses. *J Alzheimers Dis.* 2010;20(2):509–516.

412. Donnelly PS, Caragounis A, Du T, Laughton KM, Volitaskis I, Cherny RA, et al. Selective intracellular release of copper and zinc ions from bis(thiosemicarbazonato) complexes reduces levels of Alzheimer disease amyloid-beta peptide. *J Biol Chem.* 2008;283(8): 4568–4577.

413. Hung LW, Villemagne VL, Cheng L, Sherratt NA, Ayton S, White AR, et al. The hypoxia imaging agent CuII(atsm) is neuroprotective and improves motor and cognitive functions in multiple animal models of Parkinson's disease. *J Exp Med.* 2012;209(4):837–854.

414. Crapper McLachlan DR, Dalton AJ, Kruck TP, Bell MY, Smith WL, Kalow W, et al. Intramuscular desferrioxamine in patients with Alzheimer's disease. *Lancet.* 1991;337(8753):1304–1308.

16

Disease-Modifying Therapies in Neurodegenerative Disorders

JANELLE DROUIN-OUELLET AND ROGER A. BARKER

INTRODUCTION

Neurodegenerative disorders (NDDs) of the CNS all share the common feature of chronic neuronal loss. As such, what defines a given NDD is its clinical presentation, coupled with the nature of the protein pathology affecting the neurons and the most affected sites of pathology within the CNS. However, it is increasingly being recognized that many chronic NDDs have

- mixed pathology: for example, in Alzheimer's disease (AD), which is defined by its amyloid plaques and tau tangles, there is typically a degree of α-synuclein Lewy body pathology with vascular disease (1, 2);
- a wider anatomical distribution of pathology than once thought: for example, Parkinson's disease (PD) has Lewy body pathology that extends well outside the substantia nigra (3);
- a disease process that begins years before clinical features become evident: for example, Huntington's disease (HD) now seems to display imaging changes and subtle cognitive deficits over a decade before a clinical diagnosis is made (4, 5);
- a spreading pathology that may involve the transfer of a critical pathological species of protein: for example, the spread of tau between cells in a prion-like fashion has now been described in many forms of experimental tauopathies (6–8);
- a disease process that affects glial cells as much as the neurons themselves: for example, the motorneuronal loss of amyotrophic lateral sclerosis (ALS) can be induced or rescued in animal models through manipulation of the astrocytic compartment (9–12);
- an inflammatory component that seems to be common to all such diseases and that is now thought to not just be a secondary phenomenon, as was once believed (13, 14).

The realization that NDDs are not simply cell-autonomous disorders affecting specific populations of vulnerable neurons means that the development of disease-modifying therapies will need to be rethought. This will involve not only rethinking exactly what cell and what part of the pathogenic pathway should be targeted, but whether it may be more sensible to target multiple cells and a whole array of pathogenic pathways.

In this chapter, we briefly summarize the different strategies that have been tried to slow down or reverse NDDs. In addition, we also highlight new areas that may need to be more intensively studied in the future and which may also help explain the clinical trial failures of the past. Indeed, to date no disease-modifying therapy for a single NDD has been found, with the exception of multiple sclerosis (MS), where new powerful immunotherapies used early in the disease course appear to arrest the secondary phase of the illness (15, 16).

In order to help shape this discussion, we have divided the approaches to disease-modifying therapies by looking at specific targets based on what is known about the pathogenic pathways of both genetic and sporadic NDDs. This allows us to highlight where a specific therapeutic target offers hope, while also making the point that many therapies have failed in the past because of either poor target identification and engagement or an underestimation of the complexity of the disease processes.

THE PATHOGENIC PATHWAYS INVOLVED IN NEURODEGENERATIVE DISORDERS

The pathogenic cascade of events leading to the loss of cells in NDDs is summarized in Figure 16.1. These can broadly be divided up into those that are either

1. cell-autonomous and derive from an intrinsic defect within the affected cells such as protein aggregation, ubiquitin proteasome system (UPS) dysfunction, autophagy impairments, mitochondrial compromise and free radical production, axonal transport defects and so on; or

2. non-cell-autonomous and driven by processes acting on the cell from outside, such as excitotoxicity, local inflammation, protein spread from cell to cell, and so on.

Although NDDs are classically divided into those that are primarily genetic versus those that are sporadic, this distinction at a pathological level is becoming less clear-cut. Many mendelian forms of disease can have non-cell-autonomous components to their pathology (e.g., inflammation in HD); and cell-autonomous defects may drive many sporadic forms of disease (e.g., complex I dysfunction in PD). Thus, without exception, all NDDs have elements of all of these pathways in their pathophysiological makeup and must be viewed as such, with one or more playing a more dominant role.

THERAPEUTIC APPROACHES TO TREATING NEURODEGENERATIVE DISORDERS

Disease Modification at the Level of the Gene

In order for this approach to be possible, the disease must have a clear autosomal dominant origin, which would allow for the abnormal gene to be excised and corrected. It was once thought that such genetic corrections could not be done with enough fidelity, but the development of gene-editing technologies means that this now can be studied as a potential therapeutic approach. This field is in its infancy, but there are currently three approaches being used for targeted genome modification *in vivo*: zinc finger nucleases (ZFNs) (17), transcription activator-like effector nucleases (TALENs) (18),

and the clustered regularly interspaced palindromic repeats/CRISPR-associated (CRISPR/Cas) system (19). These technologies have been used to correct mutations associated with familial forms of NDDs in patient-specific derived induced pluripotent stem cells (iPSCs). For example, in iPSCs from PD patients carrying point mutations in the α-synuclein or the *LRRK2* genes, the mutation was repaired using the ZFN technology, providing an isogenic control to study the disease (20), but also reversing at least some biological features caused by the mutation (21). This correction of the phenotype associated with a mutation has also been successfully done in iPSCs from an ALS patient carrying a *SOD1* mutation using the TALEN technology (22). Importantly, ZFN technology has recently been successfully used in a transgenic mouse model of HD (23), providing a proof-of-principle that this could be used *in vivo*.

An alternative strategy has been to try to alter gene expression through changing chromatin and histones by using histone deacetylase (HDAC) inhibitors. In HD, these have been found to produce mixed results experimentally. Inhibition of HDAC 1, 2, and 4 have led to improvements in models of the disease (24–27), whereas inhibition of HDAC 6 and 7 had no effect (28, 29) and HDAC 3 inhibition has yielded mixed results (26, 30, 31). Nevertheless, one interesting feature of some of these histone deacetylase inhibitors is that they may act, at least in part, through alteration of DNA methylation, which is an epigenetic modification that can be inherited in the germ line and could thus lead to transgenerational beneficial effects on disease phenotype (32). However, the lack of selectivity of these inhibitors still remains an obstacle for their use in the clinic.

Disease Modification at the Level of mRNA

This has become a new area of therapeutic excitement in autosomal disorders of the CNS such as HD, familial forms of ALS and the spinocerebellar ataxias (SCAs). This strategy seeks to silence the abnormal mRNA that codes for the mutant protein while leaving the wild-type mRNA unaffected. This can be done using virally encoded short-hairpin RNAs (shRNAs) or microRNAs (miRNAs), as well as direct infusion of small interfering RNAs (siRNAs) or single stranded antisense oligonucleotides

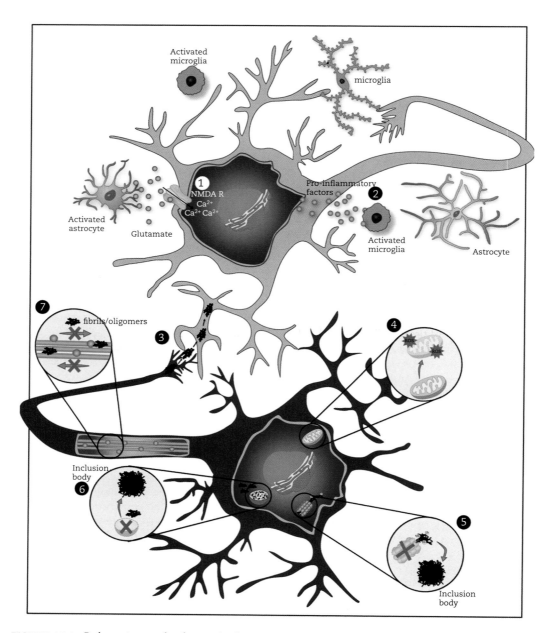

FIGURE 16.1. Pathogenic cascade of events leading to cell loss in NDDs. Schematic drawing illustrating non-cell-autonomous (1–3) as well as cell-autonomous events (4–7) leading to neuronal degeneration in NDDs. (1) Excitotoxicity caused by an overstimulation of glutamatergic receptors (e.g., NMDA), in part through poor clearance of extracellular glutamate by astrocytes. This leads to an excess of intracellular calcium, causing cellular dysfunction and death. (2) Elements involved in the pathological process, such as misfolded proteins and oxidative stress, will activate an inflammatory response predominantly driven by microglial cells. The pro-inflammatory factors generated as a result will contribute to create neuronal damage. (3) Cell-to-cell transmission of proteins involved in the pathophysiology will contribute to the spread of pathology across regions of the CNS. (4) Defects in mitochondrial function will lead to the production of reactive oxygen species, which will in turn trigger more inflammation, DNA damage, and apoptosis. (5, 6) Ubiquitin proteasome system (5) as well as lysosomal (6) dysfunction will prevent proper elimination of misfolded proteins, creating a buildup and the formation of protein oligomers and inclusions. (7) The presence of protein aggregates will disrupt the axonal protein transport, which will affect the cellular function and synaptic transmission, as well as neurotrophic factor delivery. All these events will contribute to cellular dysfunction and death.

(ASOs) to target the abnormal mRNA. In HD, this has been shown not only *in vitro*, but in some mouse models of disease as well as in non-human primates (33–38). Furthermore, it has been shown that this switching off of the mutant mRNA does not need to be permanent, as transient knock-down of it not only slows down the disease process, but actually reverses it (38), presumably by allowing the affected cells to recover back to full health before the mutant protein starts to accumulate again. As a result, several trials are now planned using this approach in HD, including ASO-HTT-Rx developed by Ionis Pharmaceuticals.

Furthermore, there is now preclinical evidence that an ASO directed against SOD1 prolonged the life span of SOD1G93A transgenic mice and that there was a widespread distribution of these ASOs throughout the CNS following cerebrospinal fluid (CSF) administration. This was associated with a reduction of SOD1 mRNA and protein in the brain and spinal cord tissues, all of which has led to a first-in-human study using this approach in a cohort of ALS patients. This phase I trial involved a single intrathecal injection of ASO directed against SOD1 (ISIS 333611) and proved to be well tolerated, although no clear efficacy was seen (39). This first trial using ASOs will lay the foundations for future studies using this same approach for other autosomal dominant neurodegenerative disorders.

Disease Modification at the Level of the Protein

Once the abnormal pathogenic form of the protein has started to be produced in the cell (for unknown reasons in the case of sporadic disease), it will start to aggregate. En route to this, it will undergo a series of conformational changes from simple oligomers to protofibrils to fibrils, and though it is debated which is the most pathogenic species, it is now generally believed that the oligomers are the most toxic moiety in most diseases. As these proteins are generated, the cell will try to remove them through either the UPS or lysosomes, often in conjunction with chaperone proteins as part of an autophagic process (Figure 16.1). As such, various therapeutic manipulations of these systems have been tried as a means to slow down the disease process. These include the following:

- *Removing the toxic species of the protein through immunization therapies*: This has been explored mostly with extracellular amyloid β (Aβ) and AD. Though preclinical studies have shown beyond doubt that this approach could successfully clear Aβ burden and lead to cognitive improvements, the clinical trials have not been successful thus far. Indeed, the first trial using active immunisation (AN1792) was halted when 6% of the vaccinated patients developed meningoencephalitis. Although autopsy results of a few patients indicated good Aβ plaque clearance (40), not all immunized patients responded with antibody production, and overall patients showed very little or no cognitive improvements (41). Trials using passive immunization have also been conducted but have also failed to show any improvements (42–44). The negative results associated with these first trials are in part due to the fact that the therapy was given late in the disease course at a stage where the pathology had already caused damage beyond repair. These disappointing findings have now resulted in approaches targeting patients with earlier disease stages such as mild cognitive impairment (MCI-AD). Furthermore, there has also been interest in using this approach to target intracellular proteins such as the tau pathology of AD, as clearing this protein may prove to be more effective than targeting Aβ pathology. Results from preclinical studies using this approach have so far shown promise (45–47) but its efficacy in patients is awaited. In addition, targeting tau would not only benefit patients with AD but also those suffering with other tauopathies and possibly those with PD. However, in the latter disorder both passive and active immunization therapies against the primary pathological protein of PD, namely α-synuclein, are being explored and have even gone to clinical trials in both PD and multiple system atrophy (MSA). In the case of PD, AFFiRis has now immunized 24 PD patients with a low- and high-dose immunization approach, and preliminary data show efficacy in those that mounted an antibody response. All of these approaches against these intracellular proteins are based on the assumption that both tauopathies and α-synucleinopathies may progress through protein spread from cell to cell. As such, the pathological protein will be released from cells into extracellular space before seeding pathology in "infected" cells in a prion-like way. Thus blocking the spreading protein when it is in the extracellular compartment should in theory arrest the disease process (48).

- *Upregulation of autophagy*: The capacity to remove proteins through the lysosomal system of the cell has been studied in many NDDs, including AD, PD, and HD. The first agent that was considered was rapamycin, a relatively selective inhibitor of the mTOR signaling pathway, which has been shown to provide beneficial effects on neuropathology and neurodegeneration in models of PD (49), AD (50, 51) and prion disease (52). However, the disease that has perhaps shown the most promising results is HD, where drugs such as rapamycin, as well as other agents known to stimulate this pathway, have been shown to be very effective in clearing mutant protein *in vitro* and in a whole range of animal models (53, 54). This approach is now entering early clinical trials with a safety assessment of rilmenidine, an anti-hypertensive drug which through its selectivity for imidazoline and α2-adrenergic receptors can upregulate autophagy (Barker, Rubinsztein: unpublished data).
- *Upregulation of the UPS system*: In addition to autophagy, the cell uses the UPS to remove abnormal proteins by ubiquitination and then proteosomal degradation. Defects in this whole pathway may underlie some genetic forms of PD, as well as other NDDs of the CNS (55), but attempts to exploit it to clear abnormal proteins to date have not been successful, as no real agents have been identified that can specifically target this system.
- *Unfolded protein response*: The abnormal production and accumulation of protein in a cell is countered by a response in which protein synthesis is switched off—the unfolded protein response. In the short term this is an effective strategy used by the cell, but when persistent, the cell loses vital components and starts to die. As such, agents that can target this pathway have been explored in prion-like disease with some success (56).
- *Modulating post-transcriptional modifications of the protein that make it more toxic, such as the phosphorylation of*

tau. To date, agents to do this are lacking, and although lithium has been proposed to work in this way, the toxicity of the drug has meant that no trials have shown it to be useful in this regard or well tolerated (e.g., in progressive supranuclear palsy [PSP]: https://clinicaltrials.gov/ct2/show/NCT00703677; Burn D: personal communication).

Disease Modification at the Level of the Mitochondria

All cells rely on the mitochondria to generate the necessary energy to maintain all of their vital functions. In neurons, this is especially the case, given their excitability and heavy reliance on ion pumps to maintain their ionic gradients. Thus anything that compromises mitochondrial function will put the cell under stress; with this comes the production of free radicals and oxidative damage, which in turn can further compromise the mitochondria. In many NDDs, mitochondria are implicated in the disease process—either directly, as in certain genetic forms of PD, or indirectly through protein accumulation within the cytoplasm. As such, this has been an area where many trials have been undertaken with therapies that are thought to target this entire process, including agents that have either a mitochondrial or an oxidative stress target. Such trials include coenzyme Q10 in PD (57–60), HD (61, 62), ALS (63, 64), and PSP (65); creatine supplementation in PD (66, 67) and HD (68, 69); selegiline and rasagailine (MAOI) (70–74), as well as MitoQ in PD (75). In all cases, the results have failed to show any great effect in the long term, in part because the agents have limited effects on mitochondria, and in part because this problem is more downstream of the major pathological problem in most NDDs. Nevertheless, there are some new agents that have been identified, including a viral non-coding RNA that specifically targets complex I of the mitochondrial respiratory chain and that has been shown to be protective in an animal model of PD (76). Moreover, other preclinical studies have identified the potential of a cell-permeable peptide antioxidant targeting mitochondria, SS-31, which protects against oxidant-induced mitochondrial dysfunction in animal models of ALS (77) and PD (78).

Disease Modification at the Level of the Cell

Ultimately the cell will die as a result of the pathogenic cascade, and although the route by which this happens is often unclear, it can broadly be thought of in terms of programmed (apoptosis) or non-programmed cell death (of which there are many different types). As such, agents have been tried that target specific components of the apoptotic pathway, although to date none has shown any lasting efficacy in animal models. An alternative approach is to try to rescue the cell through giving either agents that block those stimuli that can trigger the process from without, such as excitotoxicity and secondary calcium fluxes, or agents that are trophic to the cell. The former has led to trials of calcium antagonists and glutamate blockers, which have been shown to be ineffective in some diseases such as ALS (79, 80) and HD (81–83), but are being actively investigated in PD with agents such as the calcium channel blocker Isradipine (84, 85).

In terms of trophic factors, there have been trials of various growth factors in a range of NDDs, most of which have failed. This relates as much to technical reasons, including modes of delivery, as to the stability of the agent being given and the trial design. For example, ciliary neurotrophic factor (CNTF) has been trialed in ALS without benefit, but in this case it was administered peripherally, where it is rapidly degraded within minutes, suggesting that more efficient methods of administration are needed if it is to be used in this condition (86–88).

In HD, this agent was also tried, but in this case it was delivered by cells engineered to release CNTF. These were implanted into the lateral ventricles of patients, but without success, again because the cells released variable levels of the agent, which could not then penetrate into the striatum where it was needed to work (89). In a similar way, glial-derived neurotrophic factor (GDNF) was also tried in PD through an intraventricular delivery system, again without benefit because it could not penetrate into the nigra and thus rescue the remaining dopaminergic cells. As a result, this led to more successful open label trials in which there was intraparenchymal delivery of GDNF, which then gave way to a negative double-blind placebo-controlled trial (90, 91). The reasons that this trial produced a result at variance with the original open label studies has been disputed (92), but technical factors could not be excluded. In the last couple of years, this therapy has been re-explored, with two new trials that are ongoing in the United Kingdom and the United States involving direct GDNF infusion and viral delivery of GDNF, respectively. While these trials

were being undertaken, an alternative approach using gene delivery of neurturin (NTN), a neurotrophic factor in the GDNF family, was also being tested in PD by the company Ceregene. This also failed to show any effect on disease progression, which has been suggested to be due to the dose given and the stage of disease targeted (striatum vs. substantia nigra) (93–94). In other words, higher doses in earlier stage disease may have given very different results.

Disease Modification at the Level of a Dysfunctional Network

Although not strictly disease modifying, the ability to repair focal networks of cells with cell transplants has been tried in many diseases, most notably PD and to a lesser extent HD and ALS. In these conditions, cells have been implanted in an attempt to restore lost function through either restoration of a physiological neuronal dopamine input to the striatum in the case of PD; striatal circuitry in the case of HD (95–98); or motorneuronal rescue through astrocytic grafting in the case of ALS (for review, see 99).

In PD, this approach has had mixed success, with the best results being seen with fetal human ventral midbrain (VM) tissue grafted into the striatum (100). In some cases, patients have managed to remain off dopaminergic therapies for years post-grafting (101), although in other patients the transplants have been ineffective and have led to side effects, with graft-induced dyskinesias (102, 103). The reasons for these variable results have been widely debated and relate in part to patient selection, tissue preparation, dopamine cell distribution at the site of grafting, the immunotherapy used post-implantation, and trial design. As a result, a new trial is underway in Europe (TRANSEURO) and is seen as paving the way for the next generation of cells for use in PD, which will be of stem cell origin (104).

In HD, the number of patients allografted with fetal striatal tissue is less than that seen with PD, which makes it harder to come to any firm conclusion. However, to date the studies would suggest that such transplants have limited efficacy (97, 105, 106), in part because the environment in which the graft finds itself leads to pathology developing within the transplant (107–109). At the present time, there is a large study ongoing using this approach in France, and the result of that will determine whether there is a future in this approach, including future trials of stem-cell-derived medium spiny striatal projection neurons.

In ALS, the strategy that has been investigated most is one looking at glial cells rather than motorneurons themselves. The approach is based on the theory that in ALS there is defective glutamate clearance by the astrocytes (110), which leads to secondary loss of the motorneurons. Ergo grafting in astrocytes should rescue compromised motorneurons, and while this has been shown experimentally (111, 112), it has yet to be tried in the clinic.

Disease Modification at the Level of the Whole Brain

While the above approaches have all sought to target relatively specific aspects of the pathogenic pathway, with the possible exception of those drugs targeting mitochondrial function and free radical scavengers, an alternative therapeutic intervention involves targeting the whole body and brain. One way is through alteration in diet, as it has now been shown that altering the composition of the brain fatty acids through polyunsaturated fatty acid intake can have consequences on the loss of cells in animal models of AD (113) and PD (114, 115). While this has yet to translate to a clinical trial, at least experimentally, dietary changes influence a whole range of pathways and processes centrally, including effects on inflammation and the release of growth factors. In this respect, a few epidemiological studies have shown the protective effect of such diets in AD (116, 117), although others have not found such an association (118).

As an alternative, or in synergy with dietary changes, another area of great interest is exercise and environmental enrichment. These have been shown to alter the natural course of some animal models of NDDs, and may do so by altering central growth factor levels such as brain-derived neurotrophic factor (BDNF) (119, 120), as well as through adult neurogenesis (121, 122). However, the latter only occurs at selective sites within the adult mammalian brain—the subventricular zone and the subgranular zone in the hippocampus—and the functional capacity of these systems to repair areas of the adult human brain is yet to be determined. Nevertheless, there are now a number of studies that show that exercise may have a positive effect on disease course—at least in HD (123) and PD (124)—although whether it is truly disease modifying or simply making patients fitter and better able to cope with their neurological condition is unclear.

Sleep is essential for life, and sleep deprivation has many negative impacts on the brain. Most patients with NDDs have disorganized sleep and circadian rhythms (for reviews, see 125, 126), and it is thus hard to know whether it contributes to disease states or merely results from them and exacerbates some of their symptoms. Of late, there has been interest in investigating a more active role for sleep in disease processes. For example, there was a recent study showing a role of sleep in clearing extracellular amyloid deposits seen in experimental animal models of AD (127), as well as in maintaining and stabilizing synapses underlying many aspects of cognition that are affected in NDDs (128). Consequently, it has been suggested that restoring sleep and normal circadian rhythms may have benefits in not just improving the patient symptomatically but that it also may be disease modifying (129).

Finally, the role of inflammation has come center stage again with many NDDs, as a result of these developments:

1. the discovery that early inflammation is seen in these conditions using PET (130, 131) and at postmortem (132–134); and
2. the finding in GWAS studies that loci linked to genes for inflammation were linked to disease risk (135, 136).

This has led to epidemiological studies looking at the use of anti-inflammatory drugs and NDD incidence, as well as a slew of studies looking at markers of inflammation in these conditions (137, 138). These all suggest that inflammation may play a role and that anti-inflammatory agents may be of benefit, but unfortunately to date many trials have been undertaken that are hard to interpret due to their small size and the problem of assessing disease progression in NDDs (see, for example, 139).

CONCLUSION

In this chapter we have avoided giving a long list of diseases and all the trials of disease-modifying agents that have been undertaken in each disorder. Instead, we felt it would be more useful to look at pathogenic pathways and how agents that target elements of it have been used as possible disease-modifying therapies. This has enabled us to not only look at approaches that are highly specific and that may only treat one condition (siRNA to mutant huntingtin), but also therapeutics that could be used for a whole range of related disorders (e.g., ncRNA therapy to complex 1 of mitochondria). In addition, we have also discussed non-targeted approaches that could also be trialed in all NDDs, such as dietary manipulations and exercise/cognitive therapy programs. In all cases where clinical studies have been done, they have been difficult to interpret, not least because at the current time we have no or very few reliable and robust measures of disease progression, which are needed if the therapy is to be seen to be truly disease modifying. Even in those cases where some measures may exist (e.g., HD, ALS), the numbers needed to treat over long time frames make such studies expensive and difficult to undertake. Nevertheless, there is a growing excitement in the field as entirely new therapeutic approaches are emerging, along with a range of better biomarkers, all of which can now be better employed to treat a wide range of patients with NDDs.

REFERENCES

1. Jellinger, KA, and J Attems. 2008. Prevalence and impact of vascular and Alzheimer pathologies in Lewy body disease. *Acta Neuropathol* 115, no. 4: 427–436.
2. James, BD, DA Bennett, PA Boyle, S Leurgans, and JA Schneider. 2012. Dementia from Alzheimer disease and mixed pathologies in the oldest old. *JAMA* 307, no. 17: 1798–1800.
3. Braak, H, K Del Tredici, U Rub, RA de Vos, EN Jansen Steur, and E Braak. 2003. Staging of brain pathology related to sporadic Parkinson's disease. *Neurobiol Aging* 24, no. 2: 197–211.
4. Tabrizi, SJ, RI Scahill, G Owen, A Durr, BR Leavitt, RA Roos, B Borowsky, B Landwehrmeyer, C Frost, H Johnson, D Craufurd, R Reilmann, JC Stout, and DR Langbehn. 2013. Predictors of phenotypic progression and disease onset in premanifest and early-stage Huntington's disease in the TRACK-HD study: analysis of 36-month observational data. *Lancet Neurol* 12, no. 7: 637–649.
5. Paulsen, JS, JD Long, CA Ross, DL Harrington, CJ Erwin, JK Williams, HJ Westervelt, HJ Johnson, EH Aylward, Y Zhang, HJ Bockholt, and RA Barker. 2014. Prediction of manifest Huntington's disease with clinical and imaging measures: a prospective observational study. *Lancet Neurol* 13, no. 12: 1193–1201.
6. Clavaguera, F, H Akatsu, G Fraser, RA Crowther, S Frank, J Hench, A Probst, DT Winkler, J Reichwald, M Staufenbiel, B Ghetti, M Goedert, and M Tolnay. 2013. Brain homogenates from human tauopathies induce tau inclusions in mouse brain. *Proc Natl Acad Sci U S A* 110, no. 23: 9535–9540.
7. Clavaguera, F, J Hench, I Lavenir, G Schweighauser, S Frank, M Goedert, and M Tolnay. 2014. Peripheral administration of tau aggregates triggers intracerebral tauopathy in transgenic mice. *Acta Neuropathol* 127, no. 2: 299–301.
8. Ahmed, Z, J Cooper, TK Murray, K Garn, E McNaughton, H Clarke, S Parhizkar, MA Ward, A Cavallini, S Jackson, S Bose, F Clavaguera, M Tolnay, I Lavenir, M Goedert, ML Hutton, and MJ O'Neill. 2014. A novel in vivo model of tau propagation with rapid and progressive neurofibrillary tangle pathology: the pattern of spread is determined by connectivity, not proximity. *Acta Neuropathol* 127, no. 5: 667–683.
9. Diaz-Amarilla, P, S Olivera-Bravo, E Trias, A Cragnolini, L Martinez-Palma, P Cassina, J Beckman, and L Barbeito. 2011. Phenotypically aberrant astrocytes that promote motoneuron damage in a model of inherited amyotrophic lateral sclerosis. *Proc Natl Acad Sci U S A* 108, no. 44: 18126–18131.
10. Gallardo, G, J Barowski, J Ravits, T Siddique, JB Lingrel, J Robertson, H Steen, and A Bonni. 2014. An alpha2-Na/K ATPase/alpha-adducin complex in astrocytes triggers non-cell autonomous neurodegeneration. *Nat Neurosci* 17, no. 12: 1710–1719.
11. Rojas, F, N Cortes, S Abarzua, A Dyrda, and B van Zundert. 2014. Astrocytes expressing mutant SOD1 and TDP43 trigger motoneuron death that is mediated via sodium channels and nitroxidative stress. *Front Cell Neurosci* 8, 24.
12. Yang, C, H Wang, T Qiao, B Yang, L Aliaga, L Qiu, W Tan, J Salameh, DM McKenna-Yasek, T Smith, L Peng, MJ Moore, RH Brown Jr, H Cai, and Z Xu. 2014. Partial loss of TDP-43 function causes phenotypes of amyotrophic lateral sclerosis. *Proc Natl Acad Sci U S A* 111, no. 12: E1121-E1129.
13. Deleidi, M, and O Isacson. 2012. Viral and inflammatory triggers of neurodegenerative diseases. *Sci Transl Med* 4, no. 121: 121ps3.
14. Amor, S, LA Peferoen, DY Vogel, M Breur, P van der Valk, D Baker, and JM van Noort. 2014. Inflammation in neurodegenerative diseases: an update. *Immunology* 142, no. 2: 151–166.
15. Carrithers, MD. 2014. Update on disease-modifying treatments for multiple sclerosis. *Clin Ther* 36(12), no. 12: 1938–1945.
16. Cross, AH, and RT Naismith. 2014. Established and novel disease-modifying treatments in multiple sclerosis. *J Intern Med* 275, no. 4: 350–363.
17. Kim, H, and JS Kim. 2014. A guide to genome engineering with programmable nucleases. *Nat Rev Genet* 15, no. 5: 321–334.
18. Joung, JK, and JD Sander. 2013. TALENs: a widely applicable technology for targeted genome editing. *Nat Rev Mol Cell Biol* 14, no. 1: 49–55.

19. Haurwitz, RE, M Jinek, B Wiedenheft, K Zhou, and JA Doudna. 2010. Sequence- and structure-specific RNA processing by a CRISPR endonuclease. *Science* 329, no. 5997: 1355–1358.

20. Soldner, F, J Laganiere, AW Cheng, D Hockemeyer, Q Gao, R Alagappan, V Khurana, LI Golbe, RH Myers, S Lindquist, L Zhang, D Guschin, LK Fong, BJ Vu, X Meng, FD Urnov, EJ Rebar, PD Gregory, HS Zhang, and R Jaenisch. 2011. Generation of isogenic pluripotent stem cells differing exclusively at two early onset Parkinson point mutations. *Cell* 146, no. 2: 318–331.

21. Sanders, LH, J Laganiere, O Cooper, SK Mak, BJ Vu, YA Huang, DE Paschon, M Vangipuram, R Sundararajan, FD Urnov, JW Langston, PD Gregory, HS Zhang, JT Greenamyre, O Isacson, and B Schule. 2014. LRRK2 mutations cause mitochondrial DNA damage in iPSC-derived neural cells from Parkinson's disease patients: reversal by gene correction. *Neurobiol Dis* 62, 381–386.

22. Chen, H, K Qian, Z Du, J Cao, A Petersen, H Liu, LW 4th Blackbourn, CL Huang, A Errigo, Y Yin, J Lu, M Ayala, and SC Zhang. 2014. Modeling ALS with iPSCs reveals that mutant SOD1 misregulates neurofilament balance in motor neurons. *Cell Stem Cell* 14, no. 6: 796–809.

23. Garriga-Canut, M, C Agustin-Pavon, F Herrmann, A Sanchez, M Dierssen, C Fillat, and M Isalan. 2012. Synthetic zinc finger repressors reduce mutant huntingtin expression in the brain of R6/2 mice. *Proc Natl Acad Sci U S A* 109, no. 45: E3136-E3145.

24. Thomas, EA, G Coppola, PA Desplats, B Tang, E Soragni, R Burnett, F Gao, KM Fitzgerald, JF Borok, D Herman, DH Geschwind, and JM Gottesfeld. 2008. The HDAC inhibitor 4b ameliorates the disease phenotype and transcriptional abnormalities in Huntington's disease transgenic mice. *Proc Natl Acad Sci U S A* 105, no. 40: 15564–15569.

25. Hathorn, T, A Snyder-Keller, and A Messer. 2011. Nicotinamide improves motor deficits and upregulates PGC-1alpha and BDNF gene expression in a mouse model of Huntington's disease. *Neurobiol Dis* 41, no. 1: 43–50.

26. Jia, H, J Pallos, V Jacques, A Lau, B Tang, A Cooper, A Syed, J Purcell, Y Chen, S Sharma, GR Sangrey, SB Darnell, H Plasterer, G Sadri-Vakili, JM Gottesfeld, LM Thompson, JR Rusche, JL Marsh, and EA Thomas. 2012. Histone deacetylase (HDAC) inhibitors targeting HDAC3 and HDAC1 ameliorate polyglutamine-elicited phenotypes in model systems of Huntington's disease. *Neurobiol Dis* 46, no. 2: 351–361.

27. Mielcarek, M, C Landles, A Weiss, A Bradaia, T Seredenina, L Inuabasi, GF Osborne, K Wadel, C Touller, R Butler, J Robertson, SA Franklin, DL Smith, L Park, PA Marks, EE Wanker, EN Olson, R Luthi-Carter, H van der Putten, V Beaumont, and GP Bates. 2013. HDAC4 reduction: a novel therapeutic strategy to target cytoplasmic huntingtin and ameliorate neurodegeneration. *PLoS Biol* 11, no. 11: e1001717.

28. Benn, CL, R Butler, L Mariner, J Nixon, H Moffitt, M Mielcarek, B Woodman, and GP Bates. 2009. Genetic knock-down of HDAC7 does not ameliorate disease pathogenesis in the R6/2 mouse model of Huntington's disease. *PLoS One* 4, no. 6: e5747.

29. Bobrowska, A, P Paganetti, P Matthias, and GP Bates. 2011. Hdac6 knock-out increases tubulin acetylation but does not modify disease progression in the R6/2 mouse model of Huntington's disease. *PLoS One* 6, no. 6: e20696.

30. Moumne, L, K Campbell, D Howland, Y Ouyang, and GP Bates. 2012. Genetic knock-down of HDAC3 does not modify disease-related phenotypes in a mouse model of Huntington's disease. *PLoS One* 7, no. 2: e31080.

31. Mano, T, T Suzuki, S Tsuji, and A Iwata. 2014. Differential effect of HDAC3 on cytoplasmic and nuclear huntingtin aggregates. *PLoS One* 9, no. 11: e111277.

32. Jia, H, CD Morris, RM Williams, JF Loring, and EA Thomas. 2015. HDAC inhibition imparts beneficial transgenerational effects in Huntington's disease mice via altered DNA and histone methylation. *Proc Natl Acad Sci U S A* 112, no. 1: E56–E64.

33. Harper, SQ, PD Staber, X He, SL Eliason, IH Martins, Q Mao, L Yang, RM Kotin, HL Paulson, and BL Davidson. 2005. RNA interference improves motor and neuropathological abnormalities in a Huntington's disease mouse model. *Proc Natl Acad Sci U S A* 102, no. 16: 5820–5825.

34. Rodriguez-Lebron, E, EM Denovan-Wright, K Nash, AS Lewin, and RJ Mandel. 2005. Intrastriatal rAAV-mediated delivery of anti-huntingtin shRNAs induces partial reversal of disease progression in R6/1 Huntington's disease transgenic mice. *Mol Ther* 12, no. 4: 618–633.

35. DiFiglia, M, M Sena-Esteves, K Chase, E Sapp, E Pfister, M Sass, J Yoder, P Reeves, RK Pandey, KG Rajeev, M Manoharan, DW Sah, PD Zamore, and N Aronin. 2007. Therapeutic silencing of mutant huntingtin with siRNA attenuates striatal and cortical neuropathology and behavioral deficits. *Proc Natl Acad Sci U S A* 104, no. 43: 17204–17209.

36. Franich, NR, HL Fitzsimons, DM Fong, M Klugmann, MJ During, and D Young. 2008. AAV vector-mediated RNAi of mutant huntingtin

expression is neuroprotective in a novel genetic rat model of Huntington's disease. *Mol Ther* 16, no. 5: 947–956.

37. Drouet, V, V Perrin, R Hassig, N Dufour, G Auregan, S Alves, G Bonvento, E Brouillet, R Luthi-Carter, P Hantraye, and N Deglon. 2009. Sustained effects of nonallele-specific Huntingtin silencing. *Ann Neurol* 65, no. 3: 276–285.

38. Kordasiewicz, HB, LM Stanek, EV Wancewicz, C Mazur, MM McAlonis, KA Pytel, JW Artates, A Weiss, SH Cheng, LS Shihabuddin, G Hung, CF Bennett, and DW Cleveland. 2012. Sustained therapeutic reversal of Huntington's disease by transient repression of huntingtin synthesis. *Neuron* 74, no. 6: 1031–1044.

39. Miller, TM, A Pestronk, W David, J Rothstein, E Simpson, SH Appel, PL Andres, K Mahoney, P Allred, K Alexander, LW Ostrow, D Schoenfeld, EA Macklin, DA Norris, G Manousakis, M Crisp, R Smith, CF Bennett, KM Bishop, and ME Cudkowicz. 2013. An antisense oligonucleotide against SOD1 delivered intrathecally for patients with SOD1 familial amyotrophic lateral sclerosis: a phase 1, randomised, first-in-man study. *Lancet Neurol* 12, no. 5: 435–442.

40. Bombois, S, CA Maurage, M Gompel, V Deramecourt, MA Mackowiak-Cordoliani, RS Black, R Lavielle, A Delacourte, and F Pasquier. 2007. Absence of beta-amyloid deposits after immunization in Alzheimer disease with Lewy body dementia. *Arch Neurol* 64, no. 4: 583–587.

41. Gilman, S, M Koller, RS Black, L Jenkins, SG Griffith, NC Fox, L Eisner, L Kirby, MB Rovira, F Forette, and JM Orgogozo. 2005. Clinical effects of Abeta immunization (AN1792) in patients with AD in an interrupted trial. *Neurology* 64, no. 9: 1553–1562.

42. Salloway, S, R Sperling, S Gilman, NC Fox, K Blennow, M Raskind, M Sabbagh, LS Honig, R Doody, CH van Dyck, R Mulnard, J Barakos, KM Gregg, E Liu, I Lieburg, D Schenk, R Black, and M Grundman. 2009. A phase 2 multiple ascending dose trial of bapineuzumab in mild to moderate Alzheimer disease. *Neurology* 73, no. 24: 2061–2070.

43. Farlow, M, SE Arnold, CH van Dyck, PS Aisen, BJ Snider, AP Porsteinsson, S Friedrich, RA Dean, C Gonzales, G Sethuraman, RB DeMattos, R Mohs, SM Paul, and ER Siemers. 2012. Safety and biomarker effects of solanezumab in patients with Alzheimer's disease. *Alzheimers Dement* 8, no. 4: 261–271.

44. Sperling, R, S Salloway, DJ Brooks, D Tampieri, J Barakos, NC Fox, M Raskind, M Sabbagh, LS Honig, AP Porsteinsson, I Lieberburg, HM Arrighi, KA Morris, Y Lu, E Liu, KM Gregg, HR Brashear, GG Kinney, R Black, and M Grundman. 2012. Amyloid-related imaging abnormalities in patients with Alzheimer's disease treated with bapineuzumab: a retrospective analysis. *Lancet Neurol* 11, no. 3: 241–249.

45. Asuni, AA, A Boutajangout, D Quartermain, and EM Sigurdsson. 2007. Immunotherapy targeting pathological tau conformers in a tangle mouse model reduces brain pathology with associated functional improvements. *J Neurosci* 27, no. 34: 9115–9129.

46. Boutajangout, A, D Quartermain, and EM Sigurdsson. 2010. Immunotherapy targeting pathological tau prevents cognitive decline in a new tangle mouse model. *J Neurosci* 30, no. 49: 16559–16566.

47. Boutajangout, A, J Ingadottir, P Davies, and EM Sigurdsson. 2011. Passive immunization targeting pathological phospho-tau protein in a mouse model reduces functional decline and clears tau aggregates from the brain. *J Neurochem* 118, no. 4: 658–667.

48. Tran, HT, CH Chung, M Iba, B Zhang, JQ Trojanowski, KC Luk, and VM Lee. 2014. Alpha-synuclein immunotherapy blocks uptake and templated propagation of misfolded alpha-synuclein and neurodegeneration. *Cell Rep* 7, no. 6: 2054–2065.

49. Webb, JL, B Ravikumar, J Atkins, JN Skepper, and DC Rubinsztein. 2003. Alpha-synuclein is degraded by both autophagy and the proteasome. *J Biol Chem* 278, no. 27: 25009–25013.

50. Caccamo, A, S Majumder, A Richardson, R Strong, and S Oddo. 2010. Molecular interplay between mammalian target of rapamycin (mTOR), amyloid-beta, and Tau: effects on cognitive impairments. *J Biol Chem* 285, no. 17: 13107–13120.

51. Spilman, P, N Podlutskaya, MJ Hart, J Debnath, O Gorostiza, D Bredesen, A Richardson, R Strong, and V Galvan. 2010. Inhibition of mTOR by rapamycin abolishes cognitive deficits and reduces amyloid-beta levels in a mouse model of Alzheimer's disease. *PLoS One* 5, no. 4: e9979.

52. Cortes, CJ, K Qin, J Cook, A Solanki, and JA Mastrianni. 2012. Rapamycin delays disease onset and prevents PrP plaque deposition in a mouse model of Gerstmann-Straussler-Scheinker disease. *J Neurosci* 32, no. 36: 12396–12405.

53. Sarkar, S, B Ravikumar, RA Floto, and DC Rubinsztein. 2009. Rapamycin and mTOR-independent autophagy inducers ameliorate toxicity of polyglutamine-expanded huntingtin and related proteinopathies. *Cell Death Differ* 16, no. 1: 46–56.

54. Rose, C, FM Menzies, M Renna, A Acevedo-Arozena, S Corrochano, O Sadiq, SD Brown, and

DC Rubinsztein. 2010. Rilmenidine attenuates toxicity of polyglutamine expansions in a mouse model of Huntington's disease. *Hum Mol Genet* 19, no. 11: 2144–2153.

55. Zheng, C, T Geetha, and JR Babu. 2014. Failure of ubiquitin proteasome system: risk for neurodegenerative diseases. *Neurodegener Dis* 14, no. 4: 161–175.

56. Moreno, JA, M Halliday, C Molloy, H Radford, N Verity, JM Axten, CA Ortori, AE Willis, PM Fischer, DA Barrett, and GR Mallucci. 2013. Oral treatment targeting the unfolded protein response prevents neurodegeneration and clinical disease in prion-infected mice. *Sci Transl Med* 5, no. 206: 206ra138.

57. NINDS NET-PD Investigators. 2007. A randomized clinical trial of coenzyme Q10 and GPI-1485 in early Parkinson disease. *Neurology* 68, no. 1: 20–28.

58. Shults, CW, MF Beal, D Fontaine, K Nakano, and RH Haas. 1998. Absorption, tolerability, and effects on mitochondrial activity of oral coenzyme Q10 in parkinsonian patients. *Neurology* 50, no. 3: 793–795.

59. Shults, CW, D Oakes, K Kieburtz, MF Beal, R Haas, S Plumb, JL Juncos, J Nutt, I Shoulson, J Carter, K Kompoliti, JS Perlmutter, S Reich, M Stern, RL Watts, R Kurlan, E Molho, M Harrison, and M Lew. 2002. Effects of coenzyme Q10 in early Parkinson disease: evidence of slowing of the functional decline. *Arch Neurol* 59, no. 10: 1541–1550.

60. Muller, T, T Buttner, AF Gholipour, and W Kuhn. 2003. Coenzyme Q10 supplementation provides mild symptomatic benefit in patients with Parkinson's disease. *Neurosci Lett* 341, no. 3: 201–204.

61. Huntington Study Group. 2001. A randomized, placebo-controlled trial of coenzyme Q10 and remacemide in Huntington's disease. *Neurology* 57, no. 3: 397–404.

62. Feigin, A, K Kieburtz, P Como, C Hickey, K Claude, D Abwender, C Zimmerman, K Steinberg, and I Shoulson. 1996. Assessment of coenzyme Q10 tolerability in Huntington's disease. *Mov Disord* 11, no. 3: 321–323.

63. Ferrante, KL, J Shefner, H Zhang, R Betensky, M O'Brien, H Yu, M Fantasia, J Taft, MF Beal, B Traynor, K Newhall, P Donofrio, J Caress, C Ashburn, B Freiberg, C O'Neill, C Paladenech, T Walker, A Pestronk, B Abrams, J Florence, R Renna, J Schierbecker, B Malkus, and M Cudkowicz. 2005. Tolerance of high-dose (3,000 mg/day) coenzyme Q10 in ALS. *Neurology* 65, no. 11: 1834–1836.

64. Kaufmann, P, JL Thompson, G Levy, R Buchsbaum, J Shefner, LS Krivickas, J Katz, Y Rollins, RJ Barohn, CE Jackson, E Tiryaki, C Lomen-Hoerth, C Armon, R Tandan, SA Rudnicki, K Rezania, R Sufit, A Pestronk, SP Novella, T Heiman-Patterson, EJ Kasarskis, EP Pioro, J Montes, R Arbing, D Vecchio, A Barsdorf, H Mitsumoto, and B Levin. 2009. Phase II trial of CoQ10 for ALS finds insufficient evidence to justify phase III. *Ann Neurol* 66, no. 2: 235–244.

65. Stamelou, M, A Reuss, U Pilatus, J Magerkurth, P Niklowitz, KM Eggert, A Krisp, T Menke, C Schade-Brittinger, WH Oertel, and GU Hoglinger. 2008. Short-term effects of coenzyme Q10 in progressive supranuclear palsy: a randomized, placebo-controlled trial. *Mov Disord* 23, no. 7: 942–949.

66. Bender, A, W Koch, M Elstner, Y Schombacher, J Bender, M Moeschl, F Gekeler, B Muller-Myhsok, T Gasser, K Tatsch, and T Klopstock. 2006. Creatine supplementation in Parkinson disease: a placebo-controlled randomized pilot trial. *Neurology* 67, no. 7: 1262–1264.

67. Bender, A, W Samtleben, M Elstner, and T Klopstock. 2008. Long-term creatine supplementation is safe in aged patients with Parkinson disease. *Nutr Res* 28, no. 3: 172–178.

68. Verbessem, P, J Lemiere, BO Eijnde, S Swinnen, L Vanhees, M Van Leemputte, P Hespel, and R Dom. 2003. Creatine supplementation in Huntington's disease: a placebo-controlled pilot trial. *Neurology* 61, no. 7: 925–930.

69. Hersch, SM, S Gevorkian, K Marder, C Moskowitz, A Feigin, M Cox, P Como, C Zimmerman, M Lin, L Zhang, AM Ulug, MF Beal, W Matson, M Bogdanov, E Ebbel, A Zaleta, Y Kaneko, B Jenkins, N Hevelone, H Zhang, H Yu, D Schoenfeld, R Ferrante, and HD Rosas. 2006. Creatine in Huntington disease is safe, tolerable, bioavailable in brain and reduces serum 8OH2'dG. *Neurology* 66, no. 2: 250–252.

70. Palhagen, S, EH Heinonen, J Hagglund, T Kaugesaar, H Kontants, O Maki-Ikola, R Palm, and J Turunen. 1998. Selegiline delays the onset of disability in de novo parkinsonian patients. Swedish Parkinson Study Group. *Neurology* 51, no. 2: 520–525.

71. Rascol, O, DJ Brooks, E Melamed, W Oertel, W Poewe, F Stocchi, and E Tolosa. 2005. Rasagiline as an adjunct to levodopa in patients with Parkinson's disease and motor fluctuations (LARGO, Lasting effect in Adjunct therapy with Rasagiline Given Once daily, study): a randomised, double-blind, parallel-group trial. *Lancet* 365, no. 9463: 947–954.

72. Palhagen, S, E Heinonen, J Hagglund, T Kaugesaar, O Maki-Ikola, and R Palm. 2006. Selegiline slows the progression of the symptoms of Parkinson disease. *Neurology* 66, no. 8: 1200–1206.

73. Olanow, CW, O Rascol, R Hauser, PD Feigin, J Jankovic, A Lang, W Langston, E Melamed, W Poewe, F Stocchi, and E Tolosa. 2009. A double-blind, delayed-start trial of rasagiline in Parkinson's disease. *N Engl J Med* 361, no. 13: 1268–1278.

74. Rascol, O, CJ Fitzer-Attas, R Hauser, J Jankovic, A Lang, JW Langston, E Melamed, W Poewe, F Stocchi, E Tolosa, E Eyal, YM Weiss, and CW Olanow. 2011. A double-blind, delayed-start trial of rasagiline in Parkinson's disease (the ADAGIO study): prespecified and post-hoc analyses of the need for additional therapies, changes in UPDRS scores, and non-motor outcomes. *Lancet Neurol* 10, no. 5: 415–423.

75. Snow, BJ, FL Rolfe, MM Lockhart, CM Frampton, JD O'Sullivan, V Fung, RA Smith, MP Murphy, and KM Taylor. 2010. A double-blind, placebo-controlled study to assess the mitochondria-targeted antioxidant MitoQ as a disease-modifying therapy in Parkinson's disease. *Mov Disord* 25, no. 11: 1670–1674.

76. Kuan, WL, E Poole, M Fletcher, S Karniely, P Tyers, M Wills, RA Barker, and JH Sinclair. 2012. A novel neuroprotective therapy for Parkinson's disease using a viral noncoding RNA that protects mitochondrial complex I activity. *J Exp Med* 209, no. 1: 1–10.

77. Petri, S, M Kiaei, M Damiano, A Hiller, E Wille, G Manfredi, NY Calingasan, HH Szeto, and MF Beal. 2006. Cell-permeable peptide antioxidants as a novel therapeutic approach in a mouse model of amyotrophic lateral sclerosis. *J Neurochem* 98, no. 4: 1141–1148.

78. Yang, L, K Zhao, NY Calingasan, G Luo, HH Szeto, and MF Beal. 2009. Mitochondria targeted peptides protect against 1-methyl-4-phenyl-1,2,3,6-tetrahydropyridine neurotoxicity. *Antioxid Redox Signal* 11, no. 9: 2095–2104.

79. Bensimon, G, L Lacomblez, and V Meininger. 1994. A controlled trial of riluzole in amyotrophic lateral sclerosis. ALS/Riluzole Study Group. *N Engl J Med* 330, no. 9: 585–591.

80. Miller, RG, R Shepherd, H Dao, A Khramstov, M Mendoza, J Graves, and S Smith. 1996c. Controlled trial of nimodipine in amyotrophic lateral sclerosis. *Neuromuscul Disord* 6, no. 2: 101–104.

81. Kieburtz, K, A Feigin, M McDermott, P Como, D Abwender, C Zimmerman, C Hickey, C Orme, K Claude, J Sotack, JT Greenamyre, C Dunn, and I Shoulson. 1996. A controlled trial of remacemide hydrochloride in Huntington's disease. *Mov Disord* 11, no. 3: 273–277.

82. Verhagen Metman, L, MJ Morris, C Farmer, M Gillespie, K Mosby, J Wuu, and TN Chase. 2002.

Huntington's disease: a randomized, controlled trial using the NMDA-antagonist amantadine. *Neurology* 59, no. 5: 694–699.

83. Beister, A, P Kraus, W Kuhn, M Dose, A Weindl, and M Gerlach. 2004. The N-methyl-D-aspartate antagonist memantine retards progression of Huntington's disease. *J Neural Transm Suppl* no. 68: 117–122.

84. Parkinson Study Group. 2013. Phase II safety, tolerability, and dose selection study of isradipine as a potential disease-modifying intervention in early Parkinson's disease (STEADY-PD). *Mov Disord* 28, no. 13: 1823–1831.

85. Simuni, T, E Borushko, MJ Avram, S Miskevics, A Martel, C Zadikoff, A Videnovic, FM Weaver, K Williams, and DJ Surmeier. 2010. Tolerability of isradipine in early Parkinson's disease: a pilot dose escalation study. *Mov Disord* 25, no. 16: 2863–2866.

86. Miller, RG, WW Bryan, MA Dietz, TL Munsat, JH Petajan, SA Smith, and JC Goodpasture. 1996a. Toxicity and tolerability of recombinant human ciliary neurotrophic factor in patients with amyotrophic lateral sclerosis. *Neurology* 47, no. 5: 1329–1331.

87. Miller, RG, JH Petajan, WW Bryan, C Armon, RJ Barohn, JC Goodpasture, RJ Hoagland, GJ Parry, MA Ross, and SC Stromatt. 1996b. A placebo-controlled trial of recombinant human ciliary neurotrophic (rhCNTF) factor in amyotrophic lateral sclerosis. rhCNTF ALS Study Group. *Ann Neurol* 39, no. 2: 256–260.

88. Bongioanni, P, C Reali, and V Sogos. 2004. Ciliary neurotrophic factor (CNTF) for amyotrophic lateral sclerosis/motor neuron disease. *Cochrane Database Syst Rev* no. 3: CD004302.

89. Bloch, J, AC Bachoud-Levi, N Deglon, JP Lefaucheur, L Winkel, S Palfi, JP Nguyen, C Bourdet, V Gaura, P Remy, P Brugieres, MF Boisse, S Baudic, P Cesaro, P Hantraye, P Aebischer, and M Peschanski. 2004. Neuroprotective gene therapy for Huntington's disease, using polymer-encapsulated cells engineered to secrete human ciliary neurotrophic factor: results of a phase I study. *Hum Gene Ther* 15, no. 10: 968–975.

90. Gill, SS, NK Patel, GR Hotton, K O'Sullivan, R McCarter, M Bunnage, DJ Brooks, CN Svendsen, and P Heywood. 2003. Direct brain infusion of glial cell line-derived neurotrophic factor in Parkinson disease. *Nat Med* 9, no. 5: 589–595.

91. Lang, AE, S Gill, NK Patel, A Lozano, JG Nutt, R Penn, DJ Brooks, G Hotton, E Moro, P Heywood, MA Brodsky, K Burchiel, P Kelly, A Dalvi, B Scott, M Stacy, D Turner, VG Wooten, WJ Elias, ER Laws, V Dhawan, AJ Stoessl, J Matcham, RJ Coffey, and M Traub. 2006. Randomized controlled trial

of intraputamenal glial cell line-derived neuro-trophic factor infusion in Parkinson disease. *Ann Neurol* 59, no. 3: 459–466.

92. Barker, RA. 2006. Continuing trials of GDNF in Parkinson's disease. *Lancet Neurol* 5(4), no. 4: 285–286.

93. Bartus, RT, L Brown, A Wilson, B Kruegel, J Siffert, EM Jr Johnson, JH Kordower, and CD Herzog. 2011a. Properly scaled and targeted AAV2-NRTN (neurturin) to the substantia nigra is safe, effective and causes no weight loss: support for nigral targeting in Parkinson's disease. *Neurobiol Dis* 44, no. 1: 38–52.

94. Bartus, RT, CD Herzog, Y Chu, A Wilson, L Brown, J Siffert, EM Jr Johnson, CW Olanow, EJ Mufson, and JH Kordower. 2011b. Bioactivity of AAV2-neurturin gene therapy (CERE-120): differences between Parkinson's disease and nonhuman primate brains. *Mov Disord* 26, no. 1: 27–36.

95. Bachoud-Levi, A, C Bourdet, P Brugieres, JP Nguyen, T Grandmougin, B Haddad, R Jeny, P Bartolomeo, MF Boisse, GD Barba, JD Degos, AM Ergis, JP Lefaucheur, F Lisovoski, E Pailhous, P Remy, S Palfi, GL Defer, P Cesaro, P Hantraye, and M Peschanski. 2000a. Safety and tolerability assessment of intrastriatal neural allografts in five patients with Huntington's disease. *Exp Neurol* 161, no. 1: 194–202.

96. Bachoud-Levi, AC, P Remy, JP Nguyen, P Brugieres, JP Lefaucheur, C Bourdet, S Baudic, V Gaura, P Maison, B Haddad, MF Boisse, T Grandmougin, R Jeny, P Bartolomeo, G Dalla Barba, JD Degos, F Lisovoski, AM Ergis, E Pailhous, P Cesaro, P Hantraye, and M Peschanski. 2000b. Motor and cognitive improvements in patients with Huntington's disease after neural transplantation. *Lancet* 356, no. 9246: 1975–1979.

97. Bachoud-Levi, AC, V Gaura, P Brugieres, JP Lefaucheur, MF Boisse, P Maison, S Baudic, MJ Ribeiro, C Bourdet, P Remy, P Cesaro, P Hantraye, and M Peschanski. 2006. Effect of fetal neural transplants in patients with Huntington's disease 6 years after surgery: a long-term follow-up study. *Lancet Neurol* 5, no. 4: 303–309.

98. Reuter, I, YF Tai, N Pavese, KR Chaudhuri, S Mason, CE Polkey, C Clough, DJ Brooks, RA Barker, and P Piccini. 2008. Long-term clinical and positron emission tomography outcome of fetal striatal transplantation in Huntington's disease. *J Neurol Neurosurg Psychiatry* 79, no. 8: 948–951.

99. Thomsen, GM, G Gowing, S Svendsen, and CN Svendsen. 2014. The past, present and future of stem cell clinical trials for ALS. *Exp Neurol* 262 Pt B, 127–137.

100. Barker, RA, J Barrett, SL Mason, and A Bjorklund. 2013a. Fetal dopaminergic transplantation trials and the future of neural grafting in Parkinson's disease. *Lancet Neurol* 12, no. 1: 84–91.

101. Kefalopoulou, Z, M Politis, P Piccini, N Mencacci, K Bhatia, M Jahanshahi, H Widner, S Rehncrona, P Brundin, A Bjorklund, O Lindvall, P Limousin, N Quinn, and T Foltynie. 2014. Long-term clinical outcome of fetal cell transplantation for Parkinson disease: two case reports. *JAMA Neurol* 71, no. 1: 83–87.

102. Freed, CR, PE Greene, RE Breeze, WY Tsai, W DuMouchel, R Kao, S Dillon, H Winfield, S Culver, JQ Trojanowski, D Eidelberg, and S Fahn. 2001. Transplantation of embryonic dopamine neurons for severe Parkinson's disease. *N Engl J Med* 344, no. 10: 710–719.

103. Hagell, P, P Piccini, A Bjorklund, P Brundin, S Rehncrona, H Widner, L Crabb, N Pavese, WH Oertel, N Quinn, DJ Brooks, and O Lindvall. 2002. Dyskinesias following neural transplantation in Parkinson's disease. *Nat Neurosci* 5, no. 7: 627–628.

104. Barker, RA. 2014. Developing stem cell therapies for Parkinson's disease: waiting until the time is right. *Cell Stem Cell* 15, no. 5: 539–542.

105. Hauser, RA, S Furtado, CR Cimino, H Delgado, S Eichler, S Schwartz, D Scott, GM Nauert, E Soety, V Sossi, DA Holt, PR Sanberg, AJ Stoessl, and TB Freeman. 2002. Bilateral human fetal striatal transplantation in Huntington's disease. *Neurology* 58, no. 5: 687–695.

106. Barker, RA, SL Mason, TP Harrower, RA Swain, AK Ho, BJ Sahakian, R Mathur, S Elneil, S Thornton, C Hurrelbrink, RJ Armstrong, P Tyers, E Smith, A Carpenter, P Piccini, YF Tai, DJ Brooks, N Pavese, C Watts, JD Pickard, AE Rosser, and SB Dunnett. 2013b. The long-term safety and efficacy of bilateral transplantation of human fetal striatal tissue in patients with mild to moderate Huntington's disease. *J Neurol Neurosurg Psychiatry* 84, no. 6: 657–665.

107. Cicchetti, F, S Lacroix, G Cisbani, N Vallieres, M Saint-Pierre, I St-Amour, R Tolouei, J Skepper, R Hauser, D Mantovani, R Barker, and T Freeman. 2014. Mutant huntingtin is present in neuronal grafts in Huntington's disease patients. *Ann Neurol.* 76, no. 1: 31–42.

108. Cicchetti, F, S Saporta, RA Hauser, M Parent, M Saint-Pierre, PR Sanberg, XJ Li, JR Parker, Y Chu, EJ Mufson, JH Kordower, and TB Freeman. 2009. Neural transplants in patients with Huntington's disease undergo disease-like neuronal degeneration. *Proc Natl Acad Sci U S A* 106, no. 30: 12483–12488.

109. Cisbani, G, TB Freeman, D Soulet, M Saint-Pierre, D Gagnon, M Parent, RA Hauser, RA Barker, and F Cicchetti. 2013. Striatal allografts in patients with Huntington's disease: impact of diminished astrocytes and vascularization on graft viability. *Brain* 136, no. Pt 2: 433–443.

110. Pirooznia, SK, VL Dawson, and TM Dawson. 2014. Motor neuron death in ALS: programmed by astrocytes? *Neuron* 81, no. 5: 961–963.

111. Lepore, AC, J O'Donnell, AS Kim, T Williams, A Tuteja, MS Rao, LL Kelley, JT Campanelli, and NJ Maragakis. 2011. Human glial-restricted progenitor transplantation into cervical spinal cord of the SOD1 mouse model of ALS. *PLoS One* 6, no. 10: e25968.

112. Lepore, AC, B Rauck, C Dejea, AC Pardo, MS Rao, JD Rothstein, and NJ Maragakis. 2008. Focal transplantation-based astrocyte replacement is neuroprotective in a model of motor neuron disease. *Nat Neurosci* 11, no. 11: 1294–1301.

113. Boudrault, C, RP Bazinet, and DW Ma. 2009. Experimental models and mechanisms underlying the protective effects of n-3 polyunsaturated fatty acids in Alzheimer's disease. *J Nutr Biochem* 20, no. 1: 1–10.

114. Bousquet, M, K Gue, V Emond, P Julien, JX Kang, F Cicchetti, and F Calon. 2011. Transgenic conversion of omega-6 into omega-3 fatty acids in a mouse model of Parkinson's disease. *J Lipid Res* 52, no. 2: 263–271.

115. Bousquet, M, M Saint-Pierre, C Julien, N Jr Salem, F Cicchetti, and F Calon. 2008. Beneficial effects of dietary omega-3 polyunsaturated fatty acid on toxin-induced neuronal degeneration in an animal model of Parkinson's disease. *FASEB J* 22, no. 4: 1213–1225.

116. Morris, MC, DA Evans, JL Bienias, CC Tangney, DA Bennett, N Aggarwal, J Schneider, and RS Wilson. 2003a. Dietary fats and the risk of incident Alzheimer disease. *Arch Neurol* 60, no. 2: 194–200.

117. Morris, MC, DA Evans, JL Bienias, CC Tangney, DA Bennett, RS Wilson, N Aggarwal, and J Schneider. 2003b. Consumption of fish and n-3 fatty acids and risk of incident Alzheimer disease. *Arch Neurol* 60, no. 7: 940–946.

118. Devore, EE, F Grodstein, FJ van Rooij, A Hofman, B Rosner, MJ Stampfer, JC Witteman, and MM Breteler. 2009. Dietary intake of fish and omega-3 fatty acids in relation to long-term dementia risk. *Am J Clin Nutr* 90, no. 1: 170–176.

119. Vaynman, S, Z Ying, and F Gomez-Pinilla. 2004. Exercise induces BDNF and synapsin I to specific hippocampal subfields. *J Neurosci Res* 76, no. 3: 356–362.

120. Marais, L, DJ Stein, and WM Daniels. 2009. Exercise increases BDNF levels in the striatum and decreases depressive-like behavior in chronically stressed rats. *Metab Brain Dis* 24, no. 4: 587–597.

121. van Praag, H, T Shubert, C Zhao, and FH Gage. 2005. Exercise enhances learning and hippocampal neurogenesis in aged mice. *J Neurosci* 25, no. 38: 8680–8685.

122. Chen, L, S Gong, LD Shan, WP Xu, YJ Zhang, SY Guo, T Hisamitsu, QZ Yin, and XH Jiang. 2006. Effects of exercise on neurogenesis in the dentate gyrus and ability of learning and memory after hippocampus lesion in adult rats. *Neurosci Bull* 22, no. 1: 1–6.

123. Thompson, JA, TM Cruickshank, LE Penaililo, JW Lee, RU Newton, RA Barker, and MR Ziman. 2013. The effects of multidisciplinary rehabilitation in patients with early-to-middle-stage Huntington's disease: a pilot study. *Eur J Neurol* 20, no. 9: 1325–1329.

124. Zigmond, MJ, and RJ Smeyne. 2014. Exercise: is it a neuroprotective and if so, how does it work? *Parkinsonism Relat Disord* 20 Suppl 1, S123–S127.

125. Gagnon, JF, D Petit, V Latreille, and J Montplaisir. 2008. Neurobiology of sleep disturbances in neurodegenerative disorders. *Curr Pharm Des* 14, no. 32: 3430–3445.

126. Videnovic, A, AS Lazar, RA Barker, and S Overeem. 2014. 'The clocks that time us': circadian rhythms in neurodegenerative disorders. *Nat Rev Neurol* 10, no. 12: 683–693.

127. Xie, L, H Kang, Q Xu, MJ Chen, Y Liao, M Thiyagarajan, J O'Donnell, DJ Christensen, C Nicholson, JJ Iliff, T Takano, R Deane, and M Nedergaard. 2013. Sleep drives metabolite clearance from the adult brain. *Science* 342, no. 6156: 373–377.

128. Vorster, AP, and J Born. 2014. Sleep and memory in mammals, birds and invertebrates. *Neurosci Biobehav Rev.* 50: 103–119.

129. Hastings, MH, and M Goedert. 2013. Circadian clocks and neurodegenerative diseases: time to aggregate? *Curr Opin Neurobiol* 23, no. 5: 880–887.

130. Ouchi, Y, E Yoshikawa, Y Sekine, M Futatsubashi, T Kanno, T Ogusu, and T Torizuka. 2005. Microglial activation and dopamine terminal loss in early Parkinson's disease. *Ann Neurol* 57, no. 2: 168–175.

131. Tai, YF, N Pavese, A Gerhard, SJ Tabrizi, RA Barker, DJ Brooks, and P Piccini. 2007. Microglial activation in presymptomatic Huntington's disease gene carriers. *Brain* 130, Pt 7: 1759–1766.

132. McGeer, PL, S Itagaki, BE Boyes, and EG McGeer. 1988a. Reactive microglia are positive for HLA-DR in the substantia nigra of Parkinson's and Alzheimer's disease brains. *Neurology* 38, no. 8: 1285–1291.

133. McGeer, PL, S Itagaki, H Tago, and EG McGeer. 1987. Reactive microglia in patients with senile dementia of the Alzheimer type are positive for the histocompatibility glycoprotein HLA-DR. *Neurosci Lett* 79, no. 1–2: 195–200.

134. McGeer, PL, S Itagaki, H Tago, and EG McGeer. 1988b. Occurrence of HLA-DR reactive microglia in Alzheimer's disease. *Ann N Y Acad Sci* 540, 319–323.

135. Hamza, TH, CP Zabetian, A Tenesa, A Laederach, J Montimurro, D Yearout, DM Kay, KF Doheny, J Paschall, E Pugh, VI Kusel, R Collura, J Roberts, A Griffith, A Samii, WK Scott, J Nutt, SA Factor, and H Payami. 2010. Common genetic variation in the HLA region is associated with late-onset sporadic Parkinson's disease. *Nat Genet* 42, no. 9: 781–785.

136. Raj, T, K Rothamel, S Mostafavi, C Ye, MN Lee, JM Replogle, T Feng, M Lee, N Asinovski, I Frohlich, S Imboywa, A Von Korff, Y Okada, NA Patsopoulos, S Davis, C McCabe, HI Paik, GP Srivastava, S Raychaudhuri, DA Hafler, D Koller, A Regev, N Hacohen, D Mathis, C Benoist, BE Stranger, and PL De Jager. 2014. Polarization of the effects of autoimmune and neurodegenerative risk alleles in leukocytes. *Science* 344, no. 6183: 519–523.

137. Alzheimer's Disease Anti-inflammatory Prevention Trial Research Group. 2013. Results of a follow-up study to the randomized Alzheimer's Disease Anti-inflammatory Prevention Trial (ADAPT). *Alzheimers Dement* 9, no. 6: 714–723.

138. Samii, A, M Etminan, MO Wiens, and S Jafari. 2009. NSAID use and the risk of Parkinson's disease: systematic review and meta-analysis of observational studies. *Drugs Aging* 26, no. 9: 769–779.

139. Soulet, D, and F Cicchetti. 2011. The role of immunity in Huntington's disease. *Mol Psychiatry* 16, no. 9: 889–902.

17

Immunotherapy for Neurodegenerative Disorders

DAVID MORGAN

INTRODUCTION

Neurodegenerative diseases such as Alzheimer's disease (AD), Parkinson's disease (PD), and amyotrophic lateral sclerosis (ALS) are characterized by the accumulation of misfolded protein aggregates. In some cases, the primary localization of these proteins is outside cells (amyloid), while in other instances aggregates are found primarily inside cells (tauopathies, synucleinopathies, superoxide dismutase 1, TDP-43). *A priori*, one would not consider these disorders to be candidates for immunotherapeutic approaches. First, the proteins accumulate behind the blood–brain barrier, which reduces antibody exposure 1,000-fold. Second, they are associated in most cases with neuroinflammation, which is thought to participate in the pathogenic process. To the extent that immunotherapy would exacerbate inflammation, it may clear aggregates, but increase pathogenesis. Third, intracellular antibody targets are considered a major challenge for humoral immune interactions. In fact, cellular immune interactions, which are more frequently used to attack intracellular targets, would be expected to exacerbate neuron loss and disease pathology were cellular immune reactions to occur. In spite of all these concerns, immunotherapy has emerged as one of the leading approaches to treating the underlying cause of neurodegenerative disorders. Remarkably, in preclinical models, immunotherapy has generally been the most effective and consistent method of preventing and even reducing the deposition of misfolded protein aggregates in the brain.

How can immunotherapy, almost exclusively via active or passive immunization to increase circulating antibodies against the misfolded proteins, work to clear the deposits? The traditional mechanism would be to bind and "opsonize" the misfolded protein aggregates, form immune complexes, and induce phagocytosis of the antibody protein complex into resident microglia and/or infiltrating macrophages (the origin of phagocytes is an area of controversy and considerable research) (1). This mechanism has the advantage of not requiring 1:1 binding of antibody to antigen to clear large amounts of aggregated protein. For rapidly turning over proteins such as the Aβ peptide, a mechanism requiring equal stoichiometry of antigen and antibody would not be feasible given the miniscule amounts of antibody that enter the central nervous system (CNS). Furthermore, this mechanism using Fc receptors may enhance degradation of these complexes by trafficking them more efficiently to the degradation machinery (autophagy). The immune complexes may also "activate" microglia that have become moribund (due to senescence) into a more competent state, such as the M2b phenotype associated with immune complex stimulation (a blend of the M1 and M2a phenotypes) (2).

A second mechanism is binding the protein target and sequestering it or sterically hindering its interaction with other proteins. While of low feasibility due to stoichiometric considerations, one possibility is that the antibodies could transfer the protein complexes outside the brain, release them in plasma where the concentration is low, and recycle back into the CNS to bind and transport another protein. This could occur via the FcRn system. Golde (3) has commented how this could theoretically work, depending upon what the cycle time is for antibody influx, binding, efflux, and release. This concept underlies the mechanism referred to as the peripheral sink (4). This mechanism could be more efficient if the antibody specifically targeted toxic conformations of the protein rather than all conformational variants, both toxic and benign.

A third mechanism, alluded to in the first description of antibody effects on protein aggregates associated with neurodegeneration (5), is a catalytic action of the antibody upon the secondary structure of the target protein. Following from the prion-like nature of misfolded protein aggregation, there appear to be some conformations of the proteins that form "seeds" that can convert proteins in a non-toxic conformation into the toxic conformation. This can be observed *in vitro*, or in the propagation of pathology from one cell to another (6, 7). Demonstration that some antibodies are capable of blocking protein aggregation *in vitro* at stoichiometries of 100:1 or greater implies that at least some antibodies possess this type of activity. In this context the antibody would act somewhat like an enzyme, binding one conformation with high affinity and releasing a different conformation due to a lower affinity for it. However, unlike an enzyme, the antibody does not require covalent modification of the initially bound protein to effect its release, simply a change in conformation.

Critically, all of these mechanisms may be at work simultaneously. The most efficacious antibodies may, in fact, have all three properties and may be more effective because of these actions. However, adverse events may be associated with some mechanisms, particularly the first listed earlier, with the unintended activation of local inflammation where antibody-antigen binding and Fc receptor activation occurs.

IMMUNOTHERAPY FOR ALZHEIMER'S DISEASE

Of all neurodegenerative disorders, the use of immunotherapy as an intervention has seen the greatest effort applied to AD. While other chapters in this volume will cover the biology of AD in greater depth, the emerging consensus is that AD is an amyloid-induced tauopathy. At some level this is a tautological definition, as the pathological diagnosis of the disorder requires the presence of amyloid plaque and neurofibrillary tangle pathology. Still, the presence of other tauopathies with different brain region involvement and different clinical presentations highlights a unique role for amyloid in the initiation of AD. Inflammation also plays a role in the disorder, given recent genetic findings linking polymorphisms of inflammation related proteins to disease risk (8, 9). One possible role is that inflammation partially mediates amyloid's impact on tau deposition (10). Remarkably, there appears to be a 15–20-year

period of accumulating amyloid deposits prior to the onset of even early symptoms of the disorder (11–13). Studies in transgenic rodent models find that amyloid deposition typically causes some reversible synaptic loss and cognitive deficits, but does not result in the severe neurodegeneration and atrophy associated with AD. However, transgenic tau mice often cause degenerative changes resulting in neuron loss, atrophy, and premature mortality (14, 15).

EARLY OBSERVATIONS OF IMMUNOTHERAPY AGAINST AMYLOID

The first demonstration that antibodies might have beneficial impacts upon amyloid deposition were from Beka Solomon's group (5, 16, 17), showing that antibodies against Aβ could prevent the aggregation of Aβ into fibrils *in vitro* and could even dissociate preformed fibrils into monomers. Moreover, this could be achieved at stoichiometries of 10 moles Aß to 1 mole antibody, indicating that simple sequestration by binding was unable to explain the effect. They further found that the antibodies could protect PC12 cells from toxicity caused by high-dose Aß treatment.

Shortly thereafter, Dale Schenk and colleagues at Elan Pharmaceuticals treated the PDAPP mouse model with a vaccine against amyloid (18). The immunogen included preformed amyloid fibrils and a Freund's adjuvant, with multiple boost injections using incomplete Freunds and finally just oil. When the vaccine was administered in a prevention design (before amyloid deposition), the treatment was extremely effective in lowering amyloid loads in the mouse brains. When administered in a therapeutic design (at an age when mice already had plaques), immunization slowed the further accumulation of amyloid deposits. They further identified reduced astrocytosis in parallel with the reduced amyloid deposition. Interestingly, however, the astrocytosis per amyloid deposit was higher in the vaccinated mice. For technical reasons, the PDAPP mouse is not amenable to behavioral testing.

This surprising observation led to rapid confirmation of the effects of vaccination upon amyloid deposition in other mouse models, and extended this observation to prevention of the memory deficits (19, 20). Our own replication of these effects were prompted by concerns that the vaccination might in fact clear the amyloid, but could in the process launch an inflammatory response, resulting in bystander effects leading to deleterious outcomes. Although we failed to detect such effects in these studies in young transgenic mice, this concern—unintended deleterious outcomes from immunotherapy—continues to impact the application of amyloid immunotherapy in human populations (21–23).

ACTIVE IMMUNIZATION IN ALZHEIMER'S PARTICIPANTS

Given that there was no meaningful disease-modifying treatment for AD, Elan, in partnership with Wyeth, quickly launched an amyloid vaccination campaign in 2000. A phase I trial was conducted in the United Kingdom that enrolled 80 mild to moderate AD cases. The study used a fibrillar Aß1-42 vaccine (AN1792) with a QS21 saponin-based adjuvant, as Freund's is not permitted in human trials. About halfway through the trial, polysorbate 80 was added to the emulsified vaccine preparation to increase solubility. Although no significant adverse events resulted from this initial exposure, only half the participants elicited an antibody titer against Aß, consistent with other work examining vaccination with aging (24).

This was followed by a phase II study that intended to repeat vaccinations until participants achieved the goal of 1:2,000 plasma titers. The study planned to include 300 participants at multiple sites. In early 2002 the trial was halted because of the appearance of aseptic meningoencephalitis in roughly 5% of the cases. In at least some cases, this led to infiltration of T cells into the CNS, which was detected at autopsy (25, 26). It is believed that the adjuvant formulation chosen here led to a largely Th1-biased adaptive immune response, including humoral and cellular elements directed against the Aβ peptide, which caused an autoimmune reaction leading to T cell infiltration into the CNS in a small fraction of patients (27).

In spite of the interruption, a subset of participants did achieve anti-Aß antibody titers at the desired level. In the cohort studied in Zurich, the investigators, while still blinded to the treatment groups, measured the antibody titers using a histological approach and identified cases with high titers and cases with no antibody titers. When monitored over the first 12 months after immunization, those participants with the highest titers remained relatively stable, while those with minimal titers declined significantly more (28). This tantalizing observation served to maintain interest in finding some form of immunotherapy to reduce amyloid with a greater safety profile.

The group in Southampton, UK, has acquired 11 AD postmortem specimens from the phase I Elan trial, ranging from 4 to 111 months after the immunization. In general they report an apparent clearance of plaques in some brain regions, associated with the appearance of Aß within microglia/macrophages at early times after immunization. Moreover, the plaques appeared frayed, consistent with phagocytic activity. Associated with the clearance of the compacted plaques and diffuse parenchymal plaques, they reported an increase in amyloid angiopathy, and an increase in the presence of microhemorrhage (29, 30). There was the appearance of microglial activation, a reduction of tau in neuronal processes, but no change in tau found in neuronal somata (31). In cases examined several years after the immunization, there was little amyloid remaining, including vascular amyloid. Yet, all of this occurred in the absence of any cognitive benefits (32). Overall, the extent of Aß clearance in the brain was correlated with the extent of antibody titers developed after the immunization (32). Most recently this group has reported an apparent decrease in neurons in vaccinated cases, possibly associated with accelerated loss of neurons undergoing degeneration (23). This is consistent with the observation that immunized cases have a greater loss of hippocampal volume in the first year after the vaccination (21), and may suggest an unexpected adverse effect of anti-amyloid immunization.

An additional attempt at active immunization was performed with a vaccine designated CAD-106 from Novartis. This vaccine has multiple copies of Aß1-6 fused with a self-adjuvanting particle composed of the bacteriophage coat protein QB. These types of vaccines are hypothesized to be more effective in breaking self-tolerance and in overcoming the low titer responses associated with immunosenescence (33), both important considerations in AD. This virus-like-particle approach has been demonstrated effective in mouse models of amyloid deposition (34). From 2005 to 2007, 58 AD patients were administered 50 or 150 µg of CAD-106 three times and monitored for 12 months. No adverse events were reported that were thought to be related to the study drug, such as meningoencephalitis. Three-fourths of the cases developed antibody titers three standard deviations above baseline (approximately 1:200 half maximal titer). There was a roughly 10-fold greater IgM response than IgG response to the vaccine, which may diminish its CNS efficacy (but might still retain peripheral sink action). The antisera generated by CAD106 decorated amyloid deposits from the APP23 mouse brain tissue and labeled monomer and higher MW Aß aggregates in western blot analyses.

The agent has gone on to five phase II studies. In a presentation at the 2014 AAIC meeting, these studies in 106 mild to moderate AD individuals demonstrated prolonged elevation of antibody titers with a response rate of roughly two-thirds (up to 450 μg of vaccine), and generally continued safety after up to seven inoculations. There were four incidents of microhemorrhage development in the vaccinated cases. There was a reduction in amyloid load in a small set of responders ($n = 11$) and reduced phospho-tau ($n = 20$) compared to control cases. However, as with AN1792, there was a greater rate of whole brain shrinkage by MRI in cases with strong antibody responses (35).

Recently it was announced that CAD106 would be one of two agents tested in cognitively normal older adults at increased risk for AD due to apolipoprotein E4 homozygosity, in collaboration with the Banner Alzheimer's Institute.

Elan-Wyeth initiated a second active immunization trial with a modified vaccine, ACC-001. This was a truncated Aß peptide of aa1-7 fused with a CRM (inactivated diptheria toxin) carrier. The intention was to develop antibodies against the Aβ sequence without activating T cells against Aβ. The diptheria toxin was intended to provide the T cell "help" needed to generate the B cell response. It was injected with and without QS21. Adjuvant was indicated as necessary for the development of high antibody titers. Wyeth subsequently merged with Pfizer, and Elan's immunotherapy program was taken over by Janssen. Pfizer announced discontinuation of the vaccine program in August 2013.

An "affitope" vaccine, AD02, was developed by Affris using N-terminal amino acid mimics of Aß without the T cell antigens found in the mid-domain region of the peptide sequence. Again, the intention was to avoid a T cell response toward Aβ. In June 2014, Affris held a press conference announcing that the vaccine had no effect on the cognitive symptoms in AD cases in a phase II clinical trial. However, the adjuvant used with the vaccine did slow decline relative to the study control group and a control group model derived from placebo groups in prior AD trials. Further research is now focusing on the adjuvant/immunomodulator rather than the vaccine itself, although why the vaccine, which also contained

the adjuvant, failed to have an impact on cognition is unexplained.

ACI-24 is a vaccine constructed with Aß1-15 sequences with terminal palmitoylated lysines, which are displayed on a liposome surface as a fibrillar aggregate. The hypothesis is that this will form antibodies to a conformational epitope, rather than the linear epitope in the vaccine preparation. The vaccine further uses the lipid adjuvant MPLA. Phase I–II trials are underway.

MER5101 is a new vaccine with Aß1-15 coupled to the diptheria toxoid molecule as a carrier protein. This is combined with a novel nanoparticle adjuvant, MAS-1, and produces a strongly biased Th2 response. The hope is to avoid some of the problems that plagued the studies with QS21 as adjuvant for active anti-amyloid vaccination studies (36).

PASSIVE ANTI-Aβ IMMUNOTHERAPY

Shortly after the first reports of active immunization reducing amyloid and preventing memory deficits, Bard et al. demonstrated this effect could be mimicked by injections of monoclonal antibodies against the Aß peptide (37). Active immunization, while attractive because of cost, has certain disadvantages. In addition to variable production of autoimmune T cell reactions, the actual titer of antibody was variable and, in older adults, typically low. Moreover, it was more challenging to direct specific isotypes of antibodies to be produced, such as IgG versus IgM (a pentameric antibody complex which fails to enter the brain). While active immunization and the polyclonal antisera produced often have a primary dominant epitope, there are low levels of antibodies against many epitopes within the peptide used for immunization, which may have off-target effects and are challenging to control.

In comparison, there are several advantages of using a passive immunization approach. First, the antibody can be selected to possess specific characteristics. The epitope targeted can be specified and restricted. The immunoglobulin subtype (IgG) and isotype can be specified. The antibody affinity and epitope can be selected. Most important, the antibodies are administered like biologicals, and specific concentrations of circulating antibody can be achieved irrespective of patient age or the presence of immune senescence. The primary disadvantage is the cost of the Good Manufacturing Practice monoclonal antibodies, that often have to be humanized from antibodies that were originally murine.

Still, there are over 35 antibodies presently approved by the Food and Drug Administration (FDA) in the United States. All the required regulatory issues and manufacturing technology concerns regarding antibody therapeutics have been overcome.

Somewhat surprisingly, immunotherapy against the Aß peptide has become the first true test of the amyloid cascade hypothesis (38). In the 1990s it was suspected that drugs blocking secretases would be the most likely to reach the phase III testing phase, or possibly aggregation blockers (plaque busters). Unfortunately, these targets have proven more challenging to approach pharmacologically than anticipated (although promising agents are still being developed). A mountain of preclinical data supports the efficacy of this monoclonal antibody approach in the mouse models of amyloid deposition (reviewed in 39), in some cases reversing memory dysfunction within days of administration (40, 41). Our own work found that treating mice at advanced age (18 months) for 3 months could remove 90% of the parenchymal amyloid deposits that had accumulated for over half the mouse's life span. This was coupled with reversal of the memory deficits to the point that these mice performed as well as mice that never had amyloid deposits, and far better than mice treated with control antibodies (42). However, this rapid clearance was associated with the appearance of multiple microhemorrhages, and an increase in vascular amyloid deposits. Importantly, we subsequently demonstrated that this only occurred in aged mice. When young and old mice with comparable amyloid pathology were treated with antibodies, microhemorrhage only occurred in the old mice, in spite of comparable reductions in Aß (43). Others have reported immunotherapy-associated increases in microhemorrhage in older mouse models (44–46), although Schroeter et al. indicate that prolonged treatments can reduce vascular amyloid after hemorrhages have occurred. These data in the mouse model were predictive of the observations in the active immunization results from the Elan trial reported by Southampton group (described earlier). Immunotherapy with AN1792 caused hemorrhage shortly after starting treatment but ultimately cleared the vascular amyloid after years of exposure (29). These data from mice and the active immunotherapy trials would prove predictive of additional issues that developed in the treatment of mild to moderate AD patients with some monoclonal antibodies.

The first passive immunotherapy trials were performed with rather different antibodies. Bapineuzumab is a humanized version of the mouse monoclonal 3D6, which has an epitope in the first five amino acids of Aß. This antibody is an IgG1 isotype and known to interact with fibrillar and monomeric forms of the Aß peptide (and probably oligomeric forms as well; see Table 17.1). The phase I study examined 0.5, 1.5, and 5 mg/kg doses in a small number of AD patients (47). Cognitive assessments were made at the beginning and 16 weeks after the antibody administration. At the 5 mg/kg dose, 3 of 10 patients developed vasogenic edema and one developed a microhemorrhage. Subsequently these abnormalities became known as amyloid-related imaging abnormality E and H, respectively (ARIA-E; ARIA-H). Enticingly, exploratory analysis using MMSE scores found that there was significant improvement in patients dosed at 0.5 and 1.5 mg/kg, but not at the 5.0 mg/kg dose.

Bapineuzumab was also tested in a phase II study with 230 patients and doses ranging from 0.15 to 2 mg/kg in six infusions over 18 months (48). Although overall effects were negative, there were modest but significant cognitive benefits when non-completers were exlcuded from the analysis, or when only non-*ApoE4* cases were included. However, even at these low doses, ARIA were observed. ARIA-E were present in 17% of all participants receiving bapineuzumab (22). Half of these also had evidence of ARIA-H, which were found in 10% of all cases treated with the immunotherapy. It was further observed that these cases were dose-related and more prevalent in the *ApoE4* cases. The lack of any efficacy signal and the presence of elevated ARIA in *ApoE4* carriers led to the separate evaluation of *ApoE4* and non-*ApoE4* cases in the phase II study.

A subset of the cases from the phase II bapineuzumab study were evaluated for amyloid load using the PET imaging agent Pittsburg B (49). Approximately 30 cases divided between placebo (8) and treated (20) arms were evaluated four times over 18 months for the amyloid signal in forebrain regions relative to cerebellum. In the placebo cases there was a small but significant elevation in the amyloid signal over the 18-month study. In the treated patients there was a reduction, especially at the end of the study, such that the treated group was statistically lower than the placebo group relative to starting baseline values. This was taken as evidence that bapineuzumab had reached the CNS and had engaged the

TABLE 17.1. STATUS OF MONOCLONAL ANTIBODIES DIRECTED AGAINST AMYLOID IN CLINICAL TESTING FOR ALZHEIMER'S DISEASE

Antibody	Isotype	Epitope	Mono/Oligo/ Fibril	Raise Plasma Aβ	Status
Bapineuzumab	IgG1	aa1–5	+ /?/+	No	Ph III Negative. Discontinued
Solanezumab	IgG1	aa13–24	++/– /–	Yes	Ph III negative mild-mod AD New Ph III mild AD
Gantenerumab	IgG1	aa1–11; aa ~24	–/+?/++	No	Ph II MCI discontinued Ph III Mild AD continuing DIAN continuing
Ponezumab	IgG2a	aa28–40	+/+/+ CAA and plaque; not diffuse	Yes	Ph II Negative, discontinued Ph II Cerebral amyloid angiopathy
Crenezumab	IgG4	aa2–23; conformational	+/++/++	No	Ph II mild-mod AD, negative Ph II–III API continuing
BAN 2401	IgG1	Conformational protofibril	–/++/–	? unlikely	Ph II MCI and mild AD
Aducanumab	IgG1	conformational	–/+/+	No	Ph II moving to Ph III

aa: amino acids in Aβ sequence; Ph: phase of trial; AD: Alzheimer's disease; MCI: mild cognitive impairment; CAA: cerebral amyloid angiopathy.

amyloid target sufficiently that some clearance of amyloid was evident in the brain. Two of the cases in the treated group had developed ARIA-E during the study.

These results encouraged the launch of a phase III study of bapineuzumab. One study included 1,100 *ApoE4* carriers, and the other included 1,300 noncarriers. *ApoE4* carriers received 0.5 mg/kg bapineuzumab or placebo every 13 weeks. Non-carriers received 0.5 or 1 mg/kg after the intended 2 mg/kg doses were suspended due to the high rate of development of ARIA at this dose. These 2 mg/kg cases were transferred to 1 mg/kg dose and were included in the safety portion of the trial but not the efficacy component. The results of the trial were clearly negative with respect to the primary cognitive endpoints, ADAS-Cog 11 and Disability Assessment for Dementia scales. When examining mild AD cases in a prespecified analysis (MMSE > 20) there was a small benefit of bapineuzumab on the DAD (but not ADAS-Cog) scores ($P < 0.05$). There appeared to be a slightly greater rate of progression in the *ApoE4* carriers than the non-carriers, but this was not compared statistically. Further work with bapineuzumab has been discontinued. However, a variant of the antibody with Fc modifications designed to reduce Fc receptor interactions is evidently still being tested (AAB003).

Intriguingly, there was some evidence of target engagement in the *ApoE4* carriers in a substudy of 110 participants. Both the PET amyloid measurement and the phosphorylated tau measurement in cerebrospinal fluid indicated lower values in the cases treated with bapineuzumab. However, the PET values differed from that observed in Rinne (49), as the major change here was an increase in the placebo group and no change in the treated group (the treated group declined in Rinne et al.). In the substudy of the non-carrier group (40 cases), there was an apparent decrease in the PET amyloid measurement in the 1 mg/kg treated group, but this failed to reach significance as the placebo group also declined. The phosphorylated tau CSF measurement declined in the non-carrier group treated with 1 mg/kg bapineuzumab, but not 0.5 mg/kg relative to placebo-treated cases. From this substudy it was determined that roughly 20% of the cases examined were negative for PET amyloid, indicating that they were most likely misclassifed as having AD. This is similar to the results from the solanezumab study (see following discussion) and a study of Alzheimer's Disease Research Center autopsies, with roughly 20% of diagnoses based upon clinical criteria being incorrect (50).

A second antibody to process through to phase III testing is solanezumab. This antibody is directed at a mid-domain epitope and has considerably greater affinity for monomeric than for fibrillar amyloid deposits. It further results in a large increase in the plasma content of Aß (4). A phase I study examined doses ranging from 0.5 to 10 mg/kg (51). Although some infusion site reactions were observed, there were no ARIA-E or ARIA-H events observed after single infusions. There were also dose-dependent increases in both plasma and CSF Aß in the study participants. No changes were reported in cognitive function after these single infusions.

A second dose-ranging study (phase II) with 52 cases came to similar conclusions using multiple injections (52). Again there was no indication of ARIA-E or ARIA-H in participants infused with up to 4.8 gm of solanezumab over 12 weeks (400 mg weekly). There was also a dose-dependent increase in plasma Aß. There was a similar increase in CSF Aß at the highest doses. No changes in cognition were detected.

These safety and dose-ranging trials led to a large phase III study, conducted as two separate trials, with over 2,000 participants in total. Solanezumab was administered at a dose of 400 mg every 4 weeks for 18 months. The total antibody dose over 18 months in the solanezumab study was 17 times greater than the total dose in the 1 mg/kg bapineuzumab study, assuming a 75-kg average participant body weight. Overall, neither trial achieved the endpoint of slowing cognitive decline (ADAS-Cog) or improving activities of daily living. Subsequent substudies, however, indicated a significant benefit in mild AD patients. This was significant for ADAS-Cog in one of the two studies evaluated separately, and when the data from the two studies for mild patients were combined. There was also significantly less impairment in the ADCS ADL measurement in the second study in the mild cases. The data suggested a 25% slowing in the rate of cognitive decline for mild AD cases. There was no difference in the rate of ARIA-E or ARIA-H in the treated and control cases that participated in the study.

These results led Lilly to initiate a third trial of solanezumab focusing only on mild AD cases, which is presently underway. Solanezumab is further being tested in one arm of the Dominantly Inherited Alzheimer's Network (DIAN) study of familial AD. Solanezumab is also being tested in the Anti-Amyloid Treatment in Asymptomatic Alzheimer's Disease (A4) secondary prevention trial.

Gantenerumab is a fully human IgG1 antibody obtained using phage display technology and subsequently matured *in vitro* using CDR cassette exchange methods. The antibody has subnanomolar affinity for fibrillar Aß and associates with two domains, one N terminal (aa 8-9) and another mid-domain (residue 24 related). The antibody binds to amyloid deposits, reduces amyloid deposition in APP mice, and blocks Aß oligomer inhibition of long-term potentiation (53). The antibody facilitates macrophage phagocytosis of amyloid deposits. It does not elevate circulating levels of Aß.

A phase II study included 14 patients in a PET substudy. Participants received 60 or 200 mg gantenerumab subcutaneously every 4 weeks for up to 7 months. Treatment indicated a dose-related reduction in the change in PET signal of up to 35% compared to control cases (54). Two cases indicated appearance of ARIA-E; both were *ApoE4* carriers and in the high-dose group, similar to observations in the bapineuzumab study described earlier.

Three large trials have used gantenerumab. The first enrolled 700+ cases of MCI (prodromal) confirmed to be Aß positive using PET analysis. This study has subsequently been discontinued following a preplanned futility analysis. Part of the problem, as with bapineuzumab, may be the dose limitations required to decrease the ARIA problems (225 mg every 4 weeks). A second trial is continuing in 1,000 cases of mild AD. Ganterumab also continues to be tested in familial AD cases as part of the Dominantly Inherited Alzheimer's Disease (DIAN) study.

Ponezumab is a mutated IgG2a antibody that lacks the single carbohydrate group typically found on the Fc portion of IgG. This diminishes the affinity of the antibody for Fc receptors and for the activation of complement (55). The antibody was humanized from the murine antibody 2H6, a C terminal specific Aβ40 specific antibody, which was developed by Rinat Neuroscience, now part of Pfizer. In mouse studies, the deglycosylated 2H6 antibody was remarkably effective in removing pre-deposited amyloid from the parenchyma of the mouse brain, and did so with considerably fewer microhemorrhages than its normally glycosylated counterpart (56). The deglycosylated antibody also provoked less activation of microglia than the intact antibody. Studies with the humanized version, ponezumab, in APP mice confirmed the absence of microhemorrhage with up to 6 months of treatment, but failed to mention if the clearance of amyloid deposits was retained by the humanized version of the antibody (57). Ponezumab had no ARIA development, at least with single doses (58). However, a phase II trial resulted in no clinical benefit and no change in CSF Aß, leading Pfizer to discontinue development for AD. However, a trial is presently underway evaluating the efficacy of this Aß40 specific antibody in cerebral amyloid angiopathy, which is largely composed of Aß ending at position 40.

Crenezumab is a fully humanized IgG4 antibody that recognizes aggregated Aß with high affinity and lower affinity for monomers. This was derived from studies vaccinating mice with a liposomal-based immunogen (AC Immune) displaying multiple Aß molecules oriented to elicit conformation specific antisera (59). The IgG4 isotype was selected to try to diminish the ARIA effects of the antibody by diminishing the interaction with Fc receptors and with complement, similar to antibody deglycosylation (55). Another important feature of this antibody is that it blocks Aß aggregation at stoichiometries of 1:100 (antibody: Aß), implying the potential to use catalytic dissolution as a mechanism of amyloid clearance. The antibody has pursued two tracks clinically. The first has been in mild to moderate AD in a phase II study using either 15 mg/kg intravenous infusion monthly or 300 mg subcutaneously monthly. No issues of vasogenic edema or microhemorrhage were reported. However, the phase II study failed to meet its primary endpoints for cognition (ADAS-Cog12) or function (CDR sum of boxes). Subanalyses found a non-significant 20%–30% slowing of the rate of decline in the mildest cases at the 15 mg/kg IV dose (press release from Roche and presentation at AAIC-2015). A subsequent presentation found very little change in biomarkers associated with the treatment. Using secondary analysis methods, there was a slight trend toward slower Aß accumulation by PET in the treated group. The second approach using this agent has been in the Alzheimer's Prevention Initiative (API) treating members of a kindred in Columbia carrying a PS1 mutation. Although originally this study intended to use the subcutaneous dose, the results of the phase II study in mild to moderate AD led to changing the dose to 15 mg/kg IV in the API study.

BAN2401 is an antibody raised against Aß protofibrils produced in high abundance by the arctic APP mutation (60). It is an IgG1 antibody that has high affinity for a conformational epitope found in high molecular weight Aß aggregates referred to as protofibrils, and less affinity for other Aß forms. A phase I study found no adverse events, such as ARIA, with doses up to 10 mg/kg every 2 weeks. It is presently in phase II testing in PET-confirmed MCI and mild AD cases (22–30 MMSE).

Aducanumab is an antibody obtained from the blood of individuals who have resisted AD, in a version of reverse translational medicine. It is a fully human antibody that binds a conformational epitope of Aß with low affinity for monomers, but high affinity for fibrillar plaques. Evidently the affinity for vascular deposits is lower than that for parenchymal deposits. It successfully cleared deposited amyloid from aged APP mice without producing increased microhemorrhage. The compound has been safety tested up to 60 mg/kg in phase I studies. The antibody does not elevate plasma Aß. A phase II study designed to enroll 160 participants with mild AD (MMSE.19; CDR 0.5–1) was recently announced to advance to phase III. This announcement was made via a press release indicating cognitive benefits in patients treated for a year, without showing any results. At the 2015 AD/PD meeting in Nice, this antibody was reported to improve cognitive function in mild AD cases, and to reduce amyloid PET signals in a dose dependent manner. However, high doses were associated with increased rates of ARIA.

In summary, a great deal of effort has gone into anti-amyloid immunotherapy approaches. The results have been extremely frustrating, and one possible explanation is that the mild to moderate phase of the disease is no longer amyloid dependent. Instead, the progression of cognitive decline in symptomatic cases may result from downstream effects of amyloid, such as tau pathology or inflammation. Certainly the loss of synapses and brain mass in neurodegenerative diseases are unlikely to be recovered by removing Aß deposits (and some data suggest that this might accelerate the process of atrophy and neuron loss). Still, there are a variety of modifications being made to (a) increase the safety of the immunotherapy, (b) target forms of Aß that may be more closely linked to toxicity, and (c) apply the immunotherapy to the presymptomatic phase of the disease, when Aß deposits accumulate over a 15–20-year time frame. There is still optimism that one or more of these antibodies will slow the accumulation of Aß and subsequently delay or prevent the appearance of cognitive declines leading to dementia.

IMMUNOTHERAPY AGAINST TAU

Tau is another pathology found postmortem in AD. It appears to correlate better than amyloid with the extent of cognitive loss in AD (61). Tau is typically an axonal protein that binds to and stabilizes microtubules. During the progression of AD it becomes mislocalized to the somato-dendritic compartment of neurons and aggregates into fibrils to form what are described as neurofibrillary tangles. Associated with these tau deposits is hyperphosphorylation of the protein at numerous sites. It is unclear the degree to which this is a cause of the aggregation or secondary to the increased half-life of the protein, permitting kinases access to domains not normally phosphorylated. Although considered an intracellular cytosolic protein, tau can be detected in extracellular fluid using dialysis (62), and in human CSF (63). In CSF, levels of tau and phosphorylated tau are taken as indices of neurodegeneration, and are elevated in patients with AD.

The possibility that tau might be amenable to immunotherapy was first demonstrated in mouse models of tau deposition (64). Sigurdsson et al. used a peptide antigen that encompassed a mid-domain portion of the tau protein and overlapped the site of the widely used antibody PHF-1, thought to recognize the paired helical filaments found in neurofibrillary tangles. Treating mice for 3 months reduced the levels of insoluble tau accumulation and improved the behavioral phenotype of this tau-depositing mouse line (P301L; JNPL3). A follow-up study used a different mouse (hTauxPS1) and obtained similar reductions in both the behavioral and pathological phenotype using active immunization against a tau peptide (65). This was somewhat surprising, given the intraneuronal localization of tau. Thus, not only would antibodies need to enter the CNS, but presumably they would need to cross the neuronal plasma membrane as well. Confirming this possibility, fluorescently labeled anti-tau antibodies were found within neurons in association with tau deposits after intracarotid injections (66). No uptake of these antibodies was detected in non-transgenic mice, suggesting that the tau pathology either increased permeability or retained the small number of antibodies entering neurons. This work using active immunization has been replicated in several other models of tau deposition (67–70).

Passive immunotherapy against tau has also been demonstrated in mouse models. Again using the P301L model of tau deposition, it was found that the murine antibody PHF-1 (approximately 10 mg/kg weekly) reduced the deposition of tau histologically and neurochemically and demonstrated some behavioral benefits (71). However, the spinal cord pathology causing death of these mice (14) was unaffected and the results overall were viewed as less effective than those observed with active immunization. Others working in parallel have produced similar results (69). When compared with a conformation specific antibody, MC-1, it was found that PHF-1 was slightly more effective in reducing deposited tau, but both antibodies were effective in reducing the phenotype in two mouse models of tau deposition. MC-1 was also found effective by another research team (72). It has also been demonstrated that antibodies specific for human tau, but not mouse tau, when infused intraventricularly, reduce multiple aspects of the tau mouse phenotype (P301S; PS19) (73). The belief in this paper was that the antibody was intercepting extracellular tau and diminishing transmission of pathological tau from one cell to the next.

In this context, the work from the Kayed laboratory is potentially helpful. They have developed a monoclonal mouse antibody that recognizes oligomeric tau, but not monomeric or fibrillar tau (74). This antibody was injected either ICV or IV and showed measurable impacts on the behavioral phenotype with a single injection (75). Histopathology indicated reduction in tau oligomers, but not in monomeric or neurofibrillary forms of tau. These data argue that some of the tau behavioral phenotype, at least in P301L mice, like the amyloid phenotype, respond rapidly to clearance of intermediate aggregates, suggesting that these forms are responsible for the behavioral changes, not the deposited forms.

Tau immunotherapy is in the very earliest stages of clinical testing. AADVac1 is in phase I follow-up testing. It is a tau peptide fragment conjugated with keyhole limpet hemocyanin and an alum adjuvant. It has shown dramatic reductions in tau deposition in a rat model (76). Another vaccine, ACI-35, is being jointly developed by Johnson & Johnson and AC Immune. The vaccine is similar to the liposome-based amyloid vaccine ACI-24, except substituting multiple copies of a tau fragment including phosphorylated serines at sites corresponding to 396 and 404 of full length tau. It was demonstrated to delay death and reduce pathology in P301L mice (77).

IMMUNOTHERAPY FOR SYNUCLEINOPATHY

Alpha-synuclein (SYN) is an intraneuronal protein found largely in nerve terminals and in a monomeric form is cytosolic. However, in some circumstances it forms aggregates that can associate with the membrane fraction (78). In synucleinopathies such as PD, dementia with Lewy bodies (DLB), progressive supranuclear palsy, and multiple system atrophy, there are intracellular inclusions of aggregated proteins consisting largely of SYN. This leads to death of nigral neurons in PD and forebrain cholinergic neurons in DLB. SYN aggregates can be released from nerve terminals and become endocytosed by other cells. In a prion-like process called propagation, this can induce toxic conformations of SYN in neighboring cells (79). This type of propagation has even been observed in embryonic neuronal grafts into Parkinsonian brains (80).

The first demonstration of a potential use of anti-SYN immunotherapy used active immunization in a PDGF-SYN model (81). The investigators found that vaccination with full-length human SYN resulted in production of high-affinity antibodies that reduced SYN deposition and neurodegeneration in the transgenic mouse model of synucleinopathy. There also was a reduction of oligomeric forms of SYN, and antibodies were found in association with SYN in lysosomes of microglia (82). This occurred without the appearance of microglial activation, using Iba-1 as a marker. Subsequently a liposome-based SYN vaccine was demonstrated to reduce SYN deposition and decrease neuropathology in a mouse model of SYN deposition (83). This has now been advanced to phase I clinical testing for Parkinson's disease and multiple system atrophy (PD01).

Passive immunization against synucleinopathy has also been successful in preclinical models. A C-terminal specific antibody against SYN when administered to PDGF-SYN mice rescued memory deficits and synaptic pathology, and reduced accumulation of C-terminal truncated (calpain cleaved) SYN (84). The investigators further showed that the labeled antibody injected peripherally entered the CNS and ultimately associated with lysosomes after endocytosis. The clearance via Fc receptors more efficiently traffics SYN aggregates to the lysosomes, and blockade of autophagy prevents the SYN-lowering effects of the antibody. Intracranial administration of anti-SYN has been demonstrated to prevent propagation of SYN from neurons to astrocytes and diminishes neurodegeneration and behavioral deficits (85).

IMMUNOTHERAPY FOR PRION DISORDERS

Although a number of commonalities between prion disorders and other neurodegenerative diseases are emerging, a key distinction is that prions can be transmitted through the periphery as an infectious disease. As such, there are two conformations recognized as the normal cellular variant (PrPc), and the other being the pathogenic infectious variant, which for scrapie is known as PrPsc. Shortly after preclinical evaluation of immunotherapy approaches against amyloid, studies investigating vaccination against the PrP protein in mice found that immunotherapy could block infectivity (86), with vaccination preceding infection being more effective in delaying disease onset (87). Shortly thereafter, passive immunization was found to delay onset of the disease in mouse models (88, 89). Issues regarding vaccination as a treatment for prionoses include the possible inhibition of normal prion function and the potential for autoimmune reactions, as was apparently observed in Aß vaccination (*vide supra*).

Regarding normal cellular function, the phenotypes of prion knock-out mice appear rather minimal (90). In some cases, antibodies were generated to cryptic epitopes present in PrPsc, but were hidden in PrPC (91). Some of the antibodies "curing" prionoses in cultured cells are selective for PrPsc, but others only bind PrPC and still are effective (92). Moreover, the epitope targeted did not appear to be a critical issue. Antibodies appeared to be internalized into cells via endocytosis, leading to increased degradation of PrPC (93). However, in some instances, Fab fragments that lack internalization signals are equally effective as the cognate full-length IgG in blocking prion propagation in cultured neurons (94).

Mechanisms proposed include binding and sequestering the infectious form; binding PrPC and blocking its interaction with the infectious PrPsc or an intermediary protein; modified PrP trafficking and increased degradation; blocking replication of PrPsc by denying substrate PrPC; or stabilization of large PrPsc fibrils, slowing the rate of breakage and impairing replication (90). In spite of impressive work *in vitro* and in preclinical models, clinical trials against prionoses have yet to move forward. Part of the problem may be the relatively small number of cases to be so treated. Another concern is that the immunization would merely slow progression of the disease, which may not be a desirable outcome for the patient. It has further been shown that when injected intracranially, there was a concentration-dependent neurotoxicity observed with monoclonal anti-prion antibodies (95) and in cultured neurons (96). Nonetheless, understanding the mechanisms required and designing antibodies that can reverse the infection, rather than slow it, may lead to the first effective anti-prion therapies.

SUMMARY AND CONCLUSIONS

Although neurodegenerative diseases are unlikely targets of immunotherapeutic approaches, they have been a hotbed of activity for those developing immunotherapy. Early preclinical successes led to clinical disappointments, but when considered in the proper context of age and the types of models employed, the results could have been (and were by some) anticipated. Nonetheless, our improved understanding of presymptomatic stages of these diseases, during which abnormal conformations of misfolded protein accumulate, offers a fresh opportunity to test the hypothesis that immunotherapy may have impacts on disease risk. Moreover, they offer a unique opportunity to confirm suspicions from model systems that intermediate aggregates of proteins, so-called oligomers, are the truly toxic species and that inhibiting their actions may abrogate disease. We are learning a great deal about CNS immunotherapy from these studies, unfortunately at great expense to the pharmaceutical industry and those suffering from neurodegenerative diseases. Nonetheless, resources continue to be applied to this endeavor, and hope for its ultimate success remains high.

ACKNOWLEDGMENTS

Dr. Morgan's work on immunotherapy for neurodegenerative disorders has been supported by AG 18478 and NS 76308 from the National Institutes of Health.

REFERENCES

1. S. E. Hickman, N. D. Kingery, T. K. Ohsumi, M. L. Borowsky, L. C. Wang, T. K. Means, J. El Khoury, The microglial sensome revealed by direct RNA sequencing. *Nat Neurosci* **16**, 1896–1905 (2013).

2. T. L. Sudduth, A. Greenstein, D. M. Wilcock, Intracranial injection of Gammagard, a human IVIg, modulates the inflammatory response of the brain and lowers Abeta in APP/PS1 mice along a different time course than anti-Abeta antibodies. *J Neurosci* **33**, 9684–9692 (2013).

3. T. E. Golde, Open questions for Alzheimer's disease immunotherapy. *Alzheimers Res Ther* **6**, 3 (2014) 10.1186.

4. R. B. DeMattos, K. R. Bales, D. J. Cummins, J. C. Dodart, S. M. Paul, D. M. Holtzman, Peripheral anti-A beta antibody alters CNS and plasma A beta clearance and decreases brain A beta burden in a mouse model of Alzheimer's disease. *Proc Natl Acad Sci U S A* **98**, 8850–8855 (2001).

5. B. Solomon, R. Koppel, E. Hanan, T. Katzav, Monoclonal antibodies inhibit in vitro fibrillar aggregation of the Alzheimer beta-amyloid peptide. *Proc Natl Acad Sci U S A* **93**, 452–455 (1996).

6. L. Liu, V. Drouet, J. W. Wu, M. P. Witter, S. A. Small, C. Clelland, K. Duff, Trans-synaptic spread of tau pathology in vivo. *PLoS One* **7**, e31302 (2012) 10.1371.

7. A. de Calignon, M. Polydoro, M. Suarez-Calvet, C. William, D. H. Adamowicz, K. J. Kopeikina, R. Pitstick, N. Sahara, K. H. Ashe, G. A. Carlson, T. L. Spires-Jones, B. T. Hyman, Propagation of tau pathology in a model of early Alzheimer's disease. *Neuron* **73**, 685–697 (2012) 10.1016.

8. D. Harold, R. Abraham, P. Hollingworth, R. Sims, A. Gerrish, M. L. Hamshere, J. S. Pahwa, V. Moskvina, K. Dowzell, A. Williams, N. Jones, C. Thomas, A. Stretton, A. R. Morgan, S. Lovestone, J. Powell, P. Proitsi, M. K. Lupton, C. Brayne, D. C. Rubinsztein, M. Gill, B. Lawlor, A. Lynch, K. Morgan, K. S. Brown, P. A. Passmore, D. Craig, B. McGuinness, S. Todd, C. Holmes, D. Mann, A. D. Smith, S. Love, P. G. Kehoe, J. Hardy, S. Mead, N. Fox, M. Rossor, J. Collinge, W. Maier, F. Jessen, B. Schurmann, H. van den Bussche, I. Heuser, J. Kornhuber, J. Wiltfang, M. Dichgans, L. Frolich, H. Hampel, M. Hull, D. Rujescu, A. M. Goate, J. S. Kauwe, C. Cruchaga, P. Nowotny, J. C. Morris, K. Mayo, K. Sleegers, K. Bettens, S. Engelborghs, P. P. De Deyn, C. Van Broeckhoven, G. Livingston, N. J. Bass, H. Gurling, A. McQuillin, R. Gwilliam, P. Deloukas, A. Al-Chalabi, C. E. Shaw, M. Tsolaki, A. B. Singleton, R. Guerreiro, T. W. Muhleisen, M. M. Nothen, S. Moebus, K. H. Jockel, N. Klopp, H. E. Wichmann, M. M. Carrasquillo, V. S. Pankratz, S. G. Younkin, P. A. Holmans, M. O'Donovan, M. J. Owen, J. Williams, Genome-wide association study identifies variants at CLU and PICALM associated with Alzheimer's disease. *Nat Genet* **41**, 1088–1093 (2009).

9. J. C. Lambert, S. Heath, G. Even, D. Campion, K. Sleegers, M. Hiltunen, O. Combarros, D. Zelenika, M. J. Bullido, B. Tavernier, L. Letenneur, K. Bettens, C. Berr, F. Pasquier, N. Fievet, P. Barberger-Gateau, S. Engelborghs, P. De Deyn, I. Mateo, A. Franck, S. Helisalmi, E. Porcellini, O. Hanon, M. M. de Pancorbo, C. Lendon, C. Dufouil, C. Jaillard, T. Leveillard, V. Alvarez, P. Bosco, M. Mancuso, F. Panza, B. Nacmias, P. Bossu, P. Piccardi, G. Annoni, D. Seripa, D. Galimberti, D. Hannequin, F. Licastro, H. Soininen, K. Ritchie, H. Blanche, J. F. Dartigues, C. Tzourio, I. Gut, C. Van Broeckhoven, A. Alperovitch, M. Lathrop, P. Amouyel, Genome-wide association study identifies variants at CLU and CR1 associated with Alzheimer's disease. *Nat Genet* **41**, 1094–1099 (2009); published online EpubOct (10.1038/ng.439).

10. D. C. Lee, J. Rizer, J. B. Hunt, M. L. Selenica, M. N. Gordon, D. Morgan, Review: experimental manipulations of microglia in mouse models of Alzheimer's pathology: activation reduces amyloid but hastens tau pathology. *Neuropathol Appl Neurobiol* **39**, 69–85 (2013).

11. V. L. Villemagne, S. Burnham, P. Bourgeat, B. Brown, K. A. Ellis, O. Salvado, C. Szoeke, S. L. Macaulay, R. Martins, P. Maruff, D. Ames, C. C. Rowe, C. L. Masters, Amyloid beta deposition, neurodegeneration, and cognitive decline in sporadic Alzheimer's disease: a prospective cohort study. *Lancet Neurol* **12**, 357–367 (2013).

12. C. R. Jack, Jr., D. S. Knopman, W. J. Jagust, L. M. Shaw, P. S. Aisen, M. W. Weiner, R. C. Petersen, J. Q. Trojanowski, Hypothetical model of dynamic biomarkers of the Alzheimer's pathological cascade. *Lancet Neurol* **9**, 119–128 (2010).

13. R. J. Bateman, C. Xiong, T. L. Benzinger, A. M. Fagan, A. Goate, N. C. Fox, D. S. Marcus, N. J. Cairns, X. Xie, T. M. Blazey, D. M. Holtzman, A. Santacruz, V. Buckles, A. Oliver, K. Moulder, P. S. Aisen, B. Ghetti, W. E. Klunk, E. McDade, R. N. Martins, C. L. Masters, R. Mayeux, J. M. Ringman, M. N. Rossor, P. R. Schofield, R. A. Sperling, S. Salloway, J. C. Morris, Clinical and biomarker changes in dominantly inherited Alzheimer's disease. *N Engl J Med* **367**, 795–804 (2012).

14. J. Lewis, E. McGowan, J. Rockwood, H. Melrose, P. Nacharaju, M. Van Slegtenhorst, K. Gwinn-Hardy, M. M. Paul, M. Baker, X. Yu, K. Duff, J. Hardy, A. Corral, W. L. Lin, S. H. Yen, D. W. Dickson, P. Davies, M. Hutton, Neurofibrillary tangles, amyotrophy and progressive motor disturbance in mice expressing mutant (P301L) tau protein. *Nat Genet* **25**, 402–405 (2000).

15. K. Santacruz, J. Lewis, T. Spires, J. Paulson, L. Kotilinek, M. Ingelsson, A. Guimaraes, M. DeTure, M. Ramsden, E. McGowan, C. Forster, M. Yue, J. Orne, C. Janus, A. Mariash, M. Kuskowski, B. Hyman, M. Hutton, K. H. Ashe, Tau suppression in a neurodegenerative mouse model improves memory function. *Science* **309**, 476–481 (2005).

16. M. Arbel, I. Yacoby, B. Solomon, Inhibition of amyloid precursor protein processing by beta-secretase through site-directed antibodies. *Proc Natl Acad Sci U S A* **102**, 7718–7723 (2005).

17. B. Solomon, R. Koppel, D. Frankel, E. Hanan-Aharon, Disaggregation of Alzheimer beta-amyloid by site-directed mAb. *Proc Natl Acad Sci U S A* **94**, 4109–4112 (1997).

18. D. Schenk, R. Barbour, W. Dunn, G. Gordon, H. Grajeda, T. Guido, K. Hu, J. Huang, K. Johnson-Wood, K. Khan, D. Kholodenko, M. Lee, Z. Liao, I. Lieberburg, R. Motter, L. Mutter, F. Soriano, G. Shopp, N. Vasquez, C. Vandevert, S. Walker, M. Wogulis, T. Yednock, D. Games, P. Seubert, Immunization with amyloid-beta attenuates Alzheimer-disease-like pathology in the PDAPP mouse. *Nature* **400**, 173–177 (1999).

19. D. Morgan, D. M. Diamond, P. E. Gottschall, K. E. Ugen, C. Dickey, J. Hardy, K. Duff, P. Jantzen, G. DiCarlo, D. Wilcock, K. Connor, J. Hatcher, C. Hope, M. Gordon, G. W. Arendash, A beta peptide vaccination prevents memory loss in an animal model of Alzheimer's disease. *Nature* **408**, 982–985 (2000).

20. C. Janus, J. Pearson, J. McLaurin, P. M. Mathews, Y. Jiang, S. D. Schmidt, M. A. Chishti, P. Horne, D. Heslin, J. French, H. T. Mount, R. A. Nixon, M. Mercken, C. Bergeron, P. E. Fraser, P. George-Hyslop, D. Westaway, A beta peptide immunization reduces behavioural impairment and plaques in a model of Alzheimer's disease. *Nature* **408**, 979–982 (2000).

21. N. C. Fox, R. S. Black, S. Gilman, M. N. Rossor, S. G. Griffith, L. Jenkins, M. Koller, Effects of Abeta immunization (AN1792) on MRI measures of cerebral volume in Alzheimer disease. *Neurology* **64**, 1563–1572 (2005).

22. R. Sperling, S. Salloway, D. J. Brooks, D. Tampieri, J. Barakos, N. C. Fox, M. Raskind, M. Sabbagh, L. S. Honig, A. P. Porsteinsson, I. Lieberburg, H. M. Arrighi, K. A. Morris, Y. Lu, E. Liu, K. M. Gregg, H. R. Brashear, G. G. Kinney, R. Black, M. Grundman, Amyloid-related imaging abnormalities in patients with Alzheimer's disease treated with bapineuzumab: a retrospective analysis. *Lancet Neurol* **11**, 241–249 (2012).

23. C. Paquet, J. Amin, F. Mouton-Liger, M. Nasser, S. Love, F. Gray, R. M. Pickering, J. A. Nicoll, C. Holmes, J. Hugon, D. Boche, Effect of active Abeta immunotherapy on neurons in human

Alzheimer's disease. *J Pathology* **235**, 721–730 (2015).

24. A. J. Bayer, R. Bullock, R. W. Jones, D. Wilkinson, K. R. Paterson, L. Jenkins, S. B. Millais, S. Donoghue, Evaluation of the safety and immunogenicity of synthetic Abeta42 (AN1792) in patients with AD. *Neurology* **64**, 94–101 (2005).

25. J. A. Nicoll, D. Wilkinson, C. Holmes, P. Steart, H. Markham, R. O. Weller, Neuropathology of human Alzheimer disease after immunization with amyloid-beta peptide: a case report. *Nat Med* **9**, 448–452 (2003).

26. I. Ferrer, R. M. Boada, M. L. Sanchez Guerra, M. J. Rey, F. Costa-Jussa, Neuropathology and pathogenesis of encephalitis following amyloid-beta immunization in Alzheimer's disease. *Brain Pathol* **14**, 11–20 (2004).

27. J. M. Orgogozo, S. Gilman, J. F. Dartigues, B. Laurent, M. Puel, L. C. Kirby, P. Jouanny, B. Dubois, L. Eisner, S. Flitman, B. F. Michel, M. Boada, A. Frank, C. Hock, Subacute meningoencephalitis in a subset of patients with AD after Abeta42 immunization. *Neurology* **61**, 46–54 (2003).

28. C. Hock, U. Konietzko, J. R. Streffer, J. Tracy, A. Signorell, B. Muller-Tillmanns, U. Lemke, K. Henke, E. Moritz, E. Garcia, M. A. Wollmer, D. Umbricht, D. J. de Quervain, M. Hofmann, A. Maddalena, A. Papassotiropoulos, R. M. Nitsch, Antibodies against beta-amyloid slow cognitive decline in Alzheimer's disease. *Neuron* **38**, 547–554 (2003).

29. D. Boche, E. Zotova, R. O. Weller, S. Love, J. W. Neal, R. M. Pickering, D. Wilkinson, C. Holmes, J. A. Nicoll, Consequence of A{beta} immunization on the vasculature of human Alzheimer's disease brain. *Brain* **131**, 3299–3310 (2008).

30. J. A. Nicoll, E. Barton, D. Boche, J. W. Neal, I. Ferrer, P. Thompson, C. Vlachouli, D. Wilkinson, A. Bayer, D. Games, P. Seubert, D. Schenk, C. Holmes, Abeta species removal after abeta42 immunization. *J Neuropathol Exp Neurol* **65**, 1040–1048 (2006).

31. D. Boche, N. Denham, C. Holmes, J. A. Nicoll, Neuropathology after active Abeta42 immunotherapy: implications for Alzheimer's disease pathogenesis. *Acta Neuropathol* **120**, 369–384 (2010).

32. C. Holmes, D. Boche, D. Wilkinson, G. Yadegarfar, V. Hopkins, A. Bayer, R. W. Jones, R. Bullock, S. Love, J. W. Neal, E. Zotova, J. A. Nicoll, Long-term effects of Abeta42 immunisation in Alzheimer's disease: follow-up of a randomised, placebo-controlled phase I trial. *Lancet* **372**, 216–223 (2008).

33. B. Chackerian, D. R. Lowy, J. T. Schiller, Conjugation of self-antigen to papillomavirus-like particles allows for efficient induction of protective auto-antibodies. *J Clin Invest* **108**, 415–423 (2001).

34. Q. Li, C. Cao, B. Chackerian, J. Schiller, M. Gordon, K. E. Ugen, D. Morgan, Overcoming antigen masking of anti-Abeta antibodies reveals breaking of B cell tolerance by virus-like particles in Abeta immunized amyloid precursor protein transgenic mice. *BMC Neurosci* **5**, 21 (2004).

35. M.-E. R. Ana Graf, Angelika Caputo, Martin Rhys Farlow, Giovanni Marotta, Raquel Sanchez-Valle, Philip Scheltens, J. Michael Ryan, Rik R. Vandenberghe, Active Aβ immunotherapy CAD106 Phase II dose-adjuvant finding study: safety and CNS biomarkers. *Alzheimers Dement* **10**, Suppl 274 (2014).

36. B. Liu, J. L. Frost, J. Sun, H. Fu, S. Grimes, P. Blackburn, C. A. Lemere, MER5101, a novel Abeta1–15:DT conjugate vaccine, generates a robust anti-Abeta antibody response and attenuates Abeta pathology and cognitive deficits in APPswe/PS1DeltaE9 transgenic mice. *J Neurosci* **33**, 7027–7037 (2013).

37. F. Bard, C. Cannon, R. Barbour, R. L. Burke, D. Games, H. Grajeda, T. Guido, K. Hu, J. Huang, K. Johnson-Wood, K. Khan, D. Kholodenko, M. Lee, I. Lieberburg, R. Motter, M. Nguyen, F. Soriano, N. Vasquez, K. Weiss, B. Welch, P. Seubert, D. Schenk, T. Yednock, Peripherally administered antibodies against amyloid beta-peptide enter the central nervous system and reduce pathology in a mouse model of Alzheimer's disease. *Nat Med* **6**, 916–919 (2000).

38. J. Hardy, D. J. Selkoe, The amyloid hypothesis of Alzheimer's disease: progress and problems on the road to therapeutics. *Science* **297**, 353–356 (2002).

39. D. Morgan, Immunotherapy for Alzheimer's disease. *J Intern Med* **269**, 54–63 (2011).

40. L. A. Kotilinek, B. Bacskai, M. Westerman, T. Kawarabayashi, L. Younkin, B. T. Hyman, S. Younkin, K. H. Ashe, Reversible memory loss in a mouse transgenic model of Alzheimer's disease. *J Neurosci* **22**, 6331–6335 (2002).

41. J. C. Dodart, K. R. Bales, K. S. Gannon, S. J. Greene, R. B. DeMattos, C. Mathis, C. A. DeLong, S. Wu, X. Wu, D. M. Holtzman, S. M. Paul, Immunization reverses memory deficits without reducing brain Abeta burden in Alzheimer's disease model. *Nat Neurosci* **5**, 452–457 (2002).

42. D. M. Wilcock, A. Rojiani, A. Rosenthal, S. Subbarao, M. J. Freeman, M. N. Gordon, D. Morgan, Passive immunotherapy against Abeta in aged APP-transgenic mice reverses cognitive deficits and depletes parenchymal amyloid deposits in spite of increased vascular amyloid and microhemorrhage. *J Neuroinflammation* **1**, 24 (2004).

43. Q. Li, L. Lebson, D. C. Lee, K. Nash, J. Grimm, A. Rosenthal, M. L. Selenica, D. Morgan, M. N. Gordon, Chronological age impacts immuno- therapy and monocyte uptake independent of amyloid load. *J Neuroimmun Pharmacol* **7**, 202– 214 (2012).

44. M. Pfeifer, S. Boncristiano, L. Bondolfi, A. Stalder, T. Deller, M. Staufenbiel, P. M. Mathews, M. Jucker, Cerebral hemorrhage after passive anti- Abeta immunotherapy. *Science* **298**, 1379 (2002).

45. M. M. Racke, L. I. Boone, D. L. Hepburn, M. Parsadainian, M. T. Bryan, D. K. Ness, K. S. Piroozi, W. H. Jordan, D. D. Brown, W. P. Hoffman, D. M. Holtzman, K. R. Bales, B. D. Gitter, P. C. May, S. M. Paul, R. B. DeMattos, Exacerbation of cerebral amyloid angiopathy- associated microhemorrhage in amyloid precur- sor protein transgenic mice by immunotherapy is dependent on antibody recognition of deposited forms of amyloid beta. *J Neurosci* **19;25**, 629–636 (2005).

46. S. Schroeter, K. Khan, R. Barbour, M. Doan, M. Chen, T. Guido, D. Gill, G. Basi, D. Schenk, P. Seubert, D. Games, Immunotherapy reduces vas- cular amyloid-beta in PDAPP mice. *J Neurosci* **28**, 6787–6793 (2008).

47. R. S. Black, R. A. Sperling, B. Safirstein, R. N. Motter, A. Pallay, A. Nichols, M. Grundman, A single ascending dose study of bapineuzumab in patients with Alzheimer disease. *Alzheimer Dis Assoc Disord* **24**, 198–203 (2010).

48. S. Salloway, R. Sperling, S. Gilman, N. C. Fox, K. Blennow, M. Raskind, M. Sabbagh, L. S. Honig, R. Doody, C. H. van Dyck, R. Mulnard, J. Barakos, K. M. Gregg, E. Liu, I. Lieburg, D. Schenk, R. Black, M. Grundman, A phase 2 multiple ascend- ing dose trial of bapineuzumab in mild to moder- ate Alzheimer disease. *Neurology* **73**, 2061–2070 (2009).

49. J. O. Rinne, D. J. Brooks, M. N. Rossor, N. C. Fox, R. Bullock, W. E. Klunk, C. A. Mathis, K. Blennow, J. Barakos, A. A. Okello, S. Rodriguez Martinez de Liano, E. Liu, M. Koller, K. M. Gregg, D. Schenk, R. Black, M. Grundman, 11C-PiB PET assessment of change in fibrillar amyloid-beta load in patients with Alzheimer's disease treated with bapineuzumab: a phase 2, double-blind, placebo-controlled, ascending-dose study. *Lancet Neurol* **9**, 363–372 (2010).

50. T. G. Beach, S. E. Monsell, L. E. Phillips, W. Kukull, Accuracy of the clinical diagnosis of Alzheimer disease at National Institute on Aging Alzheimer Disease Centers, 2005–2010. *J Neuropathol Exp Neurol* **71**, 266–273 (2012).

51. E. R. Siemers, S. Friedrich, R. A. Dean, C. R. Gonzales, M. R. Farlow, S. M. Paul, R. B. Dematsos,

Safety and changes in plasma and cerebrospinal fluid amyloid beta after a single administration of an amyloid beta monoclonal antibody in subjects with Alzheimer disease. *Clin Neuropharmacol* **33**, 67–73 (2010).

52. M. Farlow, S. E. Arnold, C. H. van Dyck, P. S. Aisen, B. J. Snider, A. P. Porsteinsson, S. Friedrich, R. A. Dean, C. Gonzales, G. Sethuraman, R. B. DeMattos, R. Mohs, S. M. Paul, E. R. Siemers, Safety and biomarker effects of solanezumab in patients with Alzheimer's disease. *Alzheimers Dement* **8**, 261–271 (2012).

53. B. Bohrmann, K. Baumann, J. Benz, F. Gerber, W. Huber, F. Knoflach, J. Messer, K. Oroszlan, R. Rauchenberger, W. F. Richter, C. Rothe, M. Urban, M. Bardroff, M. Winter, C. Nordstedt, H. Loetscher, Gantenerumab: a novel human anti- Abeta antibody demonstrates sustained cerebral amyloid-beta binding and elicits cell-mediated removal of human amyloid-beta. *J Alzheimers Dis* **28**, 49–69 (2012).

54. S. Ostrowitzki, D. Deptula, L. Thurfjell, F. Barkhof, B. Bohrmann, D. J. Brooks, W. E. Klunk, E. Ashford, K. Yoo, Z. X. Xu, H. Loetscher, L. Santarelli, Mechanism of amyloid removal in patients with Alzheimer disease treated with gan- tenerumab. *Arch Neurol* **69**, 198–207 (2012).

55. N. C. Carty, D. M. Wilcock, A. Rosenthal, J. Grimm, J. Pons, V. Ronan, P. E. Gottschall, M. N. Gordon, D. Morgan, Intracranial administration of deglycosylated C-terminal-specific anti-Abeta antibody efficiently clears amyloid plaques with- out activating microglia in amyloid-depositing transgenic mice. *J Neuroinflammation* **3**, 11 (2006).

56. D. M. Wilcock, J. Alamed, P. E. Gottschall, J. Grimm, A. Rosenthal, J. Pons, V. Ronan, K. Symmonds, M. N. Gordon, D. Morgan, Deglycosylated anti- amyloid-beta antibodies eliminate cognitive deficits and reduce parenchymal amyloid with minimal vascular consequences in aged amyloid precursor protein transgenic mice. *J Neurosci* **26**, 5340–5346 (2006).

57. G. B. Freeman, T. P. Brown, K. Wallace, K. R. Bales, Chronic administration of an aglycosylated murine antibody of ponezumab does not worsen microhemorrhages in aged Tg2576 mice. *Curr Alzheimer Res* **9**, 1059–1068 (2012).

58. J. W. Landen, Q. Zhao, S. Cohen, M. Borrie, M. Woodward, C. B. Billing, Jr., K. Bales, C. Alvey, F. McCush, J. Yang, J. W. Kupiec, M. M. Bednar, Safety and pharmacology of a single intravenous dose of ponezumab in subjects with mild-to-moderate Alzheimer disease: a phase I, randomized, placebo- controlled, double-blind, dose-escalation study. *Clin Neuropharmacol* **36**, 14–23 (2013).

59. A. Muhs, D. T. Hickman, M. Pihlgren, N. Chuard, V. Giriens, C. Meerschman, I. van der Auwera, F. van Leuven, M. Sugawara, M. C. Weingertner, B. Bechinger, R. Greferath, N. Kolonko, L. Nagel-Steger, D. Riesner, R. O. Brady, A. Pfeifer, C. Nicolau, Liposomal vaccines with conformation-specific amyloid peptide antigens define immune response and efficacy in APP transgenic mice. *Proc Natl Acad Sci U S A* **104**, 9810–9815 (2007).

60. L. Lannfelt, N. R. Relkin, E. R. Siemers, Amyloid-ss-directed immunotherapy for Alzheimer's disease. *J Intern Med* **275**, 284–295 (2014).

61. P. T. Nelson, I. Alafuzoff, E. H. Bigio, C. Bouras, H. Braak, N. J. Cairns, R. J. Castellani, B. J. Crain, P. Davies, K. Del Tredici, C. Duyckaerts, M. P. Frosch, V. Haroutunian, P. R. Hof, C. M. Hulette, B. T. Hyman, T. Iwatsubo, K. A. Jellinger, G. A. Jicha, E. Kovari, W. A. Kukull, J. B. Leverenz, S. Love, I. R. Mackenzie, D. M. Mann, E. Masliah, A. C. McKee, T. J. Montine, J. C. Morris, J. A. Schneider, J. A. Sonnen, D. R. Thal, J. Q. Trojanowski, J. C. Troncoso, T. Wisniewski, R. L. Woltjer, T. G. Beach, Correlation of Alzheimer disease neuropathologic changes with cognitive status: a review of the literature. *J Neuropath Exper Neurol* **71**, 362–381 (2012).

62. K. Yamada, J. Cirrito, L. Binder, V. Lee, D. Holtzman, In vivo microdialysis reveals age-dependent decrease of brain interstitial fluid tau levels in P301S human tau transgenic mice. *J Neurosci* **14,** 13110–13117 (2011).

63. H. Hampel, K. Burger, S. J. Teipel, A. L. Bokde, H. Zetterberg, K. Blennow, Core candidate neurochemical and imaging biomarkers of Alzheimer's disease. *Alzheimers Dement* **4**, 38–48 (2008).

64. A. A. Asuni, A. Boutajangout, D. Quartermain, E. M. Sigurdsson, Immunotherapy targeting pathological tau conformers in a tangle mouse model reduces brain pathology with associated functional improvements. *J Neurosci* **27**, 9115–9129 (2007).

65. A. Boutajangout, D. Quartermain, E. M. Sigurdsson, Immunotherapy targeting pathological tau prevents cognitive decline in a new tangle mouse model. *J Neurosci* **30**, 16559 –16566 (2010).

66. E. M. Sigurdsson, Tau-focused immunotherapy for Alzheimer's disease and related tauopathies. *Curr Alzheimer Res* **6**, 446–450 (2009).

67. L. Troquier, R. Caillierez, S. Burnouf, F. J. Fernandez-Gomez, M. E. Grosjean, N. Zommer, N. Sergeant, S. Schraen-Maschke, D. Blum, L. Buee, Targeting phospho-Ser422 by active tau immunotherapy in the THYTau22 mouse model: a suitable therapeutic approach. *Curr Alzheimer Res* **9**, 397–405 (2012).

68. M. Boimel, N. Grigoriadis, A. Lourbopoulos, E. Haber, O. Abramsky, H. Rosenmann, Efficacy and safety of immunization with phosphorylated tau against neurofibrillary tangles in mice. *Exp Neurol* **224**, 472–485 (2010).

69. M. Bi, A. Ittner, Y. D. Ke, J. Gotz, L. M. Ittner, Tau-targeted immunization impedes progression of neurofibrillary histopathology in aged P301L tau transgenic mice. *PLoS One* **6**, e26860 (2011).

70. M. L. Selenica, L. Benner, S. B. Housley, B. Manchec, D. C. Lee, K. R. Nash, J. Kalin, J. A. Bergman, A. Kozikowski, M. N. Gordon, D. Morgan, Histone deacetylase 6 inhibition improves memory and reduces total tau levels in a mouse model of tau deposition. *Alzheimers Res Ther* **6**, 12 (2014).

71. A. Boutajangout, J. Ingadottir, P. Davies, E. M. Sigurdsson, Passive immunization targeting pathological phospho-tau protein in a mouse model reduces functional decline and clears tau aggregates from the brain. *J Neurochem* **118**, 658–667 (2011).

72. C. d'Abramo, C. M. Acker, H. T. Jimenez, P. Davies, Tau passive immunotherapy in mutant P301L mice: antibody affinity versus specificity. *PLoS One* **8**, e62402 (2013).

73. K. Yanamandra, N. Kfoury, H. Jiang, T. E. Mahan, S. Ma, S. E. Maloney, D. F. Wozniak, M. I. Diamond, D. M. Holtzman, Anti-tau antibodies that block tau aggregate seeding in vitro markedly decrease pathology and improve cognition in vivo. *Neuron* **80**, 402–414 (2013).

74. M. J. Guerrero-Munoz, D. L. Castillo-Carranza, R. Kayed, Therapeutic approaches against common structural features of toxic oligomers shared by multiple amyloidogenic proteins. *Biochem Pharmacol* **88**, 468–478 (2014).

75. D. L. Castillo-Carranza, U. Sengupta, M. J. Guerrero-Munoz, C. A. Lasagna-Reeves, J. E. Gerson, G. Singh, D. M. Estes, A. D. Barrett, K. T. Dineley, G. R. Jackson, R. Kayed, Passive immunization with Tau oligomer monoclonal antibody reverses tauopathy phenotypes without affecting hyperphosphorylated neurofibrillary tangles. *J Neurosci* **34**, 4260–4272 (2014).

76. E. Kontsekova, N. Zilka, B. Kovacech, P. Novak, M. Novak, First-in-man tau vaccine targeting structural determinants essential for pathological tau-tau interaction reduces tau oligomerisation and neurofibrillary degeneration in an Alzheimer's disease model. *Alzheimers Res Ther* **6**, 44 (2014).

77. C. Theunis, N. Crespo-Biel, V. Gafner, M. Pihlgren, M. P. Lopez-Deber, P. Reis, D. T. Hickman, O. Adolfsson, N. Chuard, D. M. Ndao, P. Borghgraef, H. Devijver, F. Van Leuven, A. Pfeifer, A. Muhs, Efficacy and safety of a liposome-based vaccine against protein tau, assessed in tau.P301L mice that model tauopathy. *PLoS One* **8**, e72301 (2013).

78. H. J. Lee, S. Patel, S. J. Lee, Intravesicular localization and exocytosis of alpha-synuclein and its aggregates. *J Neurosci* **25**, 6016–6024 (2005).

79. E. Angot, P. Brundin, Dissecting the potential molecular mechanisms underlying alpha-synuclein cell-to-cell transfer in Parkinson's disease. *Parkinsonism Relat Disord* **15** Suppl 3, S143–S147 (2009).

80. J. H. Kordower, Y. Chu, R. A. Hauser, T. B. Freeman, C. W. Olanow, Lewy body-like pathology in long-term embryonic nigral transplants in Parkinson's disease. *Nat Med* **14**, 504–506 (2008).

81. E. Masliah, E. Rockenstein, A. Adame, M. Alford, L. Crews, M. Hashimoto, P. Seubert, M. Lee, J. Goldstein, T. Chilcote, D. Games, D. Schenk, Effects of alpha-synuclein immunization in a mouse model of Parkinson's disease. *Neuron* **46**, 857–868 (2005).

82. I. F. Tsigelny, Y. Sharikov, M. A. Miller, E. Masliah, Mechanism of alpha-synuclein oligomerization and membrane interaction: theoretical approach to unstructured proteins studies. *Nanomedicine* **4**, 350–357 (2008).

83. A. Schneeberger, M. Mandler, F. Mattner, W. Schmidt, Vaccination for Parkinson's disease. *Parkinsonism Relat Disord* **18** Suppl 1, S11–13 (2012).

84. E. Masliah, E. Rockenstein, M. Mante, L. Crews, B. Spencer, A. Adame, C. Patrick, M. Trejo, K. Ubhi, T. T. Rohn, S. Mueller-Steiner, P. Seubert, R. Barbour, L. McConlogue, M. Buttini, D. Games, D. Schenk, Passive immunization reduces behavioral and neuropathological deficits in an alpha-synuclein transgenic model of Lewy body disease. *PLoS One* **6**, e19338 (2011).

85. E. J. Bae, H. J. Lee, E. Rockenstein, D. H. Ho, E. B. Park, N. Y. Yang, P. Desplats, E. Masliah, S. J. Lee, Antibody-aided clearance of extracellular alpha-synuclein prevents cell-to-cell aggregate transmission. *J Neurosci* **32**, 13454–13469 (2012).

86. F. L. Heppner, C. Musahl, I. Arrighi, M. A. Klein, T. Rulicke, B. Oesch, R. M. Zinkernagel, U. Kalinke, A. Aguzzi, Prevention of scrapie pathogenesis by transgenic expression of anti-prion protein antibodies. *Science* **294**, 178–182 (2001).

87. E. M. Sigurdsson, D. R. Brown, M. Daniels, R. J. Kascsak, R. Kascsak, R. Carp, H. C. Meeker, B. Frangione, T. Wisniewski, Immunization delays the onset of prion disease in mice. *Am J Pathol* **161**, 13–17 (2002).

88. E. M. Sigurdsson, M. S. Sy, R. Li, H. Scholtzova, R. J. Kascsak, R. Kascsak, R. Carp, H. C. Meeker, B. Frangione, T. Wisniewski, Anti-prion antibodies for prophylaxis following prion exposure in mice. *Neurosci Lett* **336**, 185–187 (2003).

89. A. R. White, P. Enever, M. Tayebi, R. Mushens, J. Linehan, S. Brandner, D. Anstee, J. Collinge, S. Hawke, Monoclonal antibodies inhibit prion replication and delay the development of prion disease. *Nature* **422**, 80–83 (2003).

90. T. L. Rovis, G. Legname, Prion protein-specific antibodies-development, modes of action and therapeutics application. *Viruses* **6**, 3719–3737 (2014).

91. P. D. Hedlin, N. R. Cashman, L. Li, J. Gupta, L. A. Babiuk, A. A. Potter, P. Griebel, S. Napper, Design and delivery of a cryptic PrP(C) epitope for induction of PrP(Sc)-specific antibody responses. *Vaccine* **28**, 981–988 (2010).

92. C. Feraudet, N. Morel, S. Simon, H. Volland, Y. Frobert, C. Creminon, D. Vilette, S. Lehmann, J. Grassi, Screening of 145 anti-PrP monoclonal antibodies for their capacity to inhibit PrPSc replication in infected cells. *J Biol Chem* **280**, 11247–11258 (2005).

93. V. Perrier, J. Solassol, C. Crozet, Y. Frobert, C. Mourton-Gilles, J. Grassi, S. Lehmann, Anti-PrP antibodies block PrPSc replication in prion-infected cell cultures by accelerating PrPC degradation. *J Neurochem* **89**, 454–463 (2004).

94. C. Alexandrenne, V. Hanoux, F. Dkhissi, D. Boquet, J. Y. Couraud, A. Wijkhuisen, Curative properties of antibodies against prion protein: a comparative in vitro study of monovalent fragments and divalent antibodies. *J Neuroimmunol* **209**, 50–56 (2009).

95. T. Sonati, R. R. Reimann, J. Falsig, P. K. Baral, T. O'Connor, S. Hornemann, S. Yaganoglu, B. Li, U. S. Herrmann, B. Wieland, M. Swayampakula, M. H. Rahman, D. Das, N. Kav, R. Riek, P. P. Liberski, M. N. James, A. Aguzzi, The toxicity of antiprion antibodies is mediated by the flexible tail of the prion protein. *Nature* **501**, 102–106 (2013).

96. L. Solforosi, J. R. Criado, D. B. McGavern, S. Wirz, M. Sanchez-Alavez, S. Sugama, L. A. DeGiorgio, B. T. Volpe, E. Wiseman, G. Abalos, E. Masliah, D. Gilden, M. B. Oldstone, B. Conti, R. A. Williamson, Cross-linking cellular prion protein triggers neuronal apoptosis in vivo. *Science* **303**, 1514–1516 (2004).

18

Clinical Trials and Drug Development in Neurodegenerative Diseases

Unifying Principles

JEFFREY L. CUMMINGS AND KATE ZHONG

INTRODUCTION

Neurodegenerative diseases (NDDs), including Alzheimer's disease (AD), frontotemporal dementia (FTD), dementia with Lewy bodies (DLB), multiple system atrophy (MSA), progressive supranuclear palsy (PSP), corticobasal degeneration (CBD), Huntington's disease (HD), and amyotrophic lateral sclerosis (ALS), are all gradually progressive degenerative disorders. All involve processes leading to the death of nerve cells, with concomitant decline in cognitive, behavioral, functional, and motoric aspects of function. The global burden of NDDs in terms of deaths, lost productivity, and personal and family stress is enormous. Most NDDs are age-related and will increase in the coming years as the global population ages.[1] The increase in the human, social, and economic costs of these diseases will demand huge portions of government resources if means of preventing, delaying, significantly slowing the progress, or improving the symptoms of these diseases are not found. These diseases rob individuals of their memory, personality, function, and autonomy and increase dependence on others. They represent among the greatest threats to the future of mankind.

There is an urgent need to develop meaningful new therapies for NDDs, both disease-modifying and symptomatic. The one means of developing new therapies that can eventually be advanced to market is by testing promising compounds in clinical trials. Emerging therapies for patients with an NDD may address symptoms specific to that illness (e.g., the motor abnormalities of PD), symptoms that are shared across disorders (e.g., cognitive decline), or neurodegeneration itself, with putative disease-modifying interventions. Thus far, no agents have been shown definitively to be effective in disease modification, and no agent has been approved by the US Food and Drug Administration (FDA) or other world regulatory agencies for disease modification of an NDD.

Clinical trials attempting to demonstrate disease modification face common problems across NDDs, and this chapter addresses shared features of clinical trials in NDDs. A major goal of this analysis is to identify means of improving trials across NDDs by extrapolating from one NDD to another and to assist in identifying therapies that may be applied across multiple NDDs. Discovery in one NDD may well have implications for therapies of other disorders in this class. The scientific community should be poised to exploit learnings in one NDD by rapidly extrapolating them to others.

SYMPTOMATIC VERSUS DISEASE-MODIFYING CLINICAL TRIALS

This chapter will emphasize trials for disease-modification of NDD and common features encountered in these trials, regardless of the underlying disorder. Symptomatic treatments, however, can also be used across NDDs, and features of symptomatic trials shared across NDDs will also be discussed. Trials of disease-modifying agents make different demands on sponsors and investigators and have different characteristics from trials of symptomatic agents. Table 18.1 contrasts symptomatic clinical trials with those addressing disease-modifying therapies (DMTs).

There are approved symptomatic agents in AD and PD, whereas there are no DMTs for any NDD. The goal of symptomatic treatments is the reduction of symptoms present at baseline, whereas the goal of DMTs is to prevent, delay the onset, or

TABLE 18.1. COMPARISON OF CLINICAL TRIALS AND DEVELOPMENT PROGRAMS OF SYMPTOMATIC AND DISEASE-MODIFYING THERAPIES

Trial Feature	Symptomatic	Disease-Modifying
Precedent established	Approved agents to model including cholinesterase inhibitors and memantine approved for treatment of AD	No approved agents to model
Outcome of the trial	Symptom reduction with improvement above baseline in the initial period of treatment and delay of decline for 6–9 months	Prevention, delay of onset, or slowing of progression
Trial duration	Shorter trials (3–6 months)	Longer trials (12–36 months)
Trial size	Smaller trials (100–400 per arm)	Larger trials (600–1,000 per arm)
Experience with trial instruments	Trial instrument performance established	Trial instrument performance unknown (e.g., in patients with prodromal AD or in prevention trials)
Role of biomarkers	Biomarkers used for patient selection, demonstrations of target engagement, dose selection	Biomarkers used for patient selection, demonstrations of target engagement, and dose selection, and have critical role in supporting disease modification
Experience with populations	Familiar populations (mild-severe AD dementia and similar dementias across NDDs)	Unfamiliar populations (individuals with normal cognition at risk for NDD)
Experience with targets	Familiar targets (e.g., enzymes, receptors, channels, transporters)	Unfamiliar targets (e.g., protein-protein interactions, cell-to-cell transmission)
Experience with formulations	Familiar delivery modalities (e.g., oral, patch)	Unfamiliar delivery modalities (e.g., intravenous monoclonal antibodies)
Cost of drug development	Less expensive	More expensive
Experience with payers	Approach to reimbursement known	Approach to reimbursement unknown
Regulatory pathway	Known regulatory pathway	Unknown regulatory pathway
Placebo response in trials	Placebo responses common	Placebo responses limited

AD: Alzheimer's disease; NDD: neurodegenerative diseases.

slow the progression of clinical symptoms without necessarily expecting an improvement above baseline. Trials of symptomatic agents tend to be shorter (of 3–6 months duration), whereas trials for DMTs tend to be longer (of 12–36 months duration). Symptomatic agents often have a sufficient effect size to require smaller trials (100–400 subjects per arm) compared to trials for DMTs, where smaller anticipated effect sizes typically require larger trials (600–1,000 per arm). Trials of approved symptomatic therapies have succeeded and have progressed to market. With this experience, the performance of clinical trial instruments

in symptomatic trials is better understood than in DMT trials where new, less symptomatic populations are being assessed, or where the outcome is an alteration in disease progression. In symptomatic treatment drug development programs, biomarkers have a limited role, often used only in patient selection or target engagement (e.g., receptor occupancy studies). Biomarkers have a larger role in disease-modifying trials, including patient selection, target engagement, demonstration of disease-modification, and side effect monitoring. Symptomatic trials involve familiar populations, such as mild to severe AD or other

NDD dementias, whereas disease-modifying trials increasingly involve unfamiliar populations, such as those who have no symptoms but are at increased risk because of the presence of state or trait biomarkers, or patients who have minimal symptoms and are in the very beginning phases of the symptomatic portion of the illness. In general, clinical trials of symptomatic agents are less expensive because they are shorter and smaller, whereas trials for DMTs are larger, longer, involve biomarkers, and are more expensive. There is a known regulatory pathway with previously approved symptomatic agents, whereas the regulatory requirements for DMTs are currently evolving and substantial uncertainties remain. Symptomatic agents involve familiar biological targets, such as receptors, channels, and transporters, whereas DMT trials involve unfamiliar targets such as protein-protein interactions and cell-to-cell transmission. Symptomatic agents are typically oral or administered via patch, whereas DMTs often involve less familiar delivery mechanisms such as intravenous or subcutaneous administration of monoclonal antibodies. Side effects to DMTs include unfamiliar occurrences, such as amyloid-related imaging abnormalities (ARIA), compared to more common gastrointestinal side effects encountered with symptomatic agents. Symptomatic agent trials may have a placebo response that is substantial and must be anticipated in the clinical trial design, whereas DMT trials have limited placebo responses.

SHARED TARGETS IN DISEASE-MODIFYING TRIALS OF NEURODEGENERATIVE DISORDERS

There are many shared aspects of therapeutic targets and clinical trials that are common across NDDs. Each NDD involves a culprit protein: in AD, amyloid, tau, and transactive response DNA-binding protein 43 (TDP-43) proteins aggregate; PD has aggregated neuronal alpha-synuclein, and MSA has glial cell alpha-synuclein aggregates; most FTD patients harbor either tau or TDP-43 proteins; PSP and CBD involve the tau protein; ALS involves TDP-43 and SOD-1 proteins; and DLB involves amyloid and alpha-synuclein proteins.[2] In each case, monomers are the first molecular form generated, followed by aggregation into oligomers and eventual evolution to insoluble fibrillar proteinacious forms. The aggregated oligomeric form of the protein appears to be associated with greater toxicity than either

the monomeric or insoluble fibrillar form of the protein. Autophagy and protein processing are abnormal in these disorders, leading to inefficient protein disposal and proteostasis. Proteins also appear to be transmitted from cell to cell in a prion-like fashion across these disease states.[3] The proteins spread using disorder-specific networks that can be defined using functional magnetic resonance imaging (fMRI).[4] Mitochondrial dysfunction with abnormal cellular energetics is also common across NDDs.[5] Mitochondrial abnormalities result in disturbed oxidative metabolism, reduced energy production, and increased free radical generation with oxidative injury. Heavy metals such as iron interact with these mitochondrial failures to increase oxidative injury in multiple NDDs.[6] Errors in RNA processing and epigenetic abnormalities of DNA are characteristic of NDDs. NDDs also have overlapping disease gene networks, suggesting common genetic expression patterns across NDDs.[7,8] Trophic factor abnormalities with failure to maintain cell populations normally are seen in many NDDs. Involvement of glial cells as a primary (in MSA) abnormality or through secondary mechanisms is common in NDDs. Intracellular transport abnormalities with failure to maintain synaptic integrity are also shared across NDDs.[9] All of these disturbances lead to disease-specific local changes, such as hippocampal abnormalities in AD, loss of cells in the substantia nigra in PD, neuronal loss in the motor system in ALS, and disruption of functional brain circuits unique to each disease state.[4] The shared features of NDDs suggest that some treatments may be applicable in multiple disease states, or that lessons learned from management of neurobiological abnormalities in one disease may be useful in developing therapy for other NDDs.

Common cellular abnormalities combine with unique regional vulnerabilities to produce the characteristic phenotype of each NDD (Figure 18.1). Local degeneration produces clinically distinct abnormalities that become more similar as the disease process spreads toward the end state of the disorder. The site of origin determines the first and characteristic clinical features; onset in substantia nigra leads to parkinsonism in PD; early hippocampal changes produce the episodic memory loss of AD; striatal involvement causes the chorea of HD. Symptoms become more diverse and more severe as the diseases evolve, and patients have less distinctive features in the very advanced phase of the disease.

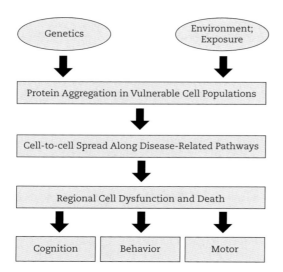

FIGURE 18.1. Summary of shared processes in the pathogenesis of NDDs.

Animal models are needed to study NDDs in laboratory settings. Animal model systems provide insight into disease mechanisms, biomarkers, behavior-pathology correlations, and potential therapies. Transgenic approaches to the creation of animal models are commonly used across different NDDs. A wide variety of transgenic model organisms have been utilized, including bacteria, nematodes, arthropods (*Drosophila melanogaster*), zebra fish, and rodents (mouse and rat).[10] Human cells may be better model systems for study, and induced pluripotent stem (iPS) cells are increasingly used to study NDDs and may enhance drug screening and development of disease treatments.[11-13]

Animal models have only modest ability to predict human side effects in drug development, and they have not predicted efficacy in humans. They do not model disease states but do provide us with insight into specific pathways and mechanisms. Each NDD is characterized by a seamless progression from asymptomatic at-risk states, to prodromal minimally symptomatic phases of the disease, to the conventional well-defined aspect of the NDD with fully expressed phenotype. They are eventually fatal, as vital functions are compromised. Terminal infections, such as pneumonia or incontinence-associated urinary tract infections, are common end-of-life events in NDDs.

NDDs have genetic and non-genetic forms of the disease. In AD, autosomal dominant forms of the disease occur with presenilin 1 (PS1), presenilin 2 (PS2), and amyloid precursor protein (APP) mutations.[14] These account for a small number of cases (approximately 3%); risk factor genes

(apolipoprotein e4 [*ApoE4*]) and non-genetic risk factors account for the majority of cases. Hereditary and environmental factors conspire in most other NDDs. HD is an exception, with only the autosomal dominant form of the disease known. Genetic causes are more prominent in FTD than in AD or PD. The genetics of familial forms of FTD involves seven recognized genes: the microtubule-associated protein tau (*MAPT*) progranulin (*GRN*), the valosin-containing protein (*VCP*), chromatin-modifying 2B (*CHMP2B*), the TDP-43 encoding gene (*TARBDP*), fused in sarcoma (*FUS*), and the open reading frame of chromosome 9 (*C9orf72*).[15] Approximately 50% of FTD patients have no recognized genetic contribution to their illness.

TRIALS OF SYMPTOMATIC TREATMENTS FOR NDD

Symptomatic treatments can be applied across NDDs. Cholinergic deficits, for example, are present in several NDDs, including AD, PD, PD dementia, and DLB.[16,17] Rivastigmine, a cholinesterase inhibitor, is approved for use in AD and in PD dementia.[18] This is the only example of an agent approved for more than one NDD and can serve as a model for cross-NDD approaches.

Other symptomatic agents may be applicable in more than one NDD. A variety of other mechanisms are being explored in cognitive-enhancement drug development programs. Mechanisms being assessed include histaminergic (H3) antagonists, serotonergic (5-HT$_6$) antagonists, cannabinoid antagonists, glutamatergic (NMDA receptor) antagonists (ampakines), and phosphodiesterase inhibitors.[19-26] In addition, AD drug development programs are investigating agents beyond the usual transmitter approaches. Synaptic support and regeneration (with drugs or medical foods), insulin and insulin sensitizers, ketogenic agents, mitochondrial agents, psychotropic drugs with cognitive-enhancing properties, and devices such as deep brain stimulation and repetitive transcranial magnetic stimulation are in clinical trials for cognitive enhancement in AD.[27-37] Success in this setting could lead to testing in other NDDs with cognitive impairment. Symptomatic agents are less dependent on specific mechanisms of cell death and may be applicable across diseases with disparate causes of neurodegeneration.

DESIGNS FOR DISEASE-MODIFYING TREATMENT TRIALS

The primary goal in the development of DMTs is to prevent or delay the onset of more severe disease in patients with no or minimal symptoms, or to slow the progression of disease in patients who have substantial symptoms. In AD, primary prevention would involve patients who have no symptoms and no state biomarkers of AD, such as changes in cerebrospinal fluid (CSF), amyloid-ß (Aß) protein, or positive amyloid imaging. Trait biomarkers such as the apolipoprotein e4 (*ApoE4*) genotype increase the risk of AD and could identify populations of patients for inclusion in primary prevention studies. Secondary prevention can be pursued in patients who are asymptomatic, but who have a positive state marker such as CSF abnormalities or positive amyloid imaging. Clinical trials in patients with prodromal AD involve subjects who have episodic memory disturbances and biomarkers indicative of the presence of AD pathology (AD CSF signature or positive amyloid imaging). Successful disease modification in prodromal trials would forestall the development of AD dementia. In AD dementia trials, DMTs can slow the progression from mild to moderate or from moderate to severe AD dementia. Similar paradigms exist for other NDDs.

A positive outcome of an NDD trial would involve demonstrating a drug-placebo difference at the end of a trial on a primary clinical outcome, plus a drug-placebo difference on a biomarker indicative of cell preservation in the treatment group (Figure 18.2). An association between the biomarker and the clinical outcome, suggesting that it had been achieved through similar drug-related mechanisms, would be expected. A

change in the slope or rate of decline is expected in trials of DMT. Likewise, an increasing drug-placebo difference over time is supportive evidence of disease-modification. Similar designs and observations would by characteristic of all DMT trials in NDDs.

Clinical trial designs that may support a disease-modifying claim without resort to a biomarker include the delayed-start and randomized-withdrawal designs. In the delayed-start design, patients are randomized to drug or placebo at baseline, and the placebo group (or a randomized subset) is transitioned to active therapy at some defined interval in the trial course. If the delayed treatment group achieves the same symptomatic benefit as the initial treatment group, a symptomatic benefit has been demonstrated (Figure 18.3). If the delayed initiation group does not catch up with the group treated at trial onset, disease modification has been demonstrated (Figure 18.4). In the randomized-withdrawal design, patients are randomized to drug or placebo at baseline. After some pre-specified interval, a randomized portion of the treatment group is withdrawn from therapy. If they decline to the level of the non-treated placebo group, then the benefits of the drug were symptomatic (Figure 18.5). If the group withdrawn from therapy continues to function above the level of the placebo group, then the trial supports disease-modification by the test agent (Figure 18.6). The ADAGIO study of rasagiline for the treatment of PD is an example of a delayed-start design to demonstrate disease-modification in an NDD.[38] Challenges to these designs include uncertainties as to how long patients must be

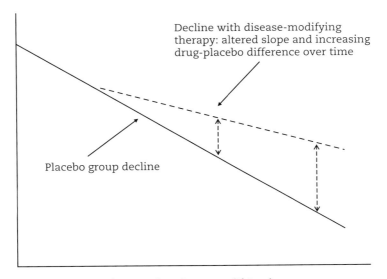

Decline with disease-modifying therapy: altered slope and increasing drug-placebo difference over time

Placebo group decline

FIGURE 18.2. Impact on the course of an NDD by a disease-modifying therapy.

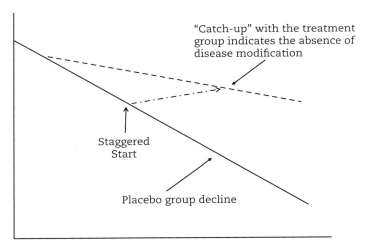

FIGURE 18.3. Delayed-start design with "catch-up" of the delayed start to the early treatment group consistent with a symptomatic treatment effect.

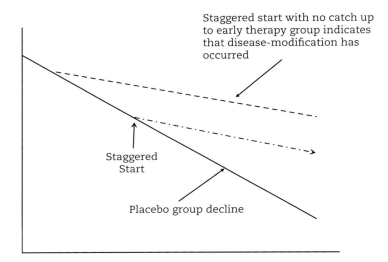

FIGURE 18.4. Delayed-start design with no "catch-up" of the delayed start to the early treatment group consistent with a disease modifying effect.

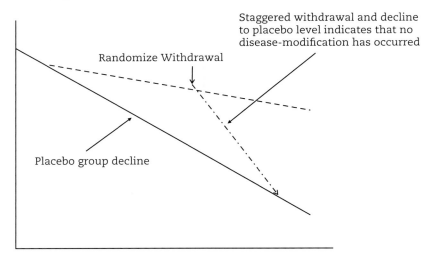

FIGURE 18.5. Staggered-withdrawal design with decline to the level of a no-treatment group and consistent with a symptomatic treatment effect.

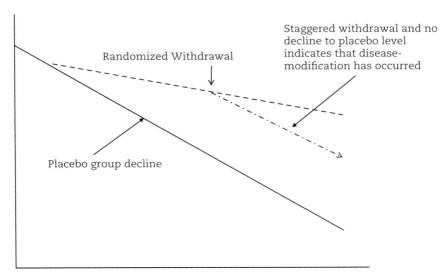

FIGURE 18.6. Staggered-withdrawal design with persistent treatment effect of a disease-modifying therapy.

treated prior to withdrawal and how long patients should be observed once treatment has been withdrawn. Such uncertainties make it difficult to estimate the sample sizes needed and the total duration of the trial. Relatively few trials of this type have been conducted.

The delay-to-milestone design (Figure 18.7) can be used to assess symptomatic or disease-modifying treatments and does not distinguish between the two types of treatment effect. A delay to clinically important milestone, such as delay of development of a Clinical Dementia Rating (CDR)[39] of 1.0 in patients with a CDR of 0.5 at baseline, could be a meaningful outcome and supportive of disease modification if used in conjunction with a biomarker supportive of a disease-modifying effect.

Adaptive clinical designs represent another approach to optimizing drug development by making maximum use of data accumulating in the course of the trial. After comprehensive pre-specification, adjustment can be made in the number of arms in the trial (eliminating a high-dose arm, for example, because of lack of tolerability or a low-dose arm for lack of efficacy), sample size, tiral duration, or entry criteria.[40]

Futility designs are another design innovation applicable to NDD trials. These trials pre-specify

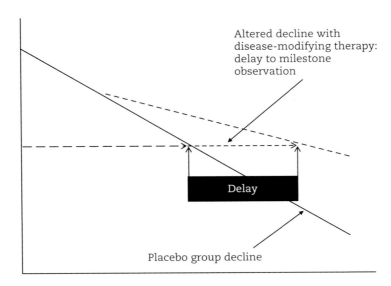

FIGURE 18.7. Delay-to-milestone trial design.

a meaningful effect size compared to a historical control group or a contemporaneous placebo
group and provide structured stopping rules if
the possibility of reaching this goal is futile.[41–43]
Conclusions regarding futility can be reached in
shorter times and with smaller sample sizes than
required for the complete trial, saving human and
economic resources. The decision to continue a
study as non-futile does not ensure that a drug-
placebo difference will be established at the end
of the study.

PRIMARY AND SECONDARY OUTCOMES FOR NDD TRIALS

Table 18.2 provides a list of typical primary outcomes for disease-modifying trials. Primary
clinical outcomes must address the core clinical
features of the disease. In AD trials and in trials of other dementia syndromes, dual outcomes
are required with one primary measure addressing the core symptoms of the disorder (e.g.,
cognitive abnormalities) and the co-primary

TABLE 18.2. COMMON FEATURES OF NEURODEGENERATIVE DISORDERS AND CLINICAL TRIALS OF DISEASE-MODIFYING AGENTS

Class	Specific Features
Shared cellular mechanisms	• Protein misfolding • Cell-to-cell spread • Energy demands and metabolic failure • Growth factor signaling abnormalities • Intracellular transport deficits • Toxic neuro-environment associated with aggregated proteins and their consequences • RNA-processing abnormalities • DNA methylation • Overlapping disease gene networks • Glial cell abnormalities • Neuronal loss
Laboratory models	• Transgenic animals with human mutations commonly used to create model systems for NDD • Primates used for pharmacokinetic studies
Progressive phases	• Asymptomatic with genetic risk factor • Asymptomatic with non-genetic state biomarkers with a positive state biomarkers • Prodromal, minimally symptomatic phase • Complete symptom complex
Genetic and non-genetic forms	• Autosomal dominant disease • Risk genes • Late-onset forms of the disease with few/no genetic risk factors
Primary outcomes	• Scores on rating scales assessing core disease symptoms
Secondary clinical trial outcomes	• Non-primary measures of cognition • Activities of daily living • Behavior • Quality of life • Pharmaco-economic outcomes • Caregiver burden and distress
Biomarker outcomes	• Target engagement biomarkers reflecting near-term mechanism of action of the test agent • Disease-modifying biomarkers reflecting alterations in processes leading to cell death • Safety biomarkers
Regulatory aspects	• No approved DMT agents for NDDs: regulatory aspects evolving

DMT: disease-modifying therapy; iPS cells: induced pluripotent stem cells; NDD: neurodegenerative disorder.

demonstrating the clinical meaningfulness of the changes in the core symptoms (functional or global assessment). In AD dementia trials, the Alzheimer's Disease Assessment Scale–Cognitive Subscale (ADAS-Cog)[44] is the typical measure of the core symptoms, and a global measure such as the CDR or a measure of activities of daily living, typically the Alzheimer's Disease Cooperative Study (ADCS) Activities of Daily Living (ADL) scale[45] or the Disability Assessment for Dementia (DAD),[46] are used to demonstrate clinical meaningfulness. Dual outcomes have been required for trials leading to the approval of rivastigmine for the treatment of PD dementia[18] and are expected in other dementing disorders, although no other agents or trials have met the requirements of the regulatory pathway.

Composite scales are commonly used as primary outcomes in clinical trials of NDDs. The PSP rating scale is a composite instrument used in PSP trials,[47] and the Unified Parkinson's Disease Rating Scale (UPDRS) is commonly used in PD trials.[38] Composite scales has been developed for use in prodromal AD (ADCOMS,[48] instrumental AD Rating Scale [ADRS]) and the CDR is a composite used in prodromal AD and AD dementia.

Tools that could be used across all NDDs would be useful to understand similarities and differences in clinical trials and drug responses. The National Institutes of Health (NIH) Toolbox Cognitive Health Battery (NIHTB-CHB) is designed to measure neurological functions that span different disciplines, apply to diverse research questions, and measure a broad range of functions across the life span from age 3 to 85 years. The NIHTB-CHB is composed of four modules: cognition, emotion, motor, and sensory.[49] Cognitive assessments of the NIHTB-CHB include measures of executive function, episodic memory, language, processing speed, working memory, and attention.[50] This instrument battery has not yet impacted clinical trials in NDD, but it represents an important unifying research direction. Similarly, the National Institute of Neurological Disease and Stroke (NINDS) supported the development of a tool for the assessment of frontosubocrtical systems, Executive Abilities: Measures and Instruments for Neurobehavioral Evaluation and Research (EXAMINER).[51] This tool includes measures of working memory, inhibition, set shifting, fluency, insight, planning, social cognition, and behavior relevant to the assessment of executive and frontal lobe function. This instrument has not yet found application in NDD clinical trials, but the psychometric properties suggest that it may be sensitive

to change over time, including changes induced by therapy. Use of the same tools across clinical trials would facilitate understanding of the common features and treatment responsiveness of cognitive domains across disease states.

If not implemented as a primary outcome, then measures of ADLs are commonly used as a secondary outcome measure. Behavioral abnormalities are also common across NDDs, and improvement in behavior from baseline and/or reduction in the emergence of new behaviors are important measures of drug benefit. The Neuropsychiatric Inventory (NPI) is the tool most commonly used to assess behavioral changes in NDD.[52]

Quality of life (QoL) measures have been developed for some NDDs and have been used in a limited number of clinical trials. Most QoL scales assess many aspects of quality of life that are not impacted by pharmacotherapy, and it has proven difficult to show changes in QoL based on pharmacologic interventions in NDDs. Caregiver burden is one aspect of caregiver quality of life, and burden scales or other means of assessing caregivers are often included in trials of NDDs.[53]

Increasingly, health maintenance organizations and other payers for pharmaceutical products are requiring a higher level of cost-utility information for decisions of whether to support new pharmacologic interventions. While clinical trials are artificial populations conducted in non-routine clinical circumstances, they can collect data relevant to pharmaco-economic decision-making. Pharmaco-economic tools have evolved for use in clinical trials, such as the Resource Utilization in Dementia (RUD), used in some AD trials.[54]

THE ROLE OF BIOMARKERS IN NEURODEGENERATIVE DISEASE TRIALS

Table 18.3 and Figure 18.8 summarize the role of biomarkers in clinical trials. Biomarkers in preclinical studies provide many types of information, including correlations with necropsy findings where animals can be sacrificed, cross-specifies fidelity of findings (e.g., from rat to monkey), increasing confidence in the extrapolation to human biomarker outcomes, systems effects such as impact on fMRI, beneficial response to treatment, and adverse event detection.[55]

Trait biomarkers such as genetic abnormalities can be used to identify trial populations of

TABLE 18.3. ROLE OF BIOMARKERS IN CLINICAL TRIALS

Biomarker Function	Example of Biomarkers Used in Clinical Trials
Subject selection	Trait biomarker such as positive amyloid imaging or positive CSF finding in AD trials
Population stratification	Risk factor genes such as *ApoE4* carrier status in AD trials
Target engagement	Amyloid synthesis and clearance in CSF using labeled leucine technology; receptor occupancy studies using PET ligands
Metabolic effects	Fluorodeoxyglucose metabolism on PET; cerebral blood flow measures on PET
Functional effects	Connectivity measures on fMRI
Disease modification	Atrophy on MRI; tau levels in CSF; tau imaging
Side effect monitoring	MRI for ARIA; ECG for cardiac effects; liver functions for hepatic effect

AD: Alzheimer's disease; ApoE: apolipoprotein E; ARIA: amyloid-related imaging abnormalities; CSF: cerebrospinal fluid; ECG: electrocardiogram; fMRI: functional magnetic resonance imaging; MRI: magnetic resonance imaging; PET: positron emission tomography.

individuals at high risk for a specific NDD. For example, the carriers of the *ApoE4* gene are at a substantially increased risk for developing AD. Likewise, *LRRK2* mutations have been associated with the occurrence of PD. Approximately 50% of FTD cases are genetic in nature and are associated with mutations of the chromosome 9 open reading frame 72 (*C9ORF72*) gene, granulin (*GRN*) gene, or microtubule associated protein tau gene (*MAPT*).[56] These genetic biomarkers can be used to identify patients at high risk for progression to symptomatic phases of NDD and to construct prevention trial populations.

State biomarkers indicative of the presence of the disease are commonly used in clinical trials targeting DMTs. In AD, for example, amyloid imaging establishes the presence of fibriller amyloid plaques in the brain, a condition that prevails for approximately 15 years prior to the onset of abnormal cognitive function.[57] Similarly, CSF changes, including low Aß 1-42 or elevated tau or hyperphosphorylated tau (p-tau), identify patients prior to the onset of symptomatic cognitive states.[58]

Target engagement biomarkers can be used to determine the near-term consequences of

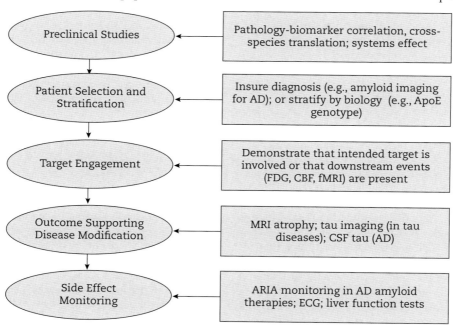

FIGURE 18.8. Biomarkers in drug development programs.

AD: Alzheimer's disease; ApoE: apolipoprotein E; ARIA: amyloid-related imaging abnormalities; CSF: cerebrospinal fluid; ECG: electrocardiogram; FDG: fluorodeoxyglucose; fMRI: functional magnetic resonance imaging; PET: positron emission tomography.

pharmacologic intervention and to determine whether the agent is having the desired effect. Relatively few target engagement biomarkers have been developed, despite the critical need for them in DMT clinical trials. Measurement of Aß-42 synthesis and clearance using labeled luceine is an example of a targeted engagement biomarker; inhibition of gamma-secretase was associated with reduced Aß synthesis.[59] Downstream biomarkers, such as fluorodeoxyglucose positron emission tomography (PET), cerebral blood flow, or effects on functional connectivity, can also support target engagement.

Biomarkers indicative of disease modification are those that support the neuro-protective effects of the intervention. Currently these are thought to include: reduced magnetic resonance imaging (MRI) atrophy, ameliorated increases in tau and p-tau, or differences in tau imaging in clinical trials of DMTs in AD or other tauopathies. MRI cortical measures could also be used to assess outcomes of DMTs in FTD and DLB; and tau imaging may perform as an outcome in trials of tauopathies. There is relatively limited experience with the performance of putative disease modification biomarkers.

Biomarkers can also be used to monitor adverse effects in clinical trials. MRI has been used to assess and track amyloid-related imaging abnormalities (ARIA) of the effusion (ARIA-E) or hemorrhagic (ARIA-H) type.[60] Electrocardiography (ECG) monitoring of cardiac effects and liver function tests assessing hepatic toxicity are also examples of biomarkers commonly used to assess adverse events in clinical trials.

DEFINITION AND REGULATORY ASPECTS OF DISEASE MODIFICATION TRIALS

There is no consensus definition of disease modification. Intervention in processes leading to cell death or delay in progression of NDD disease course have both been proposed as measures of disease modification. Combining the biological and the clinical, Cummings[61] suggested that a disease-modifying outcome would require evidence of an impact on the underlying disease process (biomarker or delayed-start or randomized-withdrawal design) plus an effect on primary clinical outcomes. No agent developed as treatment for NDD has shown disease modification, and the final regulatory approach to DMT labeling is uncertain. A refined understanding of the outcomes needed to meet criteria for regulatory approval of a DMT is required. The FDA has used the term "disease modification" in its guidelines with regard to early intervention in AD, suggesting that it may be possible to meet definitional requirements as a DMT.[62]

SUMMARY

There is a rapid increase in the understanding of NDDs. Disease mechanisms, biomarkers, clinical features and measures, and clinical trial designs are evolving rapidly. Despite this progress, no disease-modifying treatment has been approved for any NDD. For symptomatic therapies, there are approved treatments for motor symptoms of PD, delusions and hallucinations in PD (pimavanserin), and for dementia associated with PD; there are approved cognitive enhancers for AD. This is a small repertoire of therapies resulting from a huge investment in drug development programs for NDD. To best take advantage of the progress in NDDs, it is important that lessons learned in one disorder be understood and incorporated into other NDD drug-development programs. Advances in one disease may be instructive for diagnosis, monitoring, biomarker implementation, and treatment of another. Vigilance for these cross-disease learnings may accelerate the pace with which we can bring new treatments to patients with NDDs.

DISCLOSURES

Dr. Zhong has no disclosures.

Dr. Cummings has provided consultation to Abbott, Acadia, Adamas, Alzheon, Anavex, Astellas, Avanir, Avid, Eisai, Forum, GE Healthcare, Genentech, Lilly, Lundbeck, Medavante Merck, Novartis, Otsuka, Pfizer, QR, Roivant, Sanofi-Aventis, Signum, Takeda and Toyama companies. Dr. Cummings owns the copyright of the Neuropsychiatric Inventory. Dr. Cummings will discuss the use of drugs in development and not approved by the FDA.

REFERENCES

1. Reitz C, Brayne C, Mayeux R. Epidemiology of Alzheimer disease. *Nat Rev Neurol* 2011;7(3):137–152.
2. Skovronsky DM, Lee VM, Trojanowski JQ. Neurodegenerative diseases: new concepts of pathogenesis and their therapeutic implications. *Annu Rev Pathol* 2006;1:151–170.
3. Prusiner SB. Biology and genetics of prions causing neurodegeneration. *Annu Rev Genet* 2013;47:601–623.

4. Greicius MD, Kimmel DL. Neuroimaging insights into network-based neurodegeneration. *Curr Opin Neurol* 2012;25(6):727–734.

5. Guo C, Sun L, Chen X, Zhang D. Oxidative stress, mitochondrial damage and neurodegenerative diseases. *Neural Regen Res* 2013;8(21):2003–2014.

6. Ward RJ, Zucca FA, Duyn JH, Crichton RR, Zecca L. The role of iron in brain ageing and neurodegenerative disorders. *Lancet Neurol* 2014;13(10):1045–1060.

7. Forabosco P, Ramasamy A, Trabzuni D, et al. Insights into TREM2 biology by network analysis of human brain gene expression data. *Neurobiol Aging* 2013;34(12):2699–2714.

8. Novarino G, Fenstermaker AG, Zaki MS, et al. Exome sequencing links corticospinal motor neuron disease to common neurodegenerative disorders. *Science* 2014;343(6170):506–511.

9. Gouras GK. Convergence of synapses, endosomes, and prions in the biology of neurodegenerative diseases. *Int J Cell Biol* 2013;2013:141083.

10. Gama Sosa MA, De GR, Elder GA. Modeling human neurodegenerative diseases in transgenic systems. *Hum Genet* 2012;131(4):535–563.

11. Choi SH, Kim YH, Hebisch M, et al. A three-dimensional human neural cell culture model of Alzheimer's disease. *Nature* 2014;515(7526):274–278.

12. Cundiff PE, Anderson SA. Impact of induced pluripotent stem cells on the study of central nervous system disease. *Curr Opin Genet Dev* 2011;21(3):354–361.

13. Kim SU, Lee HJ, Kim YB. Neural stem cell-based treatment for neurodegenerative diseases. *Neuropathology* 2013;33(5):491–504.

14. Bertram L, Tanzi RE. The genetics of Alzheimer's disease. *Prog Mol Biol Transl Sci* 2012;107:79–100.

15. Nacmias B, Piaceri I, Bagnoli S, Tedde A, Piacentini S, Sorbi S. Genetics of Alzheimer's disease and frontotemporal dementia. *Curr Mol Med* 2014;14:993–1000.

16. Bohnen NI, Kaufer DI, Ivanco LS, et al. Cortical cholinergic function is more severely affected in parkinsonian dementia than in Alzheimer disease: an in vivo positron emission tomographic study. *Arch Neurol* 2003;60(12):1745–1748.

17. Tiraboschi P, Hansen LA, Alford M, et al. Early and widespread cholinergic losses differentiate dementia with Lewy bodies from Alzheimer disease. *Arch Gen Psychiatry* 2002;59(10):946–951.

18. Emre M, Aarsland D, Albanese A, et al. Rivastigmine for dementia associated with Parkinson's disease. *N Engl J Med* 2004;351(24):2509–2518.

19. Black MD, Stevens RJ, Rogacki N, et al. AVE1625, a cannabinoid CB1 receptor antagonist, as a co-treatment with antipsychotics for schizophrenia: improvement in cognitive function and reduction of antipsychotic-side effects in rodents. *Psychopharmacology (Berl)* 2011;215(1): 149–163.

20. Busquets-Garcia A, Gomis-Gonzalez M, Guegan T, et al. Targeting the endocannabinoid system in the treatment of fragile X syndrome. *Nat Med* 2013;19(5):603–607.

21. Francis PT. Glutamatergic approaches to the treatment of cognitive and behavioural symptoms of Alzheimer's disease. *Neurodegener Dis* 2008;5(3–4):241–243.

22. Grove RA, Harrington CM, Mahler A, et al. A randomized, double-blind, placebo-controlled, 16-week study of the H3 receptor antagonist, GSK239512 as a monotherapy in subjects with mild-to-moderate Alzheimer's disease. *Curr Alzheimer Res* 2014;11(1):47–58.

23. Haig GM, Pritchett Y, Meier A, et al. A randomized study of H3 antagonist ABT-288 in mild-to-moderate Alzheimer's dementia. *J Alzheimers Dis* 2014;42(3):959–971.

24. Heckman PR, Wouters C, Prickaerts J. Phosphodiesterase inhibitors as a target for cognition enhancement in aging and Alzheimer's disease: a translational overview. *Curr Pharm Des* 2014;21(3):317–331.

25. Upton N, Chuang TT, Hunter AJ, Virley DJ. 5-HT6 receptor antagonists as novel cognitive enhancing agents for Alzheimer's disease. *Neurotherapeutics* 2008;5(3):458–469.

26. Wilkinson D, Windfeld K, Colding-Jorgensen E. Safety and efficacy of idalopirdine, a 5-HT6 receptor antagonist, in patients with moderate Alzheimer's disease (LADDER): a randomised, double-blind, placebo-controlled phase 2 trial. *Lancet Neurol* 2014;13(11):1092–1099.

27. Bentwich J, Dobronevsky E, Aichenbaum S, et al. Beneficial effect of repetitive transcranial magnetic stimulation combined with cognitive training for the treatment of Alzheimer's disease: a proof of concept study. *J Neural Transm* 2011;118(3): 463–471.

28. Freiherr J, Hallschmid M, Frey WH, et al. Intranasal insulin as a treatment for Alzheimer's disease: a review of basic research and clinical evidence. *CNS Drugs* 2013;27(7):505–514.

29. Gonzalez-Lima F, Barksdale BR, Rojas JC. Mitochondrial respiration as a target for neuroprotection and cognitive enhancement. *Biochem Pharmacol* 2014;88(4):584–593.

30. Hescham S, Lim LW, Jahanshahi A, Blokland A, Temel Y. Deep brain stimulation in dementia-related disorders. *Neurosci Biobehav Rev* 2013;37(10 Pt 2):2666–2675.

31. Hongpaisan J, Sun MK, Alkon DL. PKC epsilon activation prevents synaptic loss, Abeta elevation, and cognitive deficits in Alzheimer's disease transgenic mice. *J Neurosci* 2011;31(2):630–643.

32. Nardone R, Tezzon F, Holler Y, Golaszewski S, Trinka E, Brigo F. Transcranial magnetic stimulation (TMS)/repetitive TMS in mild cognitive impairment and Alzheimer's disease. *Acta Neurol Scand* 2014;129(6):351–366.

33. Olde Rikkert MG, Verhey FR, Blesa R, et al. Tolerability and safety of souvenaid in patients with mild Alzheimer's disease: results of multicenter, 24-week, open-label extension study. *J Alzheimers Dis* 2015;44:471–80.

34. Scheltens P, Twisk JW, Blesa R, et al. Efficacy of Souvenaid in mild Alzheimer's disease: results from a randomized, controlled trial. *J Alzheimers Dis* 2012;31(1):225–236.

35. Shevtsova EF, Vinogradova DV, Kireeva EG, Reddy VP, Aliev G, Bachurin SO. Dimebon attenuates the Abeta-induced mitochondrial permeabilization. *Curr Alzheimer Res* 2014;11(5):422–429.

36. Xiang GQ, Tang SS, Jiang LY et al. PPARgamma agonist pioglitazone improves scopolamine-induced memory impairment in mice. *J Pharm Pharmacol* 2012;64(4):589–596.

37. Yarchoan M, Arnold SE. Repurposing diabetes drugs for brain insulin resistance in Alzheimer disease. *Diabetes* 2014;63(7):2253–2261.

38. Olanow CW, Rascol O, Hauser R, et al. A double-blind, delayed-start trial of rasagiline in Parkinson's disease. *N Engl J Med* 2009;361(13):1268–1278.

39. Morris JC. The Clinical Dementia Rating (CDR): current version and scoring rules. *Neurology* 1993;43(11):2412–2414.

40. Dragalin V. An introduction to adaptive designs and adaptation in CNS trials. *Eur Neuropsychopharmacol* 2011;21(2):153–158.

41. Elm JJ, Goetz CG, Ravina B, et al. A responsive outcome for Parkinson's disease neuroprotection futility studies. *Ann Neurol* 2005;57(2):197–203.

42. Kieburtz K, Tilley BC, Elm JJ, et al. Effect of creatine monohydrate on clinical progression in patients with Parkinson disease: a randomized clinical trial. *JAMA* 2015;313(6):584–593.

43. Tilley BC, Palesch YY, Kieburtz K, et al. Optimizing the ongoing search for new treatments for Parkinson disease: using futility designs. *Neurology* 2006;66(5):628–633.

44. Rosen WG, Mohs RC, Davis KL. A new rating scale for Alzheimer's disease. *Am J Psychiatry* 1984;141(11):1356–1364.

45. Galasko D, Bennett D, Sano M, et al. An inventory to assess activities of daily living for clinical trials in Alzheimer's disease. The Alzheimer's Disease Cooperative Study. *Alzheimer Dis Assoc Disord* 1997;11 Suppl 2:S33–S39.

46. Gelinas I, Gauthier L, McIntyre M, Gauthier S. Development of a functional measure for persons with Alzheimer's disease: the disability assessment for dementia. *Am J Occup Ther* 1999;53(5):471–481.

47. Boxer AL, Lang AE, Grossman M, et al. Davunetide in patients with progressive supranuclear palsy: a randomised, double-blind, placebo-controlled phase 2/3 trial. *Lancet Neurol* 2014;13(7):676–685.

48. Wang J, Logovinsky V, Hendrix SB, et al. ADCOMS: a composite clinical outcome for prodromal Alzheimer's disease trials. *J Neurol Neurosurg Psychiatry* doi: 10.1136/jnnp-2015-312383. [Epub ahead of print]

49 Weintraub S, Dikmen SS, Heaton RK, et al. The cognition battery of the NIH toolbox for assessment of neurological and behavioral function: validation in an adult sample. *J Int Neuropsychol Soc* 2014;20(6):567–578.

50. Weintraub S, Dikmen SS, Heaton RK, et al. Cognition assessment using the NIH Toolbox. *Neurology* 2013;80(11 Suppl 3):S54–S64.

51. Kramer JH, Mungas D, Possin KL, et al. NIH EXAMINER: conceptualization and development of an executive function battery. *J Int Neuropsychol Soc* 2014;20(1):11–19.

52. Cummings JL, Mega M, Gray K, Rosenberg-Thompson S, Carusi DA, Gornbein J. The Neuropsychiatric Inventory: comprehensive assessment of psychopathology in dementia. *Neurology* 1994;44(12):2308–2314.

53. Zarit SH. Diagnosis and management of caregiver burden in dementia. *Handb Clin Neurol* 2008;89:101–106.

54. Wimo A, Jonsson L, Zbrozek A. The Resource Utilization in Dementia (RUD) instrument is valid for assessing informal care time in community-living patients with dementia. *J Nutr Health Aging* 2010;14(8):685–690.

55. Sabbagh JJ, Kinney JW, Cummings JL. Alzheimer's disease biomarkers: correspondence between human studies and animal models. *Neurobiol Dis* 2013;56:116–130.

56. Pan XD, Chen XC. Clinic, neuropathology and molecular genetics of frontotemporal dementia: a mini-review. *Transl Neurodegener* 2013;2(1):8.

57. Fleisher AS, Chen K, Quiroz YT, et al. Florbetapir PET analysis of amyloid-beta deposition in the presenilin 1 E280A autosomal dominant Alzheimer's disease kindred: a cross-sectional study. *Lancet Neurol* 2012;11(12):1057–1065.

58. Bateman RJ, Xiong C, Benzinger TL, et al. Clinical and biomarker changes in dominantly inherited Alzheimer's disease. *N Engl J Med* 2012;367(9):795–804.
59. Bateman RJ, Munsell LY, Morris JC, Swarm R, Yarasheski KE, Holtzman DM. Human amyloid-beta synthesis and clearance rates as measured in cerebrospinal fluid in vivo. *Nat Med* 2006;12(7):856–861.
60. Sperling RA, Jack CR, Jr., Black SE, et al. Amyloid-related imaging abnormalities in amyloid-modifying therapeutic trials: recommendations from the Alzheimer's Association Research Roundtable Workgroup. *Alzheimers Dement* 2011;7(4):367–385.
61. Cummings JL. Defining and labeling disease-modifying treatments for Alzheimer's disease. *Alzheimers Dement* 2009;5(5):406–418.
62. US Food and Drug Administration. *Guidance for Industry Alzheimer's Disease: Developing drugs for the treatment of early stage disease.* 2013. Washington, DC.

19

Conclusions on Neurodegenerative Disorders

Unifying Principles

JAGAN A. PILLAI AND JEFFREY L. CUMMINGS

Neurodegenerative diseases strip individuals of their cognitive powers, functional capacity, and autonomy, while increasing their dependence on others. As such, they are an existential threat to our aging society in its ability to provide a meaningful and high quality of life to all its citizens.

The classical view of neurodegenerative disorders (NDDs) emphasized the distinctness of each NDD, with a definable clinical syndrome of neurological deficits, behavioral changes, and progressive functional decline, underpinned by inexorable neuronal loss that is pathological for the age of the subject. The view developed in this volume recognizes NDDs as sharing many commonalities:

a. The malefactors underlying inexorable progression of the diseases: These are aggregations of proteins with altered physio-chemical and neurotoxic properties. These abnormal proteins become deposited within tissues or cellular compartments, leading to early neuronal death. This has given rise to the term "conformational diseases" for NDDs.

b. Time course of changes predating the clinical syndrome: A large body of work has noted that across a variety of NDDs, the early pathological changes with abnormal protein aggregations predate the clinical syndrome, often by more than a decade. This has led to the acceptance of a general staging approach to these disorders as preclinical, mild, and fully developed clinical manifestations.

c. Genetic and molecular dysfunction leading to neuronal death among different NDDs: For example, genetic changes from *C9 ORF72* mutation and the proteinopathy of Tar DNA-binding protein –43 are shared across multiple NDD phenotypes (Alzheimer's disease [AD], frontotemporal dementia [FTD], and amyotrophic lateral sclerosis [ALS]).

d. Prion-like behavior of protein aggregation disorders: There is converging evidence across proteinopathies that aggregating proteins—amyloid, tau, alpha-synuclein—maybe transferred from cell to cell, a mechanism also observed in prion disorders.

e. Therapeutic interest in preclinical states: There has been a shift from targeting behavioral and cognitive modifications at the later stages of NDDs, when they were traditionally identified in the clinic, to finding therapeutic targets and overcoming the underlying proteinopathy before significant neuronal and functional loss has occurred in the preclinical states of the NDDs.

f. Acceptance of biomarkers: There has been a parallel shift from clinical diagnosis in later stages of the disease with classical phenotypes to concomitant use of biomarkers to aid in earlier diagnosis in preclinical and milder stages of the disease before the full disease phenotype, as classically described, has emerged.

g. Cognitive reserve: There is recognition that host factors play a role in determining the clinically observed phenotype and that greater cognitive reserve allows onset of the manifestations of the disease to be deferred. Cognitive reserve is a complex multifaceted concept that includes historical features (educational level), biological factors (genetics, developmental disorders), and environmental contributions (diet, exercise).

h. Shift in perspective on NDDs: There is an expectation that understanding a specific NDD impacts and illuminates our understanding across the spectrum of NDD

In *Neurodegenerative Disorders: Unifying Principles* we have covered each of these themes, from multiple expert domains from basic science to clinical therapeutics. This detailed overview emphasizes the recent work that has uncovered shared themes across NDDs, and further posits questions for the future.

Multiple questions about NDDs and their relationship to aging shape the future direction of this rapidly evolving field. Questions that could shape the future of this field include the following:

1. What causes the proteins to aggregate in the first place? Many of the proteinopathies are exaggerated aggregations of proteins that have normal functional roles in cellular and subcellular domains. It is still unclear what triggers these proteins to aggregate and cause downstream cell death and if there are shared triggering factors for their aggregation across NDDs.

2. Every individual is like a unique snowflake. In spite of an underlying shared proteinopathy, the clinical course of an individual is significantly variable in both temporal course and the nature of clinical and functional deficits. Some phenomena including cognitive reserve are noted across all NDDs, while others, including changes at a molecular level (e.g., chaperones, inflammation) that drive these heterogeneous individual responses, are poorly understood. Understanding molecular factors that mitigate or exacerbate the effect of abnormal protein aggregations in an individual can help us devise individually tailored therapeutic interventions.

3. Even as aging is acknowledged as a significant risk factor for the development of NDD and the biggest driver for the increasing burden of NDDs on our society, it is yet to be worked out what aspects of an aging organism are causal factors in the development of NDD in an individual. Some progress has been made in understanding the role of comorbidities (diabetes, hypertension) and molecular factors (altered ubiquitin pathway), but there is significant work yet to be done.

4. Declining cognition has been tied to functional decline among most NDDs, but as therapeutic interventions are being targeted to preclinical stages of the disease, delineating normal age-related changes from subtle early cognitive changes of NDDs when people have very different baseline performances is an area for future high-impact research.

5. Intervening in preclinical stages of NDDs also has many ethical implications that need to be worked out. Characterizing disease states before their clinical impact is noted, despite a biological rationale, may present an ethical dilemma should subjects be labeled as having a potential disease state that needs intervention when complete reversal of symptoms is not yet guaranteed.

6. Population heterogeneity: Most studies in NDDs have been done in a few developed nations. How many of these diagnostic tools and therapeutic interventions generalize across the world among pools of populations with significant genetic, economic, and cultural heterogeneity regarding aging-related diseases is unknown at this time.

We actively shape the future and drive ourselves forward by finding appropriate answers to questions that capture our imagination. The questions we raised here are being formed by our new perspective of NDDs having shared underlying themes. With the understanding of factors that trigger disease onset, drive its progression, and shape the heterogeneity of individual responses, and the unique social and cultural factors that situate an individual, distinct personalized therapeutic options may be developed for patients with NDDs in the future across the world. *Neurodegenerative Disorders: Unifying Principles* is written from the expectation that a background in this new perspective of shared features across NDDs is essential for beginning students, as well as advanced practitioners, to make the breakthroughs needed to overcome the public health challenge of the new century.

INDEX